Stuttering and Related Disorders of Fluency

Third Edition

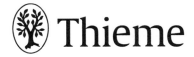

Stuttering and Related Disorders of Fluency

Third Edition

Edward G. Conture, Ph.D.
Professor and Director
Graduate Studies
Department of Hearing and Speech Sciences
Vanderbilt University
Nashville, Tennessee

Richard F. Curlee, Ph.D.
Professor Emeritus
Department of Speech and Hearing Sciences
University of Arizona
Tuscon, Arizona

Thieme
New York • Stuttgart

RC
424
.S768
2007

Thieme Medical Publishers, Inc.
333 Seventh Ave.
New York, NY 10001

Editorial Assistant: David Price
Executive Editor: Timothy Hiscock
Vice President, Production and Electronic Publishing: Anne T. Vinnicombe
Production Editor: Shannon Kerner
Associate Marketing Manager: Verena Diem
Sales Director: Ross Lumpkin
Chief Financial Officer: Peter van Woerden
President: Brian D. Scanlan
Compositor: Thomson Digital
Printer: Maple-Vail Book Manufacturing Group

Library of Congress Cataloging-in-Publication Data:

Stuttering and related disorders of fluency/[edited by] Edward G. Conture,
Richard Curlee. – 3rd ed.
    p.; cm.
    Curlee's name appears first on the earlier edition.
    Includes bibliographical references and index.
    ISBN-13: 978-1-58890-502-4 (TMP: case cover: alk. paper)
    ISBN-10: 1-58890-502-0 (TMP: case cover: alk. paper)
    ISBN-13: 978-3-13-783403-8 (GTV: case cover: alk. paper)
    ISBN-10: 3-13-783403-1 (GTV: case cover: alk. paper)   1.   Stuttering.   I. Conture, Edward G.
II. Curlee, Richard F. (Richard Frederick), 1935-
    [DNLM: 1.   Stuttering–therapy. 2.   Speech Therapy–methods.   WM 475 S9372 2007]
    RC424. S768 2007
    616.85'5–dc22

                                                                2006103498

Important note: Medical knowledge is ever-changing. As new research and clinical experience broaden our knowledge, changes in treatment and drug therapy may be required. The authors and editors of the material herein have consulted sources believed to be reliable in their efforts to provide information that is complete and in accord with the standards accepted at the time of publication. However, in view of the possibility of human error by the authors, editors, or publisher of the work herein or changes in medical knowledge, neither the authors, editors, nor publisher, nor any other party who has been involved in the preparation of this work, warrants that the information contained herein is in every respect accurate or complete, and they are not responsible for any errors or omissions or for the results obtained from use of such information. Readers are encouraged to confirm the information contained herein with other sources. For example, readers are advised to check the product information sheet included in the package of each drug they plan to administer to be certain that the information contained in this publication is accurate and that changes have not been made in the recommended dose or in the contraindications for administration. This recommendation is of particular importance in connection with new or infrequently used drugs.

Some of the product names, patents, and registered designs referred to in this book are in fact registered trademarks or proprietary names even though specific reference to this fact is not always made in the text. Therefore, the appearance of a name without designation as proprietary is not to be construed as a representation by the publisher that it is in the public domain.

Printed in United States of America

5 4 3 2 1

TMP ISBN 1-58890-502-0
TMP ISBN 978-1-58890-502-4
GTV ISBN 3-13-783403-1
GTV ISBN 978-3-13-783403-8

Contents

Preface

Failure is but one cul de sac
Not the end of all roads.

After Anna Nielsen (www.annanielsen.com)

The flip side of success is failure. Most authors in this text, after a moment's reflection, recognize that their successes have been leavened, here and there, with failure. Whether failure to help a client, failure with an experiment, or failure to publish their findings, all of us have known failure.

Stuttering, in particular, with its twists and turns of variability, within and between people who stutter, is fertile ground for failure. Failure, however, as noted above by Nielsen, is not the end, but the beginning of new explorations. Indeed, we would like to suggest that we learn far more from our failures treating and studying stuttering than we do from our successes.

Achieving even relative success with stuttering requires one to understand something about its basic characteristics. Besides its variability, another fundamental attribute of stuttering is that it is developmental. Stuttering typically begins in early childhood and then for many goes away, but for some, comes and stays. Why this is the case is still unclear. What is clear, however, is the reality that stuttering, whether viewed from a theoretical or clinical perspective, is developmental in nature. This is a reality that we believe should dampen the enthusiasm of those who try to apply adult remedies to preschool children and vice versa.

As noted in the preface to the second edition of this text, "Despite the claims of cures or that stuttering has been solved that are announced periodically, none has survived the personal experiences of those who tried them. The third edition of this text offers no such claims, and like the first two editions, includes a broad, selective range of current clinical strategies and practices that have been used successfully with children and adults who stutter". These strategies and practices however, while sometimes successful, reflect success informed by failure, a characteristic that imbues these approaches with greater longevity, wider applicability, and consequences than do those touting one-size-fits-all, with quick, easy cures.

This edition has been expanded to 18 chapters, with the first three devoted to the assessment of stuttering, the next five to the treatment of stuttering in children, the following three to the treatment of stuttering in individuals with co-occurring concerns, the next four chapters to treatments for teens and adults who stutter, and the final three chapters to related disorders of fluency, their symptoms, and treatment.

Given the widely held belief among clinicians who are experienced in treating stuttering that stuttering is best managed in childhood, this edition devotes half of its 18 chapters to children who stutter. The first two chapters focus on assessment of early childhood stuttering. Curlee provides a number of considerations, strategies, and practices for helping clinicians decide who does and does not require treatment. Zebrowski discusses and proposes strategies for dealing with various factors that may influence, to greater or lesser degrees, the therapy outcomes of children who stutter.

Following these discussions of assessing children who stutter, several chapters are devoted to the treatment of childhood stuttering. In the first such chapter, which was updated from the second edition, Harrison, Onslow, and Rousseau describe an operant-based therapy procedure that trains parents to use an approach at home that is strongly supported by evidence from therapy trials. Following that, Richels and Conture describe an indirect treatment approach to early childhood stuttering in another new chapter and report treatment outcome data of its effectiveness. Subsequently, Charles and Sara Runyan provide an updated account of their fluency rules treatment program, a well-regarded program that is used with both preschool and school-age children who stutter. After that, DiLollo and Manning present a thorough discussion, in a new chapter, of various principles and practices to consider when counseling children who stutter and their parents. In another new chapter, Langevin, Kully, and Ross-Harold describe a comprehensive treatment approach for school-age children who stutter that includes strategies for managing teasing and bullying.

In addition to the seven chapters covering assessment and treatment of childhood stuttering, three more new chapters provide both assessment and therapeutic strategies for children who have other speech-language difficulties in addition to childhood stuttering. For example, in a new chapter, Hall, Wagovich, and Bernstein Ratner discuss state of the art information regarding language and childhood stuttering. This is followed by another new chapter in which Byrd, Wolk, and Davis cover the possible role of phonology in childhood stuttering and its treatment. Next, Roberts and Shenker provide a new chapter in this area, that discusses how bilingualism may impact the onset, development, assessment, and treatment of stuttering among children as well as teens and adults.

The chapters that deal primarily with children point out, among other issues, that stuttering is a developmental problem. However, a fundamental reality of stuttering may be overlooked; stuttering is typically most apparent when the person who stutters is conversing with a listener. This is especially noticeable among older individuals who stutter, whether they're talking to classmates, teachers, employers, etc. In order for persons to exhibit stuttering reliably, most require the presence of a conversational partner. Indeed, some of stuttering variability reflects the relationship to the conversational partner, the nature of the conversational partner and/or situation and of the conversation itself. Of course, the number and nature of these variables change, over time, as a child's stuttering develops and as he or she matures into a adolescent and then, adult.

Involvement of listeners in the manifestations of stuttering suggests that the bidirectional nature of communication has an impact on stuttering. Consideration of this bidirectionality is covered in several of the chapters related to teens and adults. For example, Quesal discusses in a new chapter various traditional assessment procedures for teens and adults that take into account the totality of the communication environment as well as speech (dis)fluency. Likewise, Kully, Langevin, and Lomheim describe a comprehensive treatment approach for teens and adults who stutter that involves not only careful documentation and management of stuttering, but consideration of related behavioral and communicative issues. Next, Manning and DiLollo discuss traditional approaches to treatment of adolescents and adults who stutter, which encompasses various affective, cognitive, and behavioral aspects of stuttering. Another new chapter by Yaruss, Quesal, and Reeves describes the relatively recent growth and development of self-help, mutual aid groups as adjuncts to the treatment of stuttering. Rounding out this group of chapters, Saxon and Ludlow prepared a new chapter that thoroughly covers the principles and practices involving various pharmaceutical interventions for stuttering as well as their reported main and side effects.

Given the variable, developmental nature of stuttering (that the chapters mentioned above make quite clear), one is hard pressed to posit a static, one-source explanation for stuttering's onset and development. Indeed, it was suggested elsewhere (Conture, 2001) that stutterings most likely involves a complex interaction between the environments of persons who stutter and the skills and abilities they bring to their environment. Again, one would not be surprised to observe changes in stuttering over time because of its variable, developmental nature. For example, the manner with which nature interacts with nurture undoubtedly changes, possibly contributing to changes in stuttering across the life span. Such changes imply that as a person who stutters experiences changes in their stuttering; they learn different ways to react to and/or cope with stuttering. One might compare the way learning molds and shapes stuttering to that of an architect who designs a series of houses. While the architect leaves the basic house structure intact for each dwelling, he or she gives each house an individualized architectural expression at the same time. Thus, stuttering changes over time in ways generally similar for everyone who stutters, while still exhibiting significant degrees of variability in its expression across individuals who stutter.

Those who would deconstruct such a complex problem into one element, regardless of how objectively that element can be measured, might gain some early grasp of the behavioral escarpment that envelopes stuttering. Over time, however, this approach will likely be less than successful, as are most approaches to understanding human problem that originate from oversimplified or overly complex views. Success, on the other hand, usually comes to those who inhabit the middle ground, and who entertain and accept complexity, allowing it to inform their judgment, all the while seeking the most eloquently simple solutions to the problem.

As part of that middle ground and in consideration of the manifold elements related to stuttering, this edition ends with three chapters that expand the population of persons who stutter or have related disorders of fluency. A new chapter, by St. Louis, Myers, Bakker, and Raphael, provides state of the art conceptualizations, findings De Nil and considerations related to the often discussed, but less often understood, problem of cluttering. De Nil, Jokel, and Rochon follow this chapter with another new chapter that provides a thorough update on neurogenic stuttering, what it is, what we know about its etiology and symptoms, and what we need to know about its treatment. Last, but clearly not least, Finn provides a new chapter that presents compelling arguments and discussion of the importance of persons' assuming self-control and management of their stuttering following treatment if they want to increase the likelihood of having successful, long-term improvements in their stuttering.

Given the depth and breadth of the issues considered in this text, readers are encouraged to peruse the how to of the various treatment approaches to stuttering from the perspective that many of our clinical successes have been strongly influenced by our experiences with failure. And, as has been said, success has many fathers, but failure is an orphan. Clearly, most of us plan for success in our assessment, treatment, and study of stuttering, but failure not infrequently occurs, and it is the wise clinicians, teachers, and researchers who accept it. Furthermore, these same clinicians, teachers, and researchers should expect failure, for without it, they will be unlikely to improve their future clinical, teaching, or research endeavors.

Likewise, readers are also encouraged not to dismiss the success of others as luck, for luck favors the prepared. Instead, readers are strongly encouraged to prepare themselves for good experiences assessing, treating, and studying stuttering. Such preparation can be developed by understanding that stuttering is variable and developmental in nature, that it requires a listener to be most apparent, and most likely involves an interaction between nature and nurture. By understanding such characteristics, we can appreciate more fully some of its basic attributes. Even being prepared, however, will not protect us from failure, for failures surely will occur as we travel along our individual paths of professional development. However, such failures are only dead ends that present opportunities to travel another path, perhaps the one less traveled, as Robert Frost called it, but this time a path where our success is informed by failure.

In the end, we should not fear failure in our assessment, treatment, and study of stuttering, for it is a powerful teacher and corrector. Rather, we should cast glances askance at those who are obsessed with success, especially unbridled success that has never known the tempering hand of failure. In essence, we believe that allowing our successes to be informed by failure helps us to grow, develop, and evolve in our insight, knowledge, and wisdom, and to become better able to help people who stutter prosper, grow, develop, and improve.

Edward G. Conture, Ph.D.
Professor and Director
Graduate Studies
Department of Hearing and Speech Sciences
Vanderbilt University
Nashville, Tennessee

Contributors

Klaas Bakker, Ph.D.
Associate Professor
Department of Communication Sciences and
  Disorders
Missouri State University
Springfield, Missouri

Nan Bernstein Ratner, Ed.D.
Professor
Department of Hearing and Speech Sciences
University of Maryland
College Park, Maryland

Courtney Timpson Byrd, Ph.D.
Assistant Professor
Department of Communication Sciences and
  Disorders
University of Texas at Austin
Austin, Texas

Edward G. Conture, Ph.D.
Professor and Director
Graduate Studies
Department of Hearing and Speech Sciences
Vanderbilt University
Nashville, Tennessee

Richard F. Curlee, Ph.D.
Professor Emeritus
Department of Speech and Hearing Sciences
University of Arizona
Tuscon, Arizona

Barbara Lockett Davis, Ph.D.
Professor
Department of Communication Sciences and
  Disorders
University of Texas at Austin
Austin, Texas

Luc F. De Nil, Ph.D.
Associate Professor and Chair
Department of Speech-Language
  Pathology
University of Toronto
Toronto, Ontario, Canada

Anthony DiLollo, Ph.D
Assistant Professor
Department of Communication Sciences and
  Disorders
Wichita State University
Wichita, Kansas

Patrick Finn, Ph.D.
Associate Professor
Department of Speech, Language, and Hearing
  Sciences
University of Arizona
Tucson, Arizona

Nancy E. Hall, B.A., M.A., Ph.D.
Associate Professor and Department Chair
Department of Communication Sciences and
    Disorders
University of Maine
Orono, Maine

Elisabeth Harrison, Ph.D.
Senior Lecturer
Department of Linguistics
Macquarie University
Sydney, Australia

Regina Jokel, M.H.Sc., Ph.D. candidate
Post-Doctoral Fellow Department of
    Speech-Language Pathology
University of Toronto
Toronto, Ontario, Canada

Deborah A. Kully, M.Sc.
Executive Director and Associate Professor
Institute for Stuttering Treatment and Research
Faculty of Rehabilitation
University of Alberta
Edmonton, Alberta, Canada

Marilyn Langevin, M.Sc.
Clinical Director
Institute for Stuttering Treatment and Research
Faculty of Rehabilitation Medicine
University of Alberta
Edmonton, Alberta, Canada

Holly Lomheim, B.A., M.S.L.P. (C)
Adult Clinic and Training Coordinator
Speech Language Pathologist
Institute for Stuttering Treatment and Research
Faculty of Rehabilitation Medicine
University of Alberta
Edmonton, Alberta, Canada

Christy L. Ludlow, Ph.D.
Chief, Senior Investigator
Laryngeal and Speech Section
National Institute of Neurological Disorders and
    Stroke
Bethesda, Maryland

Walter H. Manning, Ph.D.
Professor, and Associate Dean
School of Audiology and Speech-Language
    Pathology
The University of Memphis
Memphis, Tennessee

Florence L. Myers, Ph.D.
Professor
Department of Communication Sciences and
    Disorders
Adelphi University
Garden City, New York

Mark Onslow, Ph.D.
Director
Australian Stuttering Research Centre
The University of Sydney
Lidcombe, Australia

Robert W. Quesal, Ph.D.
Professor
Department of Communication Sciences and
    Disorders
Western Illinois University
Macomb, Illinois

Lawrence J. Raphael, Ph.D.
Professor
Department of Communication Sciences and
    Disorders
Adelphi University
Garden City, New York

Corrin G. Richels, Ph.D.
Assistant Professor of Clinical Research
Hearing and Speech Sciences Department
Vanderbilt University
Nashville, Tennessee

Lee Reeves, D.V.M.
Director National Stuttering Association
Plano, Texas

Patricia M. Roberts, Ph.D., C.C.C.-S.L.P.
Associate Professor
Faculty of Health Sciences
University of Ottawa
Ottawa, Ontario, Canada

Elizabeth Rochon, Ph.D.
Associate Professor
Department of Speech-Language
    Pathology
University of Toronto
Toronto, Ontario, Canada

Beverly Ross-Harold, M.S.L.P.
Programs Coordinator and Elks Clinician
Institute for Stuttering Treatment and Research
Faculty of Rehabilitation Medicine
University of Alberta
Edmonton, Alberta, Canada

Isabelle Rousseau, Ph.D.
Doctor
Australian Stuttering Research Centre
The University of Sydney
Lidcombe, Australia

Charles M. Runyan, Ph.D.
Professor and Graduate Coordinator
Department of Communication
   Sciences and Disorders
James Madison University
Harrisonburg, Virginia

Sara Elizabeth Runyan, M.A.
Associate Professor and Director of Clinical
   Education
Department of Communication Sciences and
   Disorders
James Madison University
Harrisonburg, Virginia

Kenneth O. St. Louis, Ph.D.
Professor
Department of Speech Pathology and Audiology
West Virginia University
Morgantown, West Virginia

Keith G. Saxon, M.D.
Staff Clinician Laryngeal and Speech Section
National Institute of Neurological Disorders and
   Stroke
Bethesda, Maryland

Rosalee C. Shenker, Ph.D.
Adjunct Professor
Department of Communication Sciences and
   Disorders
Mc Gill University
Montreal, Quebec, Canada

Stacy A. Wagovich, B.S.Ed., M.A., Ph.D.
Assistant Professor
Department of Communication Science and
   Disorders
University of Missouri-Columbia
Columbia, Missouri

Lesley Wolk, Ph.D.
Adjunct Associate Professor of Speech
   Pathology
Department of Behavioral Sciences
Teachers College, Columbia University
New York, New York

J. Scott Yaruss, Ph.D.
Associate Professor
Department of Communication Sciences and
   Disorders
University of Pittsburgh
Pittsburgh, Pennsylvania

Patricia M. Zebrowski, Ph.D.
Associate Professor
Department of Speech Pathology and Audiology
University of Iowa
Iowa City, Iowa

Section I

Assessment of Stuttering

1

Identification and Case Selection Guidelines for Early Childhood Stuttering

Richard F. Curlee

The goal of this chapter is to review the findings from empirical studies of early childhood stuttering and its signs, to describe my approach to its clinical evaluation and to making clinical management decisions. Onsets of childhood stuttering are highest between a child's second and fourth birthdays, before decreasing gradually and ultimately affecting nearly 5% of the population (Andrews, 1984). Indeed, several more recent studies (Mansson, 2000; Yairi & Ambrose, 1992; Yaruss, LaSalle, & Conture, 1998) have reported that stuttering usually begins in childhood between 30 and 36 months of age. The stuttering is often episodic initially, varying from day to day and one situation to another. As a result, the child's speech may sound like that of other children in this age group much of the time (Yairi, 1981). These early onsets usually emerge gradually from a background of repetitious spoken language, much like that observed among nonstuttering children in this age group (Yairi & Ambrose, 2004). However, abrupt onsets of stuttering have been reported by about one-third of the parents in several studies (Yairi, 1983; Yairi & Ambrose, 1992). After stuttering has been present for a few years, most children who stutter can be easily distinguished from peers who are highly disfluent, even those who do not stutter (Westby, 1979; St. Louis, Hinzman, & Hull, 1985). Thus, accurate identification of early childhood stuttering, though somewhat challenging at times, seldom poses serious difficulties for experienced clinicians (Adams 1984; Conture, 2001; Curlee, 1999; Gregory, 2003; Pindzola & White, 1986).

It is widely believed that early identification and treatment of children's developmental disorders, including stuttering, is the most efficient and effective strategy for preventing such disorders from becoming chronic, long-term disabilities. Although a variety of different treatments have been reported to be successful with young children who stutter (e.g., Bloodstein, 1987; Curlee, 1999; Harrison, Onslow, & Rousseau, Chapter 4, this volume), many young preschoolers who begin to stutter stop within the first year or two of onset without having received any professional treatment (Andrews, 1984; Curlee & Yairi, 1997; Dickson, 1971; Glasner & Rosenthal, 1957; Yairi, Ambrose, Paden, & Throneburg, 1996). Nevertheless, a substantial percentage, 20 to 25% or so, continue to stutter (Andrews, 1984; Yairi and Ambrose, 2004), and if stuttering persists past puberty, it may become a lifelong disability (Curlee, 1984) that can significantly restrict adults' educational, vocational, and personal–social activities (Andrews, 1984; Yaruss, 1999). Consequently, even experienced clinicians may feel uncertain when deciding whether to defer treatment a while for young preschoolers, to see if stuttering is just a transient problem, or to begin therapy without further delay.

I believe that the clinical management of these children should be based, as much as possible, on empirical information about childhood stuttering, its onset, and remission. Such information has been substantially expanded by an ongoing longitudinal study at the University of Illinois of young children who stutter (Yairi & Ambrose, 2004). Its findings suggest that treatment may be unnecessary for many young preschoolers who recently began to stutter. This is strikingly consistent with findings from a longitudinal study completed in Great Britain some 50 years ago (Andrews, 1984) as well as the findings reported in a recent study by Mansson (2000) and a much smaller study by Ryan (1990). In addition, systematic monitoring of young children's speech soon after stuttering onset can identify most of those who will stop stuttering without receiving therapy (Yairi & Ambrose, 2004). These findings support the clinical evaluation procedures and decision-making processes described later in this chapter that I employ for identifying early childhood stuttering and determining which children are having transient fluency difficulties and which ones are at likely to continue stuttering unless therapy is initiated without unnecessary delay.

♦ Clinical Evaluation

Reliable identification of childhood stuttering relies on observing clusters of signs and symptoms that distinguish children who are stuttering from their nonstuttering peers. These signs and symptoms include qualitative and quantitative features of a child's disfluent speech and his or her reactions to it, which vary widely among this clinical population. There is no single sign or symptom that must be present, except for stuttered speech, which distinguishes stuttering from the disfluencies of nonstuttering children. However, some children who stutter may not stutter at all during their clinical evaluation. Thus, observations of a stuttering child's speech during his or her initial examination can be misleading. Signs and symptoms of childhood stuttering must occur consistently during evaluations for diagnoses of stuttering to receive sufficient support. Therefore, ongoing follow-up evaluations of a child suspected of stuttering usually will yield observations that either do or do not support a diagnosis of childhood stuttering. It is my experience, however, that clinical examinations of most of these children clearly confirm the information that I collected earlier or will collect later from parents during their case history interview.

Medical diagnoses rely on the symptoms reported by patients, clinical signs observed by physicians, and test findings to differentiate the etiology of patients' medical conditions or diseases. In contrast, diagnoses of childhood stuttering rely substantially on parents' reports and clinicians' observations of the children's speech to differentiate early signs of stuttering from the disfluencies of nonstuttering children and to determine which kinds of follow-up evaluations, treatments, or referrals may be needed. Thus, thorough evaluations of young children suspected of stuttering should provide clinicians with information that supports one of the following conclusions:

1. Few, if any, signs of childhood stuttering are present, and the child's spoken language is age-appropriate.

2. Inconsistent signs of childhood stuttering are present, making further observation and testing necessary.

3. Signs of childhood stuttering have been present less than 1 year and few negative reactions to stuttering are apparent or have been reported by parents.

4. Signs of childhood stuttering are frequently present as are one or more other speech-language problems.

5. Stuttering has been present consistently for a year or more without any signs of remission.

Although case history interviews can be conducted before, during, or following a child's evaluation, I prefer to obtain detailed case histories from parents or other caregivers prior to my clinical examination of the child, so that I know which observations and recordings I should make before deciding that a child is beginning to stutter or that parents are overreacting to normal, age-appropriate disfluent speech. In contrast, some clinicians prefer to have parents complete case history forms at home prior to a child's evaluation. In either case, the parents may also provide information suggesting other speech-language behaviors and abilities that the clinician will want to observe and test during the initial evaluation and a series of evaluations across several days, if needed, so that there will be sufficient time to make additional observations, complete further testing of the child's speech and language, analyze the video recordings and test findings acquired during the preceding sessions, and make sure there is sufficient support for a diagnosis of stuttering or normal fluency. This can be done before scheduling a meeting with the parents to review these findings, discuss their implications, and make recommendations.

Case History Interview

My interviews with parents who suspect that their child may have begun to stutter include a discussion of the child's overall development, especially his or her speech and language acquisition, as well as a careful exploration of the parents' fluency concerns. A substantial percentage of young preschoolers who stutter are later reported to have immature articulatory or phonological skills and other speech, language, or learning difficulties in school (Bloodstein, 1987; Blood, Ridenhour, Qualls, & Hammer, 2003). In some cases, these co-occurring difficulties may result in much more significant problems for a child than stuttering, and any such difficulties should be confirmed or ruled out, if possible, by further examination.

The importance of the information obtained from a thorough case history interview cannot be exaggerated. Parents are able to observe their children in a variety of circumstances that are not available to clinicians. Their repeated observations of the child in real-life situations have a validity that my observations in clinical settings can never achieve, and a case history interview provides me access to parents' recollections of key events in the child's and family's life, as well as descriptions of the child's speech that may be critical in diagnosing childhood stuttering. As I am getting to know a child through the parents' eyes, I am also learning what kinds of behaviors and reactions may be important for them to look for in their child as a result of the topics we covered and the questions I asked during the interview. Even more important, however, this interview marks the beginning of a relationship between me and the parents, which I believe significantly and positively affects the ultimate success of any professional interventions that may be needed later with them and their child.

In my experience, parents' initial descriptions of a child's speech disruptions sometimes lack the specificity to be diagnostically useful. Some simply express concern about their child's "stuttering" then seem somewhat perplexed or frustrated if I ask them to describe the child's "stuttering" in more detail. I have found, however, that most have little difficulty identifying the kinds of disfluencies that are bothering them (e.g., monosyllable whole- and part-word repetitions, sound prolongations, and tense pauses) if I simulate them. Some even recall specific examples they have observed in the child, which I believe adds to the credibility of their report. In addition, simulating specific qualitative features of stuttering can usually help parents to recall how many units of repetition they usually observe, their tempo, and whether or not increases in pitch or loudness or accessory behaviors accompany their child's speech disfluencies with some regularity. When parents can provide me detailed descriptions of their child's speech, it is much easier for me to decide which observations I need to make in determining if the child has begun to stutter or if the parents may be overreacting to their child's normal, age-appropriate disfluencies. The latter possibility seldom occurs, in my experience, however. Indeed, I can recall only a handful of parental misdiagnoses of early childhood stuttering in more than 35 years of clinical practice in its identification and treatment.

The signs and symptoms I rely on for identifying childhood stuttering and determining when to initiate treatment can be grouped into two groups of questions. Answers to the first group help me to distinguish early childhood stuttering from the disfluencies of nonstuttering children. Answers to the second group help me to distinguish children who are likely to stop stuttering without receiving treatment from those whose stuttering is likely to persist or worsen without therapy or who have co-occurring speech-language problems that also need treatment without delay. Many children, even those whose stuttering is severe, often seem unconcerned and may continue to communicate normally in spite of their stuttering, and several may also stop stuttering without treatment, as well (Andrews, 1984; Ryan, 1990; Yairi, 1997). In contrast, if stuttering is consistently present or worsens over a period of months, I believe that remission of stuttering is unlikely, at least in the short term, unless treatment is initiated without delay. This should be discussed with the parents, together with supporting references, and approved by them.

Indicators of Early Childhood Stuttering

1. *What kinds of speech disruptions are eliciting parental concern?* Children who stutter are much more disfluent than nonstuttering children, even though there is extensive overlap in the types of speech disfluencies produced by both groups (Bloodstein, 1987; Johnson & Associates, 1959; Yairi, 1997). Among those who stutter, however, monosyllabic whole- and part-word repetitions occur much more frequently and are often the first signs of early childhood stuttering (McDearmon, 1968; Yairi & Lewis, 1984; Yairi & Ambrose, 2004). Occasional sound prolongations and tense pauses, which involve fixed articulatory positions, also occur much more frequently among children who stutter and, together with single-syllable repetitions, comprise a cluster of stutter-like disfluencies (SLDs) that are obligatory signs of childhood stuttering (Adams, 1984; Johnson & Associates, 1959; Yairi & Lewis, 1984; Hubbard & Yairi, 1988; Yairi & Ambrose, 2004). Single-syllable repetitions occur frequently in the speech of most nonstuttering young children but are repeated more than twice only infrequently (Yairi, 1997; Zebrowski, 1991). On the other hand, if parents are concerned mainly about a child's revisions, interjections, and repetitions of multisyllable words and phrases, which are interruptions of speech that may reflect linguistic encoding processes (Wexler & Mysak, 1982), it is likely they are worried about the disfluencies of a child who is not yet stuttering (McDearmon, 1968).

2. *Have the child's speech disruptions changed since parents first became concerned?* Beginning stuttering is often episodic, with the frequency and severity of a child's disfluent speech varying from one day to the next and situation to situation. In fact, several days may pass with no problems being observed (Bloodstein, 1987; Van Riper, 1982; Wexler & Mysak, 1982). It is important to find out if a child's stuttering has changed since it began, whether or not it still seems to be limited to only a few situations, such as display talking at home or when excited at preschool, or if it has begun to occur throughout several of the child's conversational interactions (Adams, 1984; Curlee, 1984; Gregory & Hill, 1984; Yaruss et al., 1998). A child whose stuttering initially consisted only of effortless repetitions may begin prolonging sounds much of the time, for example (Pellowski & Conture, 2002). The longer a child stutters, it is likely that his or her stuttering will become increasingly consistent from one situation to another, whereas extended periods of fluent speech are likely to occur much less often and stuttering is likely to occur increasingly in clusters of three or more units. (Hubbard & Yairi, 1988).

3. *How long have parents been concerned about the child's fluency?* Remission of stuttering can occur at any age (Sheehan & Martyn, 1970), but at least half occur within 2 years of stuttering onset (Andrews, 1984; Yairi & Ambrose, 2004). In addition, early remissions occur more often

among young girls than boys (Yairi & Ambrose, 1990), and among those with mild rather than severe stuttering, who will have later remissions (Sheehan & Martyn, 1970; Yairi & Ambrose, 2004). Thus, if a child's stuttering persists a year beyond onset, especially if stuttering increases in frequency or severity during that period, the likelihood that an untreated remission will occur within 2 years is substantially decreased, and the need to initiate some form of treatment should be carefully reevaluated (Yaruss et al.; Pellowski & Conture, 2002).

4. *How valid do parents' concerns about stuttering appear to be?* When parents are able to describe their child's speech disruptions in detail and their patterns of occurrence with specific examples of behaviors that are commonly reported when children are beginning to stutter, it is highly unlikely their concerns are ill-founded. Such details reflect parents' careful, purposeful observations, which I believe increase the credibility of their concerns that their child has begun to stutter. Sometimes, parents or caregivers report that a child's fluency difficulties have been noticed and commented on by friends or relatives. Such reactions to their child's speech by different observers strongly support the parents' concern that the child has a fluency problem.

Indicators of Need for Treatment

1. *Is there a family history of persistent stuttering?* It has been known for several years that the incidence of stuttering is much higher in some families, extending across generations and affecting more males than females (Ambrose, Cox, & Yairi, 1997; Andrews, 1984; Felsenfeld, 1997; Kidd, 1984). This pattern of incidence is best explained by models of genetic transmission, even though environmental factors may need to be included to account for some onsets (Ambrose et al., 1997; Felsenfeld, 1997). Only recently, however, has evidence been presented that family histories of either persistence or remission of stuttering are related to the persistence or remission of childhood stuttering during the early postonset years in later generations of the family (Felsenfeld, 1997). This study also reported that preschool-age girls have early remissions of stuttering much more often than do boys, which likely accounts for the increase from a 2:1 ratio of boys to girls among young preschoolers who stutter to a 4 or 5:1 ratio among stuttering adult males and females (Felsenfeld, 1997). It is important, therefore, to have family members undertake a thorough search of their family tree, through third-degree biological relatives, for kin having current or prior stuttering problems. A child from a family with a history of persistent stuttering is much more likely to continue to stutter for at least 3 years postonset. In contrast, a family history of stuttering remissions increases the likelihood that children from a later generation of that family may have only transient stuttering difficulties. Thus, in my own clinical work, I usually discuss direct intervention options with parents sooner for young boys than for girls, as well as for those children with family histories of persistent stuttering than for those with histories of remissions, even if their postonset periods of stuttering and its severity are similar.

2. *Are the child's speech and language abilities age-appropriate?* There is a considerable body of evidence that school-age children who stutter also have other speech, language, or learning disabilities much more often than their peers who do not stutter (Blood et al., 2003; Bloodstein, 1987; Louko, Edwards, & Conture, 1990; St. Louis, Hinzman, and Mason, 1988). Most of these children, of course, have continued to stutter through the postonset period when remissions of stuttering are highest (Andrews, 1984; Yairi & Ambrose, 2004). Clearly their stuttering cannot be considered a transient difficulty, even if they do recover sometime later. I have long suspected that these children have a higher risk for persistent stuttering than if they only stuttered. Only recently, however, has some empirical support for my clinical suspicions been reported (Yairi et al., 1996). Segregation analyses by Ambrose et al (1997) suggest that persistent stuttering does not result from the genetic transmission of a more severe form of stuttering but instead may reflect the transmission of additional genetic factors. If so, these additional genetic factors may contribute to an increased incidence of other speech-language disabilities,

especially phonological disorders, among those children whose stuttering persists. It is important to keep in mind, however, that the nature of the functional relationship between stuttering and co-occurring disorders, other than a statistical correlation, is yet to be determined. I always screen preschool-age children's speech-language abilities during my initial evaluation session of their stuttering and sometimes find other speech-language problems that parents or caregivers have not noticed. Their presence, of course, necessitates further testing and presents another issue that I will need to discuss with the parents.

3. *Have the child's speech disruptions changed from predominantly two- or three-unit, seemingly effortless repetitions, to sound prolongations, tense pauses, and lengthy repetitions that are often accompanied by muscle tension and ancillary facial and body movements?* Although childhood stuttering most often begins insidiously, a substantial proportion of these young children evidence signs of severe stuttering from the very beginning (Ambrose et al., 1997; Curlee, 1984; Wexler & Mysak, 1982). Indeed, an early systematic study of a group of preschoolers post-onset of stuttering reported this (Johnson & Associates, 1959), and a later follow-up study (Ambrose et al., 1997) reported that more than one-third of their larger sample of preschoolers had abrupt onsets of stuttering. No differences were found, however, in the untreated remission rates of children having either gradual or abrupt onsets of stuttering. Nevertheless, if a child's disfluencies are accompanied increasingly by muscle tension and interruptions or cessation of articulator movement, airflow, and phonation for a year or more, the child has an increased risk that stuttering will persist, perhaps for life.

4. *Does the child often react emotionally or express concern about his or her disfluent speech?* It is not unusual for parents of young preschoolers who stutter to comment that their child seems unaware of being disfluent and has shown no signs of concern about it. As a child grows older, however, several negative emotional and cognitive reactions to stuttering are likely to emerge (Adams, 1984; Bloodstein, 1987; Vanryckeghem, Brutten, & Hernandez, 2005), especially if other children have begun to react adversely to his or her stuttering. Common, early reactions of young children include frequent blinking and breaking of eye contact during stuttering (Conture, 1997; Conture & Kelly, 1991), as well as the emergence of frustration, especially during periods when a child's stuttering is unusually severe (Curlee, 1984).

These kinds of emotional reactions ordinarily precede a child commenting about his or her disfluencies (e.g., "Mommy, I can't talk right" or "Daddy, I can't say that word") or trying to avoid talking or saying specific words, all of which are common behaviors among older children and adults who stutter. When these signs begin to appear after a child has been stuttering for several months, I view this expanding collection of affective and cognitive reactions as signs that a child's stuttering is evolving into a more severe, complex problem that may be considerably more challenging to treat successfully (Curlee, 1984).

I believe that a thorough case history interview will provide a clear impression of the kinds of fluency difficulties I am likely to observe when the child is evaluated, and I usually conclude my interview by asking the parents if there is anything else I should know about the child that hasn't been discussed or if they have other concerns that have not been mentioned. If not, I then summarize my understanding of their concerns about the child and ask if I have left out or misunderstood anything. After acknowledging any corrections or additions that I need to make and responding to any questions or further concerns they have, I give them a booklet on childhood stuttering published by the Stuttering Foundation of America, that was written specifically for parents (e.g., Conture, 2002), and I ask them to read it and to jot down any questions that arise or that they would like us to discuss at our next meeting. I usually comment at this point that the more they can learn about stuttering, the better able they will be to assist me in its treatment and remission. Finally, just before they leave, I describe the tests and observations planned for their child's evaluation and ask them to bring a video recording from home that includes the kinds of speech difficulties that are causing them concern to our next meeting. This is especially important if they have reported that the frequency and severity of the child's stuttering varies considerably.

Because I usually schedule their child's evaluation for a subsequent day, this gives me ample time to prepare a plan for screening and assessing the child's speech–language–learning abilities and to select activities that will allow me to observe the child's speech disfluencies when talking with different partners and performing tasks that involve different spoken language demands and skills.

Clinical Observations and Testing

My evaluations of children who are suspected of stuttering include observations of the child conversing with one or both parents or caregivers and later with me or another clinician while engaged in speaking tasks that vary in structure, complexity, and communicative stress. Video recordings of these conversations and tasks are analyzed subsequently to assess the child's disfluencies and language skills and are often used in follow-up meetings with the parents to display some of the child's speech and language difficulties that occurred during the evaluation. A common diagnostic plan for preschoolers whom I believe may be stuttering includes the following:

- The evaluation session usually begins by observing and making a video recording of the child and parents interacting together, often with a favorite game, puzzle, or book brought from home. This allows young preschoolers to become familiar with the clinic environment accompanied by familiar people and favorite play material so that a speech sample under relatively unstressful circumstances can be videotaped. It also allows me to observe how the parents or caregivers and child communicate with one another and their responses to the child's disfluent speech.

- After 5 to 10 minutes, I or another clinician join the child and parent and begin to interact with them. A minute or two later, the child is usually asked to help find another toy or game from a box or cabinet prepared for that purpose. If the child seems comfortable interacting and talking with me or the other clinician, the parents usually move to an adjoining observation room while the evaluation proceeds. If a child seems apprehensive, however, I think it is best to have the parents remain with the child as long as that appears to be important to the child's comfort. I believe that having a clinician in the observation room to respond to parents' questions and to discuss diagnostically significant behaviors that occur can be very helpful. I have found that subsequent discussions of diagnostic findings with parents or caregivers are much easier when they have observed the child's evaluation.

- I like to alternate administration of speech-language tests with games and play throughout a diagnostic session, but usually I assess receptive language abilities first, before a child begins to tire. I also include tests having items requiring the repetition of words, phrases, or sentences to see if the child's disfluencies increase as the length and complexity of responses increase. This can commonly occur in young children who stutter (Zackheim & Conture, 2003) and which decreases when such items are presented using slow speech models. For example, I elicit responses for later phonological or articulatory analyses using auditory models if a child's verbal responses to picture stimuli are frequently disfluent. If such modifications in test administration are likely to invalidate a test's results, I then complete additional testing during another diagnostic session if I suspect the child may have problems in that area.

- Video recordings of the child's speech talking with the clinician during unstructured play activities need to be analyzed and compared with those recorded by parents at home and during the diagnostic session to evaluate the consistency of the child's disfluencies across different speaking partners and settings under relatively unstressful circumstances. These same recordings can be used, of course, for language sample analyses, which together with the findings yielded by standardized tests of spoken language will determine if further assessment of the child's expressive language abilities is needed. If a child is obviously stuttering, I want to see if modifying speaking tasks or how the child speaks reduces the frequency or severity of the stuttering. For example, speaking tasks that require short, descriptive, concrete responses usually elicit fewer stutterings than do those requiring longer, less representative, informational narratives.

Similarly, whispering, speaking slowly with exaggerated pitch inflections, or speaking in unison with the clinician often results in reduced stuttering. In contrast, if a child has not stuttered during an evaluation, or has stuttered infrequently, I want to see if his or her stuttering increases when:

1. The child is asked to describe some past event or future plan or to retell a familiar story, such as "The Three Bears."

2. Sometimes, I interrupt or disagree with what the child says or rush his or her speech, saying we need to hurry, or use another tactic that increases the communicative stress or difficulty of the speaking task.

3. I am hoping, of course, that such tactics will allow me to observe the kinds of disfluencies that are causing parental concern but have not yet occurred during this evaluation, and to see if the child's stuttering increases substantially when he or she is stimulated emotionally or is excited.

4. I believe that a child's initial clinical examination should also include a routine audiometric screening of his or her hearing, a peroral screening of the speech production mechanism that includes speech diadochokinetic tasks, which often may trigger unambiguous instances of stuttering. These components of an examination seldom provide significant findings for diagnosing stuttering and are saved for the end of an examination, even though a child's active cooperation is likely to be more difficult to obtain.

A major goal of diagnostic evaluations of early childhood stuttering is to observe the kinds of speech problems that parents describe during their case history interview. Thus, I make sure to ask them if the child's speech during this evaluation was typical of what they have observed at home. If I am confident that a child is stuttering, I want to know if I have seen examples of the child's best, typical, or worst speech. In contrast, if I am uncertain that he or she is beginning to stutter and the parents tell me that what I have observed was atypically fluent, which happens much more often than the opposite, I schedule at least one more diagnostic session. Usually, however, parents' concerns are confirmed through observations of the child's speech, and the focus of the next evaluation shifts from problem identification to assessing the variability and severity of the child's disfluent speech and, ultimately, to deciding if treatment is needed.

The disfluencies of preschool-age children near stuttering onset can vary substantially. Consequently, it is important to record samples on different days as the child talks with different conversation partners and is engaged in different speaking tasks when assessing the consistency and severity of a child's early childhood stuttering (Costello and Ingham, 1984).

Ideally, each of these samples should approximate 500 to 1000 syllables in length (Yairi, 1997), and the parents or caregivers should confirm that the sample includes the kinds of disfluencies that are causing them concern. Unless samples are representative of a child's home speech, they are of limited value in assessing the consistency and severity of his or her problem. Samples should include consecutive conversational turns of a child until a least 500 to 1000 syllables are included, after echoes of utterances and one-word conversational responses have been excluded, unless they contain disfluencies.

After identifying the initial and final words of a sample, I count the number of words or syllables it contains. Words may yield satisfactory measures for two- and three-year-old children, but syllable measures are better for children whose utterances include a sizable percentage (e.g., >25%) of multisyllable words. I count the number of syllables or words in a sample twice. If the counts agree, I use that count for subsequent calculations of the percentage of words or syllables stuttered. If not, I make a third count and use either the modal or median count for future calculations.

There is no standardized or widely agreed upon set of procedures for counting children's stuttering or calculating percentages of their occurrence. The two procedures described below count all types of disfluencies, including those designated as stutter-like disfluencies (SLDs). It should be noted, however, that published definitions of stutterings, counting protocols, and calculation procedures often differ. Procedure A is one that I have used for several years, and Procedure B is based on those described by Yairi (1997).

- *Procedure A* Count each syllable or word as either fluent or disfluent. Each syllable or word should be counted only once, regardless of the type or number of disfluencies that accompany its production. Thus, if disfluent words are counted, no more than one disfluency should be counted for each multisyllable word. If disfluent syllables are counted, a multisyllable word can have as many disfluencies as there are syllables. I count the number of words or syllables that were disfluent twice. If both counts agree, I use that count to calculate the percentage of words or syllables that were disfluent. If the counts do not agree, I count the disfluent syllables or words in the sample again and use the modal or median count for my calculations.

- Next, I count the number of stuttering-like disfluencies (SLDs) in the sample, which means that each word or syllable is counted as either fluent or involving an SLD (i.e., within-word repetitions, monosyllabic word repetitions having two or more iterations, sound prolongations or dysrhythmic phonations, tense pauses, or any other type of disfluency that is perceived to involve excessive muscle tension or effort in its production). As before, I count the number of syllables or words that include one or more SLDs twice. If both counts agree, I use this count to calculate the percentage of syllables or words with SLDs or stutterings. If they disagree, I count a third time and use the modal or median count for calculations.

- *Procedure B* Only syllables are used in assessing a sample's disfluencies, and each sample is a multiple of 100 syllables because the disfluency counts are converted to the number occurring per 100 syllables and the overall sample must include a minimum of 500 syllables. Every disfluency is counted, regardless of type or how many were produced on a syllable. Thus, syllables may have a multiple number of disfluencies. Two counts of the number of disfluencies in a sample are made. If the counts agree, then that number is used to calculate the total number of disfluencies per 100 syllables. If the counts disagree, then another count is made to obtain a mode or median count for calculations. Next, every SLD is counted and includes as many as occur on each syllable. In this procedure, SLDs comprise part-word repetitions, monosyllabic word repetitions, dysrhythmic phonations, and tense pauses. As before, two counts are made, and if they do not agree, a third count is used to obtain a mode or median before calculating the number of SLDs observed per 100 syllables.

- Regardless of which of these two procedures is used, several other measures may need to be obtained if I am uncertain about a child's diagnosis of stuttering, or if I plan to systematically monitor the child's speech before deciding that treatment appears to be necessary. I rely on using counts of SLDs rather than stutters because these measures serve as guidelines that Yairi (1997) has used when monitoring stuttering children's speech following onset and for distinguishing those who will stop stuttering without treatment from those likely to continue stuttering unless they receive treatment. These supplementary measures usually include the following:

- The percentage of total disfluencies that were SLDs

- The percentage of stutter-like repetitions (SLRs), (i.e., those having two or more iterations)

- The average number of iterations found in 10 randomly selected SLRs, and the largest number found in one SLR

- The percentage of disfluencies clustering on the same or adjacent syllables or words, and the average number of disfluencies per cluster

- The percentage of SLDs that were accompanied by accessory behaviors in 10 randomly selected, SLDs

- If appropriate instrumentation is available, the mean duration of 10 randomly selected, dysrhythmic phonations and of 10 tense pauses can be obtained.

As was noted earlier, a substantial number of children who begin stuttering stop within 2 years of stuttering onset without receiving any professional treatment. Although it is not possible at the onset of stuttering to distinguish, with certainty, which children have only a transient stuttering problem and do not need therapy and which have stuttering that is likely to continue in the absence of treatment, Yairi (1997) and his colleagues have been highly successful, however, in making this differentiation by systematically monitoring young children's SLDs and have found that children who stop stuttering without receiving treatment within 2 years of stuttering onset evidence decreases in their SLDs during the first 15 months following stuttering onset. These finding are highly promising and may resolve this difficult prognostic task if they can be replicated in larger samples of early childhood stuttering at different clinical centers. From time to time, however, it may be apparent during a child's initial diagnostic evaluation that treatment should begin without delay.

Ordinarily, three concerns are involved in making such decisions: (1) the extent to which the child's speech presents a communication disability; (2) the distress experienced by the child or family as a result of stuttering; and (3) the child's risk of continuing to stutter unless effective intervention is begun. As before, two groups of indicators, expressed as questions, are presented. Each question should be answered on the basis of findings from observations of the child's speech and his or her reactions to disfluencies during diagnostic evaluations and from subsequent analyses of video recordings of evaluation sessions. The answers to these questions serve as guidelines for deciding if a child's chance for untreated remission is high or if therapy is needed.

Indicators of Early Childhood Stuttering

1. *Does the frequency of the speech disruptions observed place the child at risk for, or support a diagnosis of, childhood stuttering or some other fluency disorder?* Children who stutter, on average, are two to three times more disfluent than are their nonstuttering peers (Yairi, 1997). If a child's percentage of total disfluencies exceeds 10% of the words or syllables uttered, I believe, as do other clinicians (Adams, 1984; Conture, 1997), that the child has or is at risk for having a fluency disorder. The frequency of SLDs, however, is even more discriminating because children who stutter average five to six times more SLDs than do children who do not stutter (Yairi, 1997). For several years, I, like several clinicians (Adams, 1984; Conture, 1997; Curlee, 1984; Pindzola & White, 1986), have used a frequency of 3% or more stuttered words or syllables as a guideline for identifying childhood stuttering. If this guideline is exceeded substantially and consistently across samples, the child is clearly stuttering. Moreover, if only a few speech disfluencies are perceived to be unequivocal instances of severe stuttering, this may be sufficient evidence to conclude that a child has begun to stutter.

2. *Do the type, duration, and prosodic characteristics of the disfluencies observed place the child at risk for, or support a diagnosis of, childhood stuttering?* A child whose speech disruptions consist predominantly of revisions, interjections, or multisyllable word and phrase repetitions, and whose SLDs constitute fewer than half of all disfluencies, and whose disfluencies usually sound smooth, evenly paced, and effortless, probably is not beginning to stutter. In contrast, SLRs that have two or more iterations usually occur three times as often among children who stutter (Yairi, 1997), and if 25% or more of all SLRs have two or more iterations, I use this finding to support a diagnosis of childhood stuttering. The disfluencies of children who stutter also occur in clusters much more often and are longer than the disfluencies of nonstuttering peers (Yairi, 1997). If one-third or more of a child's disfluencies form clusters of three or more disfluencies in length on more than one-fourth of all clusters, I use this as a general guideline for confirming diagnoses of childhood stuttering (Yairi, 1997). Of course, several qualitative features of disfluencies can be used to support diagnoses of stuttering, as well. These qualitative signs may include unevenly paced and stressed SLRs that often sound faster in tempo, SLDs characterized by increases in loudness or pitch or interruptions in air flow or voicing, as well as such behaviors as averting the eyes or unusual posturing or movements of the face and neck that are suggestive

of muscle tension or struggle (Conture & Kelly, 1991, Curlee, 1984). If it is apparent that a child's speech disruptions are becoming more conspicuous and are occurring more frequently and consistently across settings, such changes should be monitored carefully to determine if the child needs treatment without further delay.

3. *Do observations of the child and parents in conversational interactions indicate a need for parent training or counseling?* Findings from empirical studies of parent-child conversational interactions and stuttering are largely inconsistent (Egolf, Shames, Johnson, & Kasprisin-Burelli, 1972; Meyers, 1990; Meyers & Freeman, 1985a; Meyers & Freeman, 1985b; Wilkenfeld & Curlee, 1997). The only prospective studies of such interactions involved families with children who have a high risk of beginning to stutter because one or both parents stuttered. No reliable differences were found in the communicative styles or speaking rates prior to stuttering onset of mothers whose children began to stutter, even though these mothers' mean length of utterance was shorter than that of mothers whose children continued to be fluent (Kloth, Janssen, Kraaimaat, & Brutten, 1995a). In addition, the receptive and expressive language abilities of the children who did and did not begin to stutter did not differ prior to onset. However, the articulation rates of those who began to stutter were significantly faster (Kloth, Janssen, Kraaimaat, & Brutten, 1995b). Thus, no evidence was found to support suspicions that mothers' communicative behaviors contribute to stuttering onsets. Several clinical trials and several case studies have reported positive outcomes for manipulating parents' conversational behaviors with their children who stutter (Kelly & Conture, 1991; Mallard, 1991; Rustin, 1987); however, none controlled for the high rate of untreated remission of stuttering that might be expected among such children, which occurs frequently in studies reporting treatment outcomes of children who stutter. Parent behaviors believed to be important include speaking rate, length and complexity of utterances, interruptions, and turn-switching pauses, although the evidence used to support these beliefs would also support the conclusion that these behaviors are reactions to the child's stuttering rather than precipitating factors. Nevertheless, it is reasonable to expect that some parents may interact with a child who stutters in ways that warrant attention. I can recall observing one mother, for example, who responded angrily whenever her son stuttered, even slapping his face once in my presence.

Remission of untreated childhood stuttering is relatively common, with more than two-thirds occurring within the first 24 months of onset (Yairi & Ambrose, 2004). If stuttering persists beyond a year without showing some signs of improving, clinical intervention should be discussed with parents because the child's chances of an untreated remission may be decreasing (Yairi, 1997). If stuttering persists and speech disruptions become longer, more complex, and effortful, it is increasingly likely that a child will begin to voice concern and evidence frustration, apprehension, and avoidance reactions about stuttering and speaking, which may become significant disabilities or handicaps in time (Bloodstein, 1987; Van Riper, 1982). If such signs are consistently present without amelioration a year after onset, I believe that direct clinical intervention should be initiated without delay if that child is to have a reasonable chance of stopping stuttering. Consequently, indicators of persistent stuttering focus on those signs that have been found in empirical research to be related to childhood stuttering continuing 3 years post-onset.

Indicators of Persistent Stuttering

1. *What changes have occurred in the child's disfluencies since onset?* A large proportion of the children who begin stuttering between their second and fourth birthdays and do not receive treatment begin to show decreases in their SLDs within 12 to 15 months of onset and eventually stop (Yairi, 1997). However, if SLDs have continued unabated or have worsened a year post-onset, it is likely the child will continue to stutter for at least 2 more years if treatment continues to be deferred (Yairi, 1997). In such cases I meet with parents and recommend that they reconsider initiating treatment with the child. If a child's speech has been monitored systematically at 2- to

3-month intervals using speech samples recorded both in and away from the clinic, the stability or increase in the child's SLDs in these recordings can be used to determine the need for beginning treatment. It should be kept in mind, also, that stuttering can worsen even if SLDs have decreased in frequency but have increased in duration, have begun to occur in more and longer clusters, or have become consistently associated with muscle tension and struggle.

2. *Were other speech-language skills developmentally appropriate?* Often, diagnostic evaluations of a child suspected of childhood stuttering will find that speech-language skills other than fluency test substantially below age expectation (Blood et al., 2002; Louko et al., 1990; St. Louis et al., 1988). In my experience, such difficulties most often involve failure to use age-appropriate language forms, especially phonology. Language-learning disabilities are present relatively often, also, among school-age children who stutter. Because the prevalence of these speech–language–learning problems is higher among school-age children who stutter than those who do not, it is possible that these "other" speech-language problems may hamper the remission of these children's fluency problems (Adams, 1990; Starkweather, 1997; Yairi et al., 1996). If treatment for these "other" problems is initiated, the child's fluency problems should be monitored to ensure that his or her stuttering does not worsen.

3. *Are the child's disfluencies frequently accompanied by signs of tension or struggle?* Such signs are commonly referred to as accessory behaviors and are thought to result from a child's efforts to "escape" from or avoid stuttering's involuntary disruptions of speech, which may become self-reinforcing behaviors if escape from or avoidance of stuttering is successful (Starkweather, 1997). For example, if a child's sound prolongations begin to extend beyond a second in duration, fluctuate in loudness or pitch, or terminate abruptly, a child's efforts to escape from a prolonged sound is an understandable reaction or adaptation to this difficulty, even though this behavior exacerbates the child's disfluencies. Even worse, termination of prolongations also reinforces all of the preceding tension-and-struggle behaviors that occurred. Similarly, tense pauses that precede effortful initiations of words appear to involve increased muscle tension and effort to initiate a word, which usually result in longer, more anomalous-appearing speech disruptions (Adams, 1984; Curlee, 1984; Van Riper, 1982) and increases their frequency of occurrence (Starkweather & Gottwald, 1990). Other commonly observed accessory behaviors include extraneous articulatory postures, eye blinks, turning of the head, and curling of the upper lip during stutters (Adams, 1984; Conture & Kelly, 1991; Curlee, 1984). Other adaptations to stuttering include substituting words, whispering, tapping a finger rhythmically to "get started," and slowing portions of utterances prior to anticipated stutters (Bloodstein, 1987; Van Riper, 1982). All of these behaviors indicate that stuttering is becoming more complex and severe, that a child's fluency difficulties are worsening and will become increasingly difficult to treat successfully if such behaviors are allowed to become habitual (Adams, 1984; Curlee, 1984; Starkweather & Gottwald, 1990). As tense postures and movements of the speech mechanism become persistent characteristics of a child's stuttering, his or her embarrassment, apprehension, frustration, and avoidance become frequent reactions to speaking and stuttering, and the child is much more likely to continue stuttering. I suspect that these motor, emotional, and cognitive signs and symptoms are largely self-reinforcing responses that hinder a child's production of speech that is free of stuttering and that, in time, may be only partially modifiable in stuttering adults (Curlee, 1984). Thus, the frequent and consistent occurrence of these motor, emotional, and cognitive responses may ultimately produce a chronic stuttering syndrome.

4. *Does the child display negative emotional reactions or express concern about disfluent speech?* It is not uncommon for even young preschoolers to seem embarrassed or frustrated about their fluency disruptions and to leave the impression that they often feel apprehensive about their speech. Some may exclaim, with evident emotion, "What's wrong with me?" when an especially severe stutter disrupts their efforts to communicate. When asked about their speech, some may simply state that they stutter or say that talking is difficult or that words get "stuck" sometimes. A Communication Attitude Test appropriate for school-age children has

been developed to quantify how stuttering and nonstuttering children's beliefs about speech differ (Vanryckeghem et al., 2005). Although negative emotions and attitudes commonly accompany persistent stuttering, they are not obligatory symptoms, and a substantial percentage of young preschoolers have been found to display such reactions near stuttering onset (Yairi & Ambrose, 2004). If stuttering persists into adulthood, however, reacting to speaking and stuttering with apprehension and fear, holding negative attitudes about speech, and seeing oneself as being disabled by stuttering are viewed by some clinicians as obligatory symptoms (Sheehan, 1958) that are typically present to some extent among adults who stutter. This view is consistent with my own clinical experience, and I believe that negative affective and cognitive reactions to stuttering by adults who stutter are much more likely to result in educational, vocational, or psychosocial handicaps than are the disruptions in communication produced by their stuttering.

Case Selection Criteria

Following initial observations and testing of the child, clinicians need to integrate the information obtained from their examination of the child with that from the parent interview. Most often the information from these two sources is complementary and provides a sound basis for drawing a diagnostic conclusion. Occasionally, there are substantial discrepancies, and these discrepancies need to be resolved through further interviews, observations, or testing. In my experience, however, substantial differences between parents' descriptions of a child's stuttering and what I observed during the clinical examination are usually the result of a child's inconsistent stuttering in the clinic rather than inaccurate parental descriptions. Thus, I usually assume that parents' descriptions are accurate and will be confirmed in time by direct or taped observations of a child's speech.

As was noted earlier, evaluations of children suspected of childhood stuttering result in one of five diagnostic conclusions. Each is listed below and is followed by a brief sketch of the signs and symptoms that often characterize each conclusion.

1. *Few, if any, signs of childhood stuttering are present and the child's spoken language is age-appropriate.* These children are often highly disfluent, but their interjections and repetitions of words and phrases seem to reflect efforts to maintain their speaking turns while engaged in linguistic encoding processes. Speech disfluencies of all types may exceed 10% of the syllables or words uttered, but the frequency of their SLDs usually seem to be free of excessive muscle tension and effort, and they ordinarily occur on fewer that 2 to 3% of the words or syllables uttered. Moreover, their performance on speech-language and hearing screening tests falls within normal range.

2. *Inconsistent signs of childhood stuttering are present, and further observation and testing are needed.* Some of these children may be described by parents as having stuttered severely initially, but few, if any, SLDs are present in the speech samples that were recorded and analyzed. This suggests that stuttering is not a consistent problem, which I view as a positive prognostic sign. Nevertheless, there has to be some concern that even infrequent instances of severe stuttering may be a forerunner of a significant fluency problem for a child in the future. Some preschoolers may seldom speak during their evaluation, answering questions with short utterances or a shrug of the shoulders. The result, of course, is that little stuttering is likely to occur, and other ways of observing and recording the child's speech are needed. In such cases, I have the parents videotape the child's speech several times a week at home, which they bring to the clinic for the series of follow-up evaluations I schedule. Analyses of the video recordings made at home and during the follow-up evaluations at the clinic will usually reveal whether or not the child is beginning to stutter and, if so, which clinical management approaches should be considered. It has been my experience that most of these children stop stuttering without receiving any treatment within 2 to 3 years.

3. *Signs of childhood stuttering have been present for less than 1 year, and behavioral and affective reactions to stuttering are seldom observed.* These children's speech samples usually evidence varying levels of SLDs ranging from 3 to 10%. Their speech may seldom be completely free of these disfluencies for extended periods of time. They may avert their eyes during disfluencies, some of which may also be characterized by increases in pitch, loudness, or tempo, as if excessive muscle tension were involved. If asked why he or she came to the clinic, many answer "Because of my speech" or "Because I stutter." Some seem irritated or frustrated when they are having unusual difficulty speaking but are likely to show little concern otherwise. If these signs continue unabated across multiple speech samples during follow-up monitoring evaluations for a year or more post-onset, I believe that direct clinical intervention should begin.

4. *Signs of childhood stuttering are present as well as one or more other speech-language problems.* These children consistently show signs of early stuttering and either do not pass or do not follow instructions for the speech-language screening tests that were administered. As a result, the child's speech-language skills may not be age-appropriate or fall within normal range. In such cases, I defer treatment decisions until follow-up assessments provide the information being sought about the child's speech-language skills. If the findings from these follow-up assessments indicate that therapy for a phonological or another expressive language problem is needed, I usually select treatment procedures that incorporate fluency-enhancing manners of speaking, such as speaking slowly and rhythmically, and whispering, so that the child's stuttering does not worsen during language therapy sessions. Chapters 11 and 12 describe approaches to such problems.

5. *Stuttering has been present consistently for a year or more with no signs of remitting.* Speech is often hard work for these children. Stutters occur frequently, sometimes in excess of 15% of the syllables or words uttered. The stutterers often sound effortful and are accompanied by a variety of blinks, facial twitches, lip tremors, or posturing of the articulators. Signs of frustration and avoidance are not uncommon, even among preschoolers, and usually increase with age. Although these signs may be present in some children at or soon after stuttering begins, they frequently decrease substantially within a few weeks. Typically, however, this level of severity is seldom present consistently until a child has been stuttering several years. There are several reasons why these children should be enrolled in treatment without delay. First, stuttering this severe can be a significant communication disability or handicap for most children. Second, remissions occur less frequently among persons whose severe stuttering has persisted for some time (Curlee, 1984; Sheehan & Martyn, 1970). Lastly, there is some evidence that treatment outcomes are better and that remission occurs more frequently in young children than in older teens and adults who stutter (Shearer & Williams, 1965).

It would be much more convenient, of course, if all the signs and symptoms of every stuttering child were characteristic of just one diagnostic conclusion. In actuality, many children evidence signs that are characteristic of more than one conclusion during some evaluations and then evidence different characteristics during other evaluations. If there is substantial uncertainty about which diagnostic conclusion is most appropriate, further observation and testing are needed. Many clinicians, however, believe that every child who stutters or is at risk to begin stuttering should receive some type of professional intervention and have advanced a variety of arguments for enrolling them in therapy, and sometimes with the parents, as well (Gregory, 2003; Starkweather, Gottwald, & Halfond, 1990). Some argue, for example, that early treatment of young children is more efficient and effective, even if it might be unnecessary, because no harm would be done. They are correct, however, in stating that many preschoolers stop stuttering during treatment and appear to be "cured," which seldom occurs among older teens and adults (Curlee, 1984). To date, however, studies of such treatments have not included randomly assigned, untreated comparison groups to control for the high rate of stuttering remissions among this age group of young children (Franken, Kielstra-van Der Schalk, & Boelens, 2005). Consequently, the percentage of children who stop stuttering as a result of early treatment is uncertain. Even single-subject studies, which can demonstrate that decreases in a child's stuttering are related to the treatment employed, cannot determine which of these children would have stopped stuttering sometime later without such treatment. Thus, there are several reasons why other clinicians believe that therapy is not the only management alternative that should be considered.

Some remissions may reflect a child's natural growth or maturation processes. Others might involve common sense, folk remedies employed by the parents, or the compensatory behavioral adjustments discovered through a child's efforts to cope with stuttering. Regardless, the majority of these young children, probably three-fourths or more, do not require treatment to stop stuttering. In addition, there is no evidence that postponing therapy for 6 months, 1 year, or more results in poorer treatment outcomes (Curlee & Yairi, 1997). Thus, systematic monitoring of a child's speech during the first year post-onset of stuttering is an appropriate alternative for many of these children, especially in light of all of the accompanying fees and time commitments that are usually involved in treatment. Still, the uncertainty about the necessity of treatment for a specific child who stutters may present a dilemma for some clinicians.

Dealing with Uncertainty about Need for Treatment

My preference in dealing with dilemmas like this is to support the parents' decision of whether or not to enroll a child in an early intervention program. This also introduces the parents to the kind of clinical partnership I want us to have if direct treatment of the child's stuttering is to begin. Consequently, once initial observations and testing of a child are completed, I schedule a follow-up meeting at a time when both parents can attend. This meeting provides them an opportunity to raise questions and concerns that may have arisen since our case history interview or as a result of reading the informational material that I have given them.

I like to begin this session by chatting briefly with the parents, to set them at ease, before beginning a discussion of the evaluation. I always ask how the child's speech has been at home and if more questions or concerns have arisen since we last met, then I begin my review of the evaluation findings by saying something like, "I think I have good news for you" or "I know you're interested in learning what we found, so let's get started," before launching into a careful summary of the findings. I try to relate what was observed during clinical evaluation sessions to what was reported during the case history interview. I believe that linking the diagnostic signs I observed during the evaluation with the "problems" parents have described makes it easier for them to understand and accept the conclusions I have drawn, but I am always careful to check on the parents' reactions to the information I am providing throughout the meeting. If it is clear that their child is stuttering, I review current research findings on the remission of stuttering in young children and the treatment outcomes expected for a child this age in this clinic. Once this is accomplished, I believe parents are prepared for a discussion of the clinical intervention alternatives I believe would be most appropriate for their child. If more than one alternative seems to be appropriate, which can often be the case, I assist the parents in discussing the clinical procedures and scheduling that would be involved and support whatever decision they feel is best for them and their child.

A few parents may need to be told that their child does not appear to be stuttering or does not evidence age-inappropriate or abnormal disfluencies and that there is no reason for concern on their part. However, in more than 30 years of clinical practice with childhood stuttering, I have evaluated only a handful of preschoolers whose fluency was clearly age-appropriate, even though their parents firmly believed they were stuttering. Such parents, however, usually seem relieved and very satisfied when informed that their child does not stutter. Nevertheless, a few find it difficult to accept that nothing is wrong with their child's speech, but thorough follow-up evaluations will usually convince such family members that any current or emerging problems in their child's speech will receive treatment and not be overlooked.

Most parents whose children I've seen within 6 months of stuttering onset prefer to have their child's speech carefully monitored for a while to see if their child's stuttering decreases substantially over the next few months. Many also indicate that they have tried to modify how they interact and converse with their child, in keeping with the informational material they were provided.

I believe that most of them feel less apprehensive or concerned about their child's speech if they are actively involved in trying to solve the child's problem. The decision to initiate therapy without delay is a management alternative chosen most often by parents if their child has been stuttering a year or more or is obviously upset about it. Parents who are highly concerned and upset about their child's speech usually want to begin therapy sooner than do those who are less alarmed. I also ask parents to choose between having their child seen in the clinic two or three times each week or learning how to implement a home management program for the child. Chapter 4, by Harrison, Onslow, and Rousseau, describes response-contingency procedures that parents can be trained to use successfully at home with a child who stutters.

Only a few parents, in my experience, decline to initiate therapy when no other management alternatives are suggested. At such times, I see if they will agree to my monitoring the child's speech for a while and try to understand their reluctance to begin therapy. Some families may have financial or transportation difficulties, whereas others may need additional time to accept the possibility that their child's "problem" is unlikely to be a passing phase of speech development and that professional intervention is needed. Regardless, if parents feel supported and feel that their decision is respected rather than rejected, it is usually only a few weeks until they begin to ask questions about starting therapy if their child continues to have significant stuttering problems. Although careful monitoring of the child may have only delayed the inevitable, there is no evidence that such delays are harmful in the long run, and they may, in fact, result in beginning treatment sooner than would otherwise occur in some families.

Thus, a diagnostic evaluation's concluding interview with the parents can often become a clinical session for the parents that educates them about stuttering and enlists them as partners in the clinical management of their child. They need to know that there are no guarantees, even though the odds strongly favor their child stopping stuttering, regardless of what they decide to do about therapy initially, and that some children who receive treatment continue to stutter. Such sessions may be filled with questions, long pauses, and much uncertainty. But if parents have confidence in the clinician, they are likely to leave such sessions feeling that they have made the right decision for their child and that their child's fluency difficulties will not become a severe, lifelong disability or handicap. Thus, a successful session should result in the parents feeling that, with the support and assistance of the clinician, their child's stuttering will be managed successfully.

◆ Clinical Management Decisions

As was noted in previous sections, a variety of treatment strategies have been used with apparent success with young children who are beginning to stutter (Curlee, 1984; Egolf, Shames, Johnson & Kasprisin-Burelli, 1972; Gregory, 2003; Kelly & Conture, 1991; Mallard, 1991; Peters & Guitar, 1991; Rustin, 1987; Starkweather, Gottwald, & Halfond, 1990; Van Riper, 1973). Indirect strategies are those that try to improve the child's speech by targeting the environment or changing some aspect of the child's behavior other than stuttering. At present, most indirect strategies rely on general parenting instruction, and counseling in some cases, to accomplish goals. Parent counseling, in particular, is frequently used as an adjunct to other treatment procedures for childhood stuttering (Gregory, 2003; Kloth et al., 1995; Peters & Guitar, 1991; Van Riper, 1973), and a diverse range of therapy procedures and goals have been described. Chapter 9 by DiLollo and Manning presents their views on counseling children and their parents. In contrast, direct strategies largely rely on response-contingent conditioning programs, fluency training, and other programmed learning procedures to decrease stuttering. Many clinicians, of course, use several different procedures, often in combination, in working with young children who stutter (e.g., Peters & Guitar, 1991), and subsequent chapters in this text describe a variety of procedures that are suitable for preschool through school-age children.

Systematic monitoring of a child's stuttering, both at home and in the clinic, is necessary to determine if satisfactory improvement is occurring with or without treatment. The parents need to be enlisted as active participants in monitoring the child's stuttering. There are many ways in which monitoring can be accomplished satisfactorily. What follows is one such way. Audio or video recordings of the child's speech during unstructured play with parents, siblings, or friends should be analyzed and reviewed monthly. Monitoring at the clinic should be scheduled at 2- to 3-month intervals. However, for those children whose stuttering is steadily decreasing on at-home recordings and elsewhere by parent report, I may delay follow-up visits until 6 months has passed. In contrast, children whose stuttering worsens substantially between scheduled follow-up visits should be seen during this period of heightened stuttering, if possible. During each clinic visit, samples of the child conversing with a parent and with a clinician during play or other unstructured activities should be obtained. When no stuttering is apparent in these samples, other recordings should be made of such tasks as an extended narrative or retelling of a familiar story or of the clinician speaking rapidly, frequently interrupting, and hurrying the child's speech. I use such stressful conversational interchanges to evaluate the sensitivity of a child's stuttering to stress and emotional arousal and as an indicator that in-clinic monitoring can be reduced or terminated.

When untreated remission of stuttering occurs, measures of SLDs frequency and duration gradually decrease; however, consistent, continuous decreases in stuttering across samples and time rarely occur in my experience. Typically, stuttering continues to wax and wane in frequency and severity from one day to another and situation to situation, but is usually more intermittent and less noticeable across monthly intervals. In time, at-home and in-clinic recordings become free of stuttering and parents report observing no stuttering elsewhere.

◆ Expected Outcomes

Clinical records are subject to several biases. The data from these records applies only to those families who chose to obtain assistance for a child's stuttering at a specific clinic, a university speech-language training clinic in this case. The data are always incomplete because clients stop treatment for a variety of reasons; the child begins school, the family moves, loss of employment, divorce, or illness disrupts the family's contact with the clinic, or parents decide to "stop therapy for awhile," apparently satisfied, although the child still stutters occasionally. Even those whose treatment ends only after there is no evidence of stuttering for several months may not return to the clinic if stuttering should recur. For these and other reasons, clinical records are anecdotal reports at best and their validity is always open to question. The expected outcomes summarized below are based on such records and should be interpreted accordingly.

Well over half of the children whose parents choose to defer active intervention and monitor the child's speech through recorded speaking samples at home and the clinic, supplemented by their own observations, can be expected to stop stuttering. As a group, these children have not been stuttering as long and probably evidence less frequent and less consistent stuttering at the time of their initial evaluation than do those whose parents decide to initiate therapy. Those who do not stop or show substantial decreases in stuttering in their monitored samples within 12 to 15 months of onset are enrolled in therapy, if parents permit. Children with concomitant speech-language problems are enrolled in therapy without delay as are most of those who have been stuttering 1 year or longer and whose stuttering appears likely to persist. Over half of these children are dismissed with little if any residual stuttering remaining within a year. Of those remaining, many will continue to evidence below average skills in phonology or other areas of language after a year of therapy. They may continue to stutter, even though some improvement usually has occurred. A few show little progress at first, and alternative treatment procedures should be tried or referral to another clinic considered.

◆ Conclusion

This chapter has presented information on childhood stuttering, its onset, and progression or remission, and it has summarized many of the findings from the University of Illinois longitudinal study of preschool-age children who stutter, which are a major support for clinicians wanting to monitor the disfluencies of such children during the first year post-onset. Diagnostic evaluation procedures and guidelines for identifying childhood stuttering and deciding which children have transient fluency difficulties and which appear to require treatment have been described. Such decisions, at present, rely heavily on the experience and judgment of clinicians because sufficient data from adequately controlled clinical research are not yet available. Based on the data that are available, and some 30 years of clinical experience, I have suggested that most children who begin to stutter do not require treatment and will stop stuttering within 2 years of onset. Although I believe that treatment can be deferred without harming these children or adversely affecting their later treatment, I also believe that a child's parents should make the decision of whether to defer or begin treatment without delay. In addition, systematic monitoring of a child's speech should be maintained until stuttering has stopped or it seems highly likely that stuttering will persist unless treated. Such monitoring provides empirical support for the decisions to be made and should also reduce errors of human judgment.

Deferring treatment in favor of systematic monitoring should be considered for children who are not yet 5 years of age and who have been stuttering less than a year. Deferring treatment after this period or with older stuttering children may entail greater risks. When there are other issues to consider, however, such as other speech-language problems, stuttering severe enough to handicap communication, apprehension and concern about stuttering by the parents or child, or parental wishes that the child be helped without delay, treatment should be scheduled as soon as possible. Thus, deciding whether or not to defer treatment ordinarily arises for only two of the five diagnostic conclusions that were presented in an earlier section:

1. when only inconsistent signs of childhood stuttering are present, or

2. when signs of stuttering have been present less than a year and other problems or complicating factors are absent.

References

Adams, M. (1984). The young stutterer: Diagnosis, treatment, and assessment of progress. In W. Perkins (Ed.), Stuttering disorders. New York: Thieme-Stratton Inc.

Ambrose, N. G., Cox, N. J., & Yairi, E. (1997). The genetic basis of persistence and recovery in stuttering. Journal of Speech and Hearing Research 40, 567–580.

Andrews, G. (1984). The epidemiology of stuttering. In R. Curlee & W. Perkins (Eds.), Nature and treatment of stuttering: New directions. San Diego: College-Hill Press.

Blood, G. W., Ridenour, V. J., Qualls, C. D., & Hammer, C. S. (2003). Co-occurring disorders in children who stutter. Journal of Communication Disorders 36, 427–448.

Bloodstein, O. (1987). A handbook on stuttering (4th ed). Chicago: National Easter Seal Society.

Conture, E. G. (1997). Evaluating childhood stuttering. In R. F. Curlee & G. M. Siegel (Eds.), Nature and treatment of stuttering: New directions (2nd ed.). Boston: Allyn and Bacon.

Conture, E. G. (2001). Stuttering: Its nature, diagnosis, and treatment. Needham Heights, MA: Allyn and Bacon.

Conture, E. G., Fraser J. (1989). Stuttering and your child: Questions and answers. Memphis: Speech Foundation of America.

Conture, E. G., Kelly, E. M. (1991). Young stutterers' nonspeech behavior during stuttering. Journal of Speech and Hearing Research 34, 1041–1056.

Curlee, R. (1984). A case selection strategy for young disfluent children. In W. Perkins (Ed.), Stuttering disorders. New York: Thieme-Stratton.

Curlee, R. (1999). Identification and case selection guidelines for early childhood stuttering. In R. Curlee (Ed.), Stuttering and related disorders of fluency (2nd ed.). New York: Thieme.

Curlee R., & Yairi, E. (1997). Early intervention with early childhood stuttering: A critical examination of the data. American Journal of Speech-Language Pathology 6, 8–18.

Dickson, S. (1971). Incipient stuttering symptoms and spontaneous remission of stuttered speech. Journal of Communication Disorders 4, 99–110.

Egolf, D. B., Shames, G. H., Johnson, P. R., & Kasprisin-Burrelli, A. (1972). The use of parent-child interaction patterns in therapy for young stutterers. Journal of Speech and Hearing Disorders 37, 222–232.

Felsenfeld, S. (1997). Epidemiology and genetics of stuttering. In R. Curlee & G. Siegel (Eds.), Nature and treatment of stuttering: New directions (2nd ed). Boston: Allyn and Bacon.

Franken, M. C. J., Kielstra-Van der Schalk, C. J., & Boelens, H. (2005). Experimental treatment of early stuttering: A preliminary study. Journal of Fluency Disorders 30, 189–199.

Gregory, H. H. (2003). Stuttering therapy rationale and procedures. Boston: Allyn and Bacon.

Hubbard, C., & Yairi, E. (1988). Clustering of disfluencies in the speech of stuttering and nonstuttering preschool children. Journal of Speech and Hearing Research 31, 228–233.

Johnson, W., & Associates. (1959). The onset of stuttering: Research findings and implications. Minneapolis, MN: University of Minnesota Press.

Kelly, E., & Conture E. (1991). Intervention with school-age stutterers: A parent-child fluency group approach. Seminars in Speech and Language 12, 309–321.

Kidd, K. (1984). Stuttering as a genetic disorder. In R. Curlee & W. Perkins (Eds.), Nature and treatment of stuttering: New directions. San Diego: College-Hill Press.

Kloth S., Janssen, P., Kraaimaat, F., & Brutten, G. (1995). Speech-motor and linguistic skills of young stutterers prior to onset. Journal of Fluency Disorders 20, 157–170.

Kloth, S., Janssen, P., Kraaimaat, F., & Brutten, G. (1995). Communicative behavior of mothers of stuttering and nonstuttering high-risk children prior to the onset of stuttering. Journal of Fluency Disorders 20, 365–377.

Louko, L., Edwards, M., & Conture, E. (1990). Phonological characteristics of young stutterers and their normally fluent peers. Journal of Fluency Disorders 15, 191–210.

Mallard, A. R. (1991) Family intervention in stuttering therapy. Seminars in Speech and Language 12, 265–278.

Mansson, H. (2000). Childhood stuttering: Incidence and development. Journal of Fluency Disorders 25, 41–57.

McDearmon J. R. (1968). Primary stuttering at the onset of stuttering: A re-examination of data. Journal of Speech and Hearing Research 11, 631–637.

Meyers, S. C. (1990). Verbal behaviors of preschool stutterers and conversational partners: Observing reciprocal relationships. Journal of Speech and Hearing Disorders 55, 706–712.

Meyers, S. C., & Freeman, F. J. (1985a). Interruptions as a variable in stuttering and disfluency. Journal of Speech and Hearing Research 28, 428–435.

Meyers, S. C., & Freeman, F. J. (1985b). Mother and child speech rates as a variable in stuttering and disfluency. Journal of Speech and Hearing Research 28, 436–444.

Pellowski, M. W., & Conture, E. G. (2002). Characteristics of speech disfluency and stuttering behaviors in 3- and 4-year-old children. Journal of Speech and Hearing Research 45, 20–34.

Peters T., & Guitar B. (1991). Stuttering: An integrated approach to its nature and treatment. Baltimore: Williams and Wilkins.

Pindzola, R. H., & White, D. T. (1986). A protocol for differentiating the incipient stutterer. Language, Speech, and Hearing Services in Schools 17, 2–15.

Rustin, L. (1987). Assessment and therapy programme for dysfluent children. Tucson, AZ: Communication Skill Builders.

Ryan, B. (1990). Development of stuttering: A longitudinal study presented at the Annual Convention of the American Speech-Language-Hearing Association in Seattle. ASHA 32, 144 [Abstract]

Shearer, W. M., & Williams, J. D. Self-recovery from stuttering. (1965). Journal of Speech and Hearing Disorders 30, 288–290.

Sheehan, J. G., & Martyn, M. M. Stuttering and its disappearance. (1970). Journal of Speech and Hearing Research 13, 279–289.

St. Louis, K., Hinzman, A., & Hull, F. (1985). Studies of cluttering: Disfluency and language measures in young possible clutterers and stutterers. Journal of Fluency Disorders 10, 151–172.

St. Louis, K., Hinzman, A., & Mason, N. (1988). A descriptive study of speech, language and hearing characteristics of school-age stutterers. Journal of Fluency Disorders 13, 331–356.

Starkweather, W. (1997). Learning and its role in stuttering development. In R. Curlee & G. Siegel (Eds.), Nature and treatment of stuttering: New directions (2nd ed.). Boston: Allyn and Bacon.

Starkweather, W., & Gottwald, S. (1990). The demands and capacities model II: Clinical applications. Journal of Fluency Disorders 15, 143–158.

Starkweather, W., Gottwald, S., & Halfond, M. (1990). Stuttering prevention: A clinical method. Englewood Cliffs, NJ: Prentice-Hall.

Van Riper, C. (1973). The treatment of stuttering. Englewood Cliffs, NJ: Prentice-Hall.

Van Riper, C. (1975). The stutterer's clinician. In J. Eisenson (Ed.), Stuttering: A second symposium. New York: Harper and Row.

Van Riper, C. (1982). The Nature of stuttering (2nd ed.). Englewood Cliffs, NJ: Prentice-Hall.

Vanryckeghem, M., Brutten, G. J., & Hernandez, M. (2005). A comparative investigation of the speech-associated attitude of preschool and kindergarten children who do and do not stutter. Journal of Fluency Disorders 30, 307–318.

Westby, C. E. (1979). Language performance of stuttering and nonstuttering children. Journal of Communication Disorders 12, 133–145.

Wexler, K., & Mysak, E. (1982). Disfluency characteristics of 2-, 4-, and 6-year-old males. Journal of Fluency Disorders 7, 37–46.

Wilkenfeld, J., & Curlee, R. (1997). Effects of adult questions and comments on the frequency of stuttering. American Journal of Speech-Language Pathology 6, 79–89.

Yairi, E. (1981). Disfluencies of normally speaking two-year-old children. Journal of Speech and Hearing Research 24, 490–495.

Yairi, E. (1983). The onset of stuttering in two- and three-year-old children: A preliminary report. Journal of Speech and Hearing Disorders 48, 171–177.

Yairi, E. (1997). Disfluency characteristics of childhood stuttering. In R. Curlee & G. Siegel (Eds), Nature and treatment of stuttering: New directions. (2nd ed.). Boston: Allyn and Bacon.

Yairi, E, & Ambrose, N. (1990). Onset of stuttering: Age, sex, onset type, and other factors. ASHA 32, 144.

Yairi, E., & Ambrose, N. (1992). Onset of stuttering in preschool children: Selected factors. Journal of Speech and Hearing Research 35, 782–788.

Yairi, E., & Ambrose, N. (2004). Early childhood stuttering. Austin, TX: Pro-ED.

Yairi, E., Ambrose, N., Paden, E., & Throneburg, R. (1996). Predictive factors of persistence and recovery: Pathways of childhood stuttering. Journal of Communication Disorders 29, 51–77.

Yairi, E., & Lewis, B. (1984). Disfluencies at the onset of stuttering. Journal of Speech and Hearing Research 27, 154–159.

Yaruss, J. S. (1997). Clinical implications of situational variability in preschool children who stutter. Journal of Fluency Disorders 22(4), 263–286.

Yaruss, J. S., LaSalle, L. R., & Conture, E.G. (1998). Evaluating stuttering in young children: Diagnostic data. American Journal of Speech-Language Pathology 7, 62–76.

Zackheim, C. T., & Conture, E. G. (2003). Childhood stuttering and speech disfluencies in relation to children's mean length of utterance: A preliminary study. Journal of Fluency Disorders 28, 115–142.

Zebrowski, P. M. (1991). Duration of the speech disfluencies of beginning stutterers. Journal of Speech and Hearing Research 34, 483–491.

2

Treatment Factors that Influence Therapy Outcomes of Children Who Stutter

Patricia M. Zebrowski

◆ The Efficacy of Stuttering Therapy for Children: Data and Debate

The purpose of this chapter is to describe what elements, aside from those specific to a particular treatment approach, might influence a child's responsiveness to stuttering therapy. Considering the similarities between stuttering therapy and more general counseling and psychotherapy approaches to behavioral change (e.g., both attempt to change a client's behavior through nonmedical, nonsurgical, or nonpharmacological means), it seems quite reasonable to consider the nontreatment variables that influence stuttering therapy responsiveness within the "four factors" framework described by Asay and Lambert (2004) for individuals receiving psychotherapy or counseling. Specifically, what child and parent extratherapeutic change factors and what aspects of the client-clinician relationship promote the behavioral, cognitive, and affective changes that underlie successful stuttering therapy for children? What role might expectancy or hope, either on the part of the child who stutters, his or her parents, or both, play in the child or family's responsiveness to treatment?

As the emphasis on evidence-based practice continues to flourish, researchers and clinicians in speech-language pathology have worked to verify that a particular treatment approach "works" (e.g., Hancock et al., 1998; Herder et al., 2005; Ingham, 2003; Langevin & Kully, 2003; see Bernstein Ratner, 2005a for review). Unfortunately, few, if any, studies have investigated the equally important question of why a particular treatment works when it does (Bernstein Ratner, 2005a). One of the main objectives of any treatment efficacy research is to prove the functional relationship between a particular therapy approach or technique and measurable changes in the targeted behavior of interest. As such, most therapy efficacy and effectiveness studies regarding stuttering have used pre- and post-treatment comparisons of measures of speech fluency as either the single or at least the most relevant indication of a positive outcome for adults and children who stutter. Relatively fewer reports exist in which other observations or measures of treatment achievement, in addition to increased speech fluency, are highlighted. In studies of adults who stutter, these other variables have been related to a successful therapy experience, successful long-term management of stuttering, or unassisted recovery from stuttering. These include, but are not limited to, such factors as motivation, a positive attitude toward self and communication, increased self-confidence, and changing role acceptance (DiLollo, Neimeyer, & Manning, 2002; Guitar, 1976; Guitar & Bass, 1978; Plexico, Manning, & DiLollo, 2005).

In brief, findings from empirical studies along with anecdotal reports of therapy experiences (from both the clinician and the client point of view) have provided solid evidence that successful stuttering therapy for adults can be attributed to a combination of behavioral, affective, and cognitive change. Further, it is clear that although there are commonalities among adults who stutter with regard to which variables are the most strongly related to positive change, as in all human conditions it is also the case that significant differences exist within the population. What seems to work for the group may very well be ineffective for an individual adult or child who stutters.

In contrast, relatively few data are available that indicate what "child-dependent" or "child-independent" variables are associated with therapy outcome for children who stutter. As with adults, most of the existing literature about treatment efficacy and effectiveness was designed to assess the relationship between a specific therapy approach and changes in speech fluency. The bulk of quantitative evidence supporting therapy efficacy and effectiveness for children comes from four "types" of studies. The first such approach has involved some *variation of fluency shaping*, in which the child is taught to change the entirety of speech production through the use of prolonged or "stretched" vowels or consonants, "easy" or "smooth" onset of speech, and the like. The outcome is typically a combination of both controlled and, to some extent, spontaneous fluency (e.g., Hancock et al., 1998). The second such approach has involved so-called *operant or response-contingent* approaches, in which speech fluency is increased and stuttering is decreased through systematic or prescribed implementation of schedules of reinforcement and punishment (e.g., Costello, 1975, 1983; Onslow, Andrews, & Lincoln, 1994; Ryan & Van Kirk, 1974). The third approach has involved *language-based* approaches in which spontaneous fluency in utterances of increasing length and complexity is practiced and reinforced (e.g., Costello, 1983, 1999; Ryan, 1974). Finally, the fourth approach has involved *indirect* approaches in which a reduced speech rate and/or turn-switching pauses of increased duration are used by parents and clinicians when talking with the child who stutters (e.g., Conture & Melnick, 1999; Onslow & Packman, 1999; Stephenson-Opsal & Bernstein Ratner, 1988; Zebrowski, Weiss, Savelkoul, & Hammer, 1996). In all four types of studies, measures of stuttering frequency composed the main, if not the sole, dependent variable. Of note is that few studies of treatment efficacy for stuttering in children have focused either mainly or partially on changing stuttering (i.e., "stuttering modification" or "stutter more fluently") as opposed to learning controlled fluency, or "relearning" spontaneous fluency, even though the former are widely used. This is the case for both adult and child treatment studies. As Cordes (1998) notes in a review of "recommended" and "researched" therapy approaches in the stuttering literature, "more than half (of the recommended approaches) were exclusively cognitive or relied heavily on cognitive procedures (components of stuttering modification approaches), but only 10 of 81 research reports involved cognitive/emotional procedures" (pp. 121-122). "Cognitive," in this context appears to be used to contrast these approaches to those considered "behavioral"; however, whether such approaches accurately access the cognitive processes assumed to underlie their effectiveness is still less than clear. Suffice it to say that this situation—contrasting behavioral and nonbehavioral approaches—has been the impetus for spirited debate for many years (e.g., Finn, 2004; Ingham, 2005; Ingham & Cordes, 1999; Weiss, Hall, & Leahy, 2005; Bernstein Ratner, 2005b).

This author considers with caution the argument that a lack of empirical support for any treatment means the approach is not efficacious and should not be used. In the case of stuttering modification and related approaches, it is difficult to discount the fact that all or part of this treatment paradigm has been used for many years by numerous experienced clinicians who report client success, and whose client's also report success using some of these methods (Finn, 1996; see Guitar, 1998, pp. 214–224 for discussion of various clinicians and the stuttering modification approaches they advocate). Further, most of the clinicians and researchers who developed and refined the so-called stuttering modification approach were people who stuttered themselves, and who used intense study of their own stuttering and the situations and conditions in which it varied as the basis for the approach (Gregory, 2003; Hulit, 2004; Johnson, 1929, 1931, 1961; Van Riper, 1973; Williams, 1957, 1979). This point is significant. It seems contradictory to suggest that, on the one hand, we can better understand what works in therapy (and how it works) through the subjective reports of those individuals who consider themselves to be "recovered" (Finn, 1996; Chmela, 1997; Ramig, 1997; Quesal, 1997), yet, on the other hand, we can criticize clinicians who use treatment approaches developed by scientists and clinicians who stutter (e.g., Ingham & Cordes, 1999).

Finn (2004) makes a good point in arguing that judgment heuristics (decision "rules of thumb") can bias clinical decision making, and as such, "clinical experience is an insufficient basis for determining treatment effectiveness" (p. 9). However, let's not throw out the baby with the bath water. Clinicians need to be aware of the extent to which they rely on such rules of thumb (i.e., availability, representativeness, etc.) to make treatment decisions, but at the same time, every clinical profession that involves making a diagnosis, prognosis, and recommendations for treatment requires clinical judgment, a process that by definition *requires* the use of *all* available information, *including the clinician's experience* (e.g., Grove, Zald, Lebow, Snitz, & Nelson, 2000; Records and Weiss, 1990). This is standard practice. The reality is that in clinical work, no matter what the field, the clinician's experience is a necessary piece of the decision-making process. Regardless, it remains the case that those who advocate approaches that focus on stuttering and not fluency share a responsibility to provide empirical evidence that doing so benefits their clients in some way, whether short-, medium- or long-term. The reason for lack of such evidence in both research and clinical journals is unclear, but it can be partially explained by the discussion with which this chapter began. That is, what constitutes effectiveness, and what functional relationship exists between therapy techniques or strategies and whatever variable(s) are used to measure effectiveness? In other words, what constitutes appropriate evidence and who decides? Considering the nature of stuttering modification, it is likely that the primary obstacle to efficacy research for this approach is the difficulty in operationally defining, standardizing, and measuring both the techniques used and the variables that indicate a client's responsiveness to treatment. This is in part due to the fact that although defined by guiding principles, one of the hallmarks of stuttering modification therapy is that it is client-centered, not clinician-centered, and as such it is tailored to the individual client. The inherent nature of this approach renders it difficult to uniformly describe, a necessary condition for efficacy research. Until this is done, and studies are performed, the argument that the approaches shown to be effective (fluency shaping and so-called operant approaches such as the Lidcombe procedures (Onslow, Packman, & Harrison, 2003) are the only "responsible" choices for stuttering clients will continue.

◆ Treatment Responsiveness to Psychotherapy: Application to Stuttering Therapy for Children

The biggest challenge for any clinician who attempts to bring about behavioral change in children (and adults for that matter)—speech-language pathologists, physical therapists, occupational therapists, counselors, and psychotherapists alike—is to decide what therapy approach has the highest probability of helping the particular child the most.

Within the field of psychotherapy, numerous studies have compared the effectiveness of different therapeutic approaches for the treatment of such problems as depression, anxiety, and schizophrenia in children and adults. Many of these investigations consisted of meta-analyses of the efficacy of various types of therapy (e.g., Wampold et al., 1997). Surprisingly, with rare exception this research has uncovered little significant difference in effectiveness among different psychotherapy approaches. According to Tallman and Bohart (2004), this observation has been described as "the dodo bird verdict" (Luborsky, Singer, & Luborsky, 1975; Rosenzweig, 1936) after the "caucus race" incident in *Alice in Wonderland*. Briefly, in a foot race around a circular track, where the track was unmarked by either a clear start or finish, the dodo bird declares a tie, exclaiming "*Everybody* has won, and *all* must have prizes" (Carroll, 1962). Asay and Lambert (2004) and Duncan, Miller, and Sparks (2004) suggest three possible explanations for the dodo bird verdict. The first is obvious—different therapeutic approaches use dissimilar strategies or processes to achieve the same outcome. Second, research methods may not be sensitive enough to detect differences in therapeutic effectiveness between and among approaches, or the differences are so subtle that they cannot be observed using conventional between-group research designs. Finally, it is very likely that there are common factors throughout all therapies that facilitate progress or change, factors that are separate from any specific "techniques" that define the approach.

This third reason—that there are factors separate from specific approach techniques, common across different approaches and influential in treatment outcome—has received considerable attention in the psychotherapy literature. Lambert (1992) and Asay and Lambert (2004) concluded that the lack of significant difference among treatment approaches strongly suggests that it is the similarities, rather than the differences, between approaches that account for the observation that all psychotherapeutic approaches are, in general, effective. These similarities can be collapsed into four factors or elements that are common to all forms of psychotherapy. The first of these elements is *extratherapeutic change*, and it includes those characteristics of the client and his or her environment that facilitate growth, regardless of the type of therapy or level of therapy participation. The second is the *therapeutic relationship*, which refers to those characteristics of the clinician-client liaison that promote change. The third factor is *expectancy,* also referred to as *hope* or the *placebo effect.* Expectancy relates to improvement that results from the credibility of the specific therapy strategies used, and the clinician's and the client's belief that treatment will be successful. Finally, the fourth factor, *technique,* refers to the unique strategies that characterize different therapy approaches. Lambert (1992), and Asay and Lambert (2004) went so far as to attempt to estimate the amount of contribution made by each of these four factors to the change clients undergo in therapy. They suggested that ~40% of the improvement seen as the result of psychotherapy can be attributed to client variables and extratherapeutic change, ~30% to the therapeutic relationship, and 15% each to expectancy and technique.

Although treatment of childhood stuttering and psychotherapy for children is obviously different, there are striking similarities. The specific techniques in each are directed at facilitating some type of behavioral change, and practitioners in both regard treatment outcome to be at least in part influenced by the nature of the child-clinician relationship and so-called nontreatment variables such as the child's temperament, family history, environment, and so forth (Zebrowski & Conture, 1998). Similar to psychotherapy, research in therapy effectiveness for childhood stuttering has historically focused on technique or approach, although compared with the adult literature, there is comparatively limited evidence for what approach and therapy techniques are the best when treating stuttering in children. Further, there are few studies that address other, nontreatment (or nontechnique) factors related to either positive or negative outcome in stuttering therapy for children. Perhaps more important is the absence of a clear framework for what these other factors might be.

◆ Beyond Technique: Factors That Influence Responsiveness to Stuttering Treatment for Children

Extratherapeutic Change: Child and Parent Strengths

According to Duncan, Miller, and Sparks (2004):

> "Clients have long been portrayed as the unactualized message bearers of family dysfunction, the manufacturers of resistance, and in most traditions (in psychotherapy) the targets for the presumably all-important intervention. Rarely is the client cast in the role of the chief agent of change, or even mentioned in the advertisements announcing the newest line of fashion in the therapy boutique of techniques" (p. 34).

This case has certainly been made regarding the personal characteristics and environmental variables that serve as obstacles to successful outcomes in stuttering therapy (Blood, 1993; Zebrowski & Conture, 1998). Conceptualizing the relationship between what the child and family bring to therapy from a different, perhaps opposite perspective, requires us to look at how they facilitate, rather than hinder, desired change. If we assume for a moment that in stuttering therapy, as in psychotherapy, a sizeable proportion of positive therapy outcome is determined by the child and his or her environment, what variables might be the most influential? Such factors might be considered to reflect Seligman's (2002) notion of "signature strengths," or the characteristics, skills, and abilities that the child and family inherently possess or that they have developed (or have the potential to develop) over time. According to Seligman, signature strengths are distinct characteristics that serve as paths to the practice of specific, positive behaviors that people use to cope with the realities of life (e.g., wisdom, courage, humanity, justice, temperance, and transcendence). Seligman identified 24 strengths that both children and adults possess and described them as *traits*. Traits refer to stable psychological characteristic that can be observed across time and different situations. In addition, traits hold *value in their own right, and are seen across almost every culture in the world*. Of obvious importance in a clinical relationship is that these strengths, or positive assets, can be observed, measured, and further developed. In the following section, I will discuss child and parent strengths that might be considered extratherapeutic change factors that may contribute to positive outcome in stuttering therapy with children.

Child Strengths

Temperament and Personality   Much has been written about the role that temperament plays in both the development and course of childhood stuttering (e.g., Anderson, Pellowski, Conture, & Kelly, 2003; Arnold, Conture, & Walden, 2004; Fowlie & Cooper, 1978; Glasner, 1949; Guitar, 1997; Oyler, 1996a; 1996b; Oyler & Ramig, 1995; Zebrowski & Conture, 1998). Briefly, temperament is a genetically predisposed, relatively stable over time, inherent characteristic that is manifest in our general disposition and the range of mood we experience from day to day. Further, it is thought to be associated with several basic psychological processes, such as novelty seeking or risk taking, extraversion or degree of sociability, harm avoidance, reward dependence, and persistence (Cloninger, Przybeck, Svrakic, & Wetzel, 1994). From a neurological standpoint, these psychological processes are believed to be tied to the combined influences of (1) the degree of reactivity of the nervous system to either external stimuli or one's own behavioral responses; (2) the strength of the emotional response associated with reactivity; (3) the level of physical activity and regularity of biological cycles related to both reactivity and emotional response; and (4) the number and degree of self-regulatory processes the child exhibits to either facilitate or inhibit reactive and emotional responses, for example, attention, approach versus avoidance strategies, and so forth (Arnold et al., 2004; Derryberry & Rothbart, 1984; Goldsmith, Buss, Plomin et al., 1987; Zebrowski & Conture, 1998).

Although there are few concrete distinctions between temperament and personality, temperament has been considered to be "hard-wired," whereas personality and personality traits have been regarded as "acquired patterns of thought and behavior that might be found only in organisms with sophisticated cognitive systems" (McCrae et al., 2000). Though temperament has been described as an inherited facet of a child's constitutional makeup, the development of different temperamentally linked characteristics is thought to be influenced by events and experiences across time (Rothbart & Bates, 1998). Personality traits also develop over time, as the particular temperament of an individual interacts with the environment (family patterns, cultural and societal influences, etc.) to develop characteristic adaptations. Individualistic constellations of these adaptations then come to characterize an individual's personality, and they include such traits as sociability, self-monitoring, and dominance. Though temperament and personality have been considered historically to emerge from different sources (genetic vs. genetic mediated by environment), recent analyses of studies in behavioral genetics, parent-child relationships, human and animal personality, and the long-term stability of personality and individual differences have led to the conclusion that personality may be more intrinsically or genetically predisposed than previously thought, and in fact, may be relatively immutable to environmental influences (McCrae et al., 2000).

Regardless of their similarities or differences, how can the temperament and personality of a child who stutters represent a signature strength and thus contribute to a positive outcome in therapy? There are many possibilities, but most are likely to be related to the interactions between temperament and the way the child characteristically adapts to his temperament. For example, a child may experience a strong degree of reactivity and subsequent negative emotional response to either his stuttering or the reaction of others to his stuttered speech. If the child has developed the ability to regulate his reactions to his own behavior (stuttering) or environmental reaction (e.g., routinely shift his attention onto more pleasant, positive, or facilitating stimuli, events, or people), he may fail to develop habituated avoidant speech or interaction strategies that have long been thought to characterize, and perhaps contribute to, chronic stuttering. Such resilience is the norm, not the exception, in children. Although we need to be aware of the ways in which negative experiences can affect a child, most children "can be happy and function well despite less than ideal circumstances" (Turecki & Wernick, 1994; p. 125). A child may be described as resilient when his temperament and related adaptive skills (personality traits) facilitate the ability to "bounce back" or take relatively negative stuttering-related experiences in stride. Further, a child whose levels of reactivity, emotional response, and ability to self-regulate contribute to a more dominant, extraverted, and sociable personality might be inclined to readily and positively approach various social and communication situations, including therapy (as opposed to reluctantly and negatively approaching the same). In addition, such a child might display a relatively high degree of attentional focus and risk-taking while participating in therapy and may actively seek out novel experiences while also being more apt to take risks in both social and speaking situations. The willingness and ability to take risks has long been considered a trait important to progress across all types of therapies (Yalom, 2002; Zebrowski & Kelly, 2002). Finally, preliminary research has shown that children who stutter who exhibit the temperamental substrate of rhythmicity, or temporal regularity, in eating, sleeping, and elimination may be more likely to benefit from the practice effects associated with picture naming (which might be associated with the practice effect of therapy) than do children with less rhythmic biological cycles (Arnold et al., 2004).

Self-Perception of Control and Competence   Research in youth sport participation has shown that children who perceive that they exert a relatively high level of control over what happens to them (i.e., locus of control [LOC]) also perceive themselves as more competent in athletic performance, and are more likely to seek challenging opportunities or take risks. Conversely, children who perceive that external forces (e.g., parents, coaches, "luck") are primarily responsible for events or situations perceive themselves to be less competent at sport, and are more unlikely to engage in risk-taking while playing a sport (Horn & Weiss, 1991; Wong & Bridges, 1995). Additional research has shown that a relatively high internal LOC can serve as a protective factor in children who exhibit comparatively high levels of trait anxiety or experience either harsh parental treatment or neglect (Bolger & Patterson, 2001). Finally, an internal LOC and associated self-perception of competence has been shown to characterize children who continue to be motivated to engage in a particular activity or learning task, and to maintain a relatively high level of interest in it across time (Harter, 1982). Further, while there is equivocal evidence that LOC is correlated with both short- and long-term treatment effectiveness for adults who stutter (Craig, Franklin, & Andrews, 1984; DeNil & Kroll, 1995), it appears that LOC is related to short-term, but not long-term, gains in fluency for school-age children who stutter (Madison, Budd, & Itzkowitz, 1986).

A child's perception of his or her competence, as well as the child's tendency to "own" his or her behavior, has important implications for therapy, particularly as it relates to a child's perception of competence as both a speaker, and a speaker who can change the way he or she talks (i.e., speak fluently, or stutter "easily"). There are several reports in the stuttering literature that describe the attitudes and beliefs that children who stutter exhibit about speaking in general, and stuttering in specific. Although not a measure of "perceived competence" per se, it is reasonable to speculate that children's perceptions of their speaking competence are tied to the attitudes they possess about talking. In general, most of the work in this area has shown that as a group, children who stutter possess relatively negative attitudes about speaking, and that static negative attitudes associated with talking are significantly correlated with both increased frequency of stuttering, negative emotion, and fears about speaking (e.g., Bajaj, Hodson, & Westby, 2005; Craig & Hancock, 1996; De Nil & Brutten, 1991; Vanryckeghem & Brutten, 1996; Vanryckeghem, Hylebos, Brutten, & Peleman, 2001). With specific regard to perceived competence, Blood, Blood, Tellis, and Gabel (2003) showed that teenagers who stutter possessed poorer perceptions of their communication competence and higher apprehension about communication than their nonstuttering peers. Further, there was a significant and positive relationship between stuttering severity and apprehension about verbal communication.

It is difficult, at best, to determine a causal relationship between LOC, perceived competence, negative emotion and attitudes about speaking, and stuttering, although it is likely that most if not all of these variables are the result of stuttering, and they are not related to its emergence. With regard to a child's responsiveness to stuttering therapy, considering that adults who exhibit more negative communication attitudes pre-therapy show less improvement in speech fluency following therapy (Guitar, 1976), it is likely that the same may be true for children who stutter. Further, taken together, findings from the previously described research suggest a relationship between positive communication attitudes, LOC, and perceived competence. If this relationship is valid, then it can be speculated that a positive attitude about talking can serve as a buffer or moderator between the child and either his or her own anxious feelings about stuttering, negative reactions to his or her stuttering from the environment, or both. In addition, it is not unreasonable to suggest that a child who stutters who possesses a relatively positive attitude about talking will be more likely to (1) maintain interest in therapy, (2) be motivated to actively participate in treatment, (3) actively seek communicative challenges both in and out of therapy, and (4) attend therapy consistently over time.

That being the case, it is important for clinicians to assess communication attitude as a potential harbinger for either positive or negative outcome in stuttering treatment. It may be speculated that if a stuttering child's score on the Communication Attitude Test (CAT; Brutten & Dunham, 1989; De Nil & Brutten, 1991) or the KiddyCAT (Vanryckeghem, Brutten, & Hernandez, 2005) falls within the range that typifies nonstuttering children (i.e., a more neutral or positive attitude about talking), the child's overall attitude about talking can be viewed as another signature strength that will likely be associated with success in therapy. As with the LOC, research examining the relationship between communicative attitude and treatment outcome is needed to understand the possible interaction between these constructs and therapy effectiveness for children who stutter. It should be noted as well that the clinician should be sure to acknowledge, praise, and reinforce the observation of this strength to both the child and his or her parents. Doing so will help the child and the family to recognize the abilities they possess to help and will foster feelings of competence while strengthening the relationship between the clinician, the child, and the family (Seligman, 2002).

Phonological and Language Abilities   There is ample evidence that children who stutter are more likely to exhibit articulation and phonological delay or disorder when compared with their normally fluent peers (Blood, Ridenour, Qualls, & Scheffner-Hammer, 2003; Louko, Edwards, & Conture, 1999). In fact, even when preschool children with clinically significant articulation/phonology problems are removed from both talker groups, preschool children who stutter score significantly lower on standardized tests of articulation and phonology (Pellowski, Conture, & Anderson, 2001). An additional complication is that it is common for clinicians to treat co-occurring stuttering and phonological problems sequentially, resulting in less time spent providing therapy for stuttering, and thus, longer overall treatment time (Blood, Ridenour, Qualls, & Scheffner-Hammer, 2003). This last point is of particular importance here. That is, it is likely that children who stutter, who have age-appropriate phonology and speech articulation, will not only experience a more positive treatment outcome but one that is attained more quickly than those children with coexisting communication problems.

Parent Strengths

Most, if not all therapy approaches for childhood stuttering consider parent participation to be vital for a positive outcome. Parents or primary caregivers are the main support for children, and their influence on the child's responsiveness to treatment can be observed at several levels—from the physical act of bringing the child to therapy and overseeing homework assignments, to their general response to the child and his or her stuttering and their involvement in delivering pieces of the treatment protocol with the clinician's supervision. In this section, I will discuss parent strengths within the dynamic concept of therapy. That is, what strengths do parents bring to the child's therapy experience that can impact the child's responsiveness to treatment?

Congruence   I believe that congruence is the key to our successful collaboration with the parents of the stuttering children we treat. *Congruence* is a psychological phenomenon that is thought to facilitate our effective functioning in the world (Luterman, 2001). It comprises two parts: *intellect* (or cognition) and *emotion* (or affect), and the balance or imbalance of these two components characterizes our internal level of organization. Our intellect allows us to process information, whereas emotion allows us to interpret the world and our experiences in it according to our feelings, at an "intuitive," instinctual, or "gut" level. According to Luterman, congruence is an ideal state in which we approach the world with roughly equivalent amounts of intellect and emotion. When we are congruent, we can access our rational intelligence to "process the data," and we are also able to recognize the emotional responses we generate to specific situations or events. For most of us, achieving congruence is a lifelong journey; much of the time we struggle with an imbalance, never really reaching the ideal destination of equivalency between logic and emotion. That is, we respond to a situation with either a "high-intellect" (and low-affect) or "high-affect" (and low-intellect) mode. So, to be incongruent is normal; however, clinicians can help the client and family to achieve a level of congruence that will help them make change in therapy.

For many, if not most, parents of children who stutter, the child's stuttering elicits a strong emotional response (see Zebrowski & Schum, 1993). If this emotional response continues to remain high, with concomitant, relatively low abilities to regulate that reaction, the unregulated reaction can serve to interfere with the parents' processing of information. The clinician can frequently provide parents with all sorts of excellent information about childhood stuttering and what can help, but the parents are unable to hear, listen to, or process it. In such a case, the parents may not be able to behave proactively or to participate in the child's therapy, not because they don't want to, but because their strong emotion prevents them from objectively analyzing the clinician's suggestions and their role in treatment. On the other hand, a high-intellect, low-affect response is also problematic because although the parents are good at processing and analyzing the information the clinician provides, besides a "faint knocking" (Luterman, 2001), they do not appear to be consciously aware of the nature and meaning of their feelings about the child's stuttering, or (and this is key) what they do as a result of these feelings.

Parents who are more or less congruent in general, and in their response to the child's stuttering problem in specific, have a high likelihood of being an asset to the therapy process and facilitators of positive change in their child's stuttering. There is evidence from the psychotherapy literature that parents who experience high levels of stress are more likely to discontinue their child's therapy (Armbruster & Kazdin, 1994). In these cases, it may be the case that it is not just "high stress" that contributes to dropout, but the imbalance between emotional and cognitive processing that tips the scales. Further, there is evidence that parents who are more congruent in their response to their child's problem may perceive fewer barriers to successful therapy, and therefore they are less likely to drop out of treatment. Perceived barriers may include a poor relationship with the clinician (more fully discussed later in this chapter) and the belief that therapy is too difficult or not relevant (Kazdin, Holland, & Crowley, 1997). As such, congruence might be considered a protective factor against dropout. That is because congruent parents can absorb information and objectively consider stuttering as a dynamic phenomenon. It is said that the two hallmarks of the educated mind are a tolerance for ambiguity and a devotion to a lifetime of self-education. Furthermore, congruent parents are relatively comfortable with the ambiguity surrounding causality, behavioral changes, and the like. At the same time, they can fairly easily recognize the *when* and *what* of their emotional responses, and they can talk about them with the clinician. They can be "watchers" of their own emotions and the behaviors they may generate (Tolle, 2004).

Ability to Shift the Parenting Perspective   An outcome of congruence is the ability to re-evaluate one's perspective toward a particular situation or event. For example, Turecki and Wernick (1994) argue that when children have problems, parents need to shift their perspective on how they can help. That is, instead of the typical view that parents have, that it is their responsibility to "fix" the child or "force" the child to perform or behave in a specific way, a more helpful perspective is one in which the parents "move over to the child's side" (p.14). This shift in role, from "all powerful fixer" to "ally and advocate" is thought to be one of the most effective ways to facilitate positive change in the child's behavior, and in the parent-child and parent-clinician relationship. Three basic approaches can lead to such a refocus. These include: (1) *planned communication*, in which the parents are able to recognize strong negative emotional reactions in themselves and their children, and delay either interaction or discussion until a time and place when these emotions have been diffused; (2) *objective understanding,* which refers to the ability to access observation and information processing skills as a response to the child's problem, instead of solely tapping into emotions; and (3) *active acceptance*, or the development of the parents' ability to recognize the child's special gifts and strengths, and to calibrate their expectations to the child's abilities. Hopefully, it is clear that these three approaches to the "parent-as-ally" perspective require parents to develop a basic level of congruence in the way they respond to their child. Specific to the parents' role in the treatment of stuttering, congruent parents will be more likely to develop a positive collaborative relationship with the speech-language pathologist, one in which they will be able to appreciate the relevance of therapy (or to ask questions if they don't), have an understanding of their complex role in therapy, and have reasonable expectations for therapy outcomes.

Therapeutic Relationship

In childhood stuttering, the therapeutic relationship involves the clinician, the child, and the child's parents. I have discussed specific strengths that the child and parent bring to therapy, and by extension, the relationship they form with the clinician. Presently, there are numerous resources in the literature regarding counseling and stuttering for helping clinicians develop the attributes and techniques that will support a clinical relationship that yields change (e.g., Luterman, 2001; Blood, 1993; Zebrowski, 2002). In this section, I would like to highlight three pieces of a dynamic client-clinician relationship that can promote a positive response to therapy.

Client Education and Preparation

The psychotherapy literature contains substantial evidence that when a client's understanding of the clinical process is limited, or when there is a mismatch between the client's expectations for therapy and the realities encountered, the therapeutic relationship suffers and is likely to unravel (e.g., Bachelor & Horvath, 2004; LaToore, 1977). In fact, as suggested in the previous discussion of congruence, incompatible or incongruous client-clinician expectations and inappropriate client expectations for therapy outcome are often related to a high risk for dropping out of therapy (Farley, Peterson, & Spanos, 1975). In a study of pretherapy education and preparation, Coleman and Kaplan (1990) observed that when the mothers of children who were to receive psychotherapy watched a videotape describing the specifics of the therapeutic process, they became, not surprisingly, more knowledgeable about therapy, as indicated by pre- and post-viewing measures. The same was true for the children who watched the videotape. A second, and perhaps unexpected finding, was that the mothers who received the pre-therapy education and preparation perceived their children to be producing fewer target (problem) behaviors over the course of four subsequent therapy sessions. This reduction in perceived problem behaviors across sessions was not observed for the mothers who did not receive preparation.

Coleman and Kaplan's (1990) findings have applicability to stuttering therapy for children. That is, it is likely that a child will respond positively to treatment if the clinician engages both the child and parents in an exploration of such topics as the nature of stuttering (including contemporary notions of etiology), why children who stutter come for therapy, the general structure of therapy (frequency and duration of sessions), some specifics about behavior change (i.e., what it takes to learn new behaviors so as to replace old ones), what will be taught and why, the importance of active participation, self-expression, trust, and confidentiality, and the roles of the child, the parents, and the clinician in treatment. Folded in should be some examples of positive outcomes and how they are likely to be achieved. Such examples serve as powerful motivators, especially when the clinician points out that with commitment and effort these same outcomes are possible for the child at hand (Coleman & Kaplan, 1990). As Luterman (2001) suggests, therapy should always increase the possibilities that a child and family believe are open to them.

Attending to the Client's Theory of Change   Hubble, Duncan, and Miller (1999) describe a therapeutic process in which the clinician elicits from the client his or her thoughts and beliefs about what will "work" in therapy. According to the authors, "What the client wants from treatment and how those goals can be accomplished may be the most important pieces of information that can be obtained" (p. 432). This point of view is shared by Yalom (2002), who urges psychotherapists and counselors to "create a new therapy" (p. 33) for each client by making frequent inquiries about what the client views as helpful in the therapeutic process.

The parents of children who stutter often have either fully or partially formed thoughts and beliefs about what they would like to see change as a result of stuttering therapy, and how that change is likely to occur. If the child is old enough, he or she will also have at least some rudimentary ideas about what they would like to see happen in therapy. The clinician can uncover the parent's "theory of change" by suggesting that most of the time parents have a fairly good idea of not only what is causing the stuttering problem but also of what will help. In addition, the clinician can ask parents what they see as the role that the clinician plays in attaining their (the parents') goals for the child, along with their observations of what change "looks like" for their child, in a global sense. Finally, parents should be engaged in a conversation about what they have done to try to help their child, and their observations about whether these attempts helped (or didn't), and why (Hubble et al., 1999).

Yalom (2002) describes some surprising observations as a result of frequently checking in with clients about what they think helps in therapy, and their general perceptions of how therapy is progressing. He writes that often clients believe that the quality of their relationship with the clinician, not necessarily the change in symptomatic behavior, is the most helpful piece of therapy:

> "The patient's views of helpful events in therapy are generally relational, often involving some act of the therapist that stretched outside the frame of therapy or some graphic example of the therapist's consistency and presence" (p. 37).

Obviously, the relative significance of therapeutic relationship to client satisfaction might be different in therapy for children who stutter. That is, in most cases parents surely want to see some change in the child's speech, either an increase in fluency, "easier" or shorter, less frequent, and less physically tense stutterings, or both. The desire to speak more easily is likely uppermost in the child's mind as well, although he or she is unlikely to articulate this as a personal goal for therapy. One thing we can learn from the fields of counseling and psychotherapy is that the child's and parents' observations of speech and speech change are not necessarily the sole or most important aspect of therapy. Rather, for some families, the clinician's ability and willingness to be flexible in scheduling therapy, to listen attentively and empathetically, to be readily available to the parents by phone or email, and to provide unconditional positive regard and verbal recognition that the parents love their child and are doing their best are the first things that may come to parents' minds when asked what is most helpful in intervention. The same is likely for the child who stutters. That is, when asked what he or she likes the most about therapy, or why therapy helps, the child may not mention his or her recognition of speech changes at all, but may instead comment that the clinician listens and understands what it feels like to have trouble talking. If we tie the notion that using the client's theory of change, or what helps in therapy, back to the clinical research in risks for dropping out of treatment, I suggest that when this is accomplished, perceived barriers to success in stuttering therapy are dismantled. Indeed, such barriers to progress in treatment have been studied for different types of childhood behavioral problems. Results from several studies indicate that significant risk factors for premature termination of therapy include the family's (including the child's) perception that participation in treatment is time-consuming or otherwise demanding, is of little relevance to the presenting complaint, and that the client/family-clinician relationship is poor (Kazdin et al., 1997).

Family Perception of Improvement in Therapy

Related to the family's theory of change is the significance of their perception that the child is getting better as a result of therapy, and that they and the child "feel better." "Feeling better" is a psychological phenomenon that is made up of numerous factors that are salient in different ways for different people. Feeling better, although perhaps obvious, is a relative phenomenon or condition. In the case of treatment of children who stutter and their families, this perception of relative improvement is likely related to improvements in the child speech, and a decrease in the parents' anxiety and distress, brought about through a strong relationship with the clinician.

In a related vein, clinical research in psychology has shown that the client's perception of meaningful change *within the first few visits* serves as a positive prognostic indicator for successful treatment outcomes (Duncan, Miller, Sparks, Johnson, Brown, & Anker, 2004; Haas, Hill, Lambert, & Morrell, 2002). To obtain this information, adult and child rating scales are available that allow both to rate how they perceive individual therapy sessions. In stuttering therapy, these session rating scales (Session Rating Scale [SRS V. 3.0 for adults, Johnson, Miller, & Duncan, 2000], Child Session Rating Scale [CSRS; Duncan, Miller, Sparks, & Johnson, 2003], and Young Child Session Rating Scale [YCSRS; Duncan, Miller, Huggins, & Sparks, 2003]) can be used to allow the adults (in this case, the child's parents) to rate each session on how well they felt the clinician listened and understood them, how closely the clinician focused the session in terms of what they wanted, their perception of how good the fit between the clinician's approach and their goals was, and whether or not they felt there was something missing in the session. The two children's rating scales provide the child with the opportunity to rate the session along essentially the same dimensions; the clinician's listening skills during the session (i.e., did or did not listen), personal importance of therapy focus (i.e., what was done and talked about were/were not important to the child), overall satisfaction with the session goals and activities (i.e., did/did not like), and overall satisfaction with the session (i.e., wish to do something different next time, wish to do the same kind of things next time). Yalom (2002) advocates asking the client (in this case, the child and family) at the beginning of every session how they think things are going. He encourages each client to imagine an hour or two in the future, during which time they will be looking back at the session. At those times, Yalom asks, what is the client's perception of the session? Was there anything the client wanted to say or ask that wasn't said or asked? These thoughts and feelings can then be jotted down and brought to the next session, where they can be discussed.

According to the authors of these rating scales and "checking-in" procedures, collecting these data helps clinicians to gauge the clinician-client fit early on in therapy, so as to promote early change and therefore increase the probability of a successful therapy outcome. Clearly, there is relevance here for childhood stuttering therapy. It is not unreasonable to suggest that like clinical research in counseling, research regarding stuttering therapy that uses scales like the ones just described is likely to yield similar results. Further, in the psychotherapy literature, research has shown that most of the change in this type of therapy occurs within the first seven visits (e.g., Duncan et al., 2004; Howard, Kopte, Krause, & Orlinsky, 1986). Attempts to assess this phenomenon have received limited attention in the stuttering literature (e.g., Kingston, Huber, Onslow, Jones, & Packman, 2003). Prior research suggests that both child and parent perception of "goodness of fit" in therapy early on is likely to be correlated with subjective and objective measures of stuttering, and may be a predictor of positive treatment outcome.

Hope

For people to have hope that things can change, they need to employ two types of thinking: the first has to do with their ability to develop one or two ways to accomplish change; the second is related to their ability to begin and persist in doing what is necessary to change. These two types of thought are referred to as *pathways thinking* and *agency thinking*, respectively (Barnum, Snyder, Rapoff, Mani, & Thompson, 1998; Snyder, Scott, & Cheavens, 1999). When people are unable to envision a path to change, or initiate movement toward change, they are likely to experience stress, negative emotion, and general difficulties in coping. Alternately, individuals experience positive emotion when they are able to both pursue goals and develop alternative routes to achieve them. The positive emotion that stems from the ability to successfully engage in both agency and pathway thinking is the essence of hope. Rather than considering hope to be purely an emotional phenomenon, in recent years it has been conceived of as an emotional response that is rooted in cognition.

With hope for change comes expectancy that such change can and will take place. Expectancy theory has long been used to explain the placebo effect in medicine, which is an individual's belief that a certain treatment will yield a certain effect (i.e., improved health), either triggers or correlates to that effect. Certainly, research in medicine and psychology has shown that expectancies play a key role in the placebo effect (Stewart-Williams, 2004). The relationship between proactive thought and positive emotion and expectancy is an important factor in successful therapy. Although this relationship seems obvious for the client, it is likely that the clinician's hope for change is as important. That is, a more positive treatment outcome is predicated not just on the client's hopefulness, but also on the clinician's hopefulness and expectation that the client has the ability to change, and that the clinician will be able to help the client to bring about such change (Frank & Frank, 1991; Snyder et al., 1999). Clinicians who show both the child and his or her parents that they are confident in the treatment approach they are using, have mastery over the techniques involved, and expect the child to get better are providing good models of both pathway and agency thinking. This results in a feeling of hopefulness for themselves, and in turn, for the child and family. Further, besides modeling pathway and agency thinking, the clinicians can do specific things to promote these harbingers of hope in their clients. The first way is to incorporate the child's and family's theories of what works in therapy, a key piece of what constitutes the strong client-clinician relationships discussed earlier. The second way is through assisting the child and parents in becoming good observers of change, both within and beyond the therapy session. This can be accomplished through augmented feedback from the clinician, but it is probably facilitated more strongly through implicit learning. That is, the child and parents are given limited feedback from the clinician about performance, but instead they are directed toward evaluating their own performance ("How was that?") and encouraged to "make it better" or "make it the way you want it to be" following repeated trials of a particular behavior (e.g., "easy" onset of voicing; modifying a moment of stuttering). An example here is the use of parent verbal contingencies that are the core of the Lidcombe approach to the treatment of stuttering in children, and that have been found to be related to treatment outcome (Harrison, Onslow, & Menzies, 2004). It can be argued that parental requests to "say it easy" or "try it again" immediately following a stuttered disruption, or the contingent response, "that was nice and easy" following a fluent utterance, provide the child with limited feedback (i.e., the parents do not provide the child with specific instruction about how to change a stuttered disruption or initiate/maintain fluent speech, and then evaluate the attempt) so as to facilitate self-evaluation and implicit learning on the part of the child. In addition, parents are trained to provide a limited number of verbal contingencies in the early stages of the program, gradually expanding their use in an increasing number of daily contexts. This schedule is consistent with principles of motor learning in which limited clinician feedback is associated with reduced performance in the short term but improved performance over the long term. An excellent source of information and discussion about the role of augmented clinician feedback and implicit learning in speech therapy can be found in Verdolini and Lee (2004).

So, what does the construct of hope mean for speech-language pathologists working with children who stutter and their families? If hope is built on the strength of pathways and agency thinking, then clinicians need to help both the child and the family to think about ways to accomplish the goals they have set for the child's therapy (pathways) and about strategies for maintaining consistency in doing the work needed to achieve them (agency). This can be accomplished in several ways, the first of which was discussed earlier and involves structuring therapy around the client's theory of change, or what works in therapy.

◆ Summary

The purpose of this chapter was to provide a framework for considering what works in stuttering therapy for children *besides* the specific techniques associated with different treatment approaches. This framework is based on research in psychotherapy and counseling that has consistently shown that techniques themselves are not the major agents of change in therapy. Instead, characteristics of the client, family, and environment, the therapeutic relationship, and the power of both the client's and the clinician's expectation for success (hope) appear to contribute the most to a successful outcome.

References

Armbruster, P., & Kazdin, A. (1994). Attrition in child psychotherapy. In T. H. Ollendick & R. J. Prinz (Eds.), Advances in clinical child psychology (16, pp. 81–108). New York: Plenum.

Anderson, J. D., Pellowski, M. W., Conture, E. G., & Kelly, E. M. (2003). Temperamental characteristics of young children who stutter. Journal of Speech, Language, and Hearing Research ;46(5), 1221–1233

Arnold, H., Conture, E., & Walden, T. (2004). Relation of temperamental characteristics to picture-naming practice effects in children who stutter: Preliminary findings. Poster presented at the annual meeting of the American Speech-Language-Hearing Association, Philadelphia, PA.

Asay, T. P., & Lambert, M. J. (2004). The empirical case for the common factors in therapy: Quantitative findings. In M. Hubble, B. Duncan, & S. Miller (Eds.), The heart and soul of change: What works in therapy (pp. 23–55). Washington DC: American Psychological Association.

Bachelor, A., & Horvath, A. (2004). The therapeutic relationship. In M. Hubble, B. Duncan, & S. Miller (Eds.), The heart and soul of change: What works in therapy (pp. 133–178). Washington DC: American Psychological Association.

Bajaj, A., Hodson, B., & Westby, C. (2005). Communicative ability conception among children who stutter and their fluent peers: A qualitative exploration. Journal of Fluency Disorders 30(1), 41–64.

Barnum, D., Snyder, C., Rapoff, M., Mani, M., & Thompson R. (1998) Hope and social support in the psychological adjustment of children who have survived burn injuries and matched controls. Children's Health Care 27(1), 15–30.

Bernstein Ratner, N. (2005a). Evidence-based practice in stuttering: Some questions to consider. Journal of Fluency Disorders 30(3), 163–188

Bernstein Ratner, N. (2005b). Response to Ingham (2005). Language, Speech, Hearing Services in Schools 36(2), 157–159.

Blood, G. (1993). Treatment efficacy in adults who stutter: Review and recommendations. Journal of Fluency Disorders 18, 303–318.

Blood, G. W., Blood, I. M., Tellis, G. M., & Gabel, R. M. (2003). A preliminary study of self-esteem, stigma, and disclosure in adolescents who stutter. Journal of Fluency Disorders 28(2), 143–159.

Blood, G. W., Ridenour, V. J., Qualls, C. D., & Scheffner-Hammer, C. S. (2003). Co-occurring disorders in children who stutter. Journal of Communication Disorders 36, 427–448.

Bolger, K. E., & Patterson, C. J. (2001). Pathways from child maltreatment to internalizing problems: Perceptions of control as mediators and moderators. Development and Psychopathology 13, 913–940

Brutten, G. J., & Dunham, S. (1989). The Communication Attitude Test: A normative study of grade school children. Journal of Fluency Disorders 14, 371–377.

Carroll, L. (1962). Alice's adventures in Wonderland. Harmondsworth, Middlesex: Penguin.

Chmela, K. A. (1997). Thoughts on recovery. In E. C. Healey & H. F. M. Peters (Eds.), 2nd World Congress on Fluency Disorders proceedings (pp. 376–378). San Francisco: Nijmegen University Press.

Cloninger, C. R., Przybeck, T. R., Svrakic, D. M., & Wetzel, R. D. (1994). The temperament and character inventory (TCI): A guide to its development and use. St. Louis, MO: Washington University, Center for Psychobiology of Personality.

Coleman, D. J., & Kaplan, M. S.(1990). Effects of pretherapy videotape preparation on child therapy outcomes. Professional Psychology: Research and Practice 21(3), 199–203.

Conture, E., & Melnick, K. (1999). Parent-child group approach to stuttering in preschool and school-age children. In M. Onslow & A. Packman (Eds.), Early stuttering: A handbook of intervention strategies (pp. 17–51). San Diego: Singular Press.

Cordes, A. K. (1998). Treatment procedures and outcomes. In A. K. Cordes & R. J. Ingham (Eds.), Treatment efficacy for stuttering (pp. 117–144). San Diego: Singular Publishing Group, Inc.

Costello, J. (1975). The establishment of fluency with time-out procedures: Three case studies. Journal of Speech and Hearing Disorders 40, 216–231.

Costello, J. C. (1999). Behavioral treatment of young children who stutter: An extended length of utterance method. In R. F. Curlee (Ed.), Stuttering and related disorders of fluency (2nd ed.) (pp. 80–109). New York: Thieme.

Costello, J. M. (1983). Current behavioral treatments for children. In D. Prins & R. J. Ingham (Eds.), Treatment of stuttering in early childhood (pp. 69–112). San Diego: College-Hill Press.

Craig, A., Franklin, J., & Andrews, G. (1984). A scale to measure locus of control of behavior. British Journal of Medical Psychology 57, 173–180.

Craig, A., & Hancock, K. (1996). Anxiety in children and young adolescents who stutter. Australian Journal of Human Communication Disorders 24, 28–38.

Derryberry, D., & Rothbart, M. (1984). Emotion, attention, and temperament. In C. E. Izard, J. Kagan, & R. Zajonc (Eds.), Emotion, cognition, and behavior (pp. 132–166). New York: Cambridge University Press.

De Nil, L. F., & Brutten, G. J. (1991). Speech-associated attitudes of stuttering and nonstuttering children. Journal of Speech and Hearing Research 34, 60–66.

De Nil, L. F., & Kroll, R. M. (1995). The relationship between locus of control and long-term stuttering treatment outcome in adult stutterers. Journal of Fluency Disorders 20, 345–364.

DiLollo, A., Neimeyer, R. A., & Manning, W. H. (2002). A personal construct psychology view of relapse: indications for a narrative therapy component to stuttering treatment. Journal of Fluency Disorders 27, 19–42.

Duncan B, Miller S, Huggins A, Sparks J. (2003). The Young Child Session Rating Scale. Available at: http://www.talkingcure.com/measures/htm.

Duncan, B., Miller, S., & Sparks, J. (2004). The myth of the medical model. In B. Duncan, S. Miller, & J. Sparks (Eds.), The heroic client: A revolutionary way to improve effectiveness through client-directed outcome-informed therapy (p. 32). San Francisco: John Wiley and Sons, Inc.

Duncan, B., Miller, S., Sparks, J., & Johnson, L. (2003). The Child Session Rating Scale. Available at: http://www.talkingcure.com/ measures/htm.

Duncan, B., Miller, S., Sparks, J., Johnson, L., Brown, J., & Anker, M. (2004). Becoming outcome informed. In B. Duncan, S. Miller, & J. Sparks (Eds.), The heroic client: A revolutionary way to improve effectiveness through client-directed outcome-informed therapy. San Francisco: John Wiley and Sons, Inc.

Farley, O. W., Peterson, K. D., & Spanos, G. (1975). Self-termination from a child guidance center. Community Mental Health 11, 325–334.

Finn, P. (1996). Establishing the validity of recovery from stuttering without formal treatment. Journal of Speech and Hearing Research 39, 1171–1181

Finn, P. (2004). Establishing the validity of stuttering treatment effectiveness: The fallibility of clinical experience. Perspectives on Fluency and Fluency Disorders 14(2), 9–12.

Fowlie, G., & Cooper, E. (1978). Traits attributed to stuttering and nonstuttering children by their mothers. Journal of Fluency Disorders 3, 233–246.

Frank, J. D., & Frank, J. B. (1991). Persuasion and healing: A comparative study of psychotherapy (3rd ed.). Baltimore: Johns Hopkins University Press.

Glasner, P. (1949). Personality characteristics and emotional problems in stutterers under the age of five. Journal of Speech and Hearing Disorders 14, 135–138.

Goldsmith, H. H., Buss, A. H., Plomin, R., Rothbart, M. K., Thomas, A., Chess, S., et al. (1987). Roundtable: What is temperament? Four approaches. Child Development 58, 505–529.

Gregory, H. (2003). Stuttering therapy: Rationale and procedures. Boston: Allyn and Bacon.

Grove, W. M., Zald, D. H., Lebow, B. S., Snitz, B. E., & Nelson, C. (2000). Clinical versus mechanical prediction: A meta-analysis. Psychological Assessment 12(1), 19–30.

Guitar, B. (1976). Pretreatment factors associated with the outcome of stuttering therapy. Journal of Speech and Hearing Research 19, 590–600.

Guitar B. (1998). Stuttering: An integrated approach to its nature and treatment (pp. 214–224). Baltimore, MD: Williams and Wilkins.

Guitar. B. (1997). Therapy for children's stuttering and emotions. In R.F. Curlee & G.M. Siegel (Eds.), Nature and treatment of stuttering (2nd ed.) (pp. 280–291). Needham Heights, MA: Allyn and Bacon.

Guitar. B., & Bass. C. (1978). Stuttering therapy: The relation between attitude change and long-term outcome. Journal of Speech and Hearing Disorders 43, 392–400.

Haas, E., Hill, R., Lambert, M., & Morrell, B. (2002). Do early responders to psychotherapy maintain treatment gains? Journal of Clinical Psychology 58(9), 1157–1172.

Hancock, K., Craig, A., McCready, C., McCaul, A., Costello, D., Campbell K., et al. (1998). Two to six year controlled trial stuttering outcomes for children and adolescents. Journal of Speech, Language, and Hearing Research 41, 1242–1252.

Harrison, E., Onslow, M., & Menzies, R. (2004). Dismantling the Lidcombe program of early stuttering intervention: verbal contingencies for stuttering and clinical measurement. International Journal of Language Commununication Disorders 39, 257–267.

Harter, S. (1982). The perceived competence scale for children. Child Development 53, 87–97.

Herder, C., Howard, C., Nye, C., Vanryckeghem, M., Schwartz, J., & Turner, H. (2005). Effectiveness of treatment for stuttering: A systematic review and meta-analysis. Poster presented at the annual convention of the American Speech-Language-Hearing Association, San Diego CA.

Horn, T. S., & Weiss, M. R. (1991). A developmental analysis of children's self-ability judgments in the physical domain. Pediatric Exercise Science 3, 300–326.

Howard, K. I., Kopte, S. M., Krause, M. S., & Orlinsky, D. E. (1986). The dose-effect relationship in psychotherapy. American Psychologist 41(2), 159–164.

Hubble M., Duncan B., & Miller S. (1999). Directing attention to what works. In M. Hubble, B. Duncan, & S. Miller (Eds.), The heart and soul of change: What works in therapy. Washington, DC: American Psychological Association.

Hulit, L. M. (2004). Straight talk on stuttering: Information, encouragement, counsel for stutterers, caregivers, and speech-clinicians. Springfield, IL: Charles C. Thomas.

Ingham, J. C. (2003). Evidence-based treatment of stuttering: I. Definition and application. Journal of Fluency Disorders 28(3), 197–207.

Ingham, R. J. (2005). Clinicians deserve better: Observations on a clinical forum titled "What child language research may contribute to the understanding and treatment of stuttering." Language, Speech, and Hearing Services in Schools 36(2), 152–156.

Ingham, R. J., & Cordes, A. K. (1999). On watching a discipline shoot itself in the foot: Some observations on current trends in stuttering treatment research. In N. Bernstein Ratner & E. C. Healey (Eds.), Stuttering research and practice: Bridging the gap (pp. 211–230). Mahwah, NJ: Lawrence Erlbaum Associates, Publishers.

Johnson, W. (1961). Stuttering and what you can do about it. Minneapolis: University of Minnesota Press.

Johnson, W. A. L. (1929). A stutterer's psychological study of his own case. Unpublished master's thesis, University of Iowa.

Johnson, W. A. L. (1931). The influence of stuttering on the personality. Unpublished doctoral dissertation, U. of Iowa.

Johnson, L., Miller, S., & Duncan, B. (2000). The Session Rating Scale V 3.0 [on-line]. Available at: http://www.talkingcure.com/ measures/htm.

Kazdin, A. E. , Holland, L., & Crowley, M. (1997). Family experience of barriers to treatment and premature termination from child therapy. Journal of Consulting and Clinical Psychology 65(3), 453–463.

Kingston, M., Huber, A., Onslow, M., Jones, M., & Packman, M. (2003). Predicting treatment time with the Lidcombe Program: Replication and meta-analysis. Internationl Journal of Language and Communication Disorders 38(2), 165–177.

Lambert, M. J. (1992). Implications of outcome research for psychotherapy integration. In. J. C. Norcross & M. R. Goldstein (Eds.), Handbook of psychotherapy integration (pp. 94–129). New York: Basic Books.

Langevin, M., & Kully, D. (2003). Evidence-based treatment of stuttering: III. Evidence-based practice in a clinical setting. Journal of Fluency Disorders 28(3), 219–236.

LaToore, R. A. (1977). Pretherapy role induction procedures. Can Psychol Rev 18, 308–321.

Louko, L., Edwards, M. L., & Conture, E. (1999). Treating children who exhibit co-occurring stuttering and disordered phonology. In R. F. Curlee (Ed.), Stuttering and related disorders of fluency (2nd ed.) (pp. 124–138). New York: Thieme.

Luborsky, .L, Singer, B., & Luborsky, L. (1975). Comparative studies of psychotherapies: Is it true that "everyone has won and all must have prizes?" Archives of General Psychiatry 32, 995–1008.

Luterman, D. (2001). Counseling persons with communication disorders and their families (4th ed.) Austin, TX: Pro-Ed.

Madison, L. S., Budd, K. S., & Itzkowitz, J. S. (1986). Changes in stuttering in relation to children's locus of control. Journal of Genetic Psychology 147, 233–240

McCrae, R. R., Costa, P. T. Jr., Ostendorf, F., Angleitner, A., Hrebrikova, M., Avia, M. D., et al. (2000). Nature over nurture: Temperament, personality, and life span development. Journal of Personality and Social Psychology 78(1), 173–186.

Onslow, M., Andrews, C., & Lincoln, M. (1994). A control/-experimental trial of an operant treatment for early stuttering. Journal of Speech and Hearing Research 37, 1244–1259.

Onslow, M., & Packman, A. (Eds.). (1999). Early stuttering: A handbook of intervention strategies. San Diego: Singular Press.

Onslow, M., Packman, A., &Harrison, E. (2003). The Lidcombe program of early stuttering intervention. Austin, TX: Pro-Ed.

Oyler, M. E. (1996a). Vulnerability in stuttering children. (No. 9602431). Ann Arbor, MI: UMI Dissertation Services.

Oyler, M. E. (1996b, December). Temperament: Stuttering and the behaviorally inhibited child. Seminar presented at the American Speech-Language-Hearing Association annual convention, Seattle, WA.

Oyler, M. E., & Ramig, P. R. (1995, December). Vulnerability in stuttering children. Seminar presented at the American Speech-Language-Hearing Association annual convention, Orlando, FL.

Pellowski, M., Conture, E., & Anderson J. (2001). Articulatory and phonological assessment of children who stutter. In Proceedings of the Third World Congress on Fluency Disorders, Nyborg, Denmark.

Plexico, L., Manning, W. H., & DiLollo, A. (2005). A phenomenological understanding of successful stuttering management. Journal of Fluency Disorders 30(1), 1–22.

Quesal, R. W. (1997). Knowledge, understanding, and acceptance. In E. C. Healey & H. F. M. Peters (Eds.), 2nd World Congress on Fluency Disorders Proceedings (pp. 376–378). San Francisco: Nijmegen University Press.

Ramig, P. (1997). My long-term recovery from stuttering. In E. C. Healey & H. F. M. Peters (Eds.), 2nd World Congress on Fluency Disorders Proceedings (pp. 376–378). San Francisco: Nijmegen University Press.

Records, N., & Weiss, A. (1990). Clinical judgment: An overview. Journal of Child Communication Disorders 13(2), 153–166.

Rothbart, M., & Bates J. (1998). Temperament. In N. Eisenberg (Ed.), Handbook of child psychology (5th ed.) (pp. 105–176). New York: John Wiley and Sons, Inc.

Rosenzweig, S. (1936). Some implicit common factors in diverse methods of psychotherapy. Am Journal of Orthopsychiatry 6, 412–415.

Ryan, B. (1974). Programmed therapy for stuttering in children and adults. Springfield, IL: Charles C. Thomas.

Ryan, B. P., & Van Kirk, B. (1974). The establishment, transfer, and maintenance of fluent speech in 50 stutterers using delayed auditory feedback and operant procedures. Journal of Speech and Hearing Disorders 39, 3–10.

Seligman, M. (2002). Authentic happiness: Using the new positive psychology to realize your potential for lasting fulfillment. Free Press.

Snyder, C., Scott, T., & Cheavens, J. (1999). Hope as a psychotherapeutic foundation of common factors, placebos, and expectancies. In M. Hubble, B. Duncan, & S. Miller (Eds.), The heart and soul of change: What works in therapy (pp. 179–200). Washington, DC: American Psychological Association.

Stephenson-Opsal, D., & Bernstein Ratner, N. (1988). Maternal speech rate modification and childhood stuttering. Journal of Fluency Disorders 13, 49–56.

Stewart-Williams, S. (2004). The placebo puzzle: Putting together the pieces. Health Psychology 23(2), 198–206.

Tallman, K., Bohart, A. C. (2004). The client as a common factor: Clients as self-healers. In M. Hubble, B. Duncan, & S. Miller (Eds.), The heart and soul of change: What works in therapy (pp. 91–132). Washington, DC: American Psychological Association.

Tolle, E. (2004). The power of now: A guide to spiritual enlightenment. Vancouver: Namaste Publishing.

Turecki, S., & Wernick S. (1994). Normal children have problems too. How parents can understand and help. New York: Bantam Books.

Van Riper, C. (1973). The treatment of stuttering. Englewood Cliffs, NJ: Prentice-Hall.

Vanryckeghem M., & Brutten, G. (1996). The relationship between communication attitude and fluency failure of stuttering and nonstuttering children. Journal of Fluency Disorders 21(2), 109–118.

Vanryckeghem, M., Brutten, G., & Hernandez, L. (2005). A comparative investigation of the speech-associated attitude of preschool and kindergarten children who do and do not stutter. Journal of Fluency Disorders 30(4), 307–318.

Vanryckeghem, M., Hylebos, C., Brutten, G. J., & Peleman, M. (2001). The relationship between communication attitude and emotion of children who stutter. Journal of Fluency Disorders 26(1), 1–15.

Verdolini, K., & Lee, T. (2004). Optimizing motor learning in speech interventions: Theory and practice. In C. M. Sapienza & J. K. Casper (Eds.), Vocal rehabilitation for medical speech-language pathology (pp. 403–446). Austin, TX: PRO-ED.

Wampold, B. E., Mondin, G. W., Moody, M., Stich, F., Benson, K., & Ahn, H. (1997). A meta-analysis of outcome studies comparing bona fide psychotherapies: Empirically, "all must have prizes." Psychology Bulletin 122, 203–215.

Weiss, A. L., Hall, N., Leahy, M. M. (2005). Response to "Clinicians deserve better": Observations on a clinical forum titled "What child language research may contribute to the understanding and treatment of stuttering" by Ingham (2005). Language, Speech, and Hearing Services in Schools 36(2), 156–157.

Williams, D. E. (1957). A point of view about "stuttering." Journal of Speech and Hearing Disorders 22, 390–397.

Williams, D. E. (1979). A perspective on approaches to stuttering therapy. In H. Gregory (Ed.), Controversies about stuttering therapy (pp. 241–268). Baltimore: University Park Press.

Wong, E. H., & Bridges, L. J. (1995). A model of motivational orientation for youth sport: Some preliminary work. Adolescence 30(11), 437–452.

Yalom, I. (2002). The gift of therapy. New York: Perennial; Harper Collins.

Zebrowski, P. M. (2002). Building clinical relationships with teenagers who stutter. Contemporary Issues in Communication Science and Disorders 29, 91–100.

Zebrowski, P. M., & Conture, E. G. (1998). Influence of non-treatment variables on treatment effectiveness for school-age children who stutter. In A. K.Cordes & R. J. Ingham (Eds.), Treatment efficacy for stuttering: A search for empirical bases, (pp. 293–310). San Diego: Singular Publishing Group, Inc.

Zebrowski, P. M., & Kelly, E. M. (2002). Manual of stuttering intervention. Clifton Park, NY: Singular-Thomson Learning.

Zebrowski, P. M., & Schum, R. L. (1993) Counseling parents of children who stutter. American Journal of Speech-Language Pathology 2(2), 65–73.

Zebrowski, P., Weiss, A., Savelkoul, E., & Hammer, C. (1996). The effect of maternal rate reduction on the stuttering, speech rates and linguistic productions of children who stutter: Evidence from individual dyads. Clinical Linguistics and Phonetics 10(3), 189–206.

3

Data-Based Assessment of Adolescents and Adults Who Stutter

Robert W. Quesal

The purpose of this chapter is to present strategies and techniques for assessing stuttering in adolescents and adults who stutter, and the rationale for this approach to assessment. After initial overview of the assessment of stuttering in adolescents and adults and a discussion of assessment data, the chapter provides an outline of the diagnostic process for these older clients who stutter and the things that should be done during that process. Resources to assist clinicians in assessment and the value of these resources will be discussed and examples will be provided. The goal is for the reader of this chapter to be better able to understand the principles and procedures relating to the assessment of adolescents and adults who stutter, as well as how to begin to implement these when working with adolescents and adults who stutter.

To begin, it is safe to say that like many things in the area of fluency disorders, there is no universal agreement regarding the best way to assess stuttering. The procedures discussed in this chapter are based on several basic premises about adolescents and adults who stutter, derived from several sources including reports from people who stutter. These premises direct the diagnostic process for these individuals and influence the choices we make for assessment, including the questions we ask, the assessment tools we use, and our interpretation of our findings.

Among these premises are that adolescents and adults who stutter (who hereafter will be referred to as "adults who stutter" or "people who stutter" because adolescents have more in common with adults who stutter than with children who stutter) have lived with the disorder for a decade or more. Given the relative longevity of the existence of their stuttering, we can reasonably conclude that they are unlikely to spontaneously recover from stuttering (Yairi & Ambrose, 2005). Although *improved* fluency is certainly a reasonable therapy goal for virtually all of these individuals, "normal" fluency may not be a reasonable goal for these older clients (Cooper, 1993). Instead, many may expect "less effortful stuttering" or "managed stuttering" as the optimal outcome. Their history with stuttering is likely to have led them to try various ways of dealing with the problem. These can include previous speech-language or psychologically oriented therapy, advice from well-meaning (but often misinformed) relatives and friends, information found in books, booklets, and pamphlets (and increasingly on the Internet), or self-taught strategies (e.g., Finn, Howard, & Kubala, 2005). Their experiences with stuttering may have had an impact on their educational experiences, social experiences, and vocational experiences (McClure & Yaruss, 2003; Yaruss et al., 2002). Although not all of these things will be true for all people who stutter, at least some of them will be true for most people who stutter. Thus, to determine the relevant factors for any one individual who stutters, we need to address a variety of behaviors and related issues. This suggests that our assessment of people who stutter needs to be as comprehensive as possible.

We will also assume that the individuals under consideration are "developmental" stutterers and do not suffer from cluttering, neurogenic stuttering, or psychogenic stuttering (related disorders of speech fluency that are discussed elsewhere in this volume). Many of the techniques discussed in this chapter can be used to differentially diagnose various fluency disorders (and those will be noted where relevant), but the information in this chapter focuses primarily on the assessment of the disorder of stuttering that begins in childhood. To paraphrase (Zebrowski, 2002), the question with these individuals is not *whether* they stutter. The question is *how* they stutter, and what can be done about that.

◆ Specific Considerations for Assessment of Stuttering

Assessment can be defined in several ways. For example, Yaruss (1997) describes the assessment of fluency and stuttering that takes place in the initial diagnostic evaluation as well as the ongoing assessment that occurs during treatment. The initial assessment essentially establishes a baseline, whereas the ongoing assessment during therapy helps determine change over time. In this chapter, we discuss assessment primarily in terms of the first definition—the "diagnostic process"—but, where relevant, we will also discuss the use of assessment data to support ongoing clinical decision-making during treatment. The diagnostic process is the basis of all clinical decision-making in speech-language pathology (Darley, 1978; Tomblin, 2000). It is a problem-solving process that involves gathering information about an individual so that we can determine whether treatment is needed and, if so, what the best treatment will be. The information—or data—that we gather comes from many sources: the client him or herself and results of tests that we administer. Such information also may come from, where relevant, parents, spouses, significant others, teachers, employers, previous therapy records, medical records, and so forth.

The Data We Use in Assessment

When one undertakes "data based" assessment of stuttering, one must determine the kind of "data" that will be utilized. In the currently evolving environment of evidence-based practice (EPB) in speech-language pathology, one definition of evidence (or data) is that which is published in peer-reviewed journal articles (J. C. Ingham, 2003). Of course, speech-language pathologists (SLPs) have relied on other data—clinical data—to make treatment decisions for decades. A question may be posed regarding whether "journal data" and "clinical data" have equal value. There is no question that the two types of data are different. The "clinician-researcher dichotomy" has been discussed for decades (e.g., Logemann, 2000; Ringel, 1972) and is currently re-emerging in discussions of EBP (e.g., Justice & Fey, 2004). The clinical data obtained, of course, should be based on some principles, empirical evidence, or agreement as to the basic parameters of measurement. As many authors (e.g., Tomblin, 2000) have suggested, it is not sufficient to make clinical decisions based on "instinct." To some degree that is because, as Haynes & Pindzola (2004) point out, often what is referred to as clinical intuition is nothing more than "clinical bias." Traditionally, SLPs have been viewed as "clinical scientists" who are trained to make careful, objective observations of their clients' behavior in clinical settings (e.g., Darley, 1978), and this objectivity should be paramount. However, it is important to remember that when assessing an individual who stutters, our assessment must be based on the data provided by the client we are assessing (Quesal, Yaruss, & Molt, 2004; Yaruss & Quesal, 2002), not what might be true for all, most, or the average person who stutters. That is, what that individual provides may or may not be representative of group data. In fact, it is detrimental to assume a priori that any individual client will adhere to some "group norm." For example, just because the mean IQ = 100, we would not assume that the person we are assessing or studying would also exhibit an IQ = 100. There is considerable dispersion of scores around the mean for any variable we decide to measure.

Definitions of Stuttering

A basic or at least working definition of stuttering is critical in our assessment of the disorder because it determines the variable (or variables) we will consider as we undertake the diagnostic process. On the surface, stuttering comprises breaks in speech fluency, and certainly fluency needs to be considered in assessment of stuttering. However, as many (e.g., Manning, 1999; McClure & Yaruss, 2003; Murphy, 1999) have pointed out, there is more, much more, to stuttering, particularly in older individuals, than overt or surface speech disfluency. Much of the data of interest and import associated with overt aspects of stuttering are beyond surface fluency and comes from client self-reports (Ahlbach & Benson, 1994; Bobrick, 1995; Carlisle, 1985; Hood, 1998; Jezer, 2003; Johnson, 1930; St. Louis, 2001). Although not necessarily being covert, these are less than apparent than the overt behavioral manifestations of the disorder. Many people who stutter report that the variable, involuntary nature of stuttering—or at least their belief, feeling, or sense that stuttering is involuntary—leads to a variety of coping behaviors that may become part of the problem. In fact, in more evolved cases of stuttering, there is often a dissociation between the amount of surface disfluency and the degree to which stuttering is a problem for a particular person. This clinical data—although anecdotal in nature—suggests that these under-the-surface aspects of stuttering should be investigated during our assessments.

There is evidence, over and beyond the reports of clients, to support the assessment of variables other than overt or surface aspects of speech (dis)fluency. As Yaruss (1998a, 2001) and Yaruss and Quesal (2004a) have pointed out, the World Health Organization's *International Classification of Functioning, Disability, and Health* (ICF; WHO, 2001), an updated version of the earlier *International Classification of Impairments, Disabilities, and Handicaps* (ICIDH; WHO, 1980, 1993), provides an internationally recognized framework for such a choice. The ICF takes into account the *experiences* of the individual who has any complex health condition, nor merely the overt manifestation of the condition. Furthermore, the ICF model does not suggest that all people with a specific condition will respond to that condition in the same way, but that a variety of factors both within the individual with the disorder and in his or her environment may play a role in that individual's experience. The ICF describes all health-related experiences in terms of the *structure* and *function* of the body and the *activities* a person might engage in during his or her *participation* in daily life. If a person experiences problems with body function or structure, these are termed *impairments,* and if a person experiences problems with activities or participation, these are termed activity *limitations* or participation *restrictions.* To account for individual differences among people, the WHO added an additional set of *personal* and *environmental* factors to the model. These personal/environmental factors describe the context, either within a person or around a person, that might affect the individual's ability to function effectively. The ICF framework can describe all aspects of an individual's health experience, including both normal and disordered functioning. Therefore, the ICF provides support for considering a wide range of factors that might be relevant for any one person who stutters; that is, the factors that should be assessed during an evaluation (for a more detailed discussion of stuttering and the ICF, see Yaruss & Quesal, 2004a).

◆ The Diagnostic Process for Adolescents and Adults Who Stutter

The Case History

Some information that is important in the assessment of children who stutter is less relevant for adults who stutter. That would include information such as developmental history, language and speech milestones, motor milestones, etc. That information may have some relevance for determining stuttering chronicity in children, and, as pointed out earlier, adults who stutter have a chronic problem. For that reason, our questions relate more to the evolution of the problem—after it was established, typically in later childhood—and ways in which the individual has tried to deal with the problem since that time. Below are examples of the questions we ask adults who stutter. These questions, or variations thereof, may be part of a case history questionnaire or may be asked during an interview (see Conture, 2001; Guitar, 2006).

1. Why are you here today? Tell me about your speech problem.

2. When was the problem first noticed?

3. Has your speech changed since then? How?

4. Is your speech better or worse at some times than others? Give me some examples.

5. Do you have more trouble speaking in some situations than others? Do certain words or sounds give you more trouble than others? Are some people harder to talk to than others? Give me some examples.

6. Do you avoid certain situations? Words? Sounds? Listeners? Give me some examples.

7. Can you describe or show me what happens/what you do when you stutter?

8. If you think you are going to have trouble saying a word or speaking in a particular situation, do you do anything to "help?" (Alternative: Do you use any "tricks" when you stutter?)

9. Have you ever had speech therapy? When? Where? What did you do in therapy? Did it help? Why or why not?

10. Do you have any idea why you stutter? Has anyone offered any suggestions, etc., regarding why you stutter?

11. How has your life been affected by stuttering? How would your life be different if you didn't stutter?

12. What would you like to get out of this evaluation? Are there any specific things that you are interested in or that I can do for you?

As we ask these questions, we get our first information—data—about our client. Such data help us to determine which aspects of stuttering are most important for a particular client. Open-ended questions are useful because they give the client an opportunity to state his or her concerns or questions and to provide information in his or her own words. We want to find out who referred the client. If someone else has referred the client (e.g., employer, teacher, significant other), we need to determine how interested the client is in changing his or her speech behavior. Questions relating to time since onset are relevant for a differential diagnosis of developmental stuttering versus neurogenic or psychogenic stuttering (Helm-Estabrooks, 1999). Those disorders generally are characterized by late onset, and onset is sudden, corresponding to a neurological or psychological "trauma," in contrast with developmental stuttering. We ask the client to tell us about the evolution of the problem because that may reveal changes in stuttering behavior, changes in coping with stuttering, and changes in the way that stuttering has affected his or her life. When the client reports on the variability of stuttering as it affects him or her, we begin to gain insight into situational variability and avoidance, and we can probe for more specific information about how the client copes with these aspects of stuttering. It is important to note that clients may not be willing to admit that they avoid, particularly in an initial diagnostic session. For that reason, this information may be elicited through multiple questions. It is also important to note that some people who stutter may not avoid at all.

Information about the quality and quantity of previous therapy is a very relevant consideration when initially assessing adults who stutter. Many clients have good knowledge of fluency skills or stuttering management tools from previous therapy. These can form the foundation for further therapy. Other clients bring artifacts of previous therapy—skills that have been poorly understood, mislearned, or misapplied and that are now part of the problem, such as inappropriate breathing patterns or difficulty with voicing onsets (i.e., misuse of "easy onsets"). Clients may also express less than positive opinions about previous treatment and clinicians, opinions that may influence their ability to fully participate in and/or benefit from any subsequent treatment. Clients without a formal therapy history may talk about procedures they have tried based on advice from others, or superstitious behaviors they have developed on their own. Asking the client to explain his or her theory of stuttering, or theories and ideas expressed by others, can reveal misinformation that he or she may have and/or what the client thinks "is wrong." We can use the diagnostic session (or early therapy sessions) to attempt to clarify these misunderstandings as well as to begin to orient the client toward a more current, fact-based approach to stuttering.

The client's description of how he or she stutters can provide considerable insight into that specific client's problem because the description can take many different forms. The client may demonstrate or describe the disfluent behaviors of stuttering, but many clients will describe their coping with stuttering. Clients may also report the internal feelings of discomfort or fear that accompany stuttering. A client's ability (or inability) to demonstrate or imitate his or her stuttering can reveal many things: the client's level of awareness of what he or she does when stuttering, the amount of negative emotion associated with stuttering, or the extent to which the client can objectively analyze behavior (Zebrowski, 2000). The client may reveal the extent to which he or she feels "held back" by stuttering or the extent to which stuttering has been an impediment to reaching academic, social, or vocational goals.

Allowing the client to express what he or she expects from the diagnostic session and from us helps us to focus on things that are relevant to that specific client during the evaluation. We can make sure that our goals for the evaluation align with the expectations of our client. In cases where there is a mismatch between our and the client's goals, we need to clearly state and provide the rationale for that which we do during the evaluation. We can also be sure that we do not overlook something of importance to a client.

Formal Assessment and Informal Assessment

Formal and informal assessment in stuttering often occur simultaneously. In fact, it is important to note that while we are interviewing the client, we are undertaking both formal and informal assessment. It is a formal assessment in that we are gathering a sample of the client's speech—data—that we can later analyze in detail. It is informal in that we are beginning to get an impression of the client's stuttering pattern, as well as the role stuttering plays in his or her life. Both of these will ultimately be utilized as we make our clinical decisions.

Strictly speaking, there are relatively few "formal" assessment tools for stuttering if one defines formal tools as those possessing strong psychometric characteristics: adequate random sample size, good measures of validity and reliability, etc. (Haynes & Pindzola, 2004; Tomblin, 2000). Although there are stuttering assessment protocols available commercially, the materials in these often do not meet the aforementioned psychometric critieria. Perhaps the most widely known and widely used formal measure of stuttering that is supported by some psychometric data is the *Stuttering Severity Instrument for Children and Adults,* 3rd edition (SSI-3, Riley, 1994). When using the SSI-3, the clinician measures frequency, duration, and physical concomitants of stuttering. These are converted to a numerical rating, which corresponds to the severity of stuttering.

However, if one agrees that there is more to stuttering than overt disruptions in speech fluency and that change during stuttering therapy may involve more than changes in these overt or surface aspects of speech fluency (Manning, 1999), it is necessary to assess more than speech fluency. A variety of tools have been developed over the years for assessment of stuttering beyond fluency (e.g., Ammons & Johnson, 1944; Andrews & Cutler, 1974; Crowe, Di Lollo, & Crowe, 2000; Erickson, 1969; Guitar & Grims, 1977; Lanyon, 1967; Ornstein & Manning, 1985; Riley, Riley, & Maguire, 2004; Watson, 1988; Woolf, 1967; Wright & Ayre, 2000; Yaruss & Quesal, in press).

It should be mentioned that not all of these instruments are equally strong, and not all have the same intent. Some are simply designed to describe associates of stuttering, whereas others are more helpful in discerning those who do versus those who don't stutter. A review of the measures shows that although many underwent a rigorous development process, others did not. Examples of those with stronger supporting data are the S-24 scale (Andrews & Cutler, 1974, Erickson, 1969), the Stuttering Severity scale (SS, Lanyon, 1967), and the Overall Assessment of the Speaker's Experience of Stuttering (OASES, Yaruss & Quesal, in press). The S-24, derived from Erickson's (1969) original 39-item S-Scale that was normed on 120 individuals who stutter and 144 who do not, contains 24 true-false items relating to "attitudes" toward stuttering. People who stutter score, on average, 19 (range = 9–24, SD = 4.24) on this scale, whereas those who do not stutter score, on average, 9 (range = 1–21, SD = 5.38). The SS, normed on 50 individuals who stutter and 50 who do not, is a 64-item scale containing true-false items relating to many aspects of the stuttering experience. People who stutter score ~41 (range = 7–59, SD = 11.9) on this scale, whereas those who do not stutter score ~9 (range = 1–36, SD = 6.8).

A somewhat newer test, the OASES—normed on ~300 people who stutter—contains 100 items (each on a 5-point Likert scale) divided into four related sections that are based directly on the adaptation of the ICF framework by Yaruss and Quesal (2004a). The OASES examines: (1) the speaker's perception of the stuttering *impairment*, (2) the speaker's affective, behavioral, and cognitive *reactions* to stuttering, (3) the speaker's *limitations* when communicating in daily activities (examining both activity limitation and environmental factors), and (4) the impact of stuttering on the speaker's overall *participation* in life (examining both participation restriction and environmental factors). Administration of the OASES yields a series of impact scores, which indicate the degree of negative impact experienced by the speaker. These scores are computed for each section of the OASES as well as for the overall scale. Impact scores of 20.0 to 29.9 indicate a Mild impact, scores between 30.0 and 44.9 indicate a Mild-to-Moderate impact, scores between 45.0 and 59.9 indicate a Moderate impact, scores between 60.0 and 74.9 indicate a Moderate-to-Severe impact, and scores from 75.0 to 100 indicate a Severe impact. The measures mentioned above are just a sample of those available. Some authors (e.g., Ulliana & Ingham, 1984) question whether these types of scales measure what they claim to be measuring. It is fairly easy to criticize these scales because they attempt to measure latent or covert constructs when conducting a comprehensive assessment of the stuttering disorder. These constructs, by their very definition, are less readily discernible (i.e., less auditorily/visually apparent) than overt repetitions and prolongations in speech. In essence, because these aspects are not as directly observable, they are not as easily quantified; however, difficulties with quantification do not justify lack of quantification. The authors of these scales have taken into account the human factors that affect the validity of these measures and, to the extent possible, have attempted to control those factors. Because a score can be obtained from these measures—an index that has been shown to differentiate between people who do and do not stutter as well as within the population of those who stutter—changes in that score should reflect change in a client and as such should be one of several useful measures of people who stutter. As with any test, however, these scores must be viewed in a larger context. If a client's behavior and verbal reports are in conflict with scale results, the results must be questioned (something that often happens with measures of overt behavior, e.g., where a client exhibits quite fluent speech in the clinic but reports considerable stuttering outside the clinic). For example, if a client obtains a relatively low score on one of these scales (suggesting that he or she has a good attitude about his speech or that his or her stuttering has relatively little impact on his or her life), but he or she reports things during the interview that suggest that stuttering is a problem (e.g., the client is making life decisions based on stuttering), this mismatch must be explored more fully. This exploration can occur either in the evaluation session or in early therapy sessions.

Lastly, a quasi-formal assessment procedure is a variation on the SSI-3. In this case, a clinician obtains samples of a client's speech in a variety of tasks and then analyzes those samples in a systematic way (e.g., Conture, 2001; Williams, Darley, & Spriestersbach, 1978; Zebrowski, 2000). Several concerns arise regarding this procedure and, once again, there is not universal agreement on the best way to do things. The primary areas of disagreement revolve around judges' accuracy in identifying disfluencies, the behaviors that should be counted, the procedures for quantifying fluency samples, and the influence of the variability of stuttering.

Judges' Accuracy in Identifying Disfluencies

Over the years, it has been shown that it is difficult for judges to reach high levels of agreement on measures of stuttering and disfluency in speech samples (e.g., Ham, 1989; Ingham & Cordes, 1992; Kully & Boberg, 1988). In part, the results of these studies may reflect the difficulty in "real-time" identification of stuttering, the problems that arise when "stuttering" behaviors are not clearly defined for judges, and problems that arise when different judges have different philosophies regarding "counting stutters." Indeed, it could be argued that the ultimate determiner, at least during assessment, is not whether there is a difference in point-to-point agreement between two judges but whether that difference makes a difference in terms of judging that person as someone who does versus does not stutter. However, some possible solutions for overcoming these agreement problems will be discussed later in this chapter.

Behaviors that should be Counted

Another question that arises relates to the behaviors that should be "counted" in a fluency sample. Some authors suggest that only "stutters" should be counted (e.g., Costello & Ingham, 1984), whereas others suggest that all disfluent behaviors should be counted (e.g., Williams et al, 1978). For adults who stutter, the latter of these seems to be the more reasonable for several reasons. First, it accounts for the important role of loss of control in stuttering (Perkins, 1990). Because loss of control is experienced by the speaker, there is no way that an observer can accurately determine which disfluencies are "loss of control" disfluencies and which are not. In other words, observers cannot *truly* know which disfluencies are stutters. In fact, Moore and Perkins (1990) demonstrated that when the internal cue of loss of control was eliminated, a woman who stuttered was no better at identifying her "real" versus "fake" moments of stuttering than any other judge. A second reason relates to "normal" disfluencies in the speech of people who stutter. If someone was to say, "Her name is, uh, Donna" we might assume that the speaker momentarily forgot the other person's name, was using the interjection to provide time to recall the name, or was making a selection among conflicting choices. However, if a person who stutters said, "My name is, uh, Bob" we might conclude that he was using that interjection as a postponement. (If you asked if he postponed, he might say, "I was trying to decide whether to say 'Bob' or 'Robert.'" From that point we might get into an argument about how forthcoming he was, or whether he was in denial about his use of avoidance while speaking.) If a fluency sample revealed that he frequently inserted an interjection before names or other words in his utterances (e.g., "Uh, I have to go to the uh, bookstore to uh, return this uh, textbook....") that *pattern* begins to suggest that the use of interjections may play a role in the stuttering problem. Had we made an a priori assumption that interjections—as "normal disfluencies"—were not to be counted, we would miss this element of *that particular client's* stuttering pattern. The point is that the adult who stutters has been doing so for many years, and during that time, he or she may have begun to use normal disfluencies, such as pauses or revisions, in ways that are different from that of a speaker who does not stutter. In adults, it is often very difficult to determine how these normal disfluencies contribute to the overall stuttering pattern until they are evaluated, and for that reason they should be included in the disfluency analysis.

Table 3–1   Disfluent Behaviors

Behavior	Example
Interjection	"I'll be there at, uh, five o'clock"
Revision	"I'll see you at six – five o'clock"
Phrase repetition	"We can, we can go at five o'clock"
Multisyllabic whole-word repetition	"Today, today is Friday"
Monosyllabic whole-word repetition	"I I I don't know"
Broken word	"To-day is Friday"
Sound prolongation	"Tooooooday is Friday" or "Mmmmy name is Bob"
Sound/syllable repetition	"L- let's meet at fi- fi- five o'clock"
Disrhythmic phonation	Prolongations and blocks (silent or audible)
Abandoned utterance	"I'll be there at…Where are we going?"
Insertion of schwa (neutral) vowel	"buh- buh- baseball" instead of "bay- bay- baseball"
Tense pause	"[pause] I'll be there at five o'clock" (accompanied by hard onset of phonation or signs of effort or struggle during pause)

Source: Adapted from Conture (2001), Gregory (2003), Johnson (1961), Williams et al. (1978), Yairi & Ambrose (2005).

This is not to suggest that listeners do not respond differently to some more severe disfluencies or that there are not differences between disfluency types (as discussed below). Rather, the point is that in adults, disfluencies that may be categorized as "normal" may often be used to avoid stuttering and therefore these should be included in the speech behaviors we are evaluating.

We should have some idea about what disfluencies are (**Table 3–1**), and there are several categorization schemes that have been developed over the years. One early categorization strategy was that of Johnson (1961), which categorized disfluencies as interjections, part-word repetitions, word repetitions, phrase repetitions, revisions, incomplete phrases, broken words, and prolonged sounds. Other ways of categorizing disfluencies include stutter-like disfluencies (SLDs) and other disfluencies (ODs) (Yairi & Ambrose, 2005), within-word and between-word disfluencies (Conture, 2001), or more typical–less typical (or more usual–more unusual) (Gregory, 2003). All of these categorization methods essentially expand upon the basic disfluency types and attempt to show which disfluencies are more common in people who stutter, or which are more likely to lead a speaker to be identified as one who stutters (Conture, 2001; Gregory, 2003; Yairi & Ambrose, 2005).

Procedures for Quantifying Fluency Samples

An additional consideration involves exactly how to quantify the speech disfluencies that we decide to count. Once again, a variety of measures have been proposed. Among these are stuttered words per minute, percent stuttered syllables, percent stuttering or more specific breakdowns of stuttering based on type. Certainly, stuttered words per minute by itself tells us very little without some measure of the number of words spoken. Although not without their own concerns (e.g., size and representativeness of the speaking sample), percent stuttering (percent disfluent) or percent stuttered syllables (percent disfluent syllables) appear to be fairly good overall measures. Few would disagree that 30% disfluency is more severe than 10% disfluency. However, these measures lack precision because they do not tell us what the client was doing. In other words, are 10% interjections more severe, or at least different, than 10% repetitions? If we are going to determine a baseline of disfluent behavior and then track behavioral change over time, it would seem reasonable that we would want a "fluency profile" that describes the client's speech in some detail. Consider, for example, a client whose speech is characterized by tense pauses and other hesitations. In therapy, he or she may learn to use prolongations or easy repetitions to work through those blocks. In that case, disfluency may in fact increase, at least initially. If we have not described the client's behavior, it would appear that our therapy was detrimental. If we show, however, that the original tense pauses are being replaced by an easier, more forward-moving manner of speaking, we have data that can document progress toward goals.

Variability of Stuttering

One final problem that we face in any fluency evaluation is the possibility that what we observe may not represent the client's "typical" speech. (It is not uncommon for a client to report that "My speech seems better today" during an evaluation.) To obtain a representative sample of speech, we typically try to assess fluency during at least three different tasks: conversation, monologue, and reading. As mentioned earlier, we obtain our conversational sample while obtaining case history information from the client, and during other interactions during the evaluation. The monologue is often referred to as a "job task" (Johnson, Darley, & Spriestersbach, 1963) because we may ask the client to "tell us about your job" (or school, or family, etc.)—something that will elicit a fairly long sample of uninterrupted speech. The third task is a reading task. Reading is often difficult for clients who use word substitution (or avoidance) as a "technique." Because the client has to say the words that are printed on the page, he or she is unable to substitute other words.

Even when we attempt to control for variability by using multiple speaking tasks, it is still possible that these may not be representative samples. It may be useful to try to get fluency samples with other listeners (e.g., spouse) in the therapy setting, in situations outside of the therapy room, or have the client bring an audiotape of his or her speech (see Costello & Ingham, 1984).

The Value of Recorded Fluency Samples

Video or audio recordings of our clients provide some of our most important clinical data. The recording itself could be considered the raw data. It is unlikely that others would want to review the original recording (although newer technologies such as digital video disc or digital versatile disc (DVD) or compact disc (CD) make it easier to include these archival copies), but a faithful transcription of the client's speech maintains much of the information from the original. By faithfully (i.e., carefully and specifically) transcribing the client's speech in various tasks, we provide documentation of what our client did during the assessment. The client's behavior can also be summarized in a table. Others can examine (and interpret) this documentation. Examples of these summaries are shown in **Tables 3–2 and 3–3.** Because judges do not reach perfect agreement on the behaviors exhibited in fluency samples, a transcription of a recording allows others to examine the client's speech and to see what the clinician's judgment was based on (see **Table 3–4**). There is no question that these faithful transcriptions take time (~10–15 minutes transcribing per minute of recorded speech), but SLPs who are interested in data to support their assessments should be willing to share those data with others. Indeed, and this cannot be stressed enough, evidence-based practice begins with assessment, not treatment, an observation that is as true for

Table 3–2 Pretreatment Summary Table

Disfluency Type	Number	Percent Disfluency
Part-word repetition	7	15.6%
Interjection	5	11.1%
Phrase repetition	4	8.9%
Whole-word repetition	2	4.4%
Broken word	1	2.2%
Prolongation	1	2.2%
TOTAL	20	44.4%

Time: 40; task: role-play interview.

During the role-playing activity, the client exhibited a rapid rate during disfluencies, and at times had multiple disfluency types within the same stuttered word. In two cases, the client had 16 and 17 repetitions of a word or part-word during a disfluency. Some struggle behavior was noted during more severe disfluencies.

Table 3–3   Follow-Up Summary

Disfluency Type	Number	Percent Disfluency
Interjection	8	6.0%
Part-word repetition	6	4.5%
Whole-word repetition	4	3.0%
Pause	3	2.2%
Revision	2	1.5%
Prolongation	2	1.5%
Phrase repetition	1	0.75%
Tense pause	1	0.75%
TOTAL	27	20.2%

During the interview, the client rarely repeated a word or part of a word more than one time before saying it successfully.

children who stutter as it is for adults. Because of the time involved in this procedure, however, it should be used intermittently. Other methods, such as real-time fluency tracking (e.g., Yaruss, 1998b), might be used in day-to-day tracking of client performance.

Preliminary Diagnosis

Our preliminary diagnosis evolves during the assessment. We are forming impressions about the client's speech behavior, reactions to stuttering, impact of stuttering on his or her life, etc. We are making a determination of whether the client can be meaningfully considered to be a person who stutters, if therapy would be of value, and what form that therapy might take. This information is imparted to the client at the end of the diagnostic session: "Based on what I have observed today, it appears that you do have a stuttering problem, and it is affecting you in a number of ways. From what you have told me, however, I believe that we can help you to learn a more effective way of speaking that will reduce the impact of stuttering. Once I have a chance to more completely analyze your speech samples and look over the other information you provided I will have a much

Table 3–4   Examples of Faithful Transcription of Client Speech Samples

Pretreatment Sample (time: 40; task: role-play interview)

"Well, I, um, after I got outta high school, I-I-I-I-I-I-I had a ssuh-suh-suh-sec-ret-eh-eh-s-s-sec-suh-suh-secruh-tuh-tuh-tuh-it-itarial [increased rate during 'secretarial'] j-j-j-j-j-j-j-j-j-j-j-j-j-j-j-j-j-job [increased rate during 'job'] from, uh, from fr-fr-from er from April unt-until I went I went to college in [deleted]. Um, I was, wuh-wuh-wuh, I was a, was a hostess and a, and a waitress and a-a-and I worked at [deleted] as a, as a c-, as a a-as a cashier, and...[gestures]

Sample after One Semester of Treatment (time: 1:05; task: clinical interview)

"Well, this is what happened: I was, uh, [self talk], oh, I was helping my, my mother with her hair and, and, and I was, like, right here [gestures] and the telephone was right here [gestures] and it rang and she said to me [pause], 'Answer the phone.' And I said, 'Me?' And she said, 'Yes, answer the phone.' So, um [pause] a-and and, um, sso I went and answered the phone, and I knew, everybody was, you know, was I-looking at me, which made me mmore, it um, made me really, really upset, a-and I couldn't even say hello, right? And, but then after I found out it was you, I was like, 'Phew, it's only [deleted].'" (Clinician: How did you feel when I interrupted you?) "[Hard onset] I was [pause] I don't know, I was kind of happy that that you int-interrupted me, but also, I was, I was in-annoyed at m-myself because I couldn't say hello."

Pre- and post-treatment samples are provided to illustrate the value of specific descriptions in documenting behavioral change.

more complete picture of things, and I will be sending you a formal report within a few days. In the meantime, if you have any questions you can contact me."

Formal Diagnosis and Report

The formal diagnosis is typically stated in the evaluation report, which documents the events of the assessment, the SLP's findings, and the recommendations (i.e., the need for therapy and what form that therapy might take). Evaluation reports can take many forms, from brief summaries to checklists to somewhat detailed reports. The information in the report should support the diagnosis and recommendations. Therefore, we should be sure to assess any aspect of stuttering that we address in our recommendations. For example, if we recommend that therapy address the role that stuttering plays in the client's life, we should have some data (e.g., client statements, scores on scales, etc.) to indicate that those aspects of stuttering are relevant for that client.

◆ Summary

An "ideal" assessment for an adult who stutters would begin with a thorough case history that would include both written and verbal information. This information would come from the client, previous therapy and related treatment documentation, and any other individuals who had relevant information. During the evaluation session, we obtain samples of our client's speech in conversation, reading, and monologue (job task), in multiple settings if possible. These samples are faithfully transcribed and quantified to develop a "fluency profile." This profile provides a baseline of fluency behavior that allows us to track change over time as the client progresses through treatment.

In addition to fluency measures, we administer selected scales to address less overt or "under the surface" features of stuttering. These provide a baseline of the client's reactions to stuttering, to help us determine the extent to which these factors play a role in the client's stuttering problem. These paper and pencil scales would augment the information relating to these aspects of stuttering that were elicited from the client in the interview during the evaluation.

By the end of the evaluation we have sufficient data—recordings of fluency, client statements, scores on formal measures, scores on various scales—to allow us to discuss with the client the nature of his or her problem and possible treatment options. Those are written into a formal report that is shared with the client and relevant others.

◆ Conclusion

There is no question that fluency breakdown is a major component of stuttering, and for that reason it is important to objectively assess and quantify overt disruptions in speech fluency. However, we must not let that which is most easily observed lure us into thinking that stuttering is only about fluency. Indeed, difficulties with assessment do not justify lack of assessment. We must use additional measures to assess the multidimensional nature of stuttering. Fortunately, a variety of tools exist for assessing aspects of stuttering beyond fluency. In fact, we have many types of data to support our clinical decision-making (Quesal et al., 2004; Yaruss & Quesal, 2002). We must strive to measure the panoply of our client's apparent as well as less apparent behaviors and characteristics and report these measurements in clinically relevant ways. Further, we must use those sources of data in an ongoing fashion to document change in our clients and the value of our treatments. The use of such data in the treatment process is, in the final analysis, the essence of data-based assessment and data-based treatment.

References

Ahlbach, J., & Benson, V. (Eds.). (1994). To say what is ours. Anaheim Hills, CA: National Stuttering Project.

Ammons, R., & Johnson, W. (1944). Studies in the psychology of stuttering: XVIII. Construction and application of a test of attitude toward stuttering. Journal of Speech Disorders 9, 39–49.

Andrews, G., & Cutler, J. (1974). Stuttering therapy: The relation between changes in symptom level and attitudes. Journal of Speech and Hearing Disorders 34, 312–319.

Bobrick, B. (1995). Knotted tongues: Stuttering in history and the quest for a cure. New York: Simon & Schuster.

Carlisle, J. A. (1985). Tangled tongue: Living with a stutter. Toronto: University of Toronto Press.

Conture, E. G. (2001). Stuttering: Its nature diagnosis and treatment. Needham Heights, MA: Allyn & Bacon.

Cooper, E. B. (1993). Chronic perseverative stuttering syndrome: A harmful or helpful construct? American Journal of Speech-Language Pathology 2, 11–15.

Costello, J. M., Ingham, R. J. (1984). Assessment strategies for stuttering. In R. F. Curlee & W. H. Perkins (Eds.), Nature and treatment of stuttering: New directions. San Diego: College-Hill Press.

Crowe, T. A., Di Lollo, A., Crowe, B. T. (2000). Crowe's protocols: A comprehensive guide to stuttering assessment. San Antonio, TX: The Psychological Corporation.

Darley, F. L. (1978). A philosophy of appraisal and diagnosis. In F. L. Darley & D. C. Spriestersbach (Eds.), Diagnostic methods in speech pathology. New York: Harper and Row.

Erickson, R. L. (1969). Assessing communication attitudes among stutterers. Journal of Speech and Hearing Research 12, 711–724.

Finn P., Howard R., & Kubala R. (2005). Unassisted recovery from stuttering: Self-perceptions of current speech behavior, attitudes, and feelings. Journal of Fluency Disorders 30, 281–305.

Gregory, H. H. (2003). Stuttering therapy: Rationale and procedures. Boston: Allyn & Bacon.

Guitar, B. (2006). Stuttering: An integrated approach to its nature and treatment. Philadelphia: Lippincott Williams & Wilkins.

Guitar, B., & Grims, S. (1977, November). Developing a scale to assess communication attitudes in children who stutter. Poster session presented at the American Speech-Language-Hearing Association Convention, Atlanta, GA.

Ham, R. E. (1989). What are we measuring? Journal of Fluency Disorders 14, 231–243.

Haynes, W. O., & Pindzola, R. H. (2004). Diagnosis and evaluation in speech pathology (6th ed.). Boston: Pearson Allyn & Bacon.

Helm-Estabrooks, N. (1999). Stuttering associated with acquired neurological disorders. In R.F. Curlee (Ed.), Stuttering and related disorders of fluency (2nd ed.). New York: Thieme.

Hood, S. B. (Ed.). (1998). Advice to those who stutter (2nd ed.). Memphis, TN: Stuttering Foundation of America.

Ingham, J. C. (2003). Evidence-based treatment of stuttering: I. Definition and application. Journal of Fluency Disorders 28, 197–208.

Ingham, R. J., & Cordes, A. K. (1992). Interclinic differences in stuttering-event counts. Journal of Fluency Disorders 17, 171–176.

Jezer, M. (2003). Stuttering: A life bound up in words. Brattleboro, VT: Small Pond Press.

Johnson, W. (1930). Because I stutter. New York: Appleton-Century.

Johnson, W. (1961). Measurements of oral reading and speaking rate and disfluency of adult male and female stutterers and nonstutterers. [Monograph Supplement 7] Journal of Speech and Hearing Disorders, 1–20.

Johnson, W., Darley, F. L., Spriestersbach, D. C. (1963). Diagnostic methods in speech pathology. New York: Harper & Row.

Justice, L. M., & Fey, M. E. (2004, Sept 21). Evidence-based practice in schools: Integrating craft and theory with science and data. The ASHA Leader 4–5, 30–32.

Kully, D., & Boberg, E. (1988). An investigation of inter-clinic agreement in the identification of fluent and stuttered syllables. Journal of Fluency Disorders 13, 309–318.

Lanyon, R. (1967). The measurement of stuttering severity. Journal of Speech and Hearing Research 10, 836–843.

Logemann, J. A. (2000, April). Are clinicians and researchers different? The ASHA Leader 2.

Manning, W. (1999). Progress under the surface and over time. In N. Bernstein Ratner & E. C. Healey (Eds), Stuttering research and practice: Bridging the gap (pp. 123–130). Mahwah, NJ: Lawrence Erlbaum Associates, Inc.

McClure, J. A., & Yaruss, J. S. (2003). Stuttering survey suggests success of attitude-changing treatment. The ASHA Leader 8, 19.

Moore, S. E., Perkins, & W. H. (1990). Validity and reliability of judgments of authentic and simulated stuttering. Journal of Speech and Hearing Disorders 55, 383–391.

Murphy, W. P. (1999). A preliminary look at shame, guilt, and stuttering. In N. Bernstein Ratner & E. C. Healy (Eds.), Stuttering research and practice: Bridging the gap. (pp. 131–143). Mahwah, NJ: Lawrence Erlbaum Associates.

Ornstein, A., Manning, W. H. (1985). Self-efficacy scaling by adult stutterers. J Commun Disord 18, 313–320.

Perkins, W. H. (1990). What is stuttering? Journal of Speech and Hearing Disorders 55, 370–382.

Quesal, R. W., Yaruss, J. S., & Molt, L. (2004). Many types of data: Stuttering treatment outcomes beyond fluency. In A. Packmann, A. Meltzer, & H. F. M. Peters (Eds.), Theory, research, and therapy in fluency disorders (Proceedings of the Fourth World Congress on Fluency Disorders) (pp. 218–224). Nijmegen, The Netherlands: Nijmegen University Press.

Riley, G. (1994). Stuttering severity instrument for children and adults (3rd ed.). Austin, TX: PRO-ED.

Riley, J., Riley, G., & Maguire, G. (2004). Subjective screening of stuttering severity, locus of control and avoidance: Research ed. Journal of Fluency Disorders 29, 51–62.

Ringel, R. L. (1972, July). The clinician and the researcher: An artificial dichotomy. ASHA, 351–353.

St. Louis, K. O. (2001). Living with stuttering. Morgantown, WV: Populore Publishing Company.

Tomblin, J. B. (2000). Perspectives on diagnosis. In J. B. Tomblin, H. L. Morris, & D. C. Spriestersbach (Eds.), Diagnosis in speech-language pathology (2nd ed.). San Diego: Singular Publishing Group.

Ulliana, L., & Ingham, R. J. (1984). Behavioral and nonbehavioral variables in the measurement of stutterers' communication attitudes. Journal of Speech and Hearing Disorders 49, 83–89.

Watson, J. B. (1988). A comparison of stutterers' and nonstutterers' affective, cognitive, and behavioral self-reports. Journal of Speech and Hearing Research 31, 377–385.

Williams, D. E., Darley, F. L., & Spriestersbach, D. C. (1978). Appraisal of rate and fluency. In F. L. Darley & D. C. Spriestersbach (Eds.), Diagnostic methods in speech pathology. New York: Harper and Row.

Woolf, G. (1967). The assessment of stuttering as struggle, avoidance, and expectancy. British Journal of Disorders of Communication 2, 158–171.

World Health Organization. (1980). International classification of impairments, disabilities, and handicaps: A manual of classification relating to the consequences of disease. Geneva: World Health Organization.

World Health Organization. (1993). International classification of impairments, disabilities, and handicaps: A manual of classification relating to the consequences of disease [with Foreword]. Geneva: World Health Organization.

World Health Organization. (2001). The international classification of functioning, disability, & health. Geneva: World Health Organization.

Wright, L., & Ayre, A. (2000). The Wright & Ayre stuttering self rating profile (WASSP). Bicester: Winslow Press.

Yairi E., & Ambrose N. G. (2005). Early childhood stuttering for clinicians by clinicians. Austin, TX: PRO-ED

Yaruss, J. S. (1997). Clinical measurement of stuttering behaviors. Contemporary Issues in Communication Science and Disorders 24, 33–44.

Yaruss, J. S. (1998a). Describing the consequences of disorders: Stuttering and the international classification of impairments, disabilities, and handicaps. Journal of Speech, Language, and Hearing Research 49, 249–257.

Yaruss, J. S. (1998b). Real-time analysis of speech fluency: Procedures and reliability training. American Journal of Speech-Language Pathology 7(2), 25–37.

Yaruss, J. S. (2001). Evaluating treatment outcomes for adults who stutter. Journal of Communication Disorders 34(1–2), 163–182.

Yaruss, J. S., & Quesal, R. W. (2002). Research based stuttering therapy revisited. Perspectives in Fluency and Fluency Disorders 12(2), 22–24.

Yaruss, J. S., & Quesal, R. W. (2004a). Stuttering and the international classification of functioning, disability, and health (ICF): An update. Journal of Communication Disorders 37(1), 35–52.

Yaruss, J. S., & Quesal, R. W. (2006). Overall assessment of the speaker's experience of stuttering (OASES): Documenting multiple outcomes in stuttering treatment. Journal of Fluency Disorders 31, 90–115.

Yaruss, J. S., Quesal, R. W., Reeves, L., Molt, L. F., Kluetz, B., Caruso, A. J., et al. (2002). Speech treatment and support group experiences of people who participate in the National Stuttering Association. Journal of Fluency Disorders 27, 115–135.

Zebrowksi, P. M. (2000). Stuttering. In: J. B. Tomblin, H. L. Morris, & D. C. Spriestersbach (Eds.), Diagnosis in speech-language pathology (2nd ed.). San Diego: Singular Publishing Group.

Section II

Intervention: Childhood Stuttering

4

Lidcombe Program 2007: Clinical Tales and Clinical Trials

Elisabeth Harrison, Mark Onslow, and Isabelle Rousseau

Clinicians seeking information about the Lidcombe Program of early stuttering intervention have several resources that they can use. The detailed clinician guide to the Lidcombe Program is presented by Onslow, Packman, and Harrison (2003), and the treatment manual can be downloaded from the Web site of the Australian Stuttering Research Centre (ASRC) at www.fhs.usyd.edu.au/asrc. There is a Lidcombe Program Trainers Consortium dedicated to the provision of standardized and excellent clinical training in the method in many countries, including Australia, New Zealand, Canada, the United States, the United Kingdom, and, more recently, several countries in mainland Europe (Australian Stuttering Research Centre, 2006). Consortium training emphasizes the translation of current treatment research into treatment practices.

The purpose of this chapter is to add a new resource that is intended particularly for speech-language pathologists who are not familiar with the Lidcombe Program. The only knowledge that we presume readers will have is that which is common to speech-language pathologists who treat communication disorders in young children. The first section therefore begins with an overview of the origins of the program, and a succinct description of the treatment components and how they are combined during treatment. This first section is presented without illustrative examples because we find that clinicians who are new to the program generally find it helpful to gain an overview of the treatment first, before considering how it is applied in clinical practice. In the two case studies that follow are details of Lidcombe Program treatment with two preschool-age children. Clinical issues raised by the cases are then discussed to highlight the clinician's decision-making process. This discussion also highlights typical as well as unusual features of the cases. The final section presents the program's current evidence base and concludes with information about plans for further research and development.

◆ The Origin of the Lidcombe Program

It has been suggested that there was a unique set of circumstances in Sydney during the 1980s that allowed the Lidcombe Program to develop (Onslow, & Menzies, 1996). The circumstances included what these authors described as an "Australian approach" to stuttering treatment. This was summarized as general agreement among speech pathologists of the suitability of operant approaches to stuttering treatment, and a willingness to directly target problem speech behaviors when treating stuttering in preschool children.

Another circumstance that was critical in the development of the Lidcombe Program was a speech-language pathology culture in Australia that encouraged close association between researchers and clinicians. Attanasio et al. (1996) argued that this cultural context fostered the program's development, which was largely clinician-driven and given form and substance by academic researchers. The clinicians responsible for the program were from the Stuttering Unit, Bankstown Community Health Service, Sydney. (The Stuttering Unit is based in a community health center, and it is a government-funded, public health service.) The academic researchers were from what is now the Australian Stuttering Research Centre within the Faculty of Health Sciences of The University of Sydney.

Several years earlier, single-subject laboratory experiments conducted in the United States had established remarkable information that response-contingent stimulation reduced stuttering to near zero levels in preschool children (Martin, Kuhl, & Haroldson, 1972; Reed & Godden, 1977), but these results had not immediately led to development of stuttering treatments. It is plausible that one reason for this impasse was the pervasive influence in United States speech-language pathology of Wendell Johnson's diagnosogenic theory (Johnson et al., 1942). Indeed, at the time of publication of those results, the contemporary North American approach to stuttering treatment for young children was to avoid drawing attention to stuttering and to counsel parents along the lines suggested by many prominent speech-language pathologists, for example, Van Riper (1973).

Onslow (2003) reported his unsuccessful attempts to replicate in a Sydney speech pathology clinic in 1980 Martin and colleague's (1972) methodology. Following establishment of the Stuttering Unit in 1984, its researchers and clinicians experimented clinically for a few years to determine the combination of components that might comprise an effective stuttering treatment for preschool children. Clinical data were generated and used to evaluate sequential refinements to the treatment. By 1988 the components were assembled of a near-final version of the treatment subsequently named the Lidcombe Program, and there was immediate interest from the clinical community, which wanted information about the new treatment. The first public presentations of an early version of the Lidcombe Program consisted of conference papers (Onslow, 1987; Onslow, 1988) as well as a workshop for speech pathologists (Andrews, 1989).

In the next section is a summary of the Lidcombe Program procedures, followed by two case studies that illustrate its use in clinical practice. The final section contains an outline of the empirical evidence to date of the efficacy of this treatment.

◆ The Lidcombe Program

General Principles

The Lidcombe Program is a direct treatment for stuttering in preschool children. That is, treatment is focused on children's speech and not on family relationships, parenting styles, or children's temperaments. During weekly visits with their children to the speech-language pathology clinic, parents learn how to conduct treatment and measure children's stuttering severity. Parents deliver treatment during daily conversations and measure children's stuttering severity in everyday settings. Clinicians also monitor treatment and stuttering severity measures during clinic visits and adjust parents' treatment to ensure continuing progress through the program.

The program is conducted in two stages. The goal of Stage 1 is to either eliminate children's stuttering or reduce it to a very low level and the goal of Stage 2 is to maintain that reduction for a long period. Clinic visits occur regularly each week during Stage 1, and with systematically increasing periods between each visit during Stage 2.

Child Responses

There are two child responses in the Lidcombe Program that are essential in its implementation. The first is stutter-free speech and the second is unambiguous stuttering. Both responses are produced spontaneously and without clinician instruction. In other words, the Lidcombe Program targets no change to children's customary mode of speech production.

There are two non-essential child responses in the Lidcombe Program: self-evaluation of stutter-free speech and self-correction of stuttering. Parents and children are encouraged to incorporate these responses in treatment, but they are not essential treatment components (Onslow, 2003, p. 72).

Parental Verbal Contingencies

When presenting the treatment, parents comment on episodes of children's stutter-free speech and unambiguous stuttering. In the Lidcombe Program, these comments are referred to as parental verbal contingencies. Specifically, following stutter-free speech, parents may acknowledge it (e.g., "Those words were smooth"), or praise it (e.g., "Wow, good smooth talking!"). Essentially, the difference between these contingencies is that acknowledgment of stutter-free speech is neutral—and usually briefer—whereas praise conveys affirmation. A third contingency for stutter-free speech is for parents to ask children to self-evaluate their speech (e.g., "Was that smooth?" or "Were there any bumps there?"). Following stuttering, parents may acknowledge it (e.g., "That was a bump there"), or request children to self-correct stuttered responses (e.g., "Can you say 'orange' again smoothly?"). Parental verbal contingencies for stuttering or for stutter-free speech are used intermittently so that they are neither invasive nor overwhelming for the child.

Speech Measures

The clinician uses measures of stuttering to:

◆ Prescribe treatment goals

◆ Assess the child's progress toward those goals

◆ Continuously determine the effectiveness of the treatment so that it can be adjusted as required

◆ Communicate with the child and parent about stuttering severity

◆ Determine when stuttering rate and severity are below program criteria at near-zero levels

◆ Subsequently prescribe targets for Stage 2 of the program

Parents collect two speech measures: one measure is a perceptual scaling of the severity of the child's stuttering and the other is a stutter-count measure. During all clinic visits, clinicians measure percentage of syllables stuttered in samples of children's speech. Together, these three measures are used to monitor children's responses to treatment.

The first parental speech measures are severity ratings (SRs). These ratings are made on a 10-point scale, where a rating of "1" is defined as "no stuttering," "2" means "extremely mild stuttering," and "10" means "extremely severe stuttering." Parents rate children's speech each day, write the ratings on a chart, and bring the chart to each clinic visit. The parent may assign one SR for an entire day or one SR for 10 minutes of speech each day. If the second method is used, the parent rates a variety of times and speaking situations across the week so that a representative range of the child's speech is sampled.

The second speech measure parents use occasionally is "stutters per minute of speaking time" (SMST). Whereas SRs are collected throughout Stage 1 and Stage 2, SMST is an optional measure and is collected only when an additional measure is needed to supplement parental SRs. To calculate SMST, a parent listens to the child talking in conversation. The parent measures the duration of the child's conversation and the number of unambiguous stutters during that period. SMST is calculated by dividing the number of stutters by the duration of the child's speech.

Clinicians measure the percentage of syllables stuttered (%SS) in samples of children's speech during conversations in all clinic visits. Sample sizes are commonly measured as either 300 syllables or 10 minutes of conversation. Children's speech is sampled at the beginning of clinic visits. During clinic visits early in Stage 1, when children are still adjusting to clinics and clinicians, speech samples are unlikely to be representative of children's everyday speech. Their value in early Stage 1 visits is in providing focus for discussion between parents and clinicians regarding: (1) stuttering types and frequency; (2) overall stuttering severity; and (3) comparison of clinic speech samples with children's everyday speech. Speech samples in later Stage 1 clinic visits usually reflect children's speech outside the clinic setting, reported in parents' comments and SRs, and they can indicate progress.

Clinicians check reliability of parental SRs by having parents assign SRs to recorded samples of their children's speech, and then rating them again a few weeks later. Reliability is regarded as adequate if first and second parental SRs differ by no more than one scale value. The clinician can then rely on the parental SRs that are assigned to speech samples in conversations outside the clinic.

Clinicians discuss SRs, %SS, and SMST measures with parents. Along with any other unusual features that clinicians may notice, comments would routinely be made on: (1) types of stutters observed; (2) validity of the samples; (3) stuttering severity; and (4) comparisons of speech measures with those discussed in previous clinic visits.

Clinical Protocol

Stage 1: Structured and Unstructured Treatment Conversations

During initial Stage 1 clinic visits, clinicians teach parents how to engage their child's interest in treatment and conduct treatment conversations correctly and safely. It is important that the parent applies contingencies to the target responses and not to any other speech parameter, such as vocabulary or sentence structure. Contingencies that are used constantly or with excessive focus on stuttering would be detrimental, so the parent structures treatment conversations to ensure that most of the child's responses are stutter-free and that the child enjoys the experience. Later in Stage 1, as the child's SRs decrease, treatment conversations are unstructured and the parent learns how to conduct them during everyday activities.

Early in Stage 1 the parent conducts structured treatment for 10 to 15 minutes, once or twice each day. The parent finds a quiet setting away from distractions at a time when the child is alert. Materials such as books or toys that the child enjoys are used as topics for conversation, and the parent may use a variety of linguistic cues such as sentence completion, binary choice questions, or modeling to elicit short, stutter-free responses. In fact, the parent structures motoric, linguistic and/or pragmatic aspects of the conversation to ensure that most of the child's responses are stutter-free. Typically, the parent considers location, timing, and choice of topic and stimulus materials when setting up a structured treatment conversation.

As Stage 1 continues, the child's longer stutter-free utterances become more frequent, and changes are frequently noted in the SRs. The first change noticed with many children is a *decrease in variability of SRs from one day to the next*. The next change is universal and is a *gradual decrease in SRs*. This signals that the child's increasingly frequent, longer stutter-free utterances are generalizing beyond structured treatment conversations into unstructured, everyday conversations.

Contingent stimulation for the child's spontaneous self-evaluation of stutter-free speech can be added to treatment at any time during Stage 1. This is a particularly useful contingency to promote the eventual change from treatment in structured conversations toward treatment in unstructured conversations. The clinician introduces the self-evaluation contingency during a clinic visit, either by demonstrating to the parent or explaining and then watching the parent use the contingency during treatment. After praising several consecutive stutter-free responses, the parent (or clinician) asks the child "Was that smooth?" after the next stutter-free utterance. The question is asked in a manner that makes it clear to the child that the expected response is "yes." The parent/clinician then agrees with the child and praises the stutter-free utterance. An example of this could be "Yes, I think it was smooth, too. Great talking!"

A change that commonly occurs once unstructured treatment is introduced is for children to begin spontaneous self-correction of stuttering. The child stutters, then pauses briefly and repeats the word stutter-free before continuing. Children are not taught to self-correct stutters in the Lidcombe Program because to do so would mean excessive focus on their stuttering. Rather than teaching children deliberately to become self-conscious about stuttering, it is preferable that, if anything, they become aware of how to produce effortless, stutter-free speech. The clinician monitors each child's speech for spontaneous self-correction of stutters during clinic visits and asks parents if any instances have been noticed at home. If a child spontaneously self-corrects a stutter, then the clinician and/or parent will wait until the child has finished the utterance and then praise the child with specific feedback. Examples of praise would be "Well done, you fixed up your bumpy word!" or "Great talking, you smoothed out a bumpy word by yourself!"

When a child's SRs are lower than 5 or 4, many short, stutter-free utterances will occur in his or her unstructured conversations and during both structured and unstructured treatment conversations. During each clinic visit, the clinician and parent discuss in detail the amount of structured and unstructured treatment and the frequency and types of verbal contingencies that the parent is using. The clinician ensures that contingencies for stutter-free speech are used at least five times more often than verbal contingencies for stuttering. Most commonly, the clinician asks the parent to decrease the number of structured treatment conversations by one or two each week so that, during a period of between 4 and 7 weeks, all treatment occurs during unstructured conversations. The number of parental verbal contingencies used each day will not decrease, but they will be used in many conversations rather than being concentrated in a single daily treatment conversation.

Weekly clinic visits and daily treatment continue until the clinician and parent agree that the child's speech meets Stage 2 criteria over 3 consecutive weeks. These criteria are based on speech measures made both within and outside the clinic and are:

• Less than 1.0%SS measured within the clinic

• Weekly SRs that average less than 2.0 measured outside the clinic with no more than three scores of SR2 or higher in any week

• Less than 1.5 SMST measured outside the clinic if SMST scores are used (see above)

Stage 2

The aim of Stage 2 is for parents gradually to withdraw treatment while children maintain the same level of stutter-free speech that they achieved at the end of Stage 1. Stage 2 consists of a series of half-hour clinic visits that gradually decrease in frequency contingent on the child continuing to meet criteria for speech performance. The clinician can vary the schedule of frequency for clinic visits and the speech criteria according to a child's individual needs; however, clinicians routinely use the following schedule of clinic visits, which are based on a performance-contingent procedure developed by Ingham (1980). The first two visits are 2 weeks apart, then 4 weeks, 4 weeks, 8 weeks, 8 weeks, and 16 weeks. This is not the only schedule possible, but whatever schedule is decided on, it is set by the parent and clinician and can be shorter or longer as they decide is necessary for the child.

Children's progress through the Stage 2 clinic visits is contingent on passing the speech criteria at each visit. These criteria are the same as those set for entry into Stage 2: (1) %SS less than 1.0 within the clinic; (2) SRs average less than 2.0 outside the clinic; and (3) less than 1.5 SMST outside the clinic. Within-clinic speech samples are collected during conversation between the child and the clinician or parent. Parents collect beyond-clinic speech measures during the week before their scheduled clinic visits.

In cases where children do not meet the speech criteria at a Stage 2 clinic visit, clinicians and parents confer about treatment that may still be occurring and agree on suitable strategies for the weeks ahead. According to one clinical file audit by Webber and Onslow (2003), clinicians can expect that one in two children will not meet speech criteria at a Stage 2 clinic visit, and that the majority of these situations will arise early in Stage 2. Therefore, clinicians approach the schedule with caution early in Stage 2 and, for example, schedule phone contacts if the family is unable to attend the clinic. When deciding on contingencies for stalled progress early in Stage 2, clinicians usually recommend that children stay on the same step of the Stage 2 schedule until able to meet criteria. Later in Stage 2, when clinic visits are many weeks apart, clinicians will often decide to move children back to an earlier step until either speech criteria are achieved or clinicians and parents agree to return children to Stage 1.

The expected outcomes of the Lidcombe Program are consistent, effortless stutter-free speech by the child in everyday conversations. We routinely find that by the time children are discharged from Stage 2, they have only hazy memories of ever having stuttered—nothing like outcomes typically attained with adult treatments designed to control stuttered speech. Their most enduring memories seem to be their favorite toys and games in the clinic and the stickers and stamps with which they were rewarded. A related outcome is one that is not a goal of the Program but that has been reported by many parents. Many report that their children have become confident speakers, enthusiastic participants in conversations at preschool, and willing to talk with older children and adults.

The following section contains two case studies that describe the progress of preschool-age children through Stages 1 and 2.

Case Study 1: Dominic

Background and Assessment

Dominic started to stutter rather suddenly when he was 2 years, 5 months old. A general practitioner recommended that Dominic's parents wait a short period before seeking any intervention in the expectation that the stuttering would resolve naturally. After 6 months during which there was no change, Dominic's mother–Sharon–called our speech pathology clinic for an appointment. During the initial assessment session, Dominic's stuttering was measured at 4.7%SS during a conversation with the clinician. Sharon gave that conversation a rating of 5 on the 10-point perceptual severity scale (1 = no stuttering, 2 = extremely mild stuttering, 10 = extremely severe stuttering) and said that it was typical of Dominic's speech at the time. His stutters consisted of repetitions, with three or four repeated syllables being his most common stutter. She reported that Dominic only stuttered when speaking English and did not stutter when speaking Cantonese, his second language.

A family history of stuttering was reported. Dominic's paternal uncle had stuttering treatment during his school years. Sharon and her partner had no concerns about any other aspect of Dominic's speech and language development. Sharon felt that Dominic was aware of his stuttering although was not concerned about it.

Dominic lived with his parents, maternal grandparents, and an uncle. He had an older half-sister (16 years) and brother (18 years), who lived with their father. Dominic attended preschool 2 days each week, where he spoke Cantonese and English.

Dominic's name was put on a treatment waiting list and when the family was contacted 7 months later, Sharon reported that his stuttering had remained consistent, with SRs fluctuating between 4 and 6. She also reported that Dominic had shown some signs of frustration with his stuttering on one or two occasions, throwing a toy to the floor when he was "stuck"—experiencing a fixed posture—on a word.

More speech measures were collected before the start of Stage 1. A within-clinic speech sample was measured as 7.2%SS and a conversation between Dominic and his mother recorded at home was 4.7%SS. His stuttering still consisted mostly of repeated movements, although some fixed postures without audible airflow were also noted. Dominic started the Lidcombe Program a week later when he was 3 years 6 months old, for the following reasons:

- Although stuttering severity fluctuated, his stuttering was consistently present.

- It was 13 months since stuttering onset.

- There were no signs of improvement since onset, and the appearance of fixed postures and signs of frustration suggested that stuttering severity had increased.

Stage 1

Clinic Visit 1 *Within-clinic speech measure: 4.6% SS.* The clinician explained how to measure Dominic's stuttering with SRs and recommended that Sharon collect a daily average SR during the week ahead. Dominic's SR chart is reproduced in **Fig. 4–1**. The clinician also asked Sharon to note if this daily average was a true reflection of Dominic's speech for a particular day, that is, if his stuttering severity was stable across the day. Sharon rated Dominic's stuttering in the clinic as SR5 (clinician's rating was SR5). Sharon and the clinician observed syllable repetitions and fixed postures without audible airflow, and these stutters were typical of Dominic's stuttering for that day.

The clinician explained and demonstrated a structured treatment conversation with Dominic using verbal contingencies only for stutter-free speech, and invited Sharon to do the same. A simple picture book and a token reward were used to help structure the treatment conversation. Sharon elicited mostly stutter-free speech in short phrases. The clinician recommended that Sharon conduct similar structured treatment conversations before lunchtime each day for 10 to 15 minutes. No contingencies were used for stuttering yet.

Clinic Visit 2 *Within-clinic speech measure: 5.2%SS.* Sharon reported fluctuations in Dominic's stuttering during the previous week, and this was reflected in his SRs. Although structured

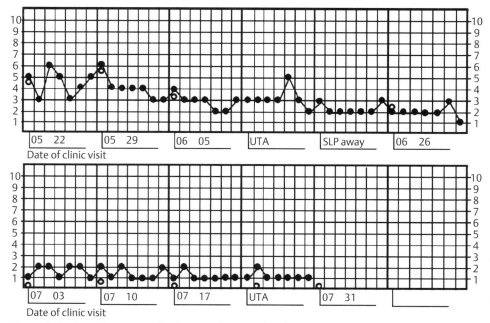

Figure 4–1 Speech measures for Dominic during Lidcombe Program Stage 1. Closed circles represent parent's daily severity ratings (SRs); open circles represent clinician's % syllables stuttered (%SS) during clinic visits.

treatment was conducted every day, Sharon reported that Dominic was rarely stutter-free during those conversations. Instead, the pictures or the token reward would distract him. The clinician spent time discussing in detail the structured treatment conducted at home, and watched while Sharon and Dominic conduct treatment in the clinic. The clinician suggested that Sharon simplify the treatment by leaving out the token reward and focusing on how she was structuring the conversation. The clinician then demonstrated treatment again and introduced the occasional contingency of requests for self-correction of stutters, which was well received by Dominic.

By the end of the clinic visit, Sharon said that she felt more comfortable conducting structured treatment, and she was able to elicit mostly stutter-free speech from Dominic and to use verbal contingencies for stutter-free speech as well as for stuttering. The clinician explained the importance of maintaining emphasis on Dominic's stutter-free speech by using contingencies for this at least five times more than contingencies for stuttering. Sharon was encouraged to continue similar procedures every day, twice a day if possible. The clinician also recommended that she start using occasional verbal contingencies for stutter-free speech during unstructured conversations—when she noticed Dominic using spontaneous, stutter-free speech at other times of the day.

Clinic Visit 3   *Within-clinic speech measure: 3.1%SS.* Sharon's rating for the within-clinic sample was SR4 and she said that this sample was typical of Dominic's speech during the previous week. She felt that his stuttering severity had generally reduced and noticed that there were relatively fewer fixed-posture stutters. The clinician's previous recommendations had been implemented successfully, and Sharon and Dominic had conducted structured treatment conversations twice a day on most days. In each conversation, Sharon had used the verbal contingency of praise for stutter-free speech four or five times and Dominic had successfully corrected one or two stutters when requested. After observing Sharon's treatment in the clinic, the clinician recommended that Sharon elicit longer responses during the treatment conversations, and make her requests for self-correction more specific. For example, rather than asking, "Would you like to try that again?" the clinician suggested that Sharon ask, "Could you try 'puppy' again?"

Dominic was clearly enjoying treatment and responding easily to all verbal contingencies. The clinician recommended that Sharon continue treatment in structured conversations at home in the same the way she had done during the clinic visit, and increase treatment in unstructured conversations.

Clinic Visit 4   *Within-clinic speech measure: 2.2%SS.* There was a 2-week break from clinic visits due to a family appointment in one week, and the clinician being unable to attend in the second week. Throughout the break, Sharon and Dominic continued daily treatment. Sharon reported generally stable SRs along with a further decrease in the number of fixed postures and a general increase in stutter-free speech. Sharon had given Dominic SR5 on one day and she attributed this to his great excitement while playing with his cousins that day. Sharon had used up to 15 verbal contingencies–mostly for stutter-free speech–during unstructured treatment conversations each day. In addition, Dominic had started spontaneously to self-correct his stutters, and Sharon had reinforced these with praise. The clinician observed Sharon conduct unstructured treatment in the clinic and recommended that most treatment should be in unstructured conversations in the week ahead, as long as Dominic sustained similar SRs. Sharon agreed to use structured treatment on days when Dominic was SR3 or higher.

Clinic Visit 5   *Within-clinic speech measure: 0%SS.* Most of the previous week's treatment was in unstructured treatment conversations, with structured treatment conducted on only two or three days. Dominic was SR1 on one of those days. Sharon said that Dominic had asked to do 'smooth talking games', several times and on one occasion pretended to stutter in an apparent attempt to persuade Sharon that they should start one on the spot. Although the clinician could see the funny side of this and was not immediately concerned about it as a one-off behavior, she wanted to ensure that it did not become more frequent. Sharon and the clinician discussed ways to continue implementing treatment when Dominic was stutter-free, and Sharon agreed to do daily treatment in unstructured conversations in the week ahead. The clinician gave a brief overview of Stage 2, and suggested that Dominic would soon move to that stage.

Clinic Visits 6 and 7   *Within-clinic speech measure: 0.4%SS and 0%SS.* Sharon reported hearing one or two stutters on SR2 days. Dominic spontaneously self-corrected most stutters and was happy to self-correct the rest when requested. Sharon continued daily, unstructured treatment and used verbal contingencies for stutter-free speech around six times each day. She reported that it was easier to conduct treatment during the school holidays, which had begun a week earlier because Dominic was at home every day. At Visit 7, Sharon reported that they would not be able to attend the following week and agreed to video-record a 10-minute speech sample with Dominic. The clinician suggested that she try to record a sample of what she expected would be Dominic's most severe stuttering.

Clinic Visit 8   *Within-clinic speech measure: 0%SS.* Dominic's ratings had been mostly SR1 and occasionally SR2, and the conversation video-recorded at home was measured as 0.1%SS. Therefore, because Dominic's speech measures met the Stage 2 criteria, the clinician explained to Sharon the schedule of clinic visits and procedures for the months ahead. She recommended that Sharon continue treatment without changes until the first Stage 2 visit, 2 weeks later.

Stage 2

Dominic progressed through the standard Stage 2 schedule and achieved criteria speech measures at each visit (SRs mostly 1 and less than 1%SS during the clinic visit). Treatment was gradually withdrawn over the first 8 weeks of Stage 2, and Sharon heard only stutter-free speech after the second Stage 2 visit. Dominic was discharged 10 months later, around 13 months since starting Stage 1.

Case Study 2: Liam

Background and Assessment

Liam was seen for a stuttering assessment at the age of 5 years, 7 months. His mother reported that the onset of his stuttering had been very gradual and his first stutters were noticed 12 months earlier. He had attended another clinic for speech therapy during the past year and that treatment had been focused on delays in his speech and language development. The treating clinician had observed stuttering in the clinic 4 months previously when Liam's stuttering became more noticeable. A within-clinic speech sample at that time was measured as 2.5%SS. Liam's mother, Olivia, had been the first person to notice Liam's stuttering. She had not been concerned about it because there had been no mention of it during the speech pathology sessions that focused on his speech-language development.

   During the stuttering assessment at the current clinic, Liam's stuttering was measured as 1.7%SS during a conversation with the clinician, and two beyond-clinic recordings of Liam talking with his parents during the previous week were measured as 6.0%SS and 4.9%SS, respectively. Liam's stuttering consisted mostly of repeated syllables, some fixed postures with audible airflow (e.g., "sssssssome"), and a superfluous "nnn" sound at the beginning of some utterances. Olivia was unsure whether Liam was aware of his stuttering because neither she nor her partner had drawn attention to it and Liam had not shown any signs of concern or frustration. No family history of stuttering was reported, although the clinician noticed that Liam's younger sister, present at the assessment, stuttered mildly. Treatment was to begin the week following the assessment, on the basis that:

• Time since onset of stuttering was 12 months.

• The stuttering appeared to have become gradually more severe.

• Stuttering onset was quite late, and Liam would soon reach school age.

Stage 1

Clinic Visit 1   *Within-clinic: 6.5%SS.* Olivia rated Liam's within-clinic speech sample as SR4 and the clinician's SR was 7. His stuttering consisted of repeated syllables and fixed postures with audible airflow, and Olivia was able to identify only Liam's most obvious stutters. The clinician explained how to collect daily SRs at home and write them on a standard SR chart. Collection of an average SR for the whole day was recommended. Liam's SR chart is reproduced in **Fig. 4–2**.

The clinician then spent time explaining to Olivia the various types of stutters and assisting her accurately to identify Liam's stutters. Treatment in structured conversations was then briefly explained to Olivia, and the clinician demonstrated the procedures while she and Liam talked about a simple picture book. The conversation was structured so that Liam's utterances would be one or two words. His initial responses were stutter-free, and the clinician used verbal contingencies of praise and acknowledgment. Olivia then continued the treatment conversation and she was able to successfully elicit short responses and provide prompt verbal contingencies for stutter-free speech. Her identification of stuttering was accurate, and she did not use any contingencies when Liam stuttered once or twice. The clinician then added occasional verbal contingencies for stuttered speech, and Liam was happy to self-correct his stutters when requested. The clinician watched while Olivia implemented similar procedures. In particular, she emphasized that Olivia should structure the conversation in such a way that most of her contingencies were for stutter-free speech, and only occasionally would she request Liam to correct a stuttered word. Olivia and Liam continued the treatment conversation and Liam remained stutter-free throughout the rest of the activity. The clinician summarized the procedures and discussed with Olivia the treatment that would be conducted at home during the week ahead.

Clinic Visit 2   *Within-clinic speech measure: 4.8%SS.* Olivia was unwell and unable to attend the next clinic visit so his father, Julian, attended with Liam. Julian was able to report on how Olivia had conducted treatment during the week and the speech measures she had collected. Julian reported that both he and Olivia felt that there had been a general improvement in Liam's stuttering over the last few days. Julian reported that he had been using verbal contingencies for Liam's stuttered speech in unstructured conversations. Although Julian confirmed that Liam was happy to self-correct stutters each time he was asked, the clinician explained that contingencies should focus on stutter-free speech and be conducted during structured conversations for the first few weeks of Stage 1. The clinician modeled treatment in a structured conversation and watched while Julian did the same. Liam's speech was mostly stutter-free, and he spontaneously self-corrected one stutter. Julian had noticed Liam self-correcting stutters occasionally during the previous week. When summarizing the procedures for the following week, the clinician recommended that Julian and Olivia praise Liam's spontaneous self-corrections of stutters and use verbal contingencies mostly for stutter-free speech. In addition to structured treatment, the clinician recommended that both parents occasionally praise Liam's spontaneously stutter-free speech during their everyday conversations. Julian and the clinician agreed that Olivia would remain the main therapy provider because Julian spent limited time with Liam due to work commitments.

Clinic Visit 3   *Within-clinic speech measures: 1.6%SS.* Liam was unable to attend one clinic visit due to illness. When he attended Visit 3, Olivia reported that very little treatment had been attempted because Liam had a high temperature for several days and had been lethargic. As a result, Liam's SR had increased a little over those 4 or 5 days. Once he recovered, daily treatment in structured conversations was conducted again, and most of Liam's sentence-length responses were stutter-free. Olivia noticed an increase in Liam's spontaneously stutter-free speech, and this change was reflected in SRs of 3 on many days. The clinician introduced treatment in unstructured conversations and recommended that Olivia praise Liam's spontaneously stutter-free speech in everyday conversations.

Clinic Visit 4   *Within-clinic speech measures: 1.6%SS.* In the few days preceding this clinic visit, Olivia had noticed that all of Liam's stutters were repeated syllables and that fixed-posture stutters had disappeared. Because the speech measures indicated that Liam was stuttering very little, the

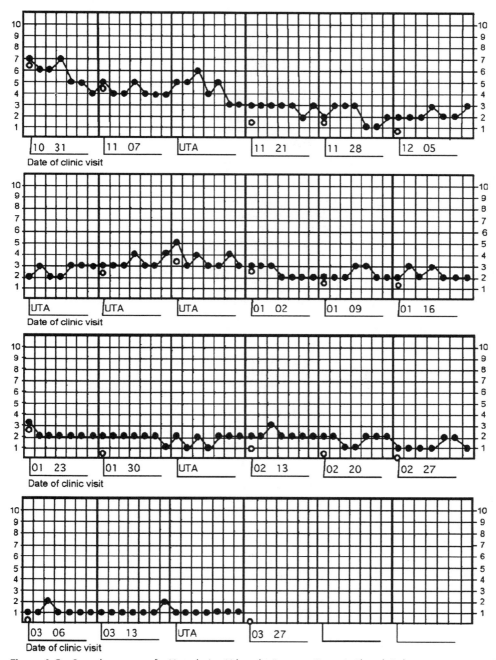

Figure 4–2   Speech measures for Liam during Lidcombe Program Stage 1. Closed circles represent parent's severity ratings (SRs); open circles represent clinician's % syllables stuttered (%SS).

contingency of requesting Liam to self-evaluate his stutter-free speech was added during this clinic visit. Olivia was instructed to continue daily structured treatment and elicit longer responses from Liam, and to increase the frequency of contingencies during unstructured conversations. The clinician explained to Olivia that these changes in treatment structure and verbal contingencies were in response to Liam's lower SRs and therefore were signs of Liam's progress.

Clinic Visit 5   *Within-clinic speech measure: 0.7%SS.* Olivia reported that she had not heard any stuttering for 2 consecutive days during the previous week, although she could only report on speech heard before and after school. Treatment on those days had consisted of praise at the end of each day for talking smoothly. The clinician emphasized the importance of continuing to deliver consistent verbal contingencies, despite the improvements made by Liam. Treatment on those days could have consisted of various types of verbal contingencies for stutter-free speech, delivered in different speaking situations. After observing Olivia conduct unstructured treatment in the clinic, during which Liam was stutter-free, the clinician recommended that the focus during the following week be on delivering consistent unstructured treatment. She also recommended that structured treatment conversations be conducted on days when Liam's SR was 2 or higher. The clinician asked Olivia to record a 10-minute sample of Liam over the Christmas period. Due to family vacations, his next visit was scheduled 4 weeks later.

Clinic Visit 6   *Within-clinic speech measure: 2.6%SS.* Olivia reported a slight increase in Liam's stuttering over the holidays and said that she was alarmed to have had to rate him SR5 on one day. Two beyond-clinic audio recordings confirmed the higher stuttering levels and were measured as 2.2%SS and 3.4%SS. The increased stuttering coincided with little treatment being conducted during the days before and after the Christmas holidays. Several relatives had been to stay and Liam's parents were fully occupied with their guests. Apart from those days, Olivia and Liam had conducted structured treatment every day and unstructured treatment on most days. The clinician explained that fluctuations in Liam's SRs when he was highly excited were not surprising and that, until stutter-free speech had generalized to all speaking situations, she could expect it to reoccur. The clinician reinforced that Olivia had done the right thing by reinstating consistent daily structured and unstructured treatment as soon as possible. She also highlighted the fact that Liam's SRs were almost back to their pre-Christmas levels. The clinician observed Olivia conduct structured treatment in the clinic, during which Liam was mostly stutter-free. The clinician noted, however, that Olivia occasionally praised what she thought was stutter-free speech but was in fact speech with mild stuttering. Again, some time was spent doing some stuttering identification during a 5-minute free-play activity. The clinician recommended that Olivia only praise utterances that she was certain were stutter-free during treatment conversations in the week ahead.

Clinic Visits 7 and 8   *Within-clinic speech measures: 1.5%SS and 1.3%SS.* Liam attended both clinic visits with his mother and his younger sister. Olivia reported that Liam's speech had been mostly stutter-free (SR2). Because Liam was still on school holidays and spending most of his time with his family, this was considered a significant and sustained improvement. On some days, Olivia rated him a SR3 and described this as "hearing around six stutters per day." She felt reasonably confident that she was identifying most stutters, although at Visit 7, attention was brought to the fact that four stutters were counted during a 10-minute within-clinic speech sample. Hence, it was possible that Liam was producing more than six stutters per day. Olivia mentioned that structured treatment was done on most days and unstructured treatment every day. In further discussion, it became clear that Olivia was prompted to do unstructured treatment whenever she heard a stutter. The clinician reiterated the importance of initiating treatment in a positive way, preferably with verbal contingencies for stutter-free speech. At Visit 8, Olivia reported she had tried to put this into practice and that Liam's stuttering severity had continued to decline. At Visits 7 and 8, Olivia conducted unstructured treatment in the clinic and involved Liam's sister in the way that she did at home on some occasions. The clinician recommended that Olivia continue daily unstructured treatment and implement structured treatment on days when Liam's SR was 3 or higher.

Clinic Visit 9   *Within-clinic speech measure: 2.5%SS.* Olivia described Liam's speech in the clinic as being typical of his most severe stuttering for the past week and rated it SR3. She reported that Liam had similar episodes of slightly increased stuttering on some days. She had conducted structured treatment on those days, as recommended previously. The clinician suggested that Olivia implement a weekly "smooth talking" chart, where Liam would get a stamp for longer periods of stutter-free speech throughout the day. The system was explained to Liam in the clinic and used following treatment in a structured conversation. Liam was very responsive to his mother's verbal contingencies for stutter-free speech, and twice he was observed spontaneously self-correcting stutters. It was agreed that Liam would get a smiley stamp for stutter-free periods of at least 5 minutes, and that up to six stamps could be awarded per day.

Clinic Visit 10   *Within-clinic speech measure: 0.2%SS.* Most of the clinic visit was taken up with discussion about treatment implemented at home during the previous week. Olivia reported that the new reward chart had been most successful. Liam was more consistently stutter-free and requested additional stamps for being "smooth" each day. Olivia found it difficult not to give Liam a stamp if he had only one stutter during a monitored period, although she was aware that Liam could routinely remain stutter-free for up to 15 minutes with one or two prompts from her. Olivia had conducted unstructured treatment conversations for a few minutes each day, up to five times a day until the end of school holidays. When Liam returned to school, treatment was confined to before and after school. Olivia also reported using one-off verbal contingencies for stutter-free speech outside her planned treatment conversations. The clinician asked Olivia whether she was able sometimes to anticipate when Liam was likely to stutter. She thought Liam was most likely to stutter when he was trying to tell a long story about something exciting, such as finding an interesting spider in the garden. The clinician recommended that Olivia increase the frequency of her contingencies for Liam's stutter-free speech before he launched into the story, and prompted him to tell her with lots of stutter-free speech.

Clinic Visit 11   *Within-clinic speech measure: 0.9%SS.* Liam's stuttering had remained stable at SR1 to SR2 over the previous 2 weeks. This was a significant improvement because one of the SR1 days occurred during the weekend, when Liam and his parents spent a lot of time together. Olivia reported that all treatment occurred during unstructured conversations, and that she had been able to anticipate Liam's periods of SR2 speech. The clinician was pleased to hear that Olivia had continued treatment on SR1 days, despite hearing no stutters. Typically, Liam could now be stutter-free for up to 2 hours at a time. The reward system was reviewed to ensure that it remained motivating and challenging for Liam.

Clinic Visit 12   *Within-clinic speech measure: 0.2%SS.* Olivia reported an overall increase in severity during the previous week, with six SR2 days and one SR3. She attributed this to Liam being unwell and reported not being able to do much treatment even though Liam stayed home from school. He responded well to unstructured treatment when his health improved and could speak consistently stutter-free for up to half a day. The clinician noticed that Olivia confused a normal disfluency with a stutter on one occasion, which prompted discussion about how to discriminate normal speech behaviors from stuttering when children were near the end of Stage 1. The clinician reassured Olivia that this uncertainty would occur infrequently, and that she should try to apply contingencies only for unambiguous stutters.

Clinic Visit 13   *Within-clinic speech measure: 0%SS.* Olivia reported decreased severity, with two SR1 days. She also was finding it difficult to remember to conduct treatment consistently because most of Liam's speech was stutter-free. The clinician suggested some modifications to the reward system previously implemented, so that Liam could receive a tangible reward if a preset goal was achieved. For example, when Liam achieved 25 stamps for the week, he would receive an additional reward. Liam was excited at the prospect of obtaining an extra "prize" and requested that they do smooth talking immediately so that he could start accumulating stamps.

The clinician explained that Stage 2 was imminent because Liam was close to Stage 2 criteria for the previous week. Olivia agreed to continue consistent, unstructured treatment, and the clinician suggested ways to help her remember to do so when Liam was SR1 for long periods. The clinician also encouraged Liam to remind his mother about treatment because he was keen to gain as many stamps as possible.

Clinic Visits 14 and 15   *Within-clinic speech measures: 0%SS and 'nil.'* Olivia reported that Liam had many SR1 days, with some occurring on weekends. Unstructured treatment was conducted every day and Liam had received a reward for achieving his speech target as negotiated with his mother. No within-clinic speech measure was available from Visit 15 because Liam was unwell and not particularly interested in talking with his mother and the clinician. The clinician recommended that Olivia use more frequent contingencies for stutter-free speech and stuttering on days when Liam was SR2.

Clinic Visit 16   *Within-clinic speech measure: 0%SS.* Liam and his mother did not attend one clinic visit because of a conflicting appointment. In Visit 16, Olivia reported that Liam had been SR1 for most of the previous fortnight. Her SR2 ratings were on days when she heard Liam stutter once or twice. The clinician confirmed that Liam had achieved the speech criteria to begin Stage 2 and recommended that Olivia continue treatment without further changes until his Stage 2 clinic visit in 2 weeks.

Stage 2

Liam progressed through the routine Stage 2 schedule uneventfully and met the criteria speech performance at each visit. Under the clinician's guidance, Olivia gradually withdrew all verbal contingencies over the first 12 weeks, and Liam was discharged 11 months after starting Stage 2.

General Observations on Case Studies

It is worthwhile reflecting briefly on these two cases and highlighting the individual case characteristics that the clinician considered when making decisions during Stage 1. It is outside the scope of this chapter to explore issues raised during Dominic's and Liam's initial evaluations such as stuttering onset, family history of stuttering, and timing of early intervention. Further information is available elsewhere about initial assessment (Rousseau & O'Brian, 2003) and the timing of early intervention with the Lidcombe Program (Packman, Onslow, & Attanasio, 2003).

Client Background

At first glance, the Dominic and Liam case studies included factors that may have complicated their stuttering treatment. Dominic spoke two languages; Liam had delayed speech and language development for which he had received therapy during the previous year. Dominic showed occasional signs of frustration about his stuttering and Liam did not show such signs, despite his stuttering being more severe. Notwithstanding these potential complications, the clinician used the Lidcombe Program as outlined in the manual and did not have to make any special adaptations for these case characteristics. With our colleagues, we have written elsewhere about using the Lidcombe Program with children who have medical problems, children from culturally and linguistically diverse backgrounds, and children who are shy or unusually sensitive to verbal feedback about their speech (Hewat, Harris, & Harrison, 2003).

Treatment Provider

Although in practice to date we have found that it is usually a mother who conducts treatment with her child, this is not an essential component of the Lidcombe Program. Therefore clinicians can be flexible when establishing who will conduct each child's treatment, as demonstrated in Liam's case when Julian became involved. Aside from parents, our experience is that child caregivers or nannies who are employed to work with children one-to-one in the home are readily able to attend weekly clinic visits, conduct daily treatment conversations, and collect SRs. On the other hand, child-care workers in preschools and all day care centers rarely have time in their schedules for weekly clinic visits and daily treatment conversations. Preschool-based caregivers are best able to contribute to Lidcombe Program treatment by collecting SRs that are passed on to the parent and clinician each week.

Clinician and Parent Collaboration

As children's SRs begin to decrease during Stage 1, treatment needs to occur during everyday, unstructured conversations, and it is the clinician's role to identify the ideal time for this change and plan the transition from structured treatment. First, the clinician ensures that the child is enjoying structured treatment conversations and that the parent is using contingencies for stutter-free and stuttered speech correctly and safely. Second, the clinician either demonstrates to the parent, or asks the parent to demonstrate, praise for stutter-free speech in an unstructured conversation during a clinic visit. When clinicians build on successful structured treatment in this way the transition to unstructured treatment occurs smoothly and without difficulty. Although most children respond to this change as readily as Liam and Dominic, it can be a little more difficult for some children. In those cases, clinicians and parents work together to find alternative ways to introduce the necessary changes. For example, if a child does not like the contingency of praise for stutter-free speech during unstructured treatment conversations, then the parent could use either acknowledgment of stutter-free speech or request self-evaluation of stutter-free speech. During the last weeks of Liam's Stage 1, there are examples of the clinician and Olivia making small adjustments to treatment conversations week by week. It is clear that there were no substantial problems in the way treatment was being conducted, neither were there any obvious changes to make. The clinician and Olivia would have discussed ways to modify the frequency and type of verbal contingencies, whether or not to add rewards, and how to monitor changes in Liam's stuttering. The outcome of these small changes is evident in Liam's SR chart, which shows that he reached the Stage 2 criteria at Clinic Visit 16.

Another example of the clinician and parent working together to solve a clinical problem—while staying within the parameters of the Lidcombe Program—occurred in the weeks following Dominic's Clinic Visit 5. At that visit, Sharon reported that Dominic had pretended to stutter in an apparent effort to have more frequent structured treatment conversations. Over preceding weeks, treatment conversations gradually had become less structured, but Dominic still particularly enjoyed structured treatment conversations with Sharon. We could speculate about which aspects of the conversations were most enjoyable for him. Perhaps he enjoyed the experience of stutter-free speech, or liked frequent praise from Sharon, or looked forward to spending one-on-one time while they played together. Or maybe it was something else that appealed to him. Whatever is the case, he wanted to continue structured treatment conversations after they had ceased to be useful stuttering treatment for him. Therefore the clinician had to take into account both his enjoyment of this now less-than-useful treatment, as well as the need to continue *unstructured* treatment conversations. The clinician knew from Dominic's SRs and Sharon's reports that he was making good progress, and she knew that Sharon was using the range of verbal contingencies safely and correctly. The clinician's decision was to suggest that Sharon increase the frequency of her contingencies for stutter-free speech and stuttering. It is worth highlighting that this was not the only possible solution in the circumstances, it was simply the one used on that occasion. Neither Sharon nor the clinician would have been sure of the outcome at the time. With hindsight, we know that it was successful because Dominic's SRs continued to decrease and he continued to enjoy unstructured treatment conversations. On the other hand, if Dominic had continued to request "smooth talking games" or his SRs had increased, then the clinician and Sharon would have tried another solution. And that brings us to a final point about clinical troubleshooting in the Lidcombe Program; if the clinician had been unable to find a successful solution after a few weeks, then she would have consulted a colleague with experience using the treatment and discussed the matter.

Children are expected to make steady progress through Stage 1 in the same manner as Liam and Dominic. The duration of Stage 1 treatment will vary among children, and clinicians will develop their preferred ways of using the Program components and troubleshooting difficulties. Despite the variations, as long as clinicians use the Program as it is outlined in the manual (Australian Stuttering Research Centre, 2004) and by Onslow et al. (2003), then they can be confident that the evidence base outlined in the following section will apply to their clients.

Quantitative Evidence for the Lidcombe Program

It seems clear now that anecdotal evidence in favor of the Lidcombe Program, in case studies such as those of Dominic and Liam, are to be found in the routine files of clinicians in many countries (Hayhow et al., 2003; Shenker & Wilding, 2003). These stories complement the growing evidence base for the Lidcombe Program. Evidence is available for the social validity of the treatment (Lincoln, Onslow & Reed, 1997), and there is evidence that it causes no changes to children's speech motor functioning (Onslow, Stocker, Packman, & McLeod, 2002) or family or child language habits (Bonelli, Dixon, Ratner, & Onslow, 2000). The Lidcombe Program has been shown to be safe, causing no anxiety in children or changes to the attachment between parent and child (Woods, Shearsby, Onslow, & Burnham, 2002). There is also experimental evidence that the Lidcombe Program provides benefits beyond those that occur with natural recovery in the short term (Harris, Onslow, Packman, Harrison, & Menzies, 2002). There are retrospective (Jones, Onslow, Harrison, & Packman, 2000) and prospective (Rousseau et al., 2005; Rousseau, Packman, Onslow, Harrison, & Jones, 2006) recovery plot data available for large cohorts of children to provide clinical benchmarks for treatment times.

The evidence base for the Lidcombe Program includes the all-important clinical trials (Robey, 2005). Phase I trials establish the safety of a treatment, and establish that those who need the treatment will comply with it, and the trials provide preliminary scientific evidence for its effectiveness. Phase II clinical trials take the process of treatment development one step further; they provide robust evidence that a sufficient number of people who receive the treatment respond to it, how long it takes for that response to occur, and establish whether the clinical response to the treatment is clinically worthwhile. Phase I and Phase II clinical trials have been completed for the Lidcombe Program (Onslow, Andrews & Lincoln, 1994; Onslow, Costa and Rue, 1990; Rousseau et al., 2005), and it is clear that the treatment is safe—in fact fun—and that the overwhelming majority of parents in such trials will comply with it, and that the overwhelming majority of children in those trials will not stutter after they have had it. For example, in the Jones et al. (2000) recovery plot study of 261 cases, 250 children and parents who began Stage 1 completed it, with stuttering below 1.0%SS and SRs of mostly 1.

Distance Intervention

There are many families who, for various reasons, are isolated from standard speech pathology treatment services (Wilson, Lincoln, & Onslow, 2002). The majority of these cases are rural dwelling families, and telehealth is a potential method to treat stuttering children in those families. Phase I trials have shown the viability of a telehealth adaptation of the treatment (Harrison, Wilson, & Onslow, 1999; Wilson, Onslow, & Lincoln, 2004). Although it is clear that this model of service delivery of the Lidcombe Program will require more time than the weekly visit format, it does look to be a solution for the many stuttering children who cannot visit a clinician each week with a parent. A Phase II trial of these telehealth procedures has been complete by Lidcombe Program researchers in Australia (Lewis, Onslow, & Packman, Manuscript).

Randomized Controlled Trial

The final stage of treatment development is the Phase III trial, or the randomized controlled trial (RCT). More recently, this "gold standard" evidence has been established for the Lidcombe Program (Jones et al, 2005). This trial compared the effectiveness of the Lidcombe Program with a control group of preschoolers who received no treatment for a 9-month period. To give it the

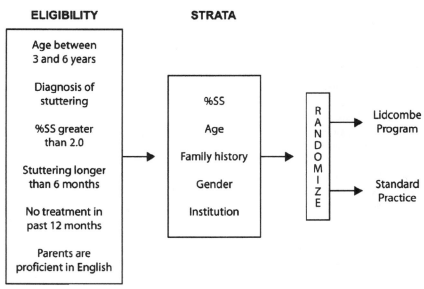

ELIGIBILITY

Age between
3 and 6 years

Diagnosis of
stuttering

%SS greater
than 2.0

Stuttering longer
than 6 months

No treatment in
past 12 months

Parents are
proficient in English

STRATA

%SS

Age

Family history

Gender

Institution

RANDOMIZE

Lidcombe
Program

Standard
Practice

Figure 4–3   Design of the randomized controlled study of the Lidcombe Program of early stuttering intervention. (From Jones et al. (2005). A randomized controlled trial of the Lidcombe Program for early stuttering. British Medical Journal 331, 659. Reprinted by permission.)

proper term, the design was a pragmatic, open plan, parallel group, RCT with blinded outcome assessment. This means that the design was intended to establish useful (pragmatic) clinical information about the value of a treatment package, that clinicians and participants alike knew whether they were in the experimental or control group ("open plan"), that there was no changing of treatments given to participants during the trial ("parallel"), and that the observers who measured stuttering severity did not know whether the participants were in the experimental or the control group ("blinded"). The design is summarized in **Fig. 4–3**. The most important feature of this design, that makes it the gold standard of clinical trials research, is the *random* allocation of participants to so-called treatment arms, in this case the Lidcombe Program and control. This randomization process ensures that the trial is free of the biases that normally affect Phase I and Phase II trials and generally lead to an over-estimate of the effect size, or how efficacious the treatment is thought to be. As it turned out, the effect size found in this RCT was large, being twice the so-called minimum worthwhile difference, which is the smallest difference between two groups that would be clinically important. Jones et al. felt justified in concluding that "the reduction in stuttering in the Lidcombe programme group was significantly and clinically greater than natural recovery" (p. 3).

The Jones et al. (2005) RCT was a landmark in the development of the Lidcombe Program evidence base. The completion of the gold standard of evidence in a RCT represents the conclusion of the basic clinical trials work of our clinical and academic group in Australia. The next stage in establishing the efficacy of the Lidcombe Program is replications of such studies by groups independent of us. There is general agreement that the ultimate goal in establishing an evidence base for health care is the completion of numerous RCTs, which allows a systematic review of that evidence and a firm conclusion to be drawn about the efficacy of an intervention. In an ideal world, in the future, Phase II trials of other treatments for early stuttering will be completed and will figure in RCTs that compare those new treatments with the Lidcombe Program. Indeed, it would be surprising if the first empirically developed treatment for early stuttering was ultimately shown to be the best of many contenders.

◆ Future Lidcombe Program Research

Improving Treatment Efficacy and Effectiveness

Our Australian research group currently is concerned with the further evidence base that needs to be developed for the Lidcombe Program. In particular, now that we await from other groups further work in demonstrating treatment *efficacy*, we are turning our research attention to the issue of treatment *effectiveness*. These often confused terms refer to two concepts that are different in an important way. *Efficacy* refers to how the treatment works under the carefully controlled conditions of an RCT, whereas *effectiveness* refers to how the treatment works at the population level where those controlled conditions do not exist. The fundamental issue here is whether clinicians who meet the professional development standards of their profession can use the Lidcombe Program to treat stuttering as well as the clinicians involved in the Jones et al. (2005) RCT. As part of the team that is developing the Lidcombe Program, we are faced with this issue regularly when parents ask our advice about finding a clinician to treat their stuttering child. We normally suggest that parents should ask whether the clinician has received Consortium training, and whether the clinician conducts the treatment according to the information pamphlet and manual at the ASRC Web site (www.fhs.usyd.edu.au/asrc). The key point here is that we simply do not know whether clinicians who have attended training and use the treatment correctly will meet established benchmarks of the number of treatment hours to complete Stage 1. Preliminary data suggest that this is an issue worthy of some serious attention (Rousseau, Packman, Onslow, Robinson, & Harrison, 2002). In particular, such data reaffirm an earlier stance that we have taken (Onslow, 1994) concerning the issue of administering the treatment in strict accordance with the manual. To us, it makes no sense to wander from such a strong database and use design variants of the Lidcombe Program with clients.

This is not to say that there is no need to change the treatment to seek improvements in treatment efficiency. To the contrary, the need to do so is dire, considering the ever present drain on public speech pathology resources in just about every country, and the considerable cost of private services. The median period required to complete Stage 1 is known to be around 12 clinical hours (Jones et al., 2000; Kingston, Huber, Onslow, Jones, & Packman, 2003; Rousseau et al., 2005). If for the sake of argument, that number could be reduced to 8 clinical hours, then each Lidcombe Program clinician would be able to have one-third more children complete Stage 1 for the same expenditure of clinical time. However, the point is that after so much careful and systematic evidence-based treatment development, any changes to treatment models need to be based on careful clinical research, such as that outlined above with a telehealth adaptation of the treatment. If clinicians make changes arbitrarily, then there is a substantial risk that any gains in treatment efficiency will be offset by the treatment becoming ineffective at the population level.

At the time of writing we have several clinical trials in progress that are designed to produce more effective means to administer the Lidcombe Program. Issues that we are exploring in that program of research deal with formats for teaching parents the basic skills of the treatments, materials used to train parents, the rates and types of parental contingencies, and a continuation of a program of research to determine exactly what components of the treatment are essential to its efficaciousness and what parts are not (Harrison, Onslow, & Menzies, 2004).

Treatment for School-Age Children Who Stutter

Although the Lidcombe Program was developed for children younger than 6 years, there are compelling reasons to contemplate whether it might be efficacious for children who are somewhat older, in the age range of 7 to 11 years. In the first instance, there is an urgent need for treatment developments with this age group, considering that some serious effects of the disorder begin during the school years. The earliest signs of its ill effects have been measured at the threshold of those years in 6- and 7-year-olds (De Nil & Brutten, 1991; Vanryckeghem & Brutten, 1997).

Virtually every adult who stutters reports experiencing the disabling effects of the condition during childhood and early adolescence (Hayhow, Cray, & Enderby, 2002). Stuttering children suffer bullying, are perceived negatively by peers, and are rejected by peers more often than children who do not stutter (Langevin, Bortnick, Hammer, & Wiebe, 1998). Further, it is quite likely that the now well-known speech-related social anxiety associated with stuttering (for an overview, see Messenger, Onslow, Packman & Menzies, 2004) has some of its origins during the school years.

In principle, the Lidcombe Program might be thought of as a first treatment of choice for children who stutter between 7 and 11 years because it is "simple" to the extent that it does not involve programmed instruction and does not require that children make any changes to their customary way of speaking. In fact, there are some data to suggest that it might be efficacious for this age group (Lincoln, Onslow, Lewis, & Wilson, 1996), however that trial was conducted prior to the evolvement of the Lidcombe Program in its current form, so we are not really sure. A recent Phase I trial of the current version of the Lidcombe Program has been completed by ourselves and colleagues (Rousseau et al., 2005). The results of that trial have prompted us to begin work, with national and international colleagues, on a Phase II clinical trial. The purpose of that trial is to determine how many school-age children respond to the Lidcombe Program, how well they respond, and how long it takes them to respond. More importantly, we have good reason from the data of Rousseau and colleagues to suspect that not all school-age children will respond favorably to the Lidcombe Program. If our suspicions are founded, then we seek to discover whether there is any discernable pattern to those non-responders.

But more importantly, we would seek to uncover some clues about whether any other treatment models involving verbal contingencies would be more viable, efficient, and efficacious for school-age children: After all, the Lidcombe Program is merely one of many possible treatment models for presenting verbal contingencies to children. In the likely event that the Lidcombe Program model is not suitable for every school-age child, we truly hope that some other model can be found involving verbal contingencies, for the alternatives known to science at present are far from compelling.

♦ Conclusion

The Lidcombe program is a stuttering treatment for preschool age children. Many children and parents have used it successfully and there is robust scientific and clinical evidence that it is an efficacious treatment. Research currently underway is designed to further develop the program, increasing its efficiency and establishing that it is effective at a population level. We expect the clinical and empirical story of the Lidcombe Program to continue to unfold in the future as it has for the past three decades.

References

Andrews, C. (1989). Response contingent stimulation treatment for preschool-age stuttering children. Workshop presented to Northern Rivers Health Service Speech Pathologists, Corakai, New South Wales, Australia.

Attanasio, J., Onslow, M., & Menzies, R. (1996). Australian and United States perspectives on stuttering in preschool children. Australian Journal of Human Communication Disorders 24, 55–61.

Australian Stuttering Research Centre. (2004). Manual for the Lidcombe Program of early stuttering intervention.

Available at: http://www3.fhs.usyd.edu.au/asrcwww/downloads/Manuals/LP_manual_English_Sep2004.pdf. Accessed September 14, 2005.

Australian Stuttering Research Centre. (2005, April). Randomised clinical trials of the Lidcombe Program. ASRC Newsletter 4(1). Available at:http://www3.fhs.usyd.edu.au/asrcwww/downloads/Newsletter/April% 202005.pdf. Accessed January 4, 2006.

Australian Stuttering Research Centre. (2006). Lidcombe Program trainers consortium. Available at: http://www3.

fhs.usyd.edu.au/asrcwww/professional/LPTC.htm. Accessed January 4, 2006.

Bonelli, P., Bernstein Ratner, N., Dixon, M., & Onslow, M. (2000). Child and parent speech and language following the Lidcombe Programme of early stuttering intervention. Clinical Linguistics and Phonetics 14, 427–446.

DeNil, L. F., & Brutten, G. J. (1991). Speech-associated attitudes of stuttering and nonstuttering children. Journal of Speech and Hearing Research 34, 60–66.

Harris, V., Onslow, M., Packman, A., Harrison, E., & Menzies, R. (2002). An experimental investigation of the impact of the Lidcombe Program on early stuttering. Journal of Fluency Disorders 27, 203–214.

Harrison, E., Onslow, M., & Menzies, R. (2004). Dismantling the Lidcombe Program of early stuttering intervention: Verbal contingencies for stuttering and clinical measurement. International Journal of Language and Communication Disorders 39, 257–267.

Harrison, E., Wilson, L., & Onslow, M. (1999). Distance intervention for early stuttering with the Lidcombe Programme. Advances in Speech-Language Pathology 1, 31–36.

Hayhow, R., Cray, A. M., & Enderby, P. (2002). Stammering and therapy views of people who stammer. Journal of Fluency Disorders 27, 1–16.

Hayhow, R., Kingston, M., & Ledzion, R. (2003). The United Kingdom. In M. Onslow, A. Packman, & E. Harrison (Eds.), The Lidcombe Program of early stuttering intervention: A clinician's guide (pp. 147–159). Austin, TX: PRO-ED.

Hewat, S., Harris, V., & Harrison, E. (2003). Special case studies. In M. Onslow, A. Packman, & E. Harrison (Eds.), The Lidcombe Program of early stuttering intervention: A clinician's guide (pp. 119–136). Austin, TX: PRO-ED.

Ingham, R. J. (1980). Modification of maintenance and generalization during stuttering treatment. Journal of Speech and Hearing Research 23, 732–745.

Johnson, W. (1942). A study of the onset and development of stuttering. Journal of Speech Disorders 7, 251–257.

Jones, M., Onslow, M., Harrison, E., & Packman, A. (2000). Treating stuttering in young children: Predicting treatment time in the Lidcombe Program. Journal of Speech, Language, and Hearing Research 43, 1440–1450.

Jones, M., Onslow, M., Packman, A., Williams S., Ormond, T., Schwartz, I., et al. (2005). Randomised controlled trial of the Lidcombe Programme of early stuttering intervention. British Medical Journal 331, 659–661.

Kingston, M., Huber, A., Onslow, M., Jones, M., & Packman, A. (2003). Predicting treatment time with the Lidcombe Program: Replication and meta-analysis. International Journal of Language and Communication Disorders 38, 165–177.

Langevin, M., Bortnick, K., Hammer, T., & Wiebe, E. (1998). Teasing/bullying experienced by children who stutter: Toward development of a questionnaire. Contemporary Issues in Communication Science and Disorders 25, 12–24.

Lincoln, M., Onslow, M., Lewis, C., & Wilson, L. (1996). A clinical trial of an operant treatment for school-age children who stutter. American Journal of Speech-Language Pathology 5, 73–85.

Lincoln, M. A., Onslow, M., & Reed, V. (1997). Social validity of the treatment outcomes of an early intervention program for stuttering. American Journal of Speech-Language Pathology 6, 77–84.

Martin, R., Kuhl, P., & Haroldson, S. (1972). An experimental treatment with two preschool stuttering children. Journal of Speech and Hearing Research 15, 743–752.

Messenger, M., Onslow, M., Packman, A., & Menzies, R. (2004). Social anxiety in stuttering: Measuring negative social expectances. Journal of Fluency Disorders 29, 201–212.

Onslow, M. (1987, February). Management of the preschool-age stutterer. Paper presented at the Annual Conference of the Australian Association of Speech and Hearing, Canberra, Australia.

Onslow, M. (1988, February). Treatment of early stuttering: What do we have to offer? Paper presented at the Annual Conference of the Australian Association of Speech and Hearing, Brisbane, Australia.

Onslow, M. (1994). The Lidcombe Programme of early stuttering intervention: The hazards of compromise. Australian Commun Q (Suppl.), 11–14.

Onslow, M. (2003). From laboratory to living room: The origins and development of the Lidcombe Program. In M. Onslow, A. Packman, & E. Harrison (Eds.), The Lidcombe Program of early stuttering intervention: A clinician's guide (pp. 21–25). Austin, TX: PRO-ED.

Onslow, M., Andrews, C., & Lincoln, M. (1994). A control/ experimental trial of an operant treatment for early stuttering. Journal of Speech and Hearing Research 37, 1244–1259.

Onslow, M., Costa, L., & Rue, S. (1990). Direct early intervention with stuttering: Some preliminary data. Journal of Speech and Hearing Disorders 55, 405–416.

Onslow, M., Packman, A., & Harrison, E. (Eds.). (2003). The Lidcombe Program of early stuttering intervention: A clinician's guide. Austin, TX: PRO-ED.

Onslow, M., Stocker, S., Packman, A., & McLeod, S. (2002). Speech timing in children after the Lidcombe Program of early stuttering intervention. Clinical Linguistics and Phonetics 16, 21–33.

Packman, A., Onslow, M., & Attanasio, J. (2003). The timing of early intervention with the Lidcombe Program. In M. Onslow, A. Packman, & E. Harrison (Eds.), The Lidcombe Program of early stuttering intervention: A clinician's guide (pp. 41–55). Austin, TX: PRO-ED.

Reed, C. G., & Godden, A. L. (1977). An experimental treatment using verbal punishment with two preschool stutterers. Journal of Fluency Disorders 2, 225–233.

Robey, R. R. (2005, May 24). An introduction to clinical trials. The ASHA Leader 10, 6–7; 22–23.

Rousseau, I., & O'Brian, S. (2003). Routine case studies. In M. Onslow, A. Packman, & E. Harrison (Eds.), The Lidcombe Program of early stuttering intervention: A clinician's guide (pp. 103–118). Austin, TX: PRO-ED.

Rousseau, I., Packman, A., & Onslow, M. (2005, June). The Lidcombe Program with school age children: A phase I trial. Paper presented at the 7th Oxford Dysfluency Conference, Oxford, UK.

Rousseau, I., Packman, A., Onslow, M., Harrison, E., & Jones, M. (2006). Language, phonology, and treatment time in the Lidcombe Program: A prospective study in a Phase II trail. Journal of Communicative Disorders.

Rousseau, I., Packman, A., Onslow, M, Robinson, R., & Harrison, E. (2002). Australian speech pathologists' use of the Lidcombe Program of early stuttering intervention. Acquiring Knowledge in Speech. Lang Hear 4, 67–71.

Shenker, R., & Wilding, J. (2003). Canada. In M. Onslow, A. Packman, & E. Harrison (Eds.), The Lidcombe Program of early stuttering intervention: A clinician's guide (pp. 161–172). Austin, TX: PRO-ED.

Van Riper, C. (1973). The treatment of stuttering. Englewood Cliffs, NJ: Prentice-Hall.

Vanryckeghem, M., & Brutten, G. J. (1997). The speech-associated attitude of children who do and do not stutter and the differential effect of age. American Journal of Speech-Language Pathology 6, 67–73.

Webber, M., & Onslow, M. (2003). Maintenance of treatment effects. In M. Onslow, A. Packman, & E. Harrison. (Eds.), The Lidcombe Program of early stuttering intervention: A clinician's guide (pp. 81–90). Austin, TX: PRO-ED.

Wilson, L., Lincoln, M., & Onslow, M. (2002). Availabilty, access, and quality of care: Inequities in rural speech pathology services and a model for redress. Advances in Speech-Language Pathology 4, 9–22.

Wilson, L., Onslow, M., & Lincoln, M. (2004). Telehealth adaptation of the Lidcombe Program of early stuttering intervention: Five case studies. American Journal of Speech-Language Pathology 13, 81–93.

Woods, S., Shearsby, J., Onslow, M., & Burnham, D. (2002). Psychological impact of the Lidcombe Program of early stuttering intervention. International Journal of Language and Communication Disorders 37, 31–40.

5

An Indirect Treatment Approach for Early Intervention for Childhood Stuttering

Corrin G. Richels and Edward G. Conture

The purpose of this chapter is to discuss a family-centered, indirect treatment approach for preschool-age children who stutter (CWS). After an initial discussion of literature pertaining to the treatment of preschool CWS, the chapter presents rationale, strategies, tactics, and outcome data regarding this treatment approach, which is in its 25th year of practice, first at Syracuse and now at Vanderbilt University. The chapter concludes with a summary of the essential aspects of the program as well as areas in need of future research and modification. We hoped that readers of this chapter will better understand the importance of including families in the treatment of young CWS, routine collection of behavioral data, and reporting such data to the child's caregivers. Additionally, we believe, clinicians should then be able to appropriately modify the approach we describe to best fit various service delivery settings.

◆ Three Treatment Paradigms for Childhood Stuttering

Historically, there have been three treatment paradigms used with stuttering: (1) direct treatment; (2) indirect treatment; and (3) a combination of direct and indirect methods (see Ramig and Bennett, 1997 for further description of these various approaches). *Direct* treatment typically involves the clinician, parent, or child identifying instances of stuttering to help the child make changes to his or her speech-language behavior. Such identification of stuttering, as well as changes to stuttering behavior, may happen with or without clinician prompting or guidance. Additionally, a direct approach to treating the child's instances of stuttering includes immediate listener feedback (e.g., from clinician or parent) regarding the child's speech-language productions (e.g., Harrison & Onslow, 1999, Chapter 4; Ingham, 1999; Runyan & Runyan, 1999, Chapter 6). Conversely, *indirect* treatment typically involves making changes to a child's environment through parent training and clinician modeling without directly or overtly identifying stutterings to the child and/or overtly attempting to change the child's speech-language production (e.g., Conture, 2001; Melnick & Conture, 1999). Obviously, a combination or hybrid treatment approach could include identification and immediate feedback of the child's speech productions along with modifications of the child's environment (e.g., Harrison & Onslow, 1999, Chapter 4). The treatment discussed in this chapter is most consistent with the tenets of *indirect* treatment of childhood stuttering, an approach whose development has been described by Conture (1982, 1990, 2001) as well as Melnick and Conture (1999).

At present, it is unclear which of these three approaches is the most efficacious for long-term improvement of stuttering in preschool children. However, there are considerable data that indicate that at least one direct approach provides significant, positive benefits for young CWS (e.g., Harrison, Onslow, & Menzies, 2004; Huber, Packman, Quine, Onslow, & Simpson, 2004; Jones et al., 2005; Lincoln & Onslow, 1997; Onslow, 2004; Onslow, Andrews, and Lincoln, 1994; Wilson, Onslow, & Lincoln, 2004). Whether direct or hybrid approaches are better, the same or worse—in the short-, medium- or long-run—than the indirect approach we describe is neither the focus nor purpose of this chapter. See Franken, van der Schalk, and Boelens (2005) for an initial attempt to make these comparisons. Indeed, it is not immediately clear *what* evidence should be used to compare these various treatment approaches and/or *who* should make these decisions. Be that as it may, this chapter provides some of the rationale, strategies, and tactics as well as outcome data pertaining to our approach, leaving it to the reader to assess its relative merits and contributions to the treatment of childhood stuttering.

◆ Rationale for the Indirect Treatment Program

The rationale for our treatment program stems from empirical findings regarding the influence of communicative/linguistic factors on instances of stuttering in young children. Our approach primarily focuses on: (1) the role of utterance complexity in the occurrence of stuttering; (2) the temporal requirements for the initiation and termination of speech-language production; (3) the rate of speech production; (4) the state as well as trait emotional/behavioral tendencies; and (5) the family's role in adapting to, addressing, and changing the preceding four items.

Based on our and others research, as well as considerable clinical experience, we believe that the utterance complexity (e.g., Zackheim & Conture, 2003), time demands and requirements for the onset and termination of speech-language production (e.g., Kelly & Conture, 1992), rate of speech production (e.g., Yaruss and Conture, 1995), and dispositional (trait) as well as situational (state) aspects of emotions and related variables (e.g., Anderson, Pellowski, Conture, & Kelly, 2003; Karrass et al., [2006]) serve as moderators of instances of childhood stuttering. Thus, these characteristics of a child's speech-language processing and production abilities, as well as a child's emotional and behavioral tendencies, can influence the quantity and quality of children's stuttering. We are not suggesting that any one of these variables is a *causal* contributor (mediator) of the stuttering behavior. However, there is increasing evidence that these variables can effect (e.g., exacerbate/influence) stuttering in children. Indeed, this supports the notion that our approach is, at least in part, "evidence-based" from the perspective of basic information about childhood stuttering. That is, we employ strategies and tactics to treat childhood stuttering that our empirical research and that of others (e.g., Bernstein-Ratner & Sih, 1987) strongly suggest impact childhood stuttering.

Role of Utterance Length and Complexity Relative to Childhood Stuttering

Empirical evidence suggests that disfluent behavior relates to a child's emerging language (e.g., Colburn & Mysak, 1982a, and 1982b). Thus, it is probably not coincidental that prominent changes in language development in some children co-occur with the onset of stuttering. One of the more dramatic changes in children's expressive language output results when a child's use of single words at 12 to 18 months of age evolves into the emergence of complex syntax by 3 years of age (Limber, 1973). Numerous empirical studies have shown that increases in utterance length and complexity influence the frequency of stuttering in children at or near the onset of stuttering (e.g., Bernstein-Ratner and Sih, 1987; Logan & Conture, 1995, 1997; Melnick & Conture, 2000; Yaruss, 1999). See Zackheim and Conture, 2003, Tables 1 and 2, for a detailed discussion of at least 15 such empirical studies of preschool-age children who do and do not stutter.

For instance, in a recent study of preschool CWS and children who do not stutter (CWNS), Zackheim and Conture (2003) reported that utterances above a child's mean length of utterance (MLU) contained disfluencies (i.e., stutter-like disfluencies [SLDs] in CWS and non-SLDs in CWNS) more frequently than utterances that were shorter than or utterances that were approximate to the child's MLU. Such findings lend support to the hypothesis that changes in utterance length and complexity—during conversational speech—may change children's speech-language planning and production in ways that support, or are less conducive to, the maintenance of speech fluency. Therefore, any difficulties with or disturbances in the efficient and rapid coordination of the multiple linguistic processes necessary to form longer, more complex utterances may contribute to increases in disfluent speech. (See Anderson, Pellowski, & Conture, 2005 for empirical data pertaining to linguistic dissociations exhibited by CWS, e.g., between expressive language and speech sound abilities.) We believe, therefore, that changes in utterance length and complexity influence the likelihood that a child's utterance will contain stuttering and that, as such, these changes are relevant to the treatment of childhood stuttering for several reasons.

First, a child who more often than not is using his or her speech-language output at maximum potential most every time he or she speaks is apt to experience disruptions in ongoing, fluent speech-language production. Second, a child who continually tries to match the length and complexity of an adult's speech-language output—for example a parent's—rather than his or her own language abilities is likely to have more disruptions in the forward flow of speech. Third, we hasten to note, here at the onset of our description of this issue, that neither our therapy nor philosophy involves the "dumbing down" of the overall length and complexity of a child's speech-language output. Rather, we encourage the parents (directly) and the child (indirectly) to *match* their speech-language output, as best they can, to the cognitive-communicative needs of the situation. This means that utterances will sometimes be short and simple, and other times long and complex, but the length and complexity of utterances should be as consistent as possible with their communicative intent. For example, when a child asks a parent for a glass of juice, this should not be used routinely by parents as another opportunity to educate. It is not necessary to explain to a 3-year-old child the various types of citrus fruits, those that yield more or less juice potential, and their relative nutritional values! Children have ample opportunities to learn complex language throughout their day's activities without the parents continually feeling they need to expand on or "improve" on their child's every utterance. Sometimes, it is perfectly acceptable for parents to respond, "Sure, here's some juice."

Again, with all of our treatment strategies and tactics, we encourage, support, and reinforce flexibility by the child and parent rather than a "one size fits all" approach. Ideally, both child and parent should routinely operate, more or less, in the mid-range of their average utterance length and complexity for many of their everyday communicative interactions. Performance roughly approximate to—sometimes higher, sometimes lower than—the child's average utterance length and complexity is preferable to performance that is either consistently at the low or the high ends of the child's length and complexity continuum. Again, both parent and child should attempt to match the "quality and quantity" of their speech-language productions to the quality and quantity of their cognitive/communicative intent. Will such matching be ideal or perfect? No, of course not; mismatches will always occur. In general, however, constantly striving to operate at psychological, cognitive, behavioral, or physical extremes will probably not lead to competent performance. Operating at the extremes of capability is unlikely to be effective across various situations that require differing, flexible strategies and approaches. Specifically, consistent performance at linguistic extremes—whether low or high—is apt to be problematic, particularly for young children's effective communication.

Time Demands and Rate of Speech-Language Production

Research indicates that when parents reduce their rate of speech with their CWS, that the child reduces his or her speech rate, which typically results in changes in the reduction of stuttering frequency or severity (e.g., Guitar & Marchinkoski, 2001; Kelly, 1994; Stephenson-Opsal, & Bernstein Ratner, 1988: Yaruss & Conture, 1995). Additionally, empirical evidence suggests that when parents reduce their communicatively interrupting behaviors, or "simultalk," the frequency of their child's stuttering also decreases (e.g., Kelly, 1994; Kelly & Conture, 1992; Livingston, Flowers, Hodor, & Ryan, 2000). We believe that appropriate reductions in speaking rates by parents and CWS allows the child the speech-language/cognitive processing *time* necessary to initiate and complete an utterance fluently (see Conture and et al., 2006, for further detail). It seems safe to say, that preschool-age children are in the beginning stages of learning to use their speech and language to communicate their intentions and thoughts effectively. Thus, the apparent desire, drive, or compulsion to get and maintain their communicative turns (and their listener's attention), for some children, have the potential to exceed their ability to efficiently and fluently manage speech-language output. By way of analogy, one might say it is the speech-language planning and production equivalent of trying to compete in the Tour de France on a bike with training wheels.

Some parents may believe that their interruptions of and simultalk with their children is helpful to the child who stutters. Parents, typically at the time of their child's initial assessment or during his or her first several treatment sessions, report that it is frustrating to see their child struggle through an utterance when they know, (or think they know) what the child is going to say. However, this kind of "help" by the parents can send the wrong message to the child on numerous levels. For example, the child may feel that the parent's interruptions are an indication that adults do not trust his or her capability to speak and finish his or her own thoughts. Additionally, a parent may guess wrong about the child's communication intent and create more frustration for the child. Indeed, when questioned about their tendency to interrupt their child and/or finish their child's utterances, some parents will freely admit that they do it because they (parent[s]) lack patience for the seemingly slow, inefficient, hesitant speech-language productions of their young child. Likewise, parents report that they do not like to wait because they "are in a hurry" or like to have "things done quickly." Indeed, a fruitful avenue of empirical research, in our opinion, would be to descriptively or experimentally assess the relative tolerance that parents of CWS have for delays, pauses, and silences during conversational speech, especially with their own children!

Although we do not know this for a fact, it is reasonable to hypothesize that the routine or consistent practice of interrupting or using overly rapid rates of speech by parents, who are the models for their children, may be problematic if it occurs routinely when they talk with their children. That is, such adult communicative behavior may encourage, or require, as well as result in the child's speech-language processing and production abilities operating at a level that exceeds what he or she is capable of efficiently and rapidly achieving. Therefore, as we will discuss below, we attempt to mitigate such parental tendencies through our own repeated modeling of a more desirable speaking rate (i.e., slow to fast normal). In so doing, we encourage—through various strategies—the child's parents to reduce their speaking rates to more appropriate levels with their child who stutters.

Role of Dispositional (Trait) and Situational (State) Aspects of Emotion and Childhood Stuttering

Perhaps no other topic relative to stuttering receives as much attention, as well as skepticism, as the role of emotions in exacerbating and causing stuttering in children, teens, or adults (e.g., Alm, 2004; Messenger, Onslow, Packman, & Menzies, 2004). However, objective evidence from our laboratory indicates that CWS are more emotionally reactive and less well regulated than are CWNS. For example, Karrass et al. (2006) found that on the basis of parents' reports on standardized questionnaires, CWS experienced and displayed more negative affect, took longer to recover to their speech baselines following their emotional upsets, and were less able to flexibly shift their attention. Subsequent research employing multiple measures of emotional reactivity and regulation replicated and extended these findings (Karrass et al, 2006). Furthermore, this subsequent study found that CWS were not as likely as CWNS to use adaptive methods to regulate emotion (e.g., appropriate distraction, avoidance, and instrumental coping) and were more likely than CWNS to use less adaptive methods, such as aggression. These findings most likely reflect situation-related or state aspects of emotions, but there is also evidence that dispositional or trait aspects of emotion may also differ between CWS and CWNS. For example, Anderson et al. (2003) reported that CWS exhibit temperamental tendencies of being less distractible (e.g., excessively vigilant), less able to adapt to change, and more irregular in their sleep, eating, and bathroom habits. Each of these temperamental characteristics can present behavioral management challenges to parents of CWS. In considering such findings, we attempt to maintain the rationale for our treatment approach current with the empirical evidence related to these characteristics of CWS. Such consideration, we believe, leads us to employ tactics that seem most conducive to meeting these issues. The following section provides details on the actual strategies, tactics, and outcomes related to our therapy, as well as the general characteristics of the children receiving this therapy.

◆ Who, When, What, Where, and How of the Indirect Treatment Program

This section provides details pertaining to: (1) *who* (e.g., in specific, the typical age range and gender composition of preschool-age children who are enrolled in our program); (2) *when* our sessions typically occur; (3) *what* a typical session looks like for both the children and their parents; and (4) *where,* or the "location" at which various components of the treatment are conducted.

To do this, we present initial diagnostic, as well as treatment outcome data, from a recent cohort of preschool-age children ($n = 32$) whom we have treated. In so doing, we are able to discuss *how* our treatment works and for whom. That is, we discuss the typical characteristics of the preschool children we treat and the treatment outcomes associated with our therapy program. We hope that such data will help readers judge, on the basis of the evidence, the nature of the preschool children we treat, as well as the successes and sometimes failures of our program.

Who: Age, Gender, and Stuttering Characteristics of Children Enrolled

Although we also provide treatment for people who stutter who are older than age 6, we focus on our work with the younger CWS, those in the preschool through kindergarten (and sometimes first grade) age range. It is important to remember that because data is based on a clinical sample the membership in this sample is relatively fluid. These children are receiving diagnostics continuously, then they are enrolled in, and subsequently discharged or dropped from, speech-language therapy in our clinic.

Given the aforementioned "fluidity" of our sample, our initial pool of participants totaled 49, but we will provide data only for those 32 preschool-age children (see **Tables 5–1A and 5–1B**) who completed 12 or more sessions of our program. In other words, of the initially available 49 children, 17 are not included. Of these 17, 16 are not included because they had completed fewer than 12 treatment sessions at the time of this writing. We excluded the remaining child from our final data corpus because she was 2 years older than the other children in her group. Occasionally, a child's chronological, as well as developmental, age is in a "gray area" of being considered ready for direct treatment only but too old for indirect treatment only.

Table 5–1A   Group Averages for Descriptive and Fluency-Related Information

	Chronological Age (months)	TSO	% Total Disfluency[†]	% SLD[‡]	% SLD to Total Disfluency[*]	SSI	TCS
N[#]	32	32	29	29	29	27	30
M	49	15.5	12.9	10.3	74.7	21.3	21.7
SD	11	9.5	7.0	7.2	17.8	8.2	5.3
Min	33	3	3.6	.6	18	6	12
Max	72	39	32	29.7	100	38	33

[†]Percent total disfluency: number of disfluencies produced divided by number of words in the sample.

[‡]Percent SLD: number of SLD divided by number of words in sample.

[*]Percent SLD to total disfluency: number of SLD divided by the total number of disfluencies in the sample.

N[#], number of CWS in each category; SSI, Stuttering Severity Instrument-3 (Riley, 1994); TCS, Temperament Characteristics Scale (Oyler, 1996); TSO, Time since reported onset of stuttering (months).

Table 5–1B   Group Averages for Six Standardized Speech and Language Measures (in standard scores)[*]

	GFTA	PPVT	EVT	TELD Receptive Subtest	TELD Expressive Subtest	TELD Spoken Language Quotient	MLU
N[#]	30	31	30	29	28	28	27
M	108.7	106.3	110.4	107.4	99.9	103.3	0.489
SD	10.1	14.5	11.9	17.8	15.1	17.5	1.4
Min	88	78	91	72	73	71	−1.43
Max	123	130	133	140	125	137	4.20

MLU, Mean length of utterance, (in standard scores) relative to norms provided in Miller (1981); PPTV, Peabody Picture Vocabulary Test; EVT, Expressive Vocabulary Test; GFTA, Goldman Fristoe Test of Articulation; TELD, Test of Early Language Development.

Characteristics of Individuals Included in the Data Analysis

Number of Sessions Completed   As we mentioned above, for a child's data to be included in these analyses, the child had to have attended at least 12 treatment sessions. The 12-session minimum was chosen because our experience has shown, among other things, that children and their families typically need ~3 months to respond adequately, as well as to adjust to the expectations of our treatment regimen. In other words, our previous work (Conture, 2001) indicated that our treatment with preschool-age children took ~12 weeks before we could reasonably assess their treatment success, failure, or progress.

Of the 32 children who met the 12-session minimum requirement, a few ($n = 9$) were in the beginning or middle stages of treatment, a larger number ($n = 17$) had completed treatment through the full maintenance phase and had been dismissed, and the smallest number ($n = 6$) had completed the 12-week minimum but had dropped out of treatment (for various reasons), usually prior to the maintenance phase of our program. Of the six children who did not complete treatment through the maintenance phase, the following reasons were apparent: (1) insurance had ceased to cover expenses ($n = 3$); (2) the family moved out of the area ($n = 2$); and (3) the family was not satisfied with the child's progress in therapy ($n = 1$).

Age and Gender The sample of the 32 preschoolers (26 males, 6 females) that we are discussing (see **Tables 5–1A and 5–1B**), is typical of the age range of the preschool-age children we treat (mean age = 4 years, 2 months; SD = 11 months; range = 2 years, 9 months to 6 years 0 months). By way of comparison, the age range we are reporting and the ratio of males to females for this sample are comparable to the second author's data for records of the children who were treated at Syracuse University. Likewise, the age range of the present sample ($n = 32$) is consistent with that of an earlier study based on preschool-age children whose stuttering was treated at Vanderbilt University (Conture, 2001, pp. 173–177). Furthermore, the age range of the current sample is comparable to that of another clinical sample ($n = 100$; Yaruss, LaSalle, & Conture, 1998) as well as to a research sample ($n = 20$; Anderson & Conture, 2000) of preschool-age children reported by the second author and colleagues (see **Fig. 5–1** for between-study comparisons of age range and other measures for Yaruss et al., Anderson & Conture, and the present study). It should be noted also that none of the preschool-age children discussed in this chapter were involved in the reports by the second author that were cited above (i.e., Anderson & Conture, 2000; Conture, 2001; Yaruss et al., 1998) (**Tables 5–1A and 5–1B**).

Stuttering Characteristics **Table 5–1A** shows that the mean frequency of stuttering among the participants described in this chapter was 10 stutterings per 100 words of conversational speech (SD = 7). These children averaged 75% stutterings per total disfluencies, (SD = 17%), which is slightly lower than the 81% reported by Pellowski and Conture (2002). They also had a mean overall score of 21.3 (SD = 8.2; rating = moderate) on the Stuttering Severity Instrument-3 (SSI-3; Riley, 1994). The calculation of the SSI-3 spanned the full range of severity classifications of very mild (n = 2), mild (n = 6), moderate (n = 12), severe (n = 4), and very severe (n = 3). The most common type of disfluency exhibited by the 32 children who stuttered in this sample was sound-syllable repetitions (69% of the sample, n = 22). Additionally, the mean time since onset of stuttering to the children's initial evaluations were scheduled to address parental concerns about stuttering was 15.5 months (SD = 9.5 months). Comparisons of the present sample's total frequency of disfluency, stuttering frequency, within-word disfluencies, and SSI scores with the data reported by Anderson and Conture (2000) and Yaruss et al. (1998) indicate performance of the preschoolers in the present sample, although involving different participants, is comparable (**Fig. 5–1**).

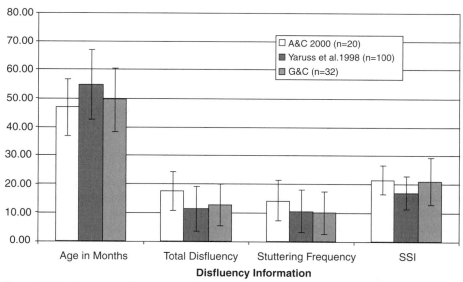

Figure 5–1 Comparison between Anderson and Conture (2000), Yaruss et al. (1998), and the present study (Graham & Conture, this chapter) participant (research and clinical) samples in terms of age and disfluency descriptors.

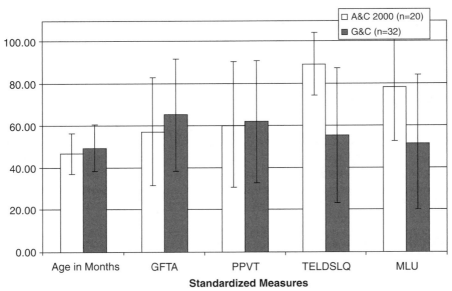

Figure 5–2   Chronological age and percentile ranks on standardized speech-language measure data: Anderson and Conture (2000) versus the present study (Graham & Conture, this chapter).

Performance on Standardized Tests of Speech-Language   The mean standard scores for the 32 participants shown in **Table 5–1B** are consistent with those of previous studies of language scores for CWS (Anderson & Conture, 2000). **Fig. 5–2** compares the percentile ranks on standardized speech-language measures of the Sounds and Words subtest of the Goldman-Fristoe Test of Articulation (GFTA, or GFTA-2; Goldman and Fristoe, 1986, 2000); the Peabody Picture Vocabulary Test-R or III (PPVT-R, or PPVT-III; Dunn and Dunn, 1981, 1997), the Test of Early Language Development-2 or 3 (TELD-2, TELD-3; Hresko, Reid, & Hamill, 1991, 1999), and MLU (Miller, 1981), thereby assessing articulation abilities, receptive vocabulary, receptive and expressive language skills, and grammatical development, respectively. It is important to note that the Anderson and Conture sample (2000) excluded children whose speech-language scores were below the 19th percentile, whereas our treatment groups include all levels of language skills. As should be expected in a clinical sample, in which all CWS are treated regardless of concomitant speech-language problems, no such exclusionary criteria were applied. Thus, of the 32 CWS there were five children ($\sim$16% of the total sample) who had low scores on either a speech (GFTA %<15), vocabulary (PPVT-III standard score<85), or language measures (TELD-3 spoken language quotient [SLQ] standard score <85). Of the 5 children with clinically significant or low scores, one child had low scores on both articulation and language measures, another had low scores on both receptive vocabulary and total language, and three children had low scores only on the total language measure (TELD-3) (**Fig. 5–2**).

Our preschool treatment groups do not enroll children of the same age in each of the groups. For example, one of the preschool groups may have an immature 5-year-old and a mature 3-year-old in the same group. The age ranges for each group are intended to include children of appropriate ages and development as well as an environment that is comfortable to each participant. Experience has shown that 3 through 5 years of age groupings work well for most children within this age range and their parents; however, exceptions do occur, for example, a child whose speech and language development is so delayed, disordered, or immature that individual treatment rather than group attention is required.

When: Scheduling Groups

The scheduling of any speech-language treatment requires a balance. That is, a balance between what a child's performances will be at a given time of day and the parents' ability to bring the child to the clinic at that time. Consequently, we schedule groups in the early afternoon and evening. Typically, groups do not start earlier than 3:00 PM or later than 5:00 PM. This time frame allows younger children an opportunity to maintain a nap schedule without becoming too tired to concentrate.

Each group meets for 50 minutes, leaving 10 minutes to discuss the child's portion of the session and for discussions with the child's family at the conclusion of therapy. Families attend therapy once a week until a consistent level of improved fluency is seen in the child and parents report improved fluency at home as well. Later in this chapter, we present examples of such consistency.

Our treatment, like other therapeutic regimens discussed in this volume (e.g., Kully & Langevin, Chapter 8), is roughly divided into three phases: (1) initial; (2) transfer; and (3) maintenance, which are described briefly in the following paragraphs.

The initial phase involves once-a-week therapy sessions. Decisions regarding changes in scheduling to any other phase of therapy rely on the data we collect during *each* weekly session, as well as parents' weekly reports regarding the status of their child's speech fluency at home, daycare, nursery school, or kindergarten. A child must begin to improve appreciably, which typically requires his or her evidencing consistent performance of stuttering frequencies that are at 5% or less for at least four consecutive therapy sessions. The child's therapy schedule then moves from a once-per-week therapy regimen to the *transfer* phase. The transfer phase begins with a biweekly schedule that is followed by sessions once every 3 weeks, and then once every 4 weeks. Transfer, in our approach, entails our continued, active involvement with the child and parents, but it also entails seeking increasingly to "move" the child's behaviors and parents' supporting thoughts and feelings into everyday situations. This phase may be viewed as a "hand-off" phase, whereby we increasingly hand over responsibility for being normally disfluent to the child and parents.

At about the time that a child switches to attending sessions once every 8 weeks, we consider him or her to be in the *maintenance* phase of treatment. Maintenance, in our approach, requires less active involvement with the child and parents. In this phase, we attempt to help, support, and encourage the parents to become more and more active in "maintaining" and expanding their child's treatment gains. Typically, attendance once every 12 weeks is reduced to once every 16 weeks, then twice a year, to once a year, and then dismissal. We believe it is important, based on our experience, to make it very clear to the family, at the time of a child's initial assessment and throughout the initial phase of treatment, that both the *transfer* and *maintenance phases are part of the overall treatment program.* In other words, we initially and continually emphasize to the parent(s) that their child's therapy will be decreased gradually as the child's fluency improves and the family seems able to consistently assist with, encourage, and support his or her improvement.

The length of our treatment plan—initial, transfer, and maintenance—as well as the timings of changes in scheduling from one phase to the next do not involve a fixed time frame. Therefore, any child and his or her family may stay on a biweekly schedule for several months before proceeding to an every-3-week schedule and then rapidly progressing from that point through to dismissal. The clinician collects measures of the child's speech-language and related behavioral performance during each treatment session. These findings, together with parental, teacher, and other professional reports, guide our decision-making every step of the way. Thus, our decisions regarding transitions from initial to transfer and transfer to maintenance are based on data that are routinely collected throughout treatment. *All* decisions are made on an individual basis with consideration for both the child's demonstrated performance during therapy and the parents' report about the child's nontherapy fluency, especially in the home setting. The goal of our scheduling is to optimize a family's ability to continue the child's improved fluency without prematurely withdrawing the support that weekly treatment sessions appear to provide. We also strive to not allow the child and his or her family to "linger" in treatment beyond the time when transfer, maintenance, or dismissal should have occurred.

Recently, we have been exploring the use of "parent data" as a supplement to the measures of stuttering and related behaviors that we collect during each treatment session. Parents are asked to rate the severity of their child's stuttering at three set times throughout the day for 7-day periods

Please Circle	
1	Mild – Rarely observed
2	Mild to Moderate – Observed sometimes
3	Moderate – Observed frequently
4	Moderate to Severe – Observed in every sentence
5	Severe – Observed in most words in sentences

Morning

Date								
	1 2 3 4 5	1 2 3 4 5	1 2 3 4 5	1 2 3 4 5	1 2 3 4 5	1 2 3 4 5	1 2 3 4 5	1 2 3 4 5
Activity								

Afternoon

Date								
	1 2 3 4 5	1 2 3 4 5	1 2 3 4 5	1 2 3 4 5	1 2 3 4 5	1 2 3 4 5	1 2 3 4 5	1 2 3 4 5
Activity								

Evening

Date								
	1 2 3 4 5	1 2 3 4 5	1 2 3 4 5	1 2 3 4 5	1 2 3 4 5	1 2 3 4 5	1 2 3 4 5	1 2 3 4 5
Activity								

Figure 5–3   Form used for parent-perceived ratings of the child's stuttering frequency for a 1-week time period.

(**Fig. 5–3**) between therapy sessions. The parent then returns the form to the clinician at the next scheduled treatment session. To date, our informal assessment indicates that parents' ratings of their child's stuttering severity do not differ substantially from the behavioral data collected during treatment sessions. However, at present, we lack sufficient evidence to arrive at a more informed conclusion.

What and Where: Format and Locations for Treatment Sessions

This section provides a general description of the organization of the treatment sessions for both the "child-treatment" and "parent-treatment" groups that are conducted simultaneously in different rooms by different clinicians, a format that defines our parent-child treatment approach.

Child-Treatment Group

We try to limit the maximum number of children in each group to no more than five. By keeping the groups relatively small, each child has a better opportunity to participate fully. Throughout each session, the clinician models a slow rate of speech, and utterances of appropriate lengths and complexity (neither overly long nor overly short). At the same time, the clinician makes sure not to interrupt, talk for, or modify the children's fluency.

Every treatment session begins with the children and clinician seated at a table or on the floor in the treatment room. Each child has an opportunity to talk with the clinician and other children. The clinician gently, but firmly, directs the topics of conversations so that they are socially appropriate (i.e., no "potty-talk"). Otherwise each child is free to discuss/relate whatever is of interest to him or her. During these conversations, counts of the disfluencies and stutterings that occur during 100 words of conversational speech will be obtained for each child. Our "100-word disfluency count" provides the data necessary to track each child's progress toward goals and to make decisions about his or her initial, transfer, or maintenance schedules. Furthermore, because conversations also occur at the beginning of each child's treatment session, they are less reflective of the immediate impact of therapy, and they seem to be more reflective of the last treatment session or perhaps a generalized influence of a child's previous treatment during intervening periods of time between sessions. These measures also provide tangible evidence of a child's improvement, or lack thereof, which are shared with parents at the end of *each* weekly treatment session using Microsoft Excel© (Redmond, Washington) charts that display their child's frequency of speech disfluencies (i.e., total speech disfluencies, stuttered disfluencies, and other disfluencies) per 100 words "across time" during each treatment session (**Fig. 5–4, Fig. 5–5, and Fig. 5–6**). Parents are trained how to read these charts and figures and the meaning of the various measures of disfluencies beginning with the child's initial diagnostic and continuing throughout treatment. Indeed, parents are given printed copies of these charts at routinely scheduled parent-clinician conferences.

Parents, like all individuals, learn such information at various rates. Thus, parents' viewing, reading, and understanding of these charts may require one parent two sessions to master and another parent two months. Our experience indicates, however, that regardless of parents' individual learning rates, they greatly appreciate being given these charts and the information they display. Many seem to use the information portrayed on these charts to reinforce and/or modify their own behavior, based on the ebb and flow of their child's behavior. It is our hope that the use of "parent-generated data" will serve the same purpose.

Following their spontaneous conversations, the children and clinician move to the floor (if they've been seated at the table), and the clinician reviews the group "rules." **Fig. 5–7** provides a pictorial illustration of the group rules. This pictorial illustration is presented to the children in

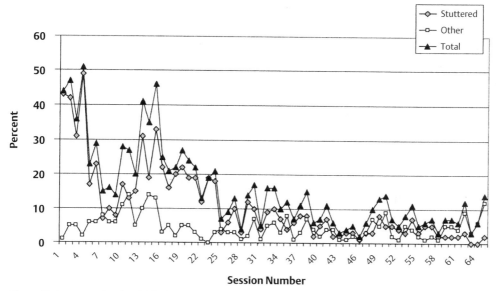

Figure 5–4   Example of a child whose treatment was successful. This individual had a 92% decrease in stutter-like disfluencies (SLDs), 23% increase in non-SLDs, and a 72% decrease in total disfluency.

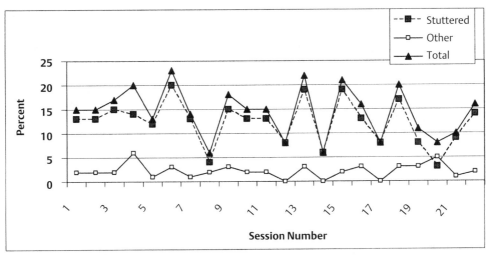

Figure 5–5 Example of a child with volatile/highly variable performance during treatment. This individual had a 6% decrease in stutter-like disfluencies (SLDs), 26% increase in non-SLDs, and a 9% decrease in total disfluency.

therapy on a piece of yellow laminated paper, and each child is asked to follow each of the three group rules during group activities:

1. Listen while others are talking.

2. Wait your turn while others are talking.

3. Be quiet while others are talking.

The rationale for these group rules is to create—during treatment sessions—a reasonably quiet, low communicative stress environment for social/communicative interaction, one in which the

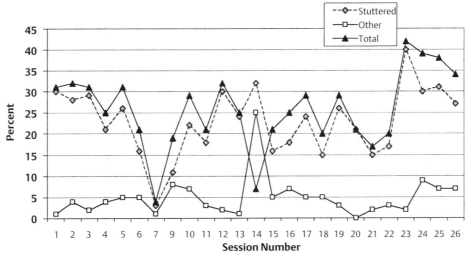

Figure 5–6 Example of a child not responding to group treatment. This individual had an 8% increase in stuttering-like disfluencies, 38% increase in non-SLDs, and a 13% increase in total disfluency.

Listen While Others Are Talking

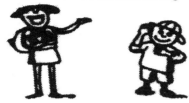

Wait your Turn While Others Are Talking

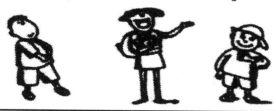

Be Quiet While Others Are Talking

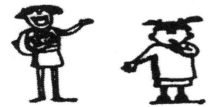

Figure 5–7 Therapy room "group rules" discussed at beginning of a session in an attempt to decrease interrupting, help with appropriate turn-taking, increase tolerance for silence/pausing/waiting, and increasing on-task speech as well as nonspeech behavior during the treatment session.

clinician and the children are listening appropriately and speaking in turn with one another (for another approach to this, see Runyan & Runyan, 1999, see Chapter 6). Clinicians enforce group rules and remind the children by pointing to the rule sheet to reinforce their appropriate behavior with such comments as, "I like the way Bob is waiting so quietly for his turn." Opportunities to practice these rules are provided throughout the remainder of the session. One of the collateral "skills" taught by this approach is a child's ability to listen, which increases his or her tolerance of remaining silent during conversations without feeling a need to talk, talk over, interrupt others, or "fill dead air." Parents routinely tell us that this skill—once learned—transfers to preschool and school situations, helping the child to be more successful during group activities that require listening and following directions.

The purposes of documenting the preceding rationale is supported by the typical long-term and short-term goals that are included in the treatment plans for CWS who are participating in our group treatment. Long-term goals are meant to be the "end product" or penultimate performance expected from a child before dismissal occurs. Conversely, short-term goals are meant to be incremental steps toward criteria of the long-term goals necessary for therapy dismissal. In our clinic, long-term goals may look like the following examples:

Long-Term Goals

Goal 1. Bob (not the client's real name) will exhibit the following characteristics during a variety of daily communication situations as measured by spontaneous samples, clinical observation, and parental report:

1. Total disfluencies less than 5% of a given sample.

2. SLDs less than 40% of total disfluencies.

Goal 2. Bob will use appropriate turn-taking skills with 80% proficiency during a variety of structured/unstructured tasks with various levels of language demands.

Goal 3. Bob's family will model the following fluency-enhancing techniques, particularly during times of apparent disfluency, in 90% of sentences for at least 5 minutes per day in targeted conversational interactions: conversational turn-taking, strategic pausing, decreased use of questions, slow-normal speaking rate, and appropriate length and complexity of utterances.

Tactics to Achieve the Above Goals

To begin, it should be noted that our experience with young children has taught us that less is more. Thus, we keep the number of tactics, activities, or tasks per session to a minimal level, which generally involve approximately three different but related tasks. By doing so, we are able to stabilize or slow down our sessions' social/communicative pace within and between a limited number of activities, rather than hurriedly "flitting" between several different, unrelated activities. Furthermore, this approach allows us to create continuity among activities (to be described below) and the child to focus in greater depth on a limited number of topics. This vertical/in-depth rather than horizontal/scattered approach to our activities and tasks contributes, we believe, a less hurried, more focused, and calmer tone to our child-clinician communicative interactions.

The *first activity* for practicing group rules (see **Fig. 5–7**) involves a book-reading activity (again, see Runyan and Runyan, 1999, for a different kind of "rules" approach to treating childhood stuttering; see Chapter 6). We attempt to select books that are read aloud to the children, which are age-appropriate and often have an abundance of rhyming words to enhance their phonological awareness skills (Justice & Schuele, 2004). This approach addresses our observations and those of others that the articulatory/phonological development of CWS can be delayed, disordered, and/or subtly inefficient (e.g., Blood, Ridenour, Qualls, & Hammer, 2003; Pellowski, Conture, Anderson, & Ohde, 2001), The clinician reads the books at a normally slow to slightly slower than normal pace and allows each child to take turns talking about, pointing to, or turning pages in the book. During this reading activity, data are collected regarding interrupting and turn-taking behaviors. A simple plus/minus system is used to designate when a child has taken his or her turn appropriately (a plus), and when he or she has interrupted the speaker (a minus). The clinician reinforces desired behaviors with such statements as, "Look how quietly John is waiting" and "It's Ted's turn to point to the squirrel." These methods are consistent with positive behavior modification approaches (Cook, Tessier, & Klein, 2000).

Following book reading, we engage in a *second activity* that involves the children returning or going to a table to participate in a craft or snack activity. These activities typically relate to the content or theme of the book (e.g., gluing farm animal cut outs to paper following a reading of "Old MacDonald"). Turn-taking and appropriate interactions are facilitated through limiting the number of materials available for an activity (e.g., two containers of glue for five kids), a strategy that helps teach the children to wait their turns. The clinician again serves as a model for normally slow utterances of appropriate length and complexity, and appropriate turn-taking. Ten minutes prior to the end of a session, parents join their children and interact with them using the techniques they are learning during the parent group.

The final 10 minutes of a session involve our *third activity,* in which parents interact with their children and share information with the clinician. The parent(s) of each child is called aside so that the clinician can discuss the child's progress based on the data from this session compared with previous sessions. As we mentioned previously, to provide parents with a visual aid, we use Microsoft Excel© to graph the fluency information (stuttering, other disfluencies, and the total number of all speech disfluencies per individual session) for each child's sessions. Examples of these graphs are provided (see **Figs. 5–4 through 5–6**).

Parent-Treatment Group

In our attempts to help prepare parents for our expectations of therapy and direct their attention to our goals and methods for the parent group, we ask them to purchase a few things at the time of the child's initial assessment/diagnostic. One is the book *Stuttering and Your Child: Questions and Answers* (Conture, 2002) from the Stuttering Foundation of America (SFA). We also ask them to purchase a videotape, *Stuttering and Your Child: A Videotape for Parents*, which is also available from the SFA (Conture, 1997). Lastly, we either give them or ask them to purchase the "talking tips" re-frigerator magnet from the SFA (Fridge Magnet for Parents; http://www.stutteringhelp.org). This magnet is a visual reminder of what we want parents to do on a daily basis.

The following list presents some of the key suggestions we provide to every family either at the time of the child's initial evaluation or his or her treatment: (1) use a normally slower rate of speech; (2) use, when appropriate, shorter and simpler sentences when explaining issues, describing events, etc.; (3) minimize answering questions for your child and/or interrupting when he or she is talking; (4) pause for a second after your child's utterances, so that you avoid "talking over" your child's utterances; and (5) also avoid any corrections, instructions, reprimands, or suggestions regarding your child's speech and language and speech disfluencies. As can be seen, these suggestions relate to our prior discussion of the rationale for our treatment approach.

As we have discussed elsewhere (e.g., Conture, 2001; Melnick & Conture, 1999), treatment for the children is occurring simultaneously with the parent portion of the parent-child treatment group. We use "parent" to broadly define the people who are primary caregivers for the CWS. Therefore, especially with single parents who cannot leave work easily to attend treatment, we may have grandparents or other family members involved as well. When this is the case, we try to ensure that the mothers, fathers, or both, who cannot attend treatment regularly, come at least once a month. Our goal is to involve people who are most influential in the child's social and communicative environment. Consequently, we want to work with those adults who are communicatively interacting with the child the most. These are the adults or primary caregivers who we try to involve in the parent training component of our treatment paradigm. It is our belief that the "child" portion of our program helps a child achieve increased speech fluency, and that the "parent" portion helps parents learn what they can do and should not do in facilitating such change outside the treatment environment.

Parents separate from their children and convene in a conference room across the hall from the room where their children are meeting. Each parent is given an opportunity to discuss issues pertinent to his or her individual child or family. Those issues are not always related specifically to the child's stuttering. In discussions of their child's speech-language development and difficulties, parents often bring up other family issues that may range from a child's difficulties with eating, to family schedules that are hectic or less than well-organized, to the child's inability to accept mistakes that he, she, or anyone else makes, and so forth. These conversations are mediated by a second clinician who attempts to direct the conversation toward topics that are relevant to a child's stuttering. It is sometimes difficult for other parents in the group to understand why, for example, Bobby's mom is talking about how much difficulty she is having getting Bobby to come in from outside, turn off television, and get ready for bed. However, such family difficulties and stresses can directly impact the family's ability to become fully engaged in the therapy process. That is, these difficulties make it a challenge for some parents to listen to and focus on what the clinician is talking about or their child's therapy program.

Our rule of thumb when dealing with parents is for them to listen to us (about their child's speech problems and what they can and cannot do to help), first, they must be listened to carefully! We must listen to what is on their minds what are the most pressing issues they have with their children, which may not be stuttering. Although we may not be able to directly or even indirectly help them with these other issues, we and other parents can listen to them sympathetically. And, often times, in so doing, they begin to listen to us, as well as to develop their own strategies for dealing with their other concerns.

Based on the principle that "before a person will listen, the person must first be listened to," the clinicians who conduct the parent groups permits and even encourages parents to discuss difficulties as mentioned above. By listening to and offering suggestions regarding such issues, our experience indicates that parents who are coping with high levels of stress are much better able to remember not to interrupt and talk for their child when he or she is stuttering and to pause appropriately and reduce their rate of speech when their child is obviously struggling to communicate with them. Additionally, understanding the family dynamics aids clinicians in anticipating possible barriers to the child's progress in therapy. Again, it is our hope that the parent data sheet (see **Fig. 5–3**) will help remind parents of what they are supposed to be doing to facilitate their child's fluency on a daily basis and how doing or not doing so is related to change or the lack of change in their child's speech (dis)fluencies.

As other clinicians have noted, parents consistently report that reducing interruptions and rate of speech is a very difficult thing. To help parents with this process, we ask them to select a specific time of day or activity to practice these procedures. Until such behavior changes are relatively easy and natural for the parents to use, we recommend that they devote only 15 minutes of concentrated practice to making these changes to reduce parental burn-out as well as increase their compliance. As the reduced speech rate, again, which should be a normally slow rate of speech (i.e., 140–160 words per minute), becomes more natural for the parents, we encourage them to try to use it "when needed," such as during periods when their child is exhibiting increased stuttering. Often the tactics we suggest to parents for slowing down their speech rate to normally slow levels aids the family in reducing the time-urgent, communicative interchanges with each other. Additionally, families report that the reduced speech rate slows the seemingly hyperkinetic activity levels that characterize many modern households. Another, perhaps secondary benefit when parents use a normally slower speaking rate is that it helps reduce the stress experienced by their children, some of whom even have difficulty adapting to their family's rapid changes in schedules, routines, etc. The parents who are the most successful at using this strategy indicate that "our whole life has slowed down and become more relaxed and, over time, our child has been much more fluent."

At first, this change in a child's stuttering occurs only during the specific time, once a day, when the parent consciously attempts to use a normally slower speaking rate, reduce interruption, avoid completing the child's sentences, etc. Most often, reductions in stuttering *both* in the clinic (clinician documented) and at home (parent reported or documented) are most apt to occur when both the child-treatment portion and the parent-treatment portions of our approach become synchronized. This synchronization or melding of our in-clinic and in-home approaches produces data showing *how* the treatment works and outcomes data for each family.

How: Treatment Outcomes

Method

Data Collected During Group Treatment Sessions   So what evidence do we have that the above procedures we just described help CWS and their families? The primary concerns here are the same for any such treatment approach: *What* is the evidence and *who* decides? Obviously, behaviors that can be easily counted and quantified may or may not be the most relevant measures for evaluating short-, medium- and long-term changes in stuttering and related behaviors. For example, what good value is increased frequency of speech fluency (or decreased frequency of speech disfluencies) if the person with increased fluency seldom talks, seldom communicates when and where appropriate, and, in essence, seldom makes use of his or her increased speech fluency? Indeed, as the second author has stated elsewhere (e.g., Conture, 2001; Conture & Guitar, 1993), the goal of treatment for people who stutter is increased and improved communication not merely increased fluency. In short, we do not engage in conversations to be fluent but to communicate!

Be that as it may, and before we have reliable, valid indexes of "communication" for people who stutter (for examples of and discussion/data pertaining to the topics related to communicative [speech] *naturalness*, see Martin & Haroldson, 1992; Martin, Haroldson, & Triden, 1984; Schiavetti, Martin, Haroldson, & Metz, 1994; for communicative [speech] *normalcy*, see Finn, Ingham, Ambrose, & Yairi, 1997; for communicative [speech] *suitability*, see Franken, van Bezooijen, & Boves, 1997), we are constrained by the measures we do have that seem to make sense, particularly those measures that seem to track at least the "fluent/disfluent" aspects of the behavioral changes that our treatments are designed to engender.

In doing so, for this chapter, using the data from the preceding 32 preschoolers who stutter, we report the number of SLDs, nonstuttering/other disfluencies, and the total disfluencies. These measures were averaged, for each of the 32 preschoolers, for the first four treatment sessions (T1) and the last four treatment sessions (T2) (after Conture, 2001; Zackheim, Conture, Ohde, Graham, & Gregory, 2003).

By comparing these first four session averages with the last four session averages for each participant and then for the group as a whole, we can calculate what we call a "change score," or an index of whether no, little, some, or significant change occurred across treatment sessions. Specifically, this change score can be calculated using this formula: % change = (T2 − T1/T1 + T2) $\times$ 100. For example, one child's average number of SLDs for the first four treatment sessions (T1) was 7.00 and his average number of SLDs for the last four treatment sessions (T2) was 1.25. Thus this child's change score was calculated as follows:

$$\% \text{ Change} = (1.25 - 7.00/7.00 + 1.25) \times 100$$

$$= (-5.75/8.25) \times 100$$

$$= -69.69$$

The resulting value, of −69.69, indicates that this child's stuttering decreased by nearly 70% over the course of his treatment in our program for stuttering. It is important to note that this formula yields negative numbers to indicate *decreases* in a behavior. Conversely, a positive number indicates an *increase* in a particular behavior.

Results

Fig. 5–8 data shows that the 32 CWS we've been describing averaged a 31% decrease in their SLDs, a 10% increase in non-SLDs, and a 17% decrease in total disfluencies. Their increase in nonstutter-like or other disfluencies reflects, in our opinion, a more normal pattern of speech-language output. That

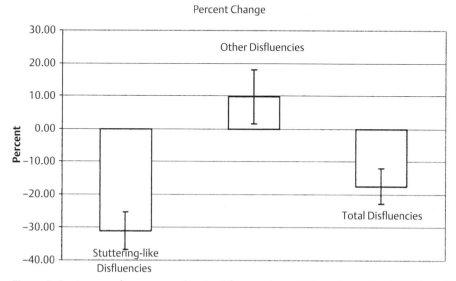

Figure 5–8   Average change scores (see text) for preschool children who stutter (CWS) (*n* = 32) in stutter-like disfluencies (SLDs), other disfluencies, and total disfluencies over the course of indirect, family-centered treatment of childhood stuttering.

Table 5–2   Select Variables at the Time of Initiation of Treatment

	Chronological Age in Months at Start of tx	Days between dx and tx	TSO[‡] at First tx	% Total Disfluency[§]	% SLD[‖]	% SLD to Total Disfluency[¶]	% Other Disfluencies
N	32	31	32	32	32	32	32
M	52.6	93.0	18.2	14.9	11.8	76.6	3.12
SD	11.8	102.5	9.2	11.0	9.7	17.0	3.43
Min	36.0	12.0	5.0	1	1	25.0	0
Max	73.0	395.0	41.0	44.5	41.3	98.0	13.3

dx, initial diagnostic; *N*, number of children for whom data were available on each measure; TSO, Time since reported onset of stuttering (months); *tx*, treatment.

[§]Percent total disfluency: number of disfluencies produced divided by number of words in the sample.

[‖] Percent SLD: number of SLDs divided by number of words in sample.

[¶]Percent SLDs to total disfluency: SLD divided by the total number of disfluencies in the sample.

is, at the beginning of treatment, the vast majority of a child's speech disfluencies are stuttered or are stutter-like; however, based on our experience, as a child begins to improve (i.e., decrease his or her stuttering), there develops an increase in the percentage of non-SLDs per the total amount of disfluency (**Fig. 5–8**).

Table 5–2 displays the means, standard deviations, minimum and maximum values for the children's chronological ages in months at the start of treatment, days between their initial diagnostic sessions and treatment sessions, the time since onset at their first treatment session, percent total disfluency, percent SLDs, proportion of SLDs to total disfluency, and percent of other disfluencies. It is important to note that at the start of treatment the average percentage of non-SLDs for these 32 CWS was around 3%. Therefore, at the conclusion of treatment, there was, on average, a 10% increase in their nonstuttered disfluencies (e.g., phrase repetitions, interjections, and revisions), together with a concomitant average decrease of 31% in stuttered disfluencies. At present, we do not know if this increase in nonstuttered disfluencies coupled with a decrease in stuttered disfluencies in preschool-age children—that we commonly see in our clinic—is a function of our treatment approach or a result of the natural course of improvement in childhood stuttering; however, it appears to be a phenomenon of interest, both at the theoretical and therapeutic levels (**Table 5–2**).

As was mentioned in the section, Characteristics of Individuals Included in the Data Analysis, there were 6 children in the dataset of 32 children who droppedout of our therapy program prior to entering the transfer or maintenance phases of treatment. Analyses of the change scores of the children who dropped out ($n = 6$) compared with the children who continued treatment ($n = 27$) found a significant difference (**Fig. 5–9**) in the changes in stuttering frequency between the two groups ($F_{(1, 30)} = 6.89$, $p < .01$). However, there were not significant differences between the continuing and drop-out groups for nonstuttering/other disfluencies ($F_{(1, 30)} = 0.25$, $p < .62$) and total disfluency ($F_{(1, 30)} = 2.43$, $p < .13$).

As mentioned previously, **Fig. 5–4** to **Fig. 5–6** are the treatment graphs (i.e., percent behavior per daily session across several sessions) for three of the CWS included in this dataset. These graphs are included to illustrate what a typical graph looks like, and what it might look like for three different profiles of therapy success.

Successful Profile

Fig. 5–4 is an example of a child who began treatment with a "very severe" SSI-3 rating and who had become, in our opinion, selectively mute. The child stuttered so severely that being silent

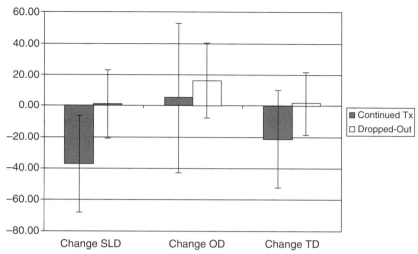

Figure 5–9   Average change scores (see text) for children who dropped out of treatment before the maintenance phase (*n* = 6) compared with children who continued in treatment (*n* = 27) for stuttering-like disfluencies (SLDs), other disfluencies, and total disfluencies. *OD*, other disfluencies; *TD*, total disfluencies.

appeared to be preferable to the difficulties/struggle that basic communication had become. Over the course of treatment her family made tremendous changes in their daily lives and the child's fluency increased. One of the challenges in the early stages of this child's treatment was convincing her that it was okay to talk no matter how it sounded when it came out. This was accomplished using the tactics discussed in the section, Child-Treatment Group. The clinician very indirectly and gently encouraged the child to talk and reinforced any and all utterances—attempts to communicate—with big smiles and positive comments. Meanwhile, the parents were encouraged to do the same. We reasoned, for this child, that positive change in stuttering during conversation could not begin until the child was communicating/talking enough for the family and the clinician to respond in fluency-enhancing ways (e.g., use a slower rate of speech, etc.). The transfer stage began at treatment session 46 with the every other week schedule. The maintenance phase began at session 59 with attendance decreasing to once a month. The once-a-month schedule was maintained until session 65, with one more follow-up session scheduled for 3 months from the date of session 65. As discussed previously, around session 46 the proportion of other/non-SLDs begins to become equal to, then exceed, the number of SLDs with a decrease also occurring in the overall disfluency. At the time of this writing, the child is in kindergarten with neither classmates nor teacher having any suspicion that she was once a very severe stutterer. Unfortunately, the therapy process does not work as smoothly for everyone as it did with this child.

Volatile Profile

Fig. 5–5 shows the graph for a child who has highly variable performance. This child's stuttering as well total disfluencies in the child group setting varied as much as 40 to 50% from one week to the next. Some of this volatility seemed to relate to the child's level of excitement at the beginning of each treatment session, the presence of new group members or absence of usual group members, and changes in family circumstances/routine (e.g., vacations, job change, etc.). This is, in our opinion, an example of a child who is highly reactive to changes in the environment and whose fluency, or lack thereof, reflects his quick as well as high level of emotional arousal (reactivity) and/or low ability to regulate that arousal. Children with this profile do make progress, as evidenced by the 5% decrease in stuttering reflected in this graph (although such change could be attributed as much to random/natural variation in stuttering as it could to the effects of treatment), but we suspect it may not be at as fast a pace as a child with a different temperament profile (Oyler, 1996). Interestingly, in the five sessions that followed, as shown in **Fig. 5–5**, the child's performance began to stabilize, and his SLDs now average around 5%. Perhaps, for children with this profile, a longer period of treatment is needed prior to determining that treatment does or does not work. Thus, although the long-term prognosis for a child with a volatile profile may be guardedly optimistic—given a sufficiently long period of treatment—for some children, as we will see immediately below, such is not the case.

Nonsuccessful Profile   **Fig. 5–6** shows the profile of a child who dropped out of the therapy program. The parents of this child sought services elsewhere. It is relevant to note that although this graph does not clearly reflect it, there were several breaks in regular attendance for this child. At times, 2 and 3 weeks would pass between sessions with subsequent volatile performance reflected in the graph when the child was in attendance. We agreed with the family that our treatment approach was not successful for this child. It was our recommendation that the family seek evaluation and possible counseling to address other issues that we believed were of concern to the child and the child's family. We believed these nonspeech concerns made it difficult for the child to receive benefit from our treatment. For example, this child was consistently being critical regarding other children, their behavior, and/or other children's seeming inability to conform to what this child thought were the rules and regulations of the group. The family eventually opted for a more direct, individualized treatment approach for the child's stuttering. At this point, the writers of this chapter have no specific knowledge regarding the outcome of the alternative treatment.

◆ Summary and Conclusion

This chapter discussed the rationale, tactics, and outcomes for a family-centered, indirect treatment approach. Its purpose has been to discuss one possible way to remediate stuttering in preschool children. Additionally, the authors attempted to emphasize the importance of systematic data collection at each and every treatment session to aid in informing treatment decisions as well as tracking and predicting possible treatment outcome.

The rationale for using this indirect approach is not only based on our combined experience working with this population, but more importantly it stems from information reported in peer-reviewed journals regarding these children's speech-language abilities. It has also been based, at least in part, on a developing literature pertaining to related behavioral and cognitive-emotional characteristics of CWS (e.g., Karrass et al., 2006).

In our experience and opinion, cognitive-linguistic-behavioral processing *speed* matters when working with young children. In essence, most preschool children - those who do, as well as do not stutter - simply lack the developmental wherewithal and life experience, on many levels, to *continuously* and *successfully* keep up with an adult's relatively rapid communicative, behavioral, emotional, or social pace. The speech fluency of young children, especially many of those who stutter, does not seem to benefit from a speech-language environment that *frequently* and *routinely* requires the child's speech-language planning, processing, and production to operate at a rate akin to that used by adults conversing with adults. Certainly, we hasten to add, from time to time, adult-paced or even rapid adult-paced communication is an acceptable as well as expected part of any child's communication environment. However, we become concerned when the important adults in the child's environment (i.e., primary caregivers) *habitually* and *pervasively* exhibit a need for speed during adult-child communication. In essence, we believe, based on considerable clinical experience and data (e.g., Kelly & Conture, 1992; Yaruss & Conture, 1995), that if the child's primary caregiver(s) need for "getting it out" (i.e., rapidly conveying their message/thoughts) *consistently* and *routinely* trumps their interest in "getting it right" (i.e., clearly, easily, and in a relaxed fashion, conveying their message/thoughts) during routine, everyday adult-child conversations, the child's speech fluency typically receives little or no benefit, if not outright hinderance.

Indeed, if speeding up the pace of such events as speech-language planning and/or production "improved" young children's speech fluency, we wager that by now such a fast-paced therapy would have been devised, developed, and employed to treat these children. However, to date, no such therapy that we know of has been so devised, and we doubt that one will be. Instead, much of the presently discussed treatment is designed to do just the opposite. The premises of the approach we describe seek to counteract the all-too-often tendency on the part of these children and their families to seemingly think, plan, and act as if microseconds/milliseconds rather than seconds/minutes were the appropriate units of temporal measure for routine, everyday conversational speech.

In passing, we'd like to note that among other interests, the desire to "work with children" seemingly leads many individuals to decide to become speech-language pathologists. Despite this desire or interest, the truth of the matter is that children come with families, with some of the more significant members of those families being adults, that is, the children's parents. Thus, in our opinion, to maximize the treatment for young children, clinicians should not disregard the possible, and many times significant, influence of adult family members (Conture & Zebrowski, 1992) on the speech-language and related behaviors of preschool-age children. Even in service delivery settings where clinicians do not have regular access to their clients families (e.g., a school setting) clinicians can engage caregivers through the use of face-to-face or phone conferences, notes, and the rating sheet seen in **Fig. 5–3**. This would seem appropriate given the fact that others in that same environment, for example, teachers and administrators, routinely set aside time to talk to and/or meet with children's parents. Likewise, clinicians and researchers should attempt to better understand how children's and their parents' behavioral, emotional, social, and related characteristics influence both the degree as well as speed of recovery during treatment. Clear, direct communication with families, repeatedly if necessary, and on a level adjusted to parental background and educational level, as well as sharing of session data will help inform both the clinician and parents of possible impediments to or facilitators of therapy progress.

In the end, of course, the present writers recognize that no one approach to the treatment of any disorder will work for everyone. Penicillin does not work for everyone; some people are allergic to penicillin and/or have infections that penicillin cannot effectively treat. Thus, recognizing that every disorder itself has variants as do the people suffering with such disorders, one searches—when attempting to treat any disorder—for a goodness rather than exactness of fit between a disorder, the people who exhibit the disorder, and the treatment of the disorder. To that end, after more than 30 years of development, we believe we are moving toward such a fit for the treatment of preschool stuttering; however, the fit is far less than exact because both people who stutter and the disorder of stuttering itself varies. Thus, our treatment must expand, contract, and change to meet the variable "needs" of CWS. Such variations, however, rather than suppress actually encourage the search for better, more comprehensive, and effective treatment.

Thus, in the present chapter we have attempted to present a cross-section, at this point in time, of our own search for effective treatment of stuttering in preschoolers. Our greatest desire has not been to persuade readers to our perspective and shun all others. Rather, we assumed that the reader's initial notion(s) about the treatment of early childhood stuttering would remain. What we desired, however, was that this initial notion would be "infused" to include a wider perspective so that the reader might better be able to consider the possible, probable, and positive that can be done to help young CWS and their families.

References

Alm, P. A. (2004). Stuttering, emotions, and heart rate during anticipatory anxiety: A critical review. Journal of Fluency Disorders 29(2), 123–133.

Anderson, J. D. & Conture E. G. (2000). Language abilities of children who stutter: A preliminary study. Journal of Fluency Disorders 25(4), 283–304.

Anderson, J. D., Pellowski, M. W., & Conture, E. M. (2005). Linguistic variables in childhood stuttering: Speech-language dissociations. Journal of Fluency Disorders 30, 219–253.

Anderson, J. D., Pellowski, M. W., Conture, E. G., & Kelly, E. M. (2003). Temperamental characteristics of young children who stutter. Journal of Speech, Language, and Hearing Research 46, 1221–1223.

Bernstein Ratner, N., & Sih, C. C. (1987). The effects of gradual increases in sentence length and complexity on children's disfluency. Journal of Speech and Hearing Disorders 52, 278–287.

Blood, G. W., Ridenour, V. J., Qualls, C. D., & Hammer, C. S. Co-occurring disorders in children who stutter. Journal of Communication Disorders 36, 427–448.

Colburn, N., & Mysak, E. D. (1982a). Developmental disfluency and emerging grammar: I. Disfluency characteristics in early syntactic utterances. Journal of Speech and Hearing Research 25, 414–420.

Colburn, N., & Mysak, E. D. (1982b). Developmental disfluency and emerging grammar: II. Co-occurrence of disfluency with specified semantic-syntactic structures. Journal of Speech and Hearing Research 25, 421–427.

Conture, E. G. (1982). Stuttering. Englewood Cliffs, NJ: Prentice-Hall, Inc.

Conture, E. G. (1990). Stuttering (2nd ed.). Englewood Cliffs, NJ: Prentice-Hall, Inc.

Conture, E. G. (1997). Stuttering and your child: A videotape for parents. Memphis, TN: Stuttering Foundation of America.

Conture, E. G. (2001). Stuttering: Its nature, diagnosis, and treatment (pp. 173–177). Boston: Allyn and Bacon.

Conture, E. (Ed.). (2002). Stuttering and your child: questions and answers. Memphis, TN: Stuttering Foundation of America.

Conture, E., & Guitar, B. (1993). Evaluating efficacy of treatment of stuttering: School-age children. Journal of Fluency Disorders 18, 253–287.

Conture, E., Walden, T., Arnold, H., Graham, C., Karrass, J., & Hartfield, K. (2006). Communicative-emotional model of stuttering. In N. Bernstein Ratner (Ed.), Stuttering: New research directions. Mahwah, NJ: Erlbaum.

Conture, E. G., & Zebrowski, P. (1992). Can childhood speech disfluencies be mutable to the influences of speech-language pathologists, but immutable to the influences of parents? Journal of Fluency Disorders 17, 121–130.

Cook, R. E., Tessier, A., & Klein, M. D. (with Carol Cole) (Eds.). (2000). Promoting social and emotional development. Adapting early childhood curricula for children in inclusive settings (5th ed.) (pp. 196–233). Englewood Cliffs, NJ: Merrill, Prentice-Hall.

Dunn, L., & Dunn, L. (1981). The Peabody Picture Vocabulary Test-Revised (PPVT-R) (2nd ed.). Circle Pines, MN: American Guidance Service, Inc.

Dunn, L., & Dunn, L. (1997). The Peabody Picture Vocabulary Test-III (PPVT-III) (3rd ed.). Circle Pines, MN: American Guidance Service, Inc.

Finn, P., Ingham, R., Ambrose, N., & Yairi E. (1997). Children recovered from stuttering without formal treatment: Perceptual assessment of speech normalcy. Journal of Speech, Language, and Hearing Research 40, 867–876.

Franken, M.C., van Bezooijen, R., & Boves, L. Stuttering and communicative suitability of speech. Journal of Speech, Language, and Hearing Research 40, 83–94.

Franken, M. C., van der Schalk, C. J. K., & Boelens, H.(2005). Experimental treatment of early stuttering: A preliminary study. Journal of Fluency Disorders 30(3), 189–199.

Goldman, R., & Fristoe, M. (1986). Goldman-Fristoe Test of Articulation (GFTA). Circle Pines, MN: American Guidance Service, Inc.

Goldman, R., & Fristoe, M. (2000). Goldman-Fristoe Test of Articulation-2 (GFTA-2) Circle Pines, MN: American Guidance Service, Inc.

Guitar, B., & Marchinkoski, L. (2001). Influence of mothers' slower speech on their children's speech rate. Journal of Speech, Language, and Hearing Research 44(4), 853–861.

Harrison, E., & Onslow, M. (1999). Early intervention for stuttering: The Lidcombe Program. In R. F. Curlee (Ed.), Stuttering and related disorders of fluency (2nd ed.) (pp. 65–79). New York: Thieme Medical Publishers, Inc.

Harrison, E., Onslow, M., & Menzies, R. (2004). Dismantling the Lidcombe Program of early stuttering intervention: Verbal contingencies for stuttering and clinical measurement. International Journal of Language and Communication Disorders 39(2), 257–267.

Hresko, W., Reid, D., & Hamill, D. (1991). Test of Early Language Development-2. Austin, TX: PRO-ED.

Hresko, W., Reid, D., & Hamill, D. (1999). Test of Early Language Development-3. Austin, TX: PRO-ED.

Huber, A., Packman, A., Quine, S., Onslow, M., & Simpson, J. (2004). Improving our clinical interventions for stuttering: Can evidence from qualitative research contribute? Advances in Speech-Language Pathology 6(3), 174–181.

Ingham, J. C. (1999). Behavioral treatment of young children who stutter: An extended length of utterance method. In R. F. Curlee (Ed.), Stuttering and related disorders of fluency (2nd ed.) (pp. 80–109). New York: Thieme Medical Publishers.

Jones, M., Onslow, M., Packman, A., Williams, S., Ormond, T., Schwarz, I., et al. (2005). Randomised controlled trial of the Lidcombe programme of early stuttering intervention. British Medical Journal 331(7518), 659

Justice, L. M., & Schuele, C. M. (2004). Phonological awareness: Description, assessment, and intervention. In J. E. Bernthal & N. W. Bankson (Eds.), Articulation and phonological disorders (5th ed.) (pp. 376–402). Boston: Pearson.

Karrass, J., Walden, T., Conture, E., Graham, C. G., Arnold, H. S., Hartfield K. N. (2006). Relation of emotional reactivity and regulation to childhood stuttering. Journal of Communication Disorders 39, 402–423.

Kelly, E. M. (1994). Speech rates and turn-taking behaviors of children who stutter and their fathers. Journal of Speech and Hearing Research 37(6), 1284–1294.

Kelly, E. M., & Conture, E. G. (1992). Speaking rates, response time latencies, and interrupting behaviors of young stutterers, nonstutterers, and their mothers. Journal of Speech and Hearing Research 35(6), 1256–1257.

Limber, J. (1973). The genesis of complex syntax. In T. E. Moore (Ed.), Cognitive development and the acquisition of language. Oxford, England: Academic Press.

Lincoln, M., & Onslow, M. (1997). Long-term outcomes of early intervention for stuttering. American Journal of Speech-Language Pathology 6, 51–58.

Livingston, L. A., Flowers, Y. E., Hodor, B. A., & Ryan, B. P. (2000). The experimental analysis of interruption during conversation for three children who stutter. Journal of Developmental and Physical Disabilities 12(4), 236–266.

Logan, K. J., & Conture, E. G. (1995). Length, grammatical complexity, and rate differences in stuttered and fluent conversational utterances of children who stutter. Journal of Fluency Disorders 20, 35–61.

Logan, K. J., & Conture, E. G. (1997). Selected temporal, grammatical, and phonological characteristics of conversational utterances produced by children who stutter. Journal of Speech, Language, and Hearing Research 40, 107–120.

Martin, R. R., & Haroldson, S. K. (1992). Stuttering and speech naturalness—Audio and audiovisual judgments. Journal of Speech and Hearing Research 35, 521–528.

Martin, R. R., Haroldson, S. K., & Triden, K.(1984). Stuttering and speech naturalness. Journal of Speech and Hearing Disorders 49, 53–58.

Melnick, K., & Conture, E. (1999). Parent-child group approach to stuttering in preschool and school-age children. In M. Onslow & A. Packman (Eds.), Early stuttering: A handbook of intervention strategies (pp. 17–51). San Diego, CA: Singular Publishing.

Melnick, K. S., & Conture, E. G. (2000). Relationship of length and grammatical complexity to the systematic and nonsystematic speech errors, and stuttering of children who stutter. Journal of Fluency Disorders 25, 21–25.

Messenger, M., Onslow, M., Packman, A., & Menzies, R. (2004). Social anxiety in stuttering: measuring negative social expanses. Journal of Fluency Disorders 29, 201–212.

Miller, J. F. (1981). Assessing language production in children: experimental procedures. Austin, TX: PRO-ED.

Onslow, M. (2004). Treatment of stuttering in preschool children. Behavior Change 21(4), 201–214.

Onslow, M., Andrews, C., & Lincoln, M. (1994). A control/experimental trial of an operant treatment for early stuttering. Journal of Speech and Hearing Research 37:1244–1259.

Oyler, M. E. (1996). Temperament: Stuttering and the behaviorally inhibited child. Seminar conducted at the meeting of the American Speech-Language-Hearing Association Annual Convention, Seattle, WA.

Oyler, M. E. (1996). Vulnerability in stuttering children. (UMI No. 9602431) Dissertation Abstracts Internationa Ann Arbon MI.

Pellowski, M., Conture, E., Anderson, J., & Ohde, R. (2001). Articulatory and phonological assessment of children who stutter. In H.-G. Bosshardt, J. Scott Yaruss, & H. F. M. Peters (Eds.), Fluency disorders: Theory, research treatment and self-help.Proceedings of the Third World Congress of Fluency Disorders (pp. 248–252). Nijmegen, The Netherlands: Nijmegen University Press.

Pellowski, M. W., & Conture, E. G. (2002). Characteristics of speech disfluency and stuttering behaviors in 3- and 4-year-old children. Journal of Speech, Language, and Hearing Research 45, 20–34.

Ramig, P. R., & Bennett, E. M. (1997). Clinical management of children: Direct management strategies. In R. F. Curlee & G. M. Siegel (Eds.), Nature and treatment of stuttering (2nd ed.) (pp. 292–312). Needham Heights, MA: Allyn & Bacon.

Riley, G. D. (1994). Stuttering Severity Instrument–3 (3rd ed.). Austin, TX: PRO-ED.

Runyan, C. M., & Runyan, S. E. (1999). Therapy for school-age stutterers: An update on the Fluency Rules Program. In R. F. Curlee (Ed.), Stuttering and related disorders of fluency, (2nd ed.) (pp. 110–123). New York: Thieme.

Schiavetti, N., Martin, R., Haroldson, S., &Metz, D. (1994). Psychophysical analysis of audiovisual judgments of speech naturalness of nonstutterers and stutterers. Journal of Speech and Hearing Research 37, 46–52.

Stephenson-Opsal, D., & Bernstein-Ratner, N. (1988). Maternal speech rate modification and childhood stuttering. Journal of Fluency Disorders 13(1), 49–56.

Wilson, L., Onslow, M., & Lincoln, M. (2004). Telehealth adaptation of the Lidcombe Program of early stuttering intervention: Five case studies. American Journal of Speech-Language Pathology 13(1):81–93.

Yaruss, J. S. (1999). Utterance length, syntactic complexity, and childhood stuttering. Journal of Speech, Language, and Hearing Research 42, 329–344.

Yaruss, J. S., & Conture, E. (1995). Mother and child speaking rates and utterance lengths in adjacent fluent utterances. Journal of Fluency Disorders 20:257–278.

Yaruss, J., LaSalle, L., & Conture, E. (1998). Evaluating young children who stutter: Diagnostic data. Journal of Speech-Language Pathology 7, 62–76.

Zackheim, C. T., Conture, E. G., Ohde, R. N., Graham, C. G., & Gregory LJ. (2003, November) Holistic (word level) vs. incremental (sound level) processing in young children who stutter: Pre- vs. post-treatment. Annual American Speech-Language Hearing Association Conference, Chicago, IL.

Zackheim, C. T., & Conture, E. G. (2003). Childhood stuttering and speech disfluencies in relation to children's mean length of utterance: A preliminary study. Journal of Fluency Disorders 28, 115–142.

6

The Fluency Rules Program for School-Age Children Who Stutter

Charles M. Runyan and Sara E. Runyan

The fluency rules program (Runyan & Runyan, 1993, 1999) is a stuttering treatment program designed for preschool and early grade-school children who stutter. The program is divided into three sections: universal rules, which are used with all clients; primary rules used when airflow and laryngeal difficulties are present; and secondary rules, which are used when concomitant behaviors are noted. To implement the rules when instances of stuttering occur, response-contingent hand gestures are used. The hand gestures are designed not to interrupt the child but to maximize clinical opportunities and treatment results. Hand gestures and treatment concepts are presented for each rule. Follow-up and carryover suggestions are discussed.

This chapter describes the rationale for, practice of, and treatment outcomes of the fluency rules program (FRP). After a brief overview of the background, development, and history of the FRP, we describe the essential elements of the program that is; the universal, primary, and secondary rules. Then we provide a step-by-step introduction to the program, using clinical examples of the application of each step. We end with a summary of the essential elements of the program, carryover and transfer suggestions, and treatment outcome data. We hope that you will learn about the principles and practices of the FRP, how to implement them and what key (non)speech behaviors of the client to monitor and consider working to establish typically fluent speech in young children who stutter (CWS).

◆ Background, History, and Development of the Fluency Rules Program

We have used the FRP to treat young CWS on a weekly basis for more than 25 years in private practice and university clinical teaching. During that period and based on these direct clinical experiences, the FRP has continually been modified and improved. Originally, the impetus for the creation and development of the FRP was threefold. First, in the late 1970s there was limited therapeutic information or materials for treating young CWS. Second, there was a need to provide public school speech-language pathologists (SLPs) with a time-efficient and clinically effective stuttering treatment program for preschool and early grade-school children. Finally, we desired to create a physiologically-based therapy paradigm that when needed would be applicable (i.e., understandable) and effective for CWS.

Our initial attempt to create a child-focused treatment program was called "Rules for Good Speech" and consisted of 10 fluency rules. Subsequent clinical experiences with this early version of the FRP indicated that two aspects of the original program needed modification. First, three rules were deemed unnecessary and were eliminated. The remaining seven rules were unchanged or slightly modified. Second, we realized it was unnecessary to teach all the "Rules for Good Speech" to every child. Instruction was only needed for the rules that would be effective in establishing fluent speech. In other words, teach the child only the rules that were "broken," thus targeting the speech behaviors that would contribute to fluent speech for each child. For example, rule 7, "Use only the 'Speech Helpers' to Talk," is intended to eliminate nonspeech behaviors (hereafter referred to as "secondary behaviors"). For CWS who demonstrate secondary behaviors, this is a very important rule. However, for children who have not developed associated secondary behaviors, this rule is unnecessary, and teaching it would not be time efficient or appropriate. This version became the FRP and was used successfully for several years until the order of rule presentation appeared to need modification. At that time, the authors realized the treatment program was being executed in a similar manner regardless of the severity of the CWS or the type of stuttering behaviors presented. Specifically, all CWS were instructed during the first treatment session to reduce the rate of speech and/or to say each word one time. These two rules became the focus of therapy and were often the only rules needed to establish fluent speech. The universal rules label was adopted for these two rules because they were used with every client. When the application of the universal rules did not eliminate all stuttering, the usual reasons were the presence of airflow and/or voicing difficulties. When this situation was noted and the universal rules did not eliminate stuttering, a more direct therapy approach focused on specific anatomic and physiological targets was required. The two rules most applicable for this aspect of therapy were: (1) "Use Speech Breathing"; and (2) "Start Mr. Voice Box Running Smoothly." These rules were thought to be "of primary importance" for the production of fluent speech and were labeled primary rules. Finally, when secondary behaviors were noted, the final three rules were used to eliminate these behaviors. These rules were only used when specific secondary behaviors were noted and therefore were categorized as secondary rules.

The seven fluency rules with the new order of presentation were the focus of our chapter published in the previous two editions of this text. Since then there has been one modification to the order of rule presentation, one name change, and one major therapy implementation change.

The modification to the order of rule presentation applies to CWS who exhibit prolongations. The secondary rule "Say It Short" (formerly "Keep the Speech Helpers Moving") was modified to become a third universal rule and is taught during the initial treatment sessions with rules 1 and 2. The above name change from "Keep the Speech Helpers Moving" to "Say It Short" clarifies the rule. The application of hand signals or gestures to the rules of the FRP was the significant change in implementation (see **Table 6–1**). The authors implemented hand gestures to avoid interrupting the child. Prior to using the hand gestures, an inordinate amount of therapy time was spent stopping the child's speech to either identify an instance of stuttering or asking the CWS whether a stuttering event or normal disfluency had just occurred. This technique halts the conversation and makes natural interactions very difficult. In fact, we sensed that using this interrupting approach caused the CWS to "shut down" and talk less, whereas the hand gestures allowed us to accomplish our therapeutic goals more efficiently.

◆ The Fluency Rules Program

The most basic principle to the speech-language therapy process with young children, even more fundamental than any individual fluency rule, is that therapy must be fun and that children must enjoy and want to come to therapy. To create this positive environment in our practices, therapy is

Table 6–1   Individual Fluency Rule with Corresponding Hand Gesture

Rule	Accompanying Hand Gesture/Nonverbal Cue
Universal Rules	
1. Speak Slowly (Turtle Speech)	Move the hand up and down in a way that traditionally means to slow down.
2. Say a Word Only Once	Hold up one finger.
3. Say It Short (formerly: Keep the Speech Helpers Moving)	Hold the thumb and forefinger close together in the child's visual field.
Primary Rules	
4. Use Speech Breathing	Begin drawing the breath curve in the air with finger, snapping silently at the moment speech should begin.
5. Start Mr. Voice Box Running Smoothly	Pull fingers apart with the one hand elevating slightly as if going up a gentle slope
Secondary Rules	
6. Touch the "Speech Helpers" Together Lightly	Touch the thumb and forefinger together lightly.
7. Use only the "Speech Helpers" to Talk	(No gesture)

usually conducted in a play atmosphere seated on the floor with toys and games, using conversational speech to implement specific fluency rules. Without happy and cooperative children, therapy will be less effective. In fact, in our private practice often children must gradually be released from therapy because they enjoy the experiences.

Universal Rules

Rule 1: Speak Slowly (Turtle Speech)

Background   This rule for speech rate reduction allows CWS additional time to monitor their speech for the presence of repetitions or prolongations. For CWS with more advanced stuttering characterized by blockages of airflow and voicing, this rule allows more time to develop self-monitoring skills necessary for the acquisition of the physiological skills required for fluent speech production.

When this rule was first considered as a component of the FRP, minimal information was available on the speaking rates of early grade-school children. This lack of information made it difficult for clinicians to determine how much to reduce a CWS's speaking rate. To obtain preliminary data on the normal speaking rates of young children, Purcell and Runyan (1980) conducted a study of students enrolled in grades 1 through 5. These results are presented in **Table 6–2**. Subsequent research has

Table 6–2   Mean and Standard Deviation of Speaking Rate of Children in Words and Syllables per Minute

Grade	Mean Words per Minute	Standard Deviation	Mean Syllables per Minute	Standard Deviation
1	124.92	12.17	147.66	13.47
2	130.44	12.05	156.72	17.14
3	133.44	10.01	158.94	14.86
4	139.32	16.33	165.66	24.58
5	141.84	16.24	170.04	23.19

Source: Adapted from Purcell, R., & Runyan, C. M. (1980). Normative study of speech rates of children. Journal of the Speech and Hearing Association of Virginia 21, 6–14. Reprinted by permission.

supported these results as well as adding new data for preschool children (Guitar, 1998; Hall, Yairi, & Amir, 1999; Kelly, 1993, 1994; Kelly & Conture 1992; Logan & Conture, 1995; Ryan, 2000).

Although this rule is labeled "speak slowly" or "turtle speech," the intent was never to encourage children to speak abnormally slowly or one word at a time. In fact, clinical experience has supported our belief that children acquiring linguistic competency are not aware of their speaking rate. The message takes precedence, and attempts to manipulate rate to one sounding abnormally slow does not have the desired therapeutic effect. Furthermore, a child is unlikely to use a dramatically reduced speaking rate or to produce speech one word at a time outside the clinical setting. In fact, during the early developmental phase of the FRP, children were instructed to produce speech by saying one word, then two words, then three words, and so on without stuttering at a slow rate. These therapeutic attempts met significant resistance from both children and parents because the resultant speech sounded abnormal, and both were reluctant to use this speech pattern outside the therapy room (see, for example, Chapter 18 in this text for the role of self-control in the treatment of stuttering).

A secondary benefit of this rule, supported by public school SLPs, is that a slow rate of speech has an overall calming effect on the child as well as on various speaking partners. This calming effect appeared to contribute to a speaking environment that was conducive to fluent speech development. Clinically, we noted that during therapy sessions in which the goal was reduction to slow, normal speaking rate, the child appeared more relaxed and therapy activities were conducted at a less frantic pace. Interestingly, during these sessions a marked reduction in stuttering was noted; however, often the speaking rate remained virtually unchanged. Therefore, the reduction in the frequency of stuttering appeared to be, on some occasions, due to the general calming effect of the therapy setting as well as possibly to be a result of the reduced speech rate.

Concept Teaching Suggestions

* *Symbolic Material*   The use of symbolic therapy materials, such as turtles and snails, to characterize slow speech has been clinically effective in teaching this concept. Cartoon characters have been used to decorate therapy rooms to create an atmosphere for slow rate and a calm environment. Smaller cartoon examples can be used on speech notebooks, refrigerators, and in other environments as reminders of this fluency rule.

* *Contrast Symbolic Material*   Here the clinician contrasts slower-moving animals (i.e., normal speech rate), with a racehorse (i.e., speech that is too fast or rapid) (Meyers and Woodford, 1992). A fun way to teach this concept is to race around the room depicting a racehorse and while "racing" stumble and fall down in a humorous manner to simulate stuttering. Explain to the child that when we run faster than the running movements can be controlled then we often stumble and/or fall. This can happen in speech when we talk faster than speech movements can be controlled, which can result in stuttering. For older children, we ask them to consider what happens when a person runs down hill. Often this causes loss of control of the movements of running resulting in a stumble or fall similar to what happens when speech is produced too rapidly and stuttering happens. Animal tracks can also be used effectively and be very entertaining for the children. Clinicians can put turtle tracks or any slow-moving-animal footprints beside racehorse tracks (i.e., horseshoes) on the floor and have the children simultaneously walk and talk symbolically like the type of animal on whose trail they are walking. As indicated above, during this activity, the therapist can act silly and fall down when going too fast on the racehorse tracks. Stumbling and falling down like this simulates stuttering, something that helps to keep the child focused on the purpose of the therapy session.

* *Slow Music/Metronome*   Earlier versions of the FRP recommended the use of a desk-level metronome set at 60 beats per minute as background during therapy to create a calm clinical atmosphere and to encourage slow speech production. However, more recently we have used soft, slow music in the background to create a calm environment.

- *Old Ears*   This concept teaching suggestion has been applied successfully with all universal rules. Constructing a pair of old ears, with wrinkles and gray hair or large rubber clown ears enhances the teaching of this rule. Tell the child your (i.e., the clinician) ears are old and tired and that if the child uses racehorse speech, your old ears will become very tired, confused, and sore. Grabbing your "sore" ears and falling to the floor in mock pain when the child talks too rapidly has been a very effective clinical strategy. An unexpected outcome of this therapy technique was having a child run to the waiting room and tell his parents that it was fun to come to therapy and to help the clinician's ears by talking slowly (i.e., following the rule). The obvious secondary value to this technique is that it places the child in the role of helper rather than a recipient of therapy.

- *Modeling*   Clinicians and parents need to adopt a more relaxed, normally slow speech-language production. Some parents are instructed to slow their speech rate, but not to prolong or use excessive pauses in their speech because these behaviors produce speech that sounds abnormal. To prevent parents from excessive reductions in speech rate, which often occurs following this instruction, a speedometer analogy is used with the suggestion that reducing speed by only 10 miles per hour (mph) will allow for better control without becoming a traffic hazard. In other words, slow down from 65 mph to 55 mph, but not to 25 mph because that is too slow and could cause a traffic problem. This analogy, coupled with the clinician modeling the intended speech rate, has proven to be successful in developing the desired speech rate in both parents and CWS.

Therapy Implementation

- *Hands Down*   The clinician gives the nonverbal cue by moving a hand up and down in a way traditionally used to mean "slow down." This visual cue does not require a direct explanation, and the child's speech rate will immediately be reduced. Clinically, the concept of slowing down speech rate is taught during the first therapy session and is implemented in all subsequent therapy activities via the hand gesture.

Rule 2: Say a Word Only Once

Background   This universal rule is the "heart" of the FRP because the dominant speech characteristics of CWS are part-word and single-syllable whole-word repetitions. Therefore, a fluency rule to help control these behavioral characteristics of stuttering is vital to treatment programs designed to help young stutterers. For this rule to be effectively implemented, clinicians must determine if the child has developed or acquired the language concepts of "once" and "word."

Concept Teaching Suggestions

- *Railroad Train*   Two different railroad trains are compared. The first train contains different cars and represents fluent speech (i.e., each car/word is different). The second train has several similar cars (e.g., box cars) placed in a row, which represents speech that contains repetitive speech samples. This technique can also be used by comparing different rows of coins, tokens, or zoo animals.

- *Different Feet*   Use the turtle or slow-animal trail to facilitate this technique (see Rule 1, Contrast Symbolic Material). Have the child say different words with each step while walking the slow-animal trail. Then explain that walking is easy and smooth when different feet are used for each step, but if the same foot is used, the child must hop on one leg, and walking becomes "hard and bumpy." During speech, if the same word is said over and over, speech gets bumpy, and people may have difficulty understanding what is being said.

- *Old Ears/Happy Ears*   Explain to the child that a person does not have to repeat words to be understood. To illustrate this point, an exaggerated, humorous, and animated example of repeating a word 10 times or more is presented and immediately the CWS is asked if the repeated word helped to better understand the message. As a follow-up therapy technique, the clinician can feign that his or her ears are hurting and can even roll on the floor in mock pain when partial word repetitions are produced by the child. This animated activity always attracts a child's attention, and carefully produced speech without repetitions usually follows. If fluent speech production continues for a reasonable period of time, the clinician can dance around with "happy ears" because no "repeating of words" has hurt the clinician's ears for the past few minutes. The combination of "happy ears" and "hurting old ears" provides constant reminders to the child to only say a word one time, and it keeps the focus on fluent speech during therapy sessions.

Therapy Implementation   The majority of therapy time with CWS is spent on this universal rule using the following implementation procedure.

- *We're Number One*   The nonverbal cue or hand gesture for this rule is the clinician holding up one finger (i.e., similar to sports fans signaling their team is number one) to indicate that a repetition has occurred. The application of this rule begins by having the CWS monitor the clinician's speech to determine when a repetition occurs. When the CWS hears the therapist repeat a word, the CWS raises a finger to indicate awareness of the repetition. In practice, if two clinicians are available (e.g., therapist and supervisor), the therapists by "playing off" each other can expedite the learning process. That is, at first have the therapists "catch" each other when one of them repeats a word by raising one finger and saying "one time." After this activity has begun, have the child join in by helping to catch (i.e., identify) the repeated word of the therapist and then turn this catching activity into a competitive contest by "seeing" who can be the first to catch the person who repeated the word. The therapists continue to frequently repeat words and the catching activity continues until the concept of identifying repeated words is firmly established.

During these initial sessions, the clinician calculates the percentage of correct identifications made by the child as well as how rapidly the child accurately identifies the repeated word. As the child's ability to correctly and rapidly identify repetitions produced by the clinician increases, the therapist will introduce the "idea" of identifying repetitions in the child's speech. The identification of repeated words in the child's speech has sometimes met resistance possibly due to the reluctance to acknowledge the repeated words, as if he or she had done "something wrong." Nevertheless, the transition can usually be accomplished by telling the child how happy the therapist is because the CWS has helped to identify repetitions in the therapist's speech, how much better the therapist's speech sounds, and that now the therapist can help the CWS's speech sound better. Again, using the competitive format the clinician and the CWS can keep score on who is first to identify any repetitions produced by either the clinician or the CWS.

Therapy Suggestion

- *The Bent Finger*   If CWS react negatively to having repeated words identified in their speech, we have been successful by raising a finger only "half way up" or slightly bent. We then ask in a questioning manner: "Did we just hear a repetition?" Although the child may deny the production of the repetition, it is easily observed in his or her nonverbal behavior such as eye movement when one was produced. Then we say: "Well, maybe we were wrong, but we did think we heard a repetition." Therefore, the therapy goal of alerting the child when a repeated word was produced was accomplished.

Once children can quickly and accurately identify part-word repetitions in their speech, clinical progress usually moves rapidly to fluent speech and dismissal from therapy.

Clinical Implementation Suggestion   As the child becomes more fluent and repetitions are less frequent, the clinician must return to frequently repeating his or her words so the child can identify these repetitions and the focus of the therapy session is not forgotten.

Several of our more dramatic treatment successes have occurred after a child has spontaneously identified instances of repeated words in his or her parents' speech. Apparently, once the concept of not repeating elements of speech is understood, a child often carries this awareness away from the clinical setting to the home and corrects the parents' nonfluent speech. Once such spontaneous generalization occurs, treatment progress can be quite rapid, usually going from a significant number of stutterings to zero in a very short period of time.

Rule 3: Say It Short (Formerly, Keep the Speech Helpers Moving)

Background   This rule was designed originally to eliminate prolongations, and in previous editions it was included with the secondary rules. This rule is not a universal rule because it is not taught to every child enrolled in therapy. However, for young CWS who exhibit prolongations, this rule becomes an integral component of the initial treatment program.

Concept Teaching Suggestions

- *Piano Fingers*   Moving the thumb to each finger or tapping the thumb and fingers on a tabletop in a sequential manner similar to Conture's thumb and opposing finger analogy (2001) has proved useful in teaching this fluency rule. This technique also demonstrates that fluent speech should move easily and smoothly from sound to sound, just like we move our thumb and fingers to tap the tabletop. With each digit representing a speech sound or syllable, the child produces short phrases, saying them and moving smoothly from sound to sound. Next, we demonstrate that if the thumb and finger stay together too long, or a finger remains on the table too long, a prolonged sound will be produced.

- *Contrast Long and Short*   Any familiar long and short objects can be used to teach this concept (e.g., pencils, pieces of string). Our best therapy success has been associated with using visual and tactile feedback, such as tracing the length of the long pencil as the therapist and CWS simultaneously exaggerate the prolongation of a word, and then saying the target word short as the length of the short pencil is traced.

Therapy Implementation   The hand gesture for this rule is holding the thumb and first finger close together in the child's visual field as a reminder to keep speech units short. Exaggerating the distance between the thumb and finger and then slowly reducing the distance illustrates the change from a prolongation to a correct "short" sound.

Primary Rules

These physiologically based rules are always taught as a unit after the clinician determines that stuttering has advanced to where airflow and laryngeal control have become affected. Conture's garden hose analogy (2001) has been used successfully to introduce these primary rules as a unit and to explain the important relationship between anatomic structures and air flow/voicing. Recall that, with several CWS who demonstrated laryngeal tension and airflow issues, the universal rules were sufficient to eliminate stuttering. Therefore, the SLP must be patient and not hurry the treatment process and too quickly assume the need to use a more direct treatment approach. Many times, for young children the reduction in stuttering is not gradual but rather abrupt, with fluency being acquired quickly. Ultimately though, the clinician must make a determination when the universal rules are not sufficient to eliminate stuttering and a more physiologically based treatment is necessary. As a clinical "rule of thumb," when CWS have demonstrated the knowledge of the concepts of the universal rules and quickly and accurately have identified when repetitions and/or prolongations occur but still demonstrate a consistent pattern of stuttering, then use of the primary rules is warranted.

Rule 4: Use Speech Breathing

Background   During the last 25 years of implementing the FRP, the primary rules have been applied whenever more direct physiological intervention has been required. During this period, our private practice achieved excellent clinical success with adolescents and adults using visual feedback of the speech-breathing curve, which assisted the speaker in coordinating speech breathing with the initiation of speech (Goebel, 1984). Because of our success with these older clients, we wanted to simulate this clinical experience and bring speech breathing to a visual and conscious level of young stutterers by utilizing visual and tactile procedures. We begin as other clinicians have successfully done (Conture, 2001; Ramig & Bennett, 1995) by explaining and illustrating (i.e., drawing a breath curve) the difference between regular and speech breathing. For speech breathing, the explanation includes: breath in, slowly let your air out, speak on the "out" breath, and keep the air moving (i.e., do not hold your breath). Also explained is the concept of pre-voiced exhalation and how important it is "to let the air out first then 'Mr. Voice Box' will vibrate and prevent laryngeal blocks" (i.e., see first concept suggestion). Following is a final clinical observation on the breathing patterns of the stutterers we have treated. As was reported in the previous editions of this text, most stuttering and vocal abuse/nodule clients seen in our practice, except for preschool and early grade-school children, were expanding or "pushing" their thoracic/diaphragmatic area outward prior to the production of speech. This exhalation pattern is in contrast to other clients or even their own nonspeech breathing, which is characterized by a steady contraction or inward movement of the thoracic/diaphragmatic area. When questioned about this unusual movement, most have reported the perception of a slight, concurrent tensing in their laryngeal area. Using the techniques described in this section has eliminated this initial irregular breathing/laryngeal pattern.

Concept Suggestions

♦ *The Breath Curve with Pre-voiced Exhalation*   Draw the typical breath curve on a chalkboard or piece of paper, illustrating inspiration with a rising line and a gradual downward slope for exhalation. Next, place an "X" on the line shortly after exhalation starts to indicate where speech should begin. Explain that the distance between the beginning of exhalation and the "X" is pre-voiced exhalation. During this portion of the breath curve it is important to open the vocal folds and allow the "air out" so the vocal folds can begin vibrating easily. Following the explanation, have the child trace the breath curve with an index finger to "feel" the breathing pattern. After the child understands the feeling of speech breathing, practice initiating speech using various vowels at the point on the breath curve where the "X" has been placed. Then, have the child count or recite days of the week or months of the year as the breathing curve is carefully traced. The clinician must be cautious at this time to make sure the child's tracing of the breath curve is in synchrony with the in and out motions of the child's breathing. Next, four- and five-syllable phrases (e.g., "Where is my toy?") are used for practicing speech breathing while the child traces the breath curve.

♦ *Tactile Feedback*   Just as the previous activity encouraged the child to visualize speech breathing and to a lesser degree feel the physiological components of speech breathing, this activity focuses on the child feeling the physiological aspects of speech breathing. To accomplish this, the clinician first positions the child's hand below his or her sternum, and then the clinician's hand is placed over the child's hand. This technique focuses the child's attention on the feeling of the in and out movements of the chest wall that accompany speech breathing. With the first concept suggestion (Breath Curve with Pre-voiced Exhalation), the child can both visualize and feel speech breathing. If needed, another clinical activity can be added. The clinician places his or her second hand around the child's upper arm and gently squeezes it to initiate speech. As the child traces the breath cycle and feels the speech breathing movements with the hand on the chest wall, the clinician squeezes the child's arm as the tracing finger passes the "X," providing a tactile cue to begin speech. These combined therapy activities have been successful and usually require only minimal therapy time to achieve a child's awareness of speech breathing, pre-voiced exhalation, and when to initiate speech.

+ *For Breath/Speech Holding*   Have the child begin a typical speech breathing cycle, and start counting from 1 to 20 at the "X." At the count of 4, ask the child to vigorously pull up on the sides of the chair until breathing and speech momentarily stops. Then, instruct the child to continue to count, pulling and tensing on every fourth count to contrast the feeling of a tense and relaxed neck and the corresponding changes that occur to the voice. Explain that if the neck is so tense that airflow stops, then speech will also stop. Finally, have the child repeat this procedure without pulling to feel how a relaxed neck facilitates the onset and maintenance of airflow and fluent speech production.

Therapy Implementation   The therapist can draw the breath curve in the air and silently snap his or her fingers when the child should begin speech (i.e., the place in the breath cycle where the "X" was placed for visual understanding). This would occur after pre-voiced exhalation and when initiating speech without airflow or voicing being compromised would be maximized. Together this hand signal and the clinical direction "Feel how your air (i.e., exhalation) carries the words out" have been very helpful.

Rule 5: Start Mr. Voice Box Running Smoothly

Background   An important modification has been made to this rule since the first publication. The original wording "Keep Mr. Voice Box Running Smoothly" was modified to "Start Mr. Voice Box Running Smoothly" to more accurately reflect the intent of this rule. This subtle change was made because of the importance for young stutterers to learn the feeling of starting their vocal folds vibrating easily and smoothly. This is often referred to as a *gentle onset* and is a major component in several fluency training programs for stutterers (Bennett, 2006; Cooper & Cooper, 1985; Costello, 1983; Culatta & Goldberg, 1995; Curlee & Perkins, 1969; Goebel, 1984; Guitar, 1998; Herring, 1986; Kully & Langevin 1999; Nielson, 1999; Neilson & Andrews, 1993; Pindzola, 1987; Ramig & Bennet, 1995; Riley & Riley, 1984; Schwartz, 1999; Shine, 1988; Wall & Myers, 1994; Webster, 1979, 1980; Zebrowski & Kelly, 2002). Although this is a commonly used therapeutic activity with stutterers, there does not appear to be a universally accepted definition of gentle onset. In our therapy program, it is defined as *the gradual increase of intensity over time that occurs at the beginning of an utterance or after a pause.* Therapeutic success has been achieved using this definition particularly with those children who pointed to their neck and indicated this is where they get "stuck," as illustrated in Conture's text (2001, p. 196).

Concept Suggestions

+ *Awareness*   A variety of caricatures have been used to represent "Mr. Voice Box" to show children that "he lives" in the neck, and that when Mr. Voice Box is running they can feel the vibration. Have the child hum while touching the neck area with his or her hand to locate where Mr. Voice Box lives. Clinicians can further illustrate that Mr. Voice Box lives in the neck by "shaking" the larynx gently with their fingers while the CWS is vocalizing, causing Mr. Voice Box to make funny noise.

+ *The Laryngeal Lips*   Because Mr. Voice Box "lives" in the neck and cannot be seen, there seems to be a certain kind of mystery about the larynx for many young children (Conture, 2001, p. 189). To help the children visualize the vocal folds and understand "how the larynx and vocal folds work," clinicians can use their lips as a model. By producing what is often called a "raspberry sound" (i.e., blowing air between and vibrating the lips), the clinician can demonstrate the principals of air flow and medial vocal fold compression. Clinicians also can demonstrate that air flow stops if we press our lips together too tightly, which may be similar to what some children do with their vocal folds when they feel tension in their neck. These demonstrations and an age-appropriate explanation of these principals can greatly help CWS understand the larynx and this therapeutic goal.

♦ *Gentle Not Soft*   In our early attempts to teach gentle onset, some children misinterpreted this therapy technique as soft onset (i.e., reduced intensity), and they would begin speech at a very low intensity. To illustrate that the therapy goal is a gentle, not a soft, onset, two horizontal lines are drawn on a chalkboard or paper with a sloping line, drawn at a 45-degree angle, connecting the lower to the upper line. The lower horizontal line is marked as zero intensity, which we refer to as silence; the upper horizontal line, as the child's normal speaking intensity; and the 45-degree connecting line, as gentle onset. Using this drawing, the child is asked to begin speech with an easy onset of phonation as he or she traces the sloping line while initiating speech with exaggerated slowness. As soon as the clinician believes the concept has been learned, the child is instructed to reduce the exaggerated slow onset to normal-sounding speech, albeit with a slightly prolonged initiation of speech.

Therapy Implementation   The hand signal for this rule is touch the fingers of both hands together and then slowly pull the finger tips apart with one hand elevating slightly as if going up a gentle slope.

Secondary Rules

These rules are used as needed to eliminate secondary or concomitant behaviors presented by CWS, and they should be applied as soon as such behaviors are observed. When secondary behaviors are observed, we explain that these are not necessary for speech production and could actually be "working against fluent speech production."

Rule 6 Touch the "Speech Helper" Together Lightly

Background   The "speech helpers" (i.e., lips, tongue, and teeth) have been depicted as cartoon characters that are parts of the mouth that are important in the production of "speech sounds." Several public school SLPs have used these cartoon "speech helpers" to decorate the walls of their therapy rooms/offices, which increases the awareness of children to these anatomic structures. CWS are instructed to touch the speech helpers together very lightly because if they press them together too hard, speech breathing and speech will stop.

Concept Suggestions

♦ *The Hard Contact*   Instruct the child to attempt a bilabial plosive (e.g., "buh") by pressing the lips together tightly "until a word pops out." Some older children have been encouraged by well-intentioned parents to "just try harder" and their speech will improve. Therefore, clinical explanations and demonstrations are used to show that easier not harder efforts and contacts are necessary for producing fluent speech. To illustrate, practice hard contacts in front of a mirror with the CWS using a great deal of animated effort while pointing out, humorously, the futility of trying to produce speech with excessive effort. For example, the clinician can press his or her lips together with a great deal of effort and a contorted face while jumping up and down to demonstrate that no matter how hard the clinician tries a word will just not "pop out." Then the clinician can demonstrate that by just lightly touching the lips together, fluent speech is produced with ease, not effort. Children usually enjoy practicing these contrasting methods of speech production and quickly learn the importance of easy contacts of the articulators for fluent speech.

♦ *Can I Hold Your Arm?*   Another treatment technique that illustrates the goal of light contact of the speech helpers involves squeezing the child's arm as he or she speaks, as described in Rule 4 (Tactile Feedback). As the child speaks fluently, the clinician holds one arm lightly, but as soon as a hard contact occurs, the clinician squeezes the child's arm gently but firmly. The amount of pressure applied by the squeeze should be roughly proportional to the amount of tension perceived in the hard contact.

Rule 7: Use Only the "Speech Helpers" to Talk

Background   This rule explains that fluent speech is produced by moving only the speech helpers, and it is not necessary or helpful to move other muscles or body parts when speaking.

Concept Suggestions

• *The Mirror*   A mirror may be all that is needed for some CWS to eliminate secondary behaviors. Frequently, CWS are unaware of the extraneous body movements or other secondary behaviors that accompany their stuttering behaviors, and once these secondary behaviors are visually pointed out, they are often quickly eliminated.

• *Too Much of a Bad Thing*   The mirror is again used with this technique. For example, if a CWS turns his or her head when speech begins, we explain that turning the head does not help anyone produce speech. Standing with the child in front of the mirror and using animated humor, we say and then demonstrate that "We are going to turn our heads as hard and as frequently as possible until a word comes out." Obviously nothing happens, and it is clear that turning the head to start speech is not helpful and should be eliminated. This therapy technique can be used to demonstrate to a child with any inappropriate motor responses that speech does not begin until airflow begins and the speech helpers move smoothly.

Summary of the Fluency Rules Program

The suggested order of implementation for the fluency rules program:

1. Determine which fluency rule(s) is/are broken.

2. Teach language concepts (e.g., one, short) if necessary for clear understanding of therapy instructions for the universal rules. If prolongations are present include the third universal rule.

3. Apply the universal rules. Practice fluent speech production implementing the universal rules and the accompanying gestures. Incorporate hand gestures as quickly as possible to avoid interrupting the child. This will improve the therapy process by maximizing the clinical opportunities for the CWS to practice the fluency rules and fluent speech.

    a. For clinical expediency, and again to expedite therapy, all disfluencies are targeted for therapeutic intervention. Early in the development of the FRP, we spent a significant amount of treatment time discussing with the client whether a disfluent event was a stutter or a normal disfluency. Now, our clinical rule is that all disfluencies are identified and scored as behaviors to be eliminated. This identification procedure and the use of the hand gestures have improved the CWS's ability to monitor the occurrence of disfluencies and have been demonstrated to be efficient and effective in eliminating all disfluencies.

4. Develop the child's self-monitoring to accelerate therapy. Focusing "on the moment" of speech production is an important concept for CWS because of their tendency to mentally scan ahead for previously difficult sounds rather than to focus on "the present" and the physiological concepts necessary to produce fluent speech. With older children we have discussed the difficulty of this duel attention process (De Nil & Bosshardt, 2001) of scanning ahead and searching for difficult sounds/words while simultaneously trying to learn and apply a fluency rule. They reported that these combined activities are very difficult to execute and scanning ahead is difficult to stop. To understand the difficult nature of this task we have challenged our SLP students to try for a day not to say words beginning with a particular sound. None were successful in this task.

5. Be patient and allow the CWS time to incorporate the universal rules into their speech production. Remember, for some children the elimination of stuttering can be abrupt. The most dramatic success we experienced was a preschooler who stuttered on more than 80% of his words.

After several therapy sessions, minimal progress had been achieved. After we discovered he was fascinated by puzzles and we incorporated them into the therapy program using just the universal rules in conversational speech, stuttering decreased to zero in 1 week. The dramatic decrease in stuttering occurred between two therapy sessions and by the parents' report happened when the child practiced fluency rule 2 ("Say a Word Only Once") at home and spontaneously corrected his parents when they repeated a word. He returned to therapy for three more sessions and did not repeat a word. Fifteen years later, he has remained a fluent speaker.

6. Apply primary rules, if necessary, when CWS continue to stutter even after mastery of the universal rules.

   a. Demystify stuttering, explain speech production, and teach treatment concepts with age-appropriate analogies. Sports or physical activity examples work well to explain the following (Manning, 1991): speech is a motor act, feeling fluency, controlling speaking rate (i.e., do not play "out of control" because that is when errors occur), the ability to self-monitor muscle movements, planned practice, controlling stress, and staying focused.

   b. Drill on perceived "difficult sounds." As in the previous step, we demystify difficult sounds. Our explanation is that if the CWS practices the fundamentals of speech fluency by utilizing the primary rules of focusing on speech breathing, pre-voiced exhalation, light contact, and starting the vocal folds vibrating gently, then it does not matter what word or sound is attempted, it will be produced fluently. A sports analogy (i.e., explained above) and basketball example we have used successfully is telling the CWS that it does not matter if he or she shoots a new ball, old ball, rubber ball, or a leather ball—when the fundamental motor mechanics of shooting the basketball are correct, any one of the balls will go in the basket. Therefore, if fundamental speech mechanics are correct, any sound or word can be produced fluently.

   c. Have the client focus on the feeling of fluency. As new motor skills of fluency are acquired it is important that CWS feel the ease of fluent speech production.

7. Carry over procedures for the home and classroom (see next section).

♦ Carryover and Transfer

The final phase of the FRP involves the carryover or transfer of the fluency rules to the child's home and classroom. Obviously, for transfer to be effective, the child must remember the rules in new speaking environments. The most effective procedure we have found to facilitate such carryover has been to place a discriminative stimulus in each environment. In school, the SLP, the classroom teacher, the subject teacher, and the student meet to select a small unobtrusive item to be placed in each room as a reminder of the fluency rule (e.g., sticker on notebooks or refrigerator magnets on the edge of chalkboards). Only the teacher and the CWS need be aware of the item and its significance. Then, if the CWS forgets to use a fluency rule, the teacher can provide a reminder by glancing in the direction of or touching the designated item.

At home, the same procedure can be used with the same or different discriminative stimuli. The family places reminders (e.g., symbolic elephants are effective because "elephants never forget") in conversation areas (e.g., the family room, kitchen, bedroom, and dining room) and family members call attention as needed. The subtle nature of these stimuli and how they are used also provides a secondary benefit. The stimuli eliminate the need for direct confrontations when fluency rules are not used, which reduces family conflicts that may arise from frequent verbal reminders, particularly during the early stages of transfer. Ideally, the transfer segment of therapy will result in the fluency rules being generalized to areas away from the therapy room and, ultimately, will lead to fluent speech in all environments.

An effective treatment strategy that we use clinically as discriminative stimuli and reinforcements involves electronic games, toys, and other games. These materials have considerable motivational appeal for children and can be used to motivate children to use the fluency rules in therapy, at home, and at school. During scheduled therapy sessions, usually when drill activities on difficult words is the focus of therapy, computer games or other play-time breaks are a regularly scheduled aspect of therapy and are used to reinforce correct application of the fluency rules. However, during these play breaks the fluency rules must be practiced. To facilitate carry over of fluency rules at home, we have a lending library arrangement that allows children to check out one computer game until the next therapy session. Toys and games are used with younger children and work in the same way. A board game, toy, or stuffed animal can be loaned until the next treatment session. The parents' agreement to play with their child and the borrowed toy and to encourage use of the fluency rules is pre-arranged. To check out a game or toy, the CWS must agree to use the fluency rules at home, especially when playing the game. An additional positive effect of the lending library is that it stimulates more parental involvement at a point in the therapeutic process where parents can make positive contributions toward their child's progress. Equally impressive is the motivational value of these games in the clinic with children. When our lending library was started, there were two difficult children on the caseload. Their renewed interest and subsequent increased cooperation in therapy because of the inclusion of the video games and their ability to "borrow the games" was impressive. Both children successfully completed therapy, which we feel was due in part to the use of the library and the interest these games brought to the therapy process.

Lastly, we also used telephone calls as a discriminative stimulus to help carry over fluency to the home environment. We begin, typically, near the end of therapy, when the child is using the fluency rules effectively in therapy sessions. At this point, we encourage the CWS to think about and use the rules at home. To assist in keeping awareness high, we call the child at home and ask about his or her speech and if the fluency rules are being used. At first, with the parents' permission, these calls are frequent, several calls a night. This frequency of calls is continued for about 1 week, and then calls are gradually reduced until they occur infrequently, about once a month. Periodically, however, we again call several times on randomly selected nights. The intended outcome of this procedure is to have the CWS think that every time the phone rings "the therapist is calling again," which serves as a reminder to use the fluency rules. Since the creation of the lending library, calls are longer and more effective because conversations can also be directed toward the use of the toys or games and not just directed toward checking up on speech. These calls also provide an excellent opportunity to evaluate the child's fluency in a different setting than the clinic.

◆ Outcomes

In our first publication of the FRP, therapeutic results based on nine children were reported. The children consisted of five males and four females, with an average age of 5 years, 5 months. Based on Riley's (1994) severity scale, three were mild, four were moderate, and two were severe stutterers. Five of these children were followed for 2 years after therapy, whereas four were followed for 1 year. All had been treated in a public-school setting, receiving therapy two or three times a week for 30 or 40 minutes. The data indicated that all of the children evidenced a significant improvement in fluency while maintaining a normal speaking rate and eliminating all secondary behaviors. Further inspection of the data revealed that the improvement in fluent speech production that occurred in the first year of therapy was maintained during follow-up. However, a lingering concern remained. Although each child demonstrated marked improvement in fluent speech production, each child's speech also contained slight, residual signs of the stuttering. These residual effects were mild part-word repetitions of two or less iterations and no secondary behaviors. Unfortunately, these children could not be followed for longer periods of time, and no additional data are available. Also of note is that these CWS were treated with an early version of the FRP when all rules were taught and before the order of presentation was modified.

In the previous edition of this text we reported on 17 CWS who we have personally treated in our private practice, and it is the information from these stutterers that follows. This group consisted of 3 female and 14 male stutterers whose ages at the beginning of therapy averaged slightly less than 7 years of age. Based on the Stuttering Prediction Instrument (Riley, 1981), there were 2 severe, 8 moderate, and 7 mild stutterers. Nine of these children demonstrated secondary behaviors. The mild stutterers and 1 moderate stutterer did not exhibit accessory behavior. All of the 17 children's speech was judged by the authors to be within the acceptable range on the naturalness scale at the release from therapy. Average length of therapy was 9 months, with a range of 3 to 20 months. Recently we became aware that one of the female early grade-school subjects who was released from therapy as a fluency success is now a high-school-age stutterer. Unfortunately, we lost contact with the family and do not know the history of the relapse.

Since the last edition we have data on six additional CWS. They were six males whose average age was 5 years, 11 months, with two being preschoolers. Four of the CWS were judged to be of moderate severity and two severe. The oldest CWS, a second grader, continues in therapy, and although he is still rated as severe, he has improved markedly by dramatically reducing secondary behaviors. Unfortunately, because of logistical factors he can only attend therapy once a month. The remaining five children have been released from therapy following the elimination of stuttering behavior. Length of therapy for one preschooler was 23 months, the remaining four averaged 9 months in therapy.

Efficiency and adaptability were important factors in the design of the FRP because of the typical public-school treatment format. Results of the first group of children treated using this program demonstrated that it was effective in reducing stuttering when treatment was conducted in the public schools. Six of the 17 children in the second group reported received services in the public schools in addition to private practice therapy, as well as all 6 of the most recent group reported. Therefore, it appears that the FRP can be implemented successfully in combined effort between the public school and the private sector.

♦ Conclusion

Finally, we again encourage clinicians in all therapeutic environments to use the FRP and to share the results, techniques, and experiences with us and their colleagues at professional meetings. The ultimate effectiveness and utility of the FRP can only be demonstrated when larger and more diverse groups of stuttering children are treated by different therapists in different settings and followed over longer periods of time.

References

Bennett, E. M. (2006). Working with people who stutter: A lifespan approach. Upper Saddle River, NJ: Pearson Education, Inc.

Conture, E, G. (2001). Stuttering:Its nature, diagnosis, and treatment. Boston: Allyn & Bacon.

Cooper, E. B., & Cooper, C. S. (1985). Cooper personalized fluency control therapy. Allen, TX: DLM.

Costello, J. M. (1983). Current behavioral treatments for children. In D. Prins & R. J. Ingham (Eds.), Treatment of stuttering in early childhood: Methods and issues. San Diego: College-Hill Press.

Culatta, R., & Goldberg, S. A. (1995). Stuttering therapy: An integrated approach to theory and practice. Boston: Allyn & Bacon.

Curlee, R. F., & Perkins, W. H. (1969). Conversational rate control therapy for stutterers. Journal of Speech and Hearing Disorders 34, 245–250.

De Nil, L. F., & Bosshardt, H.-G. (2001). Studying stuttering from a neurological and cognitive information processing perspective. In H.-G. Bosshardt, J. S. Yaruss, & H. F. M. Peters (Eds.), Stuttering: Research, therapy, and self-help. Proceedings of the Third World Congress on Fluency Disorders (pp. 53–58). Nijmegen: Nijmegen University Press.

Goebel, M. D. (1984, November). A computer-aided fluency treatment program for adolescents and adults. Paper presented at the ASHA, San Francisco.

Guitar, B. (1998). Stuttering: An integrated approach to its nature and treatment. Baltimore: Williams and Wilkins.

Hall, K. D., Yairi, E., & Amir, O. (1999). A longitudinal investigation of speaking rate in preschool children who stutter. Journal of Speech Language and Hearing Research, 42, 1367–1377.

Herring, J. P. (1986). Fluency criterion program: A stuttering management system for children and adults. Tucson, AZ: Communication Skill Builders, Inc.

Kelly, E. M. (1993). Speech rates and turn-taking behaviors of children who stutter and their parents. Seminars in Speech and Language 14, 203–214.

Kelly, E. M. (1994). Speech rates and turn-taking behaviors of children who stutter and their fathers. Journal of Speech and Hearing Research 37, 1284–1294.

Kelly, E. M., & Conture, E. G. (1992). Speaking rates, response time latencies, and interrupting behaviors of young stutterers, nonstutterers, and their mothers. Journal of Speech and Hearing Research 35, 1256–1267.

Kully, D., & Langevin, M. (1999). Intensive treatment for stuttering adolescents. In R. Curlee (Ed.), Stuttering and related disorders of fluency (pp. 139–159). New York: Theime.

Logan, K., & Conture, E. (1995). Length, grammatical complexity, and rate differences in stuttered and fluent conversational utterances of children who stutter. Journal of Fluency Disorders 20, 35–62.

Manning, W. H. (1991). Sports analogies in the treatment of stuttering: Taking the field with your client. Public School Caucus 10(2), 1,10–11.

Meyers, S., & Woodford, L. (1992). The fluency development system for young children. Buffalo, NY: United Educational Services.

Neilson, M., & Andrews, G. (1993). Intensive fluency training of chronic stutterers. In R. Curlee (Ed.), Stuttering and related disorders of fluency (pp. 139–165). New York: Thieme.

Neilson, M. D. (1999). Cognitive-behavioral treatment of adults who stutter: The process and the art. In R. Curlee (Ed.), Stuttering and related disorders of fluency 2nd ed. (pp. 188–191). New York: Theime.

Pindzola, R. (1987) Stuttering intervention program. Austin, TX: PRO-ED.

Purcell, R., & Runyan, C. M. (1980). Normative study of speech rates of children. Journal of the Speech and Hearing Association of Virginia 21, 6–14.

Ramig, P. R., & Bennett, E. M. (1995). Working with 7- to 12- year-old children who stutter: Ideas for intervention in the public schools. Language, Speech, and Hearing Services in Schools 26(2), 138–149.

Riley, G. (1981). Stuttering prediction instrument for young children (rev. ed.). Austin, TX: PRO-ED.

Riley, G. (1994). Stuttering severity instrument for children and adults (3rd. ed.) (SSI-3). Austin, TX: PRO-ED.

Riley, G. D., & Riley, J. (1984). A component model for treating stuttering in children. In M. Peins (Ed.), Contemporary approaches in stuttering therapy (pp. 123–171). Boston: Little, Brown and Co.

Riley, J., & Riley, G. (1999). Speech motor training. In M. Onslow & A. Packman (Ed.), The handbook of early stuttering intervention. (pp. 139–158). San Diego: Singular.

Runyan, C. M., & Runyan, S. E. (1993). Therapy for school-aged stutterers: An update on the fluency rules program. In R. Curlee (Ed.), Stuttering and related disorders of fluency (pp. 101–123). New York: Theime.

Runyan, C. M., & Runyan, S. E. (1999). Therapy for school-aged stutterers: An update on the fluency rules program. In R. Curlee (Ed.), Stuttering and related disorders of fluency (pp. 101–123). New York: Theime.

Ryan, B. P. (2000). Speaking rate, conversational speech acts, interruption, and linguistic complexity of 20 preschool stuttering and non-stuttering children and their mothers. Clinical Linguistics and Phonetics 14(1), 25–51.

Schwartz, H. D. (1999). A primer for stuttering therapy. Boston: Allyn & Bacon.

Shine, R. E. (1988). Symmetric fluency training for young children (3rd ed.). Austin, TX: PRO-ED.

Wall, M., & Myers, F. (1994). Clinical management of childhood stuttering. Austin, TX: PRO-ED.

Webster, R. L. (1979). Empirical consideration regarding stuttering therapy. In H. H. Gregory (Ed.), Controversies about stuttering therapy. Baltimore: University Park Press.

Webster, R. L. (1980). Evolution of a target-based behavioral therapy for stuttering. Journal of Fluency Disorders 5, 303–320.

Zebrowski, P. M., & Kelly, E. M. (2002). Manual of stuttering intervention. New York: Singular.

7

Counseling Children Who Stutter and Their Parents

Anthony DiLollo and Walter H. Manning

The purpose of this chapter is to provide a specific framework around which speech-language pathologists might structure their approach to counseling both preschool and school-age children who stutter and their parents. After a review of the background issues relevant to counseling children who stutter and their families, the chapter outlines a general, constructivist framework for counseling, followed by an application of that framework to the problem of stuttering. Specific discussions of constructivist counseling with preschool and school-age children who stutter are also presented. It concludes with an application of constructivist counseling with parents of children who stutter. We hope that the reader of this chapter will develop a better appreciation of the importance of counseling children who stutter and their families and will be better able to effectively engage children and parents in counseling that is grounded in a specific theoretical framework.

The topics of counseling children who stutter and their parents, two related but very distinct topics, have received relatively minimal attention in the stuttering literature. Most of what has been written on these topics has focused on parent counseling, with some useful and insightful contributions helping to guide speech-language pathologists in this area (e.g., Bloom and Cooperman, 1999; Conture, 2001; C. B. Gregory, 2003; H. H. Gregory, 1986; Manning, 2001; Starkweather, 1986). Relatively few sources exist, however, that specifically describe counseling with children who stutter, Perhaps this is due to the greater success of behavioral treatments with young children who stutter, or perhaps because it is assumed that children are too young—cognitively/socially/emotionally—to meaningfully engage in and receive benefit from counseling. Or as others have suggested, this relative lack of information may reflect a general discomfort that many speech-language pathologists have with regard to counseling, particularly with young children and their parents (Luterman, 2001; Shames, 2000). Whatever the reason, speech-language pathologists who wish to engage a child who stutters in counseling have, at the present time, few published resources to turn to for guidance.

The counseling framework that we present in this chapter is intended to provide a consistent means for interpreting issues and problems raised by the experience of stuttering, living with stuttering, and the process of treating stuttering. This framework can be useful when working with preschool children who stutter, who have had relatively brief experiences with stuttering, as well as when working with older, school-age children who stutter, who have a much longer, more intricate relationship with stuttering. Of course, this is by no means the only way in which stuttering and counseling with persons who stutter can be approached, but it is one specific framework that we have found to be useful in our endeavors with children who stutter and their parents.

◆ Counseling and the Treatment of Stuttering

Before we begin discussing applications of counseling in the treatment of children who stutter and their parents, a working definition of counseling might be helpful. It goes without saying, of course, that the relationship between counseling and psychotherapy is very strong. In fact, Crowe (1997) suggested that counseling is a type of psychotherapy intended for assisting persons with interpersonal problems that are seen as less severe than those associated with mental illness (e.g., depression, schizophrenia, etc.), the latter typically requiring more in-depth psychotherapy.

Among various definitions of counseling, Rollin (2000) has suggested that "counseling is a dynamic process that involves a complex interaction between and among people" (p. 2). Similarly, Webster (1977) stated that "the term counseling is a very broad one, but it simply refers to a number of situations in which people communicate" (p. 1). More specifically, Luterman (2001) referred to the act of counseling as "a clinician trying to help a client *manage change*" (p. 9). Further, it has been suggested by numerous authors that the relationship or alliance between those involved in counseling is central to the process (e.g., Manning, 2001; Wampold, 2001). In fact, Patterson (1985) stated that counseling not only *involves* the relationship, it *is* the relationship. Interestingly, several authors (e.g., Benson & Epstein, 1975; Benson & McCallie, 1979) even point to the client-clinician relationship as a major mechanism of change in the placebo effect, suggesting that this may be an important aspect of the *entirety* of our treatment of persons who stutter, not just the "counseling" aspect.

Given these views on counseling, it might be suggested that counseling children who stutter and their parents should involve a therapeutic relationship that is interactive, communicative, and directed toward facilitating long-term management of the desired changes that traditional therapy for stuttering might produce. It is our belief that successful, long-term behavioral change cannot occur without accompanying emotional and cognitive adjustments, and that many (but not all!) persons who stutter (including children) will need at least some help in making those appropriate personal changes. Therefore, our "working" definition of counseling in the context of this chapter is that counseling is an *interactive, communicative* process that involves a *relationship between clinician and client,* and that is focused on *facilitating effective change.*

Psychotherapy and the Treatment of Stuttering

Given the close association between psychotherapy and counseling, it may be useful for us to next consider what we may learn from psychotherapeutic approaches to the treatment of stuttering. Although we are not suggesting that counseling alone might be the preferred approach to the treatment of stuttering, research regarding the effectiveness of psychotherapy with adult persons who stutter can provide us with some useful insights into the role that counseling might play in an integrated therapy approach for both adults and children who stutter.

For example, Nystul and Muszynska (1976) employed an *Adlerian* psychotherapy approach to the treatment of "a classical case of stuttering" in an adult, with reportedly excellent results. These authors argued that "the person's attitude toward self is the major force in determining his/her speech fluency and social participation" (p. 195). Similarly, Kaplan and Kaplan (1978), working from a *Gestalt* psychotherapy perspective, defined stuttering as occurring when the person who stutters "plugs into his fears, his expectations, and his self-percept as inferior, incompetent, or helpless" (p. 3). Gestalt therapy was aimed at changing the "I am a stutterer" system by facilitating greater awareness of how adults who stutter hold back themselves and how they can get in touch with the resources within themselves that are not a part of the stuttering system. Garber (1973) applied *psychodramatic* techniques in working with a 30-year-old person who stuttered, Lentz, who had tried and failed numerous "traditional" treatments for his problem. Through the use of psychodrama, Lentz was reportedly able to differentiate a nonstuttering self from a stuttering self and to examine the roles that these selves would play in his life. Garber reported that Lentz decided not to "wipe out" his "stuttering self" but to maintain his life-long relationship with stuttering while not allowing it to control him.

What is evident from these published reports of psychotherapeutic intervention with stuttering is that the focus of counseling is *not* on the *speech behaviors* but on the associated psychodynamics of the person who stutters. Specifically, such intervention focuses on the individual's attitude toward self, his or her fears and expectations, the concept of "self-as-a-stutterer," the activation of untapped resources, and the idea that the individual may have a "relationship" with "stuttering," all aspects of the individual's psychosocial dynamics that clinicians with a psychotherapeutic orientation believe may need to change. This set of foci for counseling intervention, then, would appear to be highly *complementary* to the goals of traditional approaches to stuttering therapy. Furthermore, applying these concepts to counseling children who stutter suggests important areas that may be targeted in a *prevention* model of treatment for young children who stutter. For example, counseling with children who stutter may focus on improving attitudes toward self, diminishing the concept of "self-as-a-stutterer," building and activating personal strengths and resources, and guiding the child's "relationship" with stuttering so that it is the child, not "stuttering," who is in control.

In the following section, we describe a counseling model that we have found useful in working with both adults and children who stutter. This model is helpful in addressing issues such as self-concept, activation of resources, and reconstructing the child's "relationship" with stuttering.

◆ Constructivist Counseling for Children Who Stutter

Constructivist Theory

To provide one reasonable, widely used, and current theoretical framework for our discussion of counseling of young children who stutter and their families, we will employ constructivist theory, an area of clinical psychology that is exemplified by George Kelly's (1955) seminal work, *The Psychology of Personal Constructs*, and a growing body of applied and theoretical research (e.g., Applegate, 1990; Fransella, 2003; Raskin, 2002; Winter, 2003). Constructivist theory emphasizes the belief that humans create their own reality; constructing personal meanings which develop in an individual's narratives and are influenced by, and changed in, social contexts (Neimeyer, 1999). Kelly (1955) proposed a comprehensive constructivist model that posited personal constructs, meanings composed of bipolar aspects (e.g., good-bad, happy-sad, etc.), which individuals create to interpret their environment. The personal constructs people develop give structure and meaning to how they interpret the world. That is, an individual looks at the world "through transparent patterns or *templets* which he creates and then attempts to fit over the realities of which the world is composed" (Kelly, p. 8). Thus, how a person interprets or construes events is determined by his or her individual constructs or meanings.

Kelly (1955) believed that people act as scientists in their lives and use their constructs to predict and hypothesize about events, people, and experiences. These hypotheses are then tested through further experience and either confirmed or discounted. Through repetition of these outcomes, personal constructs are strengthened, changed, or expanded, and a personal world view emerges.

When experience contrasts with a strongly held personal construct (what Kelly called "core" constructs), *however, individuals may subconsciously choose to protect those constructs by denying, ignoring, or trivializing the invalidating experience* (This is a key point that will be repeatedly emphasized over the course of this discussion).

Constructivism also accounts for how emotional reactions such as fear, threat, anxiety, and guilt may be generated when individuals are faced with experience that contrasts with their core constructs. For example, Landfield and Leitner (1980) described *fear* as "the awareness of imminent incidental change in one's core structures" (p. 12) and *threat* as "an awareness of an imminent and *comprehensive* change in core structure" (p. 12). Importantly, such imminent changes need not be negative, suggesting that even positive, therapeutic change might generate such emotional reactions. As Landfield and Leitner stated, "if a person has defined his life-role in terms of sickness, the prospect of successful therapy could be traumatizing" (p. 12).

The concept of "anxiety" has a long history in stuttering theory and research (Bloodstein, 1995 Menzies, Onslow, & Packman, 1999), including studies that have investigated several different definitions of the concept such as "social anxiety" (Messenger, Onslow, Packman, & Menzies, 2004), "cognitive anxiety" (DiLollo, Manning, & Neimeyer, 2003), "state" and "trait" anxiety (Miller & Watson, 1992), and "emotional reactivity" (Conture, Walden, Graham, Arnold, Hartfield, & Karrass, in press). Kelly (1955) described a constructivist take on anxiety, defining it as an awareness that a person's constructs are not relevant to the events he or she is experiencing. In such a case, the person has no way of effectively predicting the course of such events. This reaction, then, may occur when a person experiences *new* events, or when an individual experiences invalidating events that have previously been denied or ignored. For example, a child on his first ski-trip getting on a chairlift for the first time may be anxious as he has no constructs relevant to this experience. Over the course of a few rides, however, the child develops constructs that allow him to predict the event (and his safety) and anxiety decreases.

Guilt, in personal construct terms, may occur when a person acts in a way that is contradictory to his or her *core constructs* (Landfield & Leitner, 1980). For example, an individual might feel *guilt* if he or she were to do something that violated a strongly held belief about him- or herself as a person.

Narrative Therapy

Subsumed under the general category of "constructivism," *narrative therapy* provides an additional constructivist perspective on the process of personal change and may have particular relevance to working with persons who stutter. Wendell Johnson, one of the pioneers of stuttering therapy, was greatly influenced by the writings of Alfred Korzybski (1933) on the topic of "general semantics," the concept that the words we use both reflect and influence our thoughts, and which is often referred to as an early example of "constructivist" thinking (Neimeyer, 1999).

Narrative therapy (Parry & Doan, 1994; White, 1995; White & Epston, 1990) is based on the concept of people as "storytellers" and that the stories they tell about themselves, and that others tell about them, significantly shape their behavior and sense of self (Madigan & Goldner, 1998; Neimeyer, 1999; Winslade & Monk, 1999). The term *narrative* is commonly used in speech-language pathology to refer to a type of discourse that has certain linguistic properties (McCabe & Bliss, 2003). Within this chapter, the term *narrative* has a more narrow focus, referring to an individual's personal story that influences how events and experiences are interpreted, consolidates self-understanding, and guides behavior. These personal narratives serve to create meaning from experience in much the same way as Kelly (1955) described the role of personal constructs. As such, narratives are used for anticipating events, planning actions, and orienting the self in the world (Dimaggio, Salvatore, Azzara, & Catania, 2003).

Importantly, however, we are not the sole author of our stories as we continually receive "input" from significant others and our sociocultural and sociopolitical environments (Winslade & Monk, 1999), essentially imposing subplots to our stories that are sometimes unwanted and personally limiting (Drewery & Winslade, 1997; McKenzie & Monk, 1997). These personally limiting subplots can come to dominate the narratives of individuals and, as such, cause them to interpret their world primarily in ways that maintain the dominant story. In such cases, experiences that might invalidate the dominant story are denied, ignored, or trivialized, in much the same way as described by Kelly (1955) for the protection of core constructs.

A Constructivist Approach to Stuttering

To build a platform for discussing counseling for both preschool and school-age children who stutter, we first briefly outline the application of constructivist theory to the problem of stuttering in a more general sense, and follow it with a description of how this approach to understanding stuttering might be used with specific age groups. As such, some aspects of the general theory may not appear to specifically apply to all age groups of children who stutter. As we shall see, however, constructivist theory does provide implications for working with all ages of children who stutter, with the focus with preschool children being "prevention" compared with the "treatment" orientation with older children.

Fransella (1972) proposed a "theory of stuttering" based on Kelly's (1955) personal construct theory in which she suggested that persons who stutter develop construct systems based on the experience of stuttering, effectively blocking experiences of fluent speech from meaningful integration into their world view. She suggested that, for persons who stutter, a *fluent speaker role* tends to lack any meaningful, predictive quality, whereas a *stutterer role* tends to be more "meaningful" in that it facilitates accurate prediction of internal and external reactions to, and consequences of, speaking. Fransella concluded that a person continues to stutter "because it is in this way that he can anticipate the greatest number of events; it is by behaving in this way that life is most meaningful to him" (p. 58).

Our own research has indicated support for Fransella's (1972) theory and has demonstrated that adult persons who stutter report more cognitive anxiety, or inability to adequately construe events, associated with fluent rather than disfluent episodes (DiLollo et al., 2003), and that they also have a less complex cognitive representation of themselves in a fluent as opposed to stuttering role (DiLollo, Manning, & Neimeyer, 2005).

We have also proposed that Fransella's (1972) theory might also be framed in terms of narrative therapy (DiLollo, Neimeyer, & Manning, 2002; Manning, 2005). By so doing, we further clarify the position that one of the primary problems for persons who stutter is the lack of a meaningful *fluent speaker role*. In this construction, the person who stutters is seen as having developed a "dominant narrative" based on his or her experiences with stuttering, with the consequence being that he or she denies or trivializes any experiences of fluent speech.

Therefore, a constructivist conceptualization of stuttering helps us—at least in terms of treatment—to focus on some key issues in counseling children who stutter and their parents. In this next section, we examine how the constructivist framework can guide our approach to counseling children who stutter, with specific reference to preschool and school-age children.

Constructing a Meaningful Fluent Speaker Role for Preschool-Age Children

For young children who stutter, constructs relating to their role as a speaker tend to be weakly formed or, for many, not formed at all. Consequently, in contrast to adults who have developed and strengthened their personal constructs over the course of many years, children's constructs remain loose and permeable—relatively easily influenced by experience. At this point in time, two factors are important for the child in developing constructs: (1) that events are repeated; the more repetitions of an event, the greater the chance for the child to extract consistent themes; and (2) that events have something that clearly stands out to the child, such as a consequence or outcome, so that it may be abstracted across repetitions of that event.

Yairi and Ambrose (2005) have demonstrated that children who stutter are aware of their stuttering at or shortly following onset (mean age of 33 months). As such, young children who stutter may be faced with the difficult task of trying to create a meaningful speaker role from two competing sets of stimuli. Unfortunately, for most children who stutter, fluent speech, being the "expected" or "normal" behavior, will have few outcomes that stand out. Stuttered speech, however, may produce reactions from parents, siblings, peers, and others, along with consequences that may often be penalizing to the child. These events, then, stand out to the child and are easily abstracted across repetitions of the event (i.e., stuttering) to produce constructs about the child's role as a speaker and predictions about how such events will unfold. Therefore, at this crucial time, experiences that focus on stuttering and its social consequences can have a powerful effect on the constructs that the child finds meaningful and predictive.

The implications of the above description of early childhood stuttering for treatment and counseling would appear to be clear—the majority of attention (therapeutic and parental/social) needs to be on the child's *fluent* speech productions rather than his or her disfluent productions. Such an approach can facilitate the development of a meaningful speaker role for the child that is primarily based on experiences and consequences of fluent speech. As the child experiences fluent speech, this experience can be made "meaningful" by being brought to the child's attention and commented on by parents and other caregivers in the child's environment.

In addition, from a narrative perspective, therapy and attention focused on the child's stuttering may contribute to the development for the child of a story of "a stutterer," whereas overt, gently repeated focus on the child's fluent speech productions can contribute to the development of a story more closely aligned to that of a fluent speaker.

Reconstructing a Meaningful Fluent Speaker Role for School-Age Children

For older children who stutter, their constructs or personal narratives about themselves as speakers have become, generally speaking, more firmly developed than those of preschool children; older children who stutter, in general, are more resistant to the influences of invalidating experiences such as fluent speech production. Therefore, counseling with these children needs to focus more on *changing* or *reconstructing* their personal narrative rather than merely establishing a meaningful fluent speaker role as we described for younger children. In addition, traditional treatment specific to increasing the amount of fluent speech experienced by the child is important, as this will provide the foundation against which counseling will "push" on the dominant "I am a stutterer" narrative.

Reconstructing Speaking: Beyond Behavior Change

As the older child who stutters begins to experience increases in the amount of fluent speech he or she produces, emotional responses may occur. Emotions such as fear, threat, anxiety, and guilt may increase as the child acts in a way that is in contrast to, and threatens, his or her "stutterer" construct system (see also, Jezer, 1997; Kuhr & Rustin, 1985, who describe emotional difficulties near the completion of successful stuttering treatment). If the clinician can help the child develop more meaningful constructs based on fluent rather than stuttered speech, these emotional responses can be decreased.

One approach to facilitating this reconstruction may be to encourage the child to *experiment* with new behaviors. Although speech-language pathologists already do this during traditional treatment for stuttering, incorporating a constructivist counseling component into this existing activity significantly changes the focus of the activity from a *behavioral* level to a *meaning* level. That is, a child can perform a new behavior, such as speaking fluently, but ignore or trivialize the act to protect his or her existing constructs by saying, for example, "It wasn't me, it was just the techniques" or "I was just lucky this time" or "Yes, I guess I was fluent in the conversation, but I really messed up when I introduced myself later." In this case, the behavior was successfully practiced, but the experience was not meaningfully integrated on a cognitive and/or emotional level; it didn't impact the speaker in terms of his or her self concept as a speaker. Alternatively, prior to the experiment, the child may be asked to *predict* the likely outcome of the activity, and to write his or her predictions in a notebook. Then, the child is instructed to pay attention to *all* aspects of the event—both internal (feelings and emotional reactions) and external (environment, people's reactions, outcomes, etc.)—so that he or she can report back to the clinician in detail what happened. Following completion of the experiment, the clinician and child discuss the experiment and compare what actually happened with what the child predicted would happen. This has the effect of (1) elaborating or increasing the child's ability to construe "being a fluent speaker" as he or she will usually report *more* observations from the experiment than were initially predicted; and (2) contrasting the child's current constructs (i.e., the predictions) with actual outcomes, in essence *forcing* meaningful consideration of an event that might have previously been ignored or trivialized.

Narrative Therapy

Additionally, speech pathologists working with older children who stutter might find it useful to engage the child in counseling based on the concepts of narrative therapy described earlier. The way children interpret the experience of stuttering can have a profound impact on their stories about themselves. As previously described, these children are at risk for developing negative stories that are dominated by the experience of stuttering and that would prevent them from activating positive resources, capabilities, and talents. A narrative therapy approach attempts to facilitate a client's discovery of new stories that are based on strengths, preferences, and new possibilities (Sax, 1997).

Telling the "Problem-Saturated Story"   Children who stutter come to therapy with a story to tell. They are often anxious, confused, afraid, or feeling defeated by their problem-saturated story of stuttering (Payne, 2000). Clinicians can begin the counseling process by simply asking to hear the child's story. With some children—those who simply do not talk—this can be a difficult task and may take some time to get started. The clinician must be patient and allow such children to tell their story on their own terms. Of course, the clinician can engage in rapport-building activities to help the child develop a level of comfort and trust that might facilitate participation. In addition, the clinician can model the storytelling mode of communication, even throwing in some easy disfluencies in the narrative production, suggesting to the child that fluent speech is not the goal of the interaction. When the child does tell his or her story, the clinician takes the role of interested listener, curiously asking clarifying questions and inviting as detailed a description of the problem as the child can provide. It is important that the clinician accept the child's story and take it seriously, while at the same time understanding that it is not likely to be "the whole story" (Payne). As the child tells the problem-saturated story over one or more meetings, he or she will almost always provide the clinician with "clues" to an ignored or overlooked alternative storyline—one that is resistant to the problem and its effects on the child (Payne). It is from these brief, mentioned-in-passing clues that an alternative story might emerge.

Externalizing Language   After listening to the client's initial narrative, the therapist might invite the client to give the problem a name (White & Epston, 1990). Naming the problem allows clients to position themselves differently in relation to the problem. For children who stutter, this may afford them the opportunity to, for the first time, consider stuttering as something "external" to themselves as opposed to an enduring, internal trait (Payne, 2000; White & Epston, 1990). In other words, it gives the children the sense of being separated from stuttering. This can facilitate the stance of the child being an *active* participant in *resisting* the problem rather than being the passive *recipient* of treatment.

After naming the problem, the clinician and child can engage in "externalizing language" (White & Epston, 1990) that portrays the problem as a separate entity, with its own feelings, motivations, strengths, and weaknesses. For example, following a stuttering event, the clinician might say to the child, "I wonder why "Stuttering" decided to come to visit you just then?" Similarly, the child and the clinician might talk about the things "Stuttering" is telling the child when he or she chooses not to answer a question in class, or how powerful "Stuttering" felt when it convinced the child not to order what he or she really wanted at a restaurant. Thus, not only does this approach help children to separate themselves from their problem, but it often promotes a "lighter," more "playful" atmosphere during therapy (Freeman, Epston, & Lobovits, 1997).

An interesting contrast to this approach was suggested by Williams (1957) in his classic article, "A Point of View about Stuttering." In this discussion of stuttering, Williams identified the difficulties that can occur when a person who stutters thinks of stuttering as a "part of him or her" in a way similar to the way that White and Epston (1990) talked about the "problem person." Williams also suggested, however, that "animistic" thinking, thinking of stuttering as a "thing that lies inside him,"or her, may be a significant part of the stuttering problem and should be discouraged, implying a contrast to our previous discussion of externalizing language. On closer consideration, however, Williams' discussion of animistic thinking is actually supportive of the use of externalizing language with persons who stutter. Williams' argument against "animistic" thinking is that it prevents the person from recognizing his or her alternative ways of behaving by handing over control of behavior to the "thing." The purpose of using externalizing language in narrative therapy is to make the animistic thinking overt and more real to clients so that they can then deal with its influence in their thinking—effectively neutralizing its effect, as suggested by Williams.

Unique Outcomes and Redescription   Once "clues" to the alternative story have been identified, the clinician can invite the client to elaborate on the topic, using externalizing language, and expanding the clue to a "unique outcome" (White & Epston, 1990) that describes the basis for a preferred, alternative narrative to the problem-saturated one. The clinician again takes the stance of a curious listener, sometimes even feigning misunderstanding to encourage the child to re-state and expand on his or her description of the alternative story (Freeman et al., 1997).

Following the identification of unique outcomes that have facilitated the development of an alternative story, children can be invited to explore how their alternative story will affect their relationships with themselves, others, and the problem (White & Epston, 1990). Clinicians might consider "unique redescription questions" (Epston & White, 1999) that can be used to aid clients in this process (See DiLollo et al., 2002 for these and other questions), although such questions would need to be adapted for use with children. For example, the clinician might ask a child to think of him or herself as a "superhero" and to describe his or her "superpowers" that enabled him or her to battle "Stuttering." The goal is to facilitate the ability of children who stutter to resist stuttering's influence, undermining it, and altering the relationship between the child and the problem so that "Stuttering" is no longer "in control."

Elaboration of Alternative Stories through Creative Play   Creative endeavors can play an important role in counseling with both preschool and school-age children who stutter. Barragar-Dunne (1997) described how the use of drama and play in therapy with children can serve to "open rather than close or narrow the therapeutic space" (p. 74). When children (and adults, for that matter) engage in a creative process, they can often express emotions, thoughts, and insights that may not have been available to them at a more conscious level (Neimeyer, 2000). In addition, children might find it easier to express some events and experiences in a creative or dramatic form rather than talking about them face-to-face with the clinician (Barragar-Dunne, 1997). Therefore, it might be through creative play that the child might provide a "clue" to a unique outcome, or creative play might provide the child with a safe way to experiment with new behaviors and try out an alternative story.

Cattanach (1992, 1994) described three kinds of play that could be useful in expanding a child's experiences:

1. *Embodiment play*, which involves the child exploring the world through the senses and utilizes such items as play-dough, slime, clay, and other tactile materials that can be manipulated. Particularly for young children who stutter, embodiment play might provide a safe, playful environment in which further exploration of their fluent speaker role can occur.

2. *Progressive play*, which involves children discovering and exploring the world outside of themselves through the use of toys, dolls, and other objects. Progressive play might be used to help children to better understand the concept of "externalization" and to explore alternative stories. For example, a child and clinician might agree that a certain doll or toy will represent "Stuttering." Then, when they use externalizing language, they will talk *to* the doll or toy and also provide it with *its own voice* to talk about its motivations and feelings. Similarly, puppets might be used to act out alternatives to an experience that didn't go well for the child or an experiment that the child is going to eventually try out.

3. *Role play*, which involves the child first playing himself or herself in a familiar situation but then switching to take on the role of someone else. This type of play might aid in externalization by allowing the child to take on the role of "Stuttering" and to talk about how and why it likes to push the child around. Alternatively, once the child has developed some skill at controlling stuttering, the clinician might ask the child to act "as if" he or she were a fluent speaker. Barragar-Dunne (1997) emphasized the powerful, transformational effects that role play can generate for children, even suggesting that children may "experience these changes on a bodily, kinesthetic level" (p. 76).

Importantly, "creative play" can also include various forms of artistic expression such as drawing, painting, sculpture, collage, mask making, poetry, and other forms of creative writing. Therefore, children can be invited to gain meaning from their experiences through different forms of expressive art. For example, a child could be encouraged to create a mask for "Stuttering"—creatively representing on the mask various images, colors, patterns, and/or icons that reflect the child's feelings about, and understanding of, this lifelong "companion." The mask, then, might become the basis for further externalizing conversations and might even be used in conjunction with a role-playing activity.

Supporting the Alternative Story   *Management of change* was one of the important aspects of counseling that we derived in our "working definition" at the start of this chapter, and this may be particularly important when counseling persons who stutter. The process of facilitating *meaningful* change requires that the clinician be involved in supporting and promoting the child's emerging alternative story. This may be accomplished in several ways.

Many narrative therapists (e.g., Payne, 2000; White & Epston, 1990; Winslade & Monk, 1999) recommend the use of *therapeutic documents* as one way to promote meaningful change. Although sounding rather intimidating, therapeutic documents are simply tangible and durable retellings of part, or all, of a child's alternative story. These may take the form of letters, emails, certificates, pictures, or video that provide the child with specific feedback regarding his or her alternative story (See **Appendix 7–1** for examples). Therapeutic documents may be used at various stages of treatment to reflect on significant accomplishments, changes, or insights that might be occurring and to provide a voice to the alternative story that is outside that of the child's. These documents should be creative and fun, particularly when using them with children, and they may often reflect a theme or topic that is of special interest to the child. Furthermore, therapeutic documents may be used with young, pre-literate children, provided appropriate materials are used. For example, most young children will recognize the concept of a certificate with a gold star, a trophy, or a medal as a sign of successful achievement.

Payne (2000) also emphasized the importance of sharing the alternative story with important people in the child's life. This can help challenge secrecy and isolation and invites others to interact with the child in a supportive manner. Furthermore, Payne suggested that it is important to encourage the significant others in the child's life to tell and re-tell the alternative story – providing the child with the opportunity to hear others tell the story; to hear himself or herself being "cast" in this alternative role.

Summary

We have attempted to present a framework for engaging children who stutter in counseling that has the specific goal of supporting the change process that is the focus of traditional treatments for stuttering. This constructivist approach to counseling specifically aims to help children who stutter change their stuttering-dominated self narratives and can help address as well as mitigate issues such as fear, anxiety, guilt, and helplessness. In addition, this approach to counseling can provide clinicians with a theoretical framework that can organize and guide their counseling interactions with children who stutter.

◆ Constructivist Counseling for Parents of Children Who Stutter

Emotional Reactions of Parents

Parents of children who stutter often find themselves in a world that looks very different from the one in which they are accustomed to living. As the concept of a potentially chronic stuttering problem for their child becomes a reality for these parents, emotional reactions are very likely to occur (Crowe, 1997). In fact, parents of young children just beginning to stutter have reported emotions of grief, fear, anxiety, guilt, and isolation (Crowe, 1997; Manning, 2001).

The Grieving Process

Although the parents of children with speech, language, and hearing problems are typically not facing the *physical* loss of their child, many authors have pointed out that such parents still experience emotional reactions associated with *grieving* (Crowe, 1997; Moses, 1985; Tanner, 1980). Parents of children who stutter can exhibit many of the "classic" grieving reactions such as denial, anger, bargaining, depression, and acceptance (Kubler-Ross, 1969). Importantly, though, recent thought on the topic of grieving has moved away from a "stage" model such as that of Kubler-Ross, and more toward an individualized, personal model of grieving that focuses on the usefulness of grief as a way of creating meaningful transition into a new world view (Neimeyer, 2000; 2001).

Consequently, clinicians working with parents of children who stutter who are experiencing grief need to listen to, and acknowledge, the grief, and then to encourage the parents to re-focus that energy toward involvement in treatment and support of the child. Clinicians should point out to parents that grief in this situation may be a normal reaction, but that feeling bad about the grief, or becoming focused on this reaction to the exclusion of more "constructive" reactions, might be less than helpful. In other words, parents faced with the unanticipated world of having a child who stutters, can take action and create meaning from their new situation by using their grief to motivate them to become "experts" on stuttering, finding out all they can of the topic, participating in treatment, and providing the necessary support for their child. One danger in this approach may be that some parents may get overly involved in the cognitive/logical/factual aspects of stuttering and eschew the emotional realities of the problem, leading to inappropriate degrees of intellectualization. It is the responsibility of the clinician to facilitate a "balanced" understanding of the problem of stuttering for the parents. Given their active participation in programs such as the Lidcombe program (Onslow, Packman, & Harrison, 2003) and Demands and Capacities (Starkweather, 1997) approaches to treatment, parents are apt to experience a reduction of anxiety and increased parental locus of control that may also facilitate favorable changes in the child (Ratner & Guitar, 2005). Parental participation in a support group at a local or national level can also have an empowering effect on parents and facilitate both understanding and support for the child (Manning, 2001).

Other Emotional Reactions

The constructivist philosophy described earlier and applied to counseling children who stutter may also be considered as a possible approach for counseling the parents of children who stutter. Recall that emotional reactions such as *fear* and *threat* can be related to a perceived change in one's core constructs. For parents of children who stutter, their constructs related to parenting a child and having a "perfect child" are being severely challenged.

Furthermore, *guilt* was described as a situation in which a person was acting in contrast to his or her core constructs. Many parents of children who stutter fear that *they* have done something to cause their child to stutter, a notion often still reinforced by references to Wendell Johnson and Associates' (1959) *diagnosogenic* theory of stuttering. Consequently, such misinformation can, quite naturally, lead parents to feel guilty, as they would seem to have acted in a way that is in contrast to their core constructs of themselves as caring, protective parents.

Similarly, anxiety was defined as occurring when an individual possessed insufficient constructs to accurately predict the unfolding of events. Parents of children who stutter often have little knowledge about stuttering, how it will develop, or what stuttering therapy might mean for their child (as well as the time, energy, and money commitment entailed for them). In addition, parents frequently have few experiences to inform them of what to expect for their child's educational, social, and vocational future. With such a lack of constructs related to stuttering, it is not surprising that many parents present with significant levels of anxiety and concern related to their child's stuttering.

Elaborating Parents' Construct Systems Related to Stuttering

From a constructivist perspective, clinicians working with parents of children who stutter need to facilitate an increase in the constructs that these parents have about stuttering and stuttering treatment. This understanding of the potential emotional reactions of parents underscores the importance of *education* and *information giving* in counseling parents of children who stutter. By providing parents with information regarding the onset, development, and course of stuttering and the types and potential outcomes of stuttering treatments, clinicians can facilitate the elaboration of the parents' construct systems about stuttering and their child's future, helping to reduce fear, anxiety, and guilt, even if the information is not what the parents were hoping to learn. Such education can be done verbally, with video and audio recordings, through pamphlets and books, or, in some instances, via the internet (a list of useful resources for clinicians can be found in **Appendix 7–2**). By accessing such material, parents can integrate the information at their own pace, perhaps avoiding the "overload" that sometimes occurs when clinicians try to provide relevant information to parents. Of course, as we noted in our working definition, counseling needs to be *interactive* and *communicative*, so it is the responsibility of the clinician not only to provide parents with access to this information but also to discuss it with them, facilitating their understanding of the material and the integration of it as a meaningful part of their construct system related to their child. Providing such information to parents may require judiciously repetitive, redundant coverage for many parents, to ensure they are understanding and/or implementing necessary behavioral, cognitive, emotional, and social changes.

Another way that parents of children who stutter can be helped to develop constructs about stuttering and what their child is dealing with is through real and pseudo experiences of stuttering. The real experiences of stuttering, of course, come from the children, and parents should be encouraged to pay close attention to what happens when their child stutters. Many parents fear their child's stuttering and attempt to ignore it as much as possible. This can result in them having little understanding of what their child's experience with stuttering is like, while also suggesting to the child that stuttering is something to be feared and ashamed of. With the clinician modeling pseudo-stuttering, parents can be encouraged to role play and "experiment" with stuttering in a variety of settings to get a glimpse of what stuttering is like for their child. Parents may also choose to share these experiences with older children, discussing feelings and reactions, and even attempting some joint experiments with stuttering in public. These experiences will help parents to understand that their school-age child's participation in daily speaking situations, in spite of some stuttering, indicates real courage. Parents begin to understand that participation (versus avoidance of speaking) is a primary goal of treatment. And finally, experimenting by the parents with easier forms of stuttering also helps parents to alter the categorical view that stuttering is "bad" and fluency is "good."

Parents as Audience and Storytellers

Earlier in this chapter we discussed the development of a meaningful fluent speaker role for children who stutter, the concept of facilitating an alternative self-narrative, based on experiences of fluent speech as opposed to stuttered speech. Recall that Payne (2000) emphasized the need for an *audience* of significant others in the child's life to listen to, accept, and support the child's emerging alternative story. Parents (or the primary caregiver) are the most important "audience" for the child's story. Furthermore, Payne indicated that others in the child's environment needed to become *tellers* of the alternative story so that the child becomes not just author and narrator, but audience to his or her own story. This is a very important role that parents play in strengthening and facilitating the emergence of the alternative story due to their significant influence on the child at this time.

The Lidcombe Program: An Example of Constructivist Counseling?

One recent treatment program that appears to be producing favorable outcomes with young children who stutter is the Lidcombe Program (Onslow, et al., 2003). The fundamental treatment procedure of the program is "parental verbal contingencies during everyday conversations" (Onslow et al., 2003, p. 6), with parents commenting on and praising "stutter-free" speech, while also occasionally acknowledging a moment of stuttering. Importantly, the recommended ratio of commenting on and praising stutter-free speech compared with stuttered speech is *5 to 1.*

Onslow et al. (2003) described the Lidcombe Program as an *operant conditioning* program, and this may be one mechanism relating to the success of the program. It may also be possible, however, that there are *multiple mechanisms* contributing to the observed outcomes (Ratner & Guitar, 2005). Another mechanism may be the *construction of a meaningful fluent speaker role* for the children, based on the increased attention given to stutter-free speech by the child's parents. In addition, the Lidcombe Program is also reported to be less successful with older children who stutter, which could be interpreted as indicating that once a child's constructs (or "stories") about being a "stutterer" have had time to develop and strengthen, it is more difficult for experiences of fluent speech to impact his or her self-concept.

♦ Conclusion

The process of helping people who stutter, in terms of long-term, meaningful change, involves far more than changing speech fluency. We are treating the person rather than simply treating what appears to be the obvious communication problem. This is clearly the case for older children, adolescents, and adults who, for many years, have done their best to survive as someone who stutters and have had time to firmly develop their personal narratives. We have improved our understanding about how very young children who are beginning to stutter are aware of their fluency and realize that speaking is often unpleasant (Vanryckeghem, Brutten, & Hernandez, 2005). This understanding requires our response to the child's cognitive-emotional reactions as well as the more obvious behavioral features of the child's situation. Regardless of the treatment protocol, counseling occurs in many forms during the process of change. Whether intended or not, there are common principles of counseling that take place during treatment including understanding, empathy, and the development of a therapeutic relationship that facilitates change. In this chapter we have described a therapeutic/counseling response based on principles of a constructivist-narrative approach that emphasizes experimentation with the child's constructs about his or her ability to communicate. The primary emphasis is on altering the meaningfulness of the child's current story to reconstrue a preferred story using a variety of narrative therapy procedures. Parents, as the child's primary caregivers, are invited to understand the stuttering experience on a basic level to appreciate the nature of the child's current and alternative narratives. This understanding allows parents to play an active role in helping to change how the child construes him or herself and facilitates decreased anxiety and increased locus of control for both the child and the parents.

References

Applegate, J. L. (1990). Constructs and communication: A pragmatic integration. In G.J. Neimeyer, & R. A. Neimeyer (Eds.), Advances in Personal Construct Psychology: A Research Annual (Vol. 4). (pp.203–230). Greenwich, CT: JAI Press.

Barragar-Dunne P. (1997). "Catch the little fish": Therapy utilizing narrative, drama, and dramatic play with young children. In C. Smith & D. Nylund (Ed.), Narrative therapies with children and adolescents (pp. 71–110). New York: The Guilford Press.

Benson, H., & Epstein, M. D. (1975). The Placebo effect: a neglected asset in the care of patients. Journal of the American Medical Association, 232, 1225–1227.

Benson, H., & Mcallie, D. F. (1979). Angina pectoris and the placebo effect. The New England Journal of Medicine, 300, 1424–1429.

Bloodstein, O. (1995). A handbook on stuttering. San Diego, CA: Singular.

Bloom, C, & Cooperman, D. K. (1999). Synergistic stuttering therapy: A holistic approach. Woburn, MA: Butterworth-Heinemann.

Cattanach, A. (1992). Play therapy with abused children. London: Jessica Kingsley.

Cattanach, A. (1994). Where the sky meets the underworld. London: Jessica Kingsley.

Conture, E. G. (2001). Stuttering: Its nature, diagnosis, and treatment. Needham Heights, MA: Allyn & Bacon.

Conture, E. G., Walden, T. A., Arnold, H. S., Graham, C. G., Hartfield, K. N., & Karrass, J. (2006). Communicative-Emotional Model of Developmental Stuttering. In N. Bernstein Ratner & J. Tetnowski (Eds.) Current issues in stuttering research and practice. Mahwah, NJ: Lawrence Erlbaum Assoc.

Crowe, T. A. (Ed.). (1997). Applications of counseling in speech-language pathology and audiology. Philadelphia: Williams & Wilkins.

DiLollo, A., Manning, W. H., & Neimeyer, R. A. (2003). Cognitive anxiety as a function of speaker role for fluent speakers and persons who stutter. Journal of Fluency Disorders 28(3), 167–186.

DiLollo, A., Manning, W. H., & Neimeyer, R. A. (2005). Cognitive complexity as a function of speaker role for adult persons who stutter. Journal of Constructivist Psychology 18, 215–236.

DiLollo, A., Neimeyer, R. A., & Manning, W. H. (2002). A personal construct psychology view of relapse: Indications for a narrative therapy component to stuttering treatment. Journal of Fluency Disorders 27, 19–42.

Dimaggio, G., Salvatore, G., Azzara, C., & Catania, D. (2003). Rewriting self-narratives: The therapeutic process. Journal of Constructivist Psychology 16, 155–181.

Drewery, W., & Winslade, J. (1997). The theoretical story of narrative therapy. In G. Monk, J. Winslade, K. Crocket, & D. Epston (Eds.), Narrative therapy in practice: The archaeology of hope. San Francisco: Jossey-Bass Publishers.

Epston, D., & White, M. (1999). Termination as a right of passage: Questioning strategies for a therapy of inclusion. In R. A. Neimeyer, & R. J. Mahoney (Eds.), Constructivism in psychotherapy. Washington, DC: American Psychological Association.

Fransella, F. (1972). Personal change and reconstruction. London: Academic Press.

Fransella, F. (2003). International Handbook of Personal Construct Psychology. West Sussex, England: John Wiley & Sons.

Freeman, J., Epston, D., & Lobovits, D. (1997). Playful approaches to serious problems. New York: W.W. Norton & Company, Inc.

Garber, A. (1973). Psychodramatic treatment of a stutterer. Group Psychotherapy and Psychodrama 26, 34–47.

Gregory, C. B. (2003). Counseling and stuttering therapy. In H. H. Gregory (Ed.), Stuttering therapy: Rationale and procedures. (pp. 263–296). Boston: Allyn & Bacon.

Gregory, H. H. (1986). Environmental manipulation and family counseling. In G. H. Shames & H. Rubin (Eds.), Stuttering then and now (pp. 273–291). Columbus, OH: Charles E. Merrill Publishing.

Jezer, M. (1997). Stuttering: a life bound up in words. New York: Basic Books.

Johnson, W., & Associates. (1959). The onset of stuttering. Minneapolis, MN: University of Minnesota Press.

Kaplan, N. R., & Kaplan, M. L. (1978) The Gestalt approach to stuttering. Journal of Communication Disorders 11:1–9.

Kelly, G. A. (1955). The psychology of personal constructs (Vol. 1). New York: Norton.

Korzybski, A. (1933), Science and sanity. New York: International Non-Aristotelian Library.

Kubler-Ross, E. (1969). On death and dying. New York: Macmillan.

Kuhr, A.,& Rustin, L.(1985). The maintenance of fluency after intensive inpatient therapy: Long-term follow-up. Journal of Fluency Disorders 10, 229–236.

Landfield, A. W., & Leitner, L. M. (1980). Personal construct psychology. In A. W. Landfield & L. M. Leitner (Eds.), Personal construct psychology. New York: John Wiley & Sons.

Luterman, D. M. (2001). Counseling persons with communication disorders and their families (4th ed.). Austin, TX: PRO-ED.

Madigan, S. P., & Goldner, E. M. (1998). A narrative approach to anorexia. In M. F. Hoyt (Ed.), The handbook of constructive therapies: Innovative approaches from leading practitioners. San Francisco: Jossey-Bass Publishers.

Manning, W. H. (2001). Clinical decision making in fluency disorders (2nd ed.). Vancouver, Canada: Singular.

Manning, W. H. (2006). Therapeutic change and the nature of our evidence: improving our ability to help. In N. Bernstein Ratner & J. Tetnowski (Eds.). Current issues in stuttering research and practice. Mahwah, NJ: Lawrence Erlbaum Assoc.

McCabe, A., & Bliss, L. S. (2003). Patterns of narrative discourse: A multicultural lifespan approach. Boston, MA: Allyn and Bacon.

McKenzie, W., & Monk, G. (1997). Learning and teaching narrative ideas. In G. Monk, J. Winslade, K. Crocket, & D. Epston (Eds.), Narrative therapy in practice: The archaeology of hope. San Francisco: Jossey-Bass Publishers.

Menzies, R. G., Onslow, M., & Packman, A. (1999). Anxiety and stuttering: Exploring a complex relationship. American Journal of Speech-Language Pathology, 8, 3-10.

Messenger, M., Onslow, M., Packman, A., & Menzies, R. (2004). Social anxiety in stuttering: Measuring negative social expectancies. Journal of Fluency Disorders, 29, 201-212.

Miller, S., & Watson, B. G. (1992). The relationship between communication attitude, anxiety, and depression in stutterers and nonstutterers. Journal of Speech and Hearing Research, 35,789-798.

Moses, K. L. (1985). Dynamic intervention with families. In E. Cherow (Ed.), Hearing impaired children and youth with disabilities. Washington, DC: Galludet College Press.

Neimeyer, R. A. (1999). An invitation to Constructivist psychotherapies. In R. A. Neimeyer & M. J. Mahoney (Eds.), Constructivism in Psychotherapy. Washington, DC: American Psychological Association.

Neimeyer, R. A. (2000). Lessons of loss. Keystone Heights, FL: PsychoEducational Resources, Inc.

Neimeyer, R. A. (2001). The language of loss. In R. A. Neimeyer (Ed.), Meaning reconstruction and the experience of loss. Washington, DC: American Psychological Association.

Nystul, M. S., & Muszynska, E. Adlerian treatment of a classical case of stuttering. Journal of Individual Psychology 32, 194–202.

Onslow, M., Packman, A., & Harrison, E. (2003). The Lidcombe Program of early stuttering intervention. Austin, TX: PRO-ED.

Parry, A., & Doan, R. E. (1994). Story re-visions: Narrative therapy in the postmodern world. New York: Guilford Press.

Patterson, C. H. (1985). The therapeutic relationship: Foundations for an eclectic psychotherapy. Pacific Grove, CA: Brooks/Cole.

Payne, M. (2000). Narrative therapy: An introduction for counsellors. Thousand Oaks, CA: SAGE Publications.

Raskin, J. D. (2002). Constructivism in psychology: Personal Construct Psychology, Radical Constructivism, and Social Constructivism. In J. D. Raskin & S. K. Bridges (Eds). Studies in Meaning: Exploring constructivist psychology, (pp.l-26). New York: Pace University Press.

Ratner, N. B., & Guitar, B. (2005). Treatment of very early stuttering and parent-administered therapy: The state of the art. In N. Bernstein Ratner & J. Tetnowski (Eds.) Current issues in stuttering research and practice. Mahwah, NJ: Lawrence Erlbaum Assoc.

Rollin, W. J. (2000). Counseling individuals with communication disorders: Psychodynamic and family aspects (2nd ed.). Boston: Butterworth-Heinemann.

Sax, P. (1997). Narrative therapy and family support: Strengthening the mother's voice in working with families with infants and toddlers. In C. Smith & D. Nylund (Eds.), Narrative therapies with children and adolescents. (pp. 111–146). New York: The Guilford Press.

Shames, G. H. (2000). Counseling the communicatively disabled and their families. Needham Heights, MA: Allyn & Bacon.

Starkweather, C. W. (1986). Talking with the parents of young stutterers. In E. C. Healey (Ed.), Readings in stuttering. (pp.145–154). New York: Longman.

Starkweather, C. W. (1997). Therapy for younger children. In R. R. Curlee & G. M. Siegel (Eds.), Nature and treatment of stuttering, 2nd edition (pp. 257–279). Boston: Allyn and Bacon.

Tanner, D. C. (1980). Loss and grief: Implications for the speech-language pathologist and audiologist. ASHA 22, 916–928.

Vanryckeghem, M., Brutten, G. J., & Hernandez, L. H. (2005). A comparative investigation of the speech-associated attitude of preschool and kindergarten children who do and do not stutter. Journal of Fluency Disorders, 30, 307-318.

Wampold, B. E. (2001). The great psychotherapy debate: Models, methods, and findings. Mahwah, NJ: Lawrence Erlbaum Associates.

Webster, E. J. (1977). Counseling with parents of handicapped children. San Diego, CA: College-Hill Press.

White, M. (1995). Re-authoring lives: Interviews and essays. Adelaide, Australia: Dulwich Centers Publications.

White, M., & Epston, D. (1990). Narrative means to therapeutic ends. New York: W.W. Norton & Company.

Williams, D. E. (1957). A point of view about stuttering. Journal of Speech and Hearing Disorders, 22, 390-397.

Winslade, J., & Monk G. (1999). Narrative counseling in schools: Powerful and brief. Thousand Oaks, CA: Corwin Press, Inc.

Yairi, E., & Ambrose, N. G. (2005). Early childhood stuttering: For clinicians by clinicians. Austin, TX: PRO-ED.

Appendix 7.1

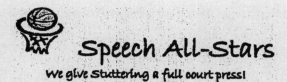

Speech All-Stars

We give Stuttering a full court press!

June 31, 2005

Dear "David,"

What an exciting couple of weeks we've had! Over these past two weeks, we have talked a lot about the three "tough guys" on Stuttering's team: Stuttering, Teasing, and Fear. You know how these guys play the game—they're tough, sometimes they even play "dirty"! And now you have shown that you know how to stand up to them and beat them at their own game. By writing your story about how Stuttering, Teasing, and Fear try to take over your life, you explained that they are nothing but "bullies and wimps" who like to make you feel like you are weak. But guess what David? In this game, you are the MVP! By blocking Fear and learning to be your own self advocate, you were able to slam-dunk Stuttering and steal the ball from his good friend Teasing! You stood up to them many times in the games we played and you didn't let them stop you from getting to the basket!

Not only do you know how to stand up to Teasing and how to beat Fear, but you also know how to take the game away from Stuttering. As you told us, you have certain moves that Stuttering can't handle, like slowing down you're speech, starting out your sentences with a "light touch," and "stretching out your sounds." We talked about how these moves make Stuttering mad because YOU are controlling the game. Remember David: even though Stuttering can seem huge at times, you know how to beat him. YOU can control the game!

Enclosed, you will find a certificate that celebrates what you have accomplished these past two weeks. I hope that you will enjoy what it has to say and that you will take time to look at it often.

Take care,

Coach Mike

Speech All-Stars

We give Stuttering a Full-Court Press!

Congratulations "David"!

Over these past two weeks, you have demonstrated the exceptional ability to:

Slam-dunk Stuttering!
Block fear!
Post-up against Teasing!
And
Take control of the game!

Way to go "David"!

June 31, 2005

Appendix 7.2

Resources on Stuttering and Child Development for Parents and Clinicians
of Children Who Stutter

Stuttering and Counseling

1. Stuttering Foundation of America: Ph. 1–800–992–9392 (www. stutteringhelp.org)

    Books:

    - The school-age child who stutters: Working effectively with attitudes and emotions (Publication No. 5)

    - If your child stutters: A guide for parents, 6th edition (Publication No. 11)

    - Stuttering and your child: Questions and answers (3rd ed.) (Publication No. 22)

    Videos:

    - Listening to and talking with parents of children who stutter (Video No. 0122)

    - The school-age child who stutters: Working effectively with attitudes and emotions (Video No. 0085)

    - The school-age child who stutters: Dealing effectively with guilt and shame (Video No. 0086)

    - Counseling parents of children who stutter (Video No. 0090)

2. The Stuttering Home Page (http://www.mnsu.edu/comdis/kuster/) provides extensive links to resources for clinicians and parents.

3. Payne, M. (2000). Narrative therapy: An introduction for counsellors. Thousand Oaks, CA: SAGE Publications (Primarily for clinicians interested in the narrative approach to counseling)

4. Home page of the Dulwich Centre (http://www.dulwichcentre.com.au/), a primary source for narrative therapy training and information

Child development

Books:

Phelan, T. W. (2003). 1–2–3– Magic: Effective discipline for children 2–12. Parentmagic Inc.

Zrzour, K. (2000). Facing the schoolyard bully. Firefly Books.

Stein, M. B., & Walker, J. R. (2003). Triumph over shyness. McGraw-Hill.

Faber, A., & Mazlish, E. (1999). How to talk so kids will listen & listen so kids will talk. HarperResource.

Support groups

National Stuttering Association (NSA). Ph. 800–937–8888 (www.nsastutter.org)

Friends, National Association of Young People Who Stutter. Ph. 866–866–8335 (www.friendswhostutter.org)

8

The Comprehensive Stuttering Program for School-Age Children with Strategies for Managing Teasing and Bullying

Marilyn Langevin, Deborah A. Kully, and Beverly Ross-Harold

The purpose of this chapter is to describe the Comprehensive Stuttering Program for School-Age Children (CSP-SC) and the strategies for managing teasing and bullying that are embedded in the program. The CSP-SC has been developed at the Institute for Stuttering Treatment and Research (ISTAR) at the University of Alberta (Canada) over a 20-year period (see Kully & Boberg, 1991). In developing the program we drew from the work of many clinicians and researchers[1] (see Langevin & Kully, 2003). Before describing the program in detail, we begin with a brief overview of its focus and the age group for which it was developed. We hope that the reader will acquire an understanding of the goals and components of the CSP-SC and the differing needs and responses of children treated with the program.

◆ Overview

The CSP-SC is an integrated treatment program that addresses both overt stuttering and the attitudinal-emotional consequences of stuttering. It is designed for children 7 to 12 years of age for whom comprehensive therapy is warranted. This is a broad age range with great differences in cognitive, emotional, social, and academic development. Thus, it is critical that treatment goals be adjusted to match the child's capabilities in these domains. Such adjustments will be illustrated in four case examples that are included to illustrate clinical decision making as well as variations in treatment response and outcomes in the CSP-SC. The procedures described herein represent the current status of the CSP-SC as it is delivered in a 4-week intensive format with six to eight children. However, the components and procedures represent the core set of therapy principles, concepts, and techniques that are drawn on to design therapy for children who participate in other formats delivered in the clinic or via telehealth (Kully, 2002).

---

[1]Due to space limitations in this chapter and because these references have been cited in Langevin and Kully (2003), we have opted to refer readers to that publication. This is in no way intended to undervalue the contributions of the work of these researchers and clinicians, and we again acknowledge their contributions that have influenced our work and the development of the CSP-SC.

◆ Treatment Goals and Components

The four basic treatment goals of the CSP-SC are as follows:

1. *Speech-related goals* include: (1) the ability to use fluency-enhancing skills in all speaking environments with approximately normal sounding prosody and rate; (2) the ability to manage residual stuttering; and (3) improved communication skills.

2. *Attitudinal-emotional goals* include development of: (1) positive attitudes toward communication; (2) comfort with and openness about stuttering and fluency enhancing skills; (3) reduced avoidance behavior; (4) the ability to manage fear and anxiety; (5) the ability to handle regression (i.e., increased frequency of stuttering) and recognize when relapse (i.e., return to pretreatment stuttering frequency) is occurring (to the extent that it is possible for children); (6) improved social skills and confidence; and (7) the ability to deal with teasing, bullying, and negative listener reactions.

3. *Self-management goals* include development of: (1) problem-solving skills; (2) self-monitoring, self-evaluation, and self-reinforcement skills (see Chapter 18, this volume); (3) the ability to manage the environment to support needs (e.g., asking peers to not interrupt); and (4) the ability to plan practice activities.

4. *Environmental* goals include development of parental understanding of: (1) the etiology and development of stuttering; (2) the process of speech and attitudinal change; (3) how to manage environmental variables that support or disrupt the child's fluency; (4) how to participate in and deliver therapy; (5) how to deal with regression and relapse; and (6) bullying management principles and strategies.

To achieve the aforementioned goals, the CSP-SC employs three main components. The first component teaches fluency-enhancing skills, the second addresses attitudes and emotions, and the third incorporates parents and family into therapy. **Table 8–1** outlines the concepts, strategies, and techniques that constitute each of the components. Although the components are delivered in an integrated way, they will be discussed separately.

Table 8–1 Components of the Comprehensive Stuttering Program for School-Age Children (CSP-SC)

1. Teaching Fluency-Enhancing Skills		
Acquisition	Identification or Speech Production Awareness	Discuss speech processes and Identify locus of occlusion
	Introduction to Fluency Enhancing Skills Tension modification Prolongation (Stretch) Easy breathing (EB) Gentle Starts (GS) Smooth Blending (SB) Light touches (LT) Self-correction (Fixes; re-breathe) 3-T's (Think, Take a breath, Talk)	⟷ Training Steps for Introduction to Each Skill* 1. Discuss rationale (goal) for skill 2. Describe and model skill 3. Describe, model, and have child identify errors in skill production 4. Shape and practice skill 5. Develop self-evaluation 6. Apply criterion step 7. Check comprehension 8. Design and execute home practice
	Prolongation Rate and Skill Refinement Slow stretch (40–60 SPM) Medium stretch (60–90 SPM)	⟷ Cycle Through Skills Sessions* Stretch → EB → GS → SB → LT → All Skills

(Continued)

Slight stretch (90–120+ SPM)   → Fixes (re-breathes; pull-outs; rate
                                              change†) → 3-T's → Self-Evaluation
                                              ↓
                                              Criterion Step

Transfer   Preparation for Transfer   → Beyond Clinic Transfers
               Fluency skills in off-task talking   Simulated school day
               "Remembers"   Field trips
               "Forgets"   Shopping trips
               Stretch zones   Track and field (sports)
               Reinforcement for naturally   Usual life activities, e.g., going to library,
                 occurring fluent speech   ordering food, telephone, shopping

Maintenance   Home Practice   ↔ SLP Sessions
               Sit-down practice   Contingency based, or as requested
               Remembers   by parents
               Planned transfers
               Severity ratings

	2. Attitude-Emotions	**3. Involving Parent/Family in Therapy**

Acquisition ↕ **Transfer**	Feelings about stuttering
	Cause of stuttering
	Acceptance of stuttering
	Acceptance of fluency skills
	Openness
	Avoidance/coping skills
	Listeners who interrupt
	Effective communication strategies
	Self-perceptions and self-talk
	Teasing and bullying
	  Bullying behaviors
	  Hurtful teasing – Non-hurtful teasing
	  Differences, self-acceptance, respecting
	    and celebrating differences
	  Feelings
	  Why kids bully
	  How kids who bully can be helped to
	    stop bullying
	  Coping strategies: Helpful and not-helpful
	    strategies and conflict resolution strategies
	  Reasons why children don't report bullying
	  Tattling vs responsible reporting
	  Maintaining or re-gaining power
		Model and reinforce fluency skills
		Sequence speech practice
		Reinforce naturally occurring fluent speech
		Reinforce self-corrections of stutters
		Primary agents for reinforcement in
		  beyond-clinic transfers
		Daily home practice (speech and
		  attitude-emotional)
		Severity ratings
		Parent Meeting Topics
		  Cause and development of stuttering
		  Environmental fluency facilitators and
		    disruptors
		  Maintenance
		  Preparing family and friends
		  Educating teachers
		  Teasing and bullying
		  Bullying behaviors
		  Frequency and nature of bullying
		Role of bystanders
		  Coping strategies
		  Principles of intervention
		  Working with school personnel

Maintenance	Continued attention to attitude and emotional issues	Home practice activities (described above) Seek support from SLP as needed Liaise with school personnel

*Naturalness (i.e.,vocal quality, pitch, and prosody) is shaped throughout fluency skill practice sessions as needed.

†Rate changes are introduced at the medium stretch rate of prolongation.

SPM, syllables per minute.

As depicted in **Table 8–1**, therapy involves several interdependent phases: (1) *acquisition*: children and parents acquire the skills to manage the child's speech and relevant attitudinal-emotional issues; (2) *transfer*: skills learned in acquisition are transferred to everyday life situations and environments; and (3) *maintenance*: fluency, attitudinal-emotional, and environmental management goals are monitored and supported through ongoing practice. Transition from one phase to the next is fluid. For example, throughout acquisition children and parents are being prepared for transfer and maintenance.

During acquisition and transfer, fluency-enhancing skill sessions are delivered in small groups of 2 children to 1 clinician. There are also large-group activities to promote generalization of fluency skills. In the attitudinal-emotional component, therapy is delivered in large-group, small-group, and individual sessions. In the parent/family component, both large-group and individual meetings are undertaken.

◆ Case Examples

Prior to describing the components of the CSP-SC, we present the case examples to which references are made throughout this chapter. **Table 8–2** presents: (1) pretreatment age and stuttering severity; (2) distinguishing stuttering behaviors; (3) response to therapy in terms of: levels of utterance length and complexity achieved at each rate of prolongation, percentage of utterances prolonged in transfer, and post-treatment speech outcome for each case. All case patient examples are boys. Cases 1 to 3 are typical of girls and boys treated in the program. Case Patient 4 is a boy with profoundly severe stuttering who had an atypical response to therapy in that he did not become stutter-free during prolongation.

◆ Components

Fluency Enhancing Skills

As shown in **Table 8–1**, acquisition comprises identification, introduction to fluency enhancing skills, and prolongation rate and skill refinement stages. In the introduction to fluency skills stage, eight training steps are used to introduce each fluency skill. In the prolongation rate and skill refinement stage, increases in prolongation rates and utterance length and complexity are achieved in "Cycle Through Skills sessions" that comprise nine steps. Movement from one prolongation rate to another is marked by a criterion step. Transfer comprises strategies that prepare the children for transfer, followed by beyond-clinic transfers. Finally, maintenance comprises home practice and speech-language pathologist (SLP) sessions.

Speech practice is designed to move children from short, simple, and highly structured speaking tasks to increasingly complex and natural exchanges while ensuring that high levels of skill production and fluency are attained. Naturalness is shaped throughout all practice. (See **Table 12–3** in Kully, Langevin and Lomhein [chapter 12] for presentation of variables manipulated in this program).

Acquisition

In this chapter, references to "fluency enhancing skills" include fluency skills (e.g., easy onsets, soft contacts) and stuttering management techniques (e.g., pull-outs, Van Riper, 1973).

Identification (Speech Production Awareness)   Clinicians guide children through an exploration of the physiological systems involved in speech (i.e., respiration, phonation, and articulation; e.g., see Conture, 2001). Clinicians model stutters and have children identify the place of occlusion. Children then identify where their own stutters ("sticks" and "bumps") occur. It is thought that this activity demystifies stuttering and helps children learn that stuttering is a physical interference of the smooth flow of speech.

Introduction to Fluency-Enhancing Skills   The fluency-enhancing skills outlined in **Table 8–1** are described in detail below. Children who participate in the intensive program generally learn all of

Table 8–2 Presenting Stuttering Profile, Utterance Length and Complexity at Criterion Steps, Percentage Utterances Prolonged in Transfer, and Speech Outcomes for Four Case Examples

Case (initials; age)	Case 1 (ST; 7 y)	Case 2 (MA; 8 y, 7 mo)	Case 3 (JS; 9 y)	Case 4 (CH; 11 y)
Presenting Stuttering Profile				
Stuttering severity	Moderate-severe	Moderate-severe	Moderate-severe	Profoundly severe
Distinguishing stuttering behaviors	Lengthy prolonged repetitions; multiple final consonant repetitions	Pitch rises; pressurized articulatory contacts	Multiple within word sound repetitions (e.g., hi-i-i-t); silent prolongations of 4–6 seconds	Pronounced oral tension; audible and silent prolongations
Utterance Length and Complexity Achieved in Criterion Steps at Each Rate of Prolongation				
Slow stretch	5 BG in R; 8 BG in PD	25 BG in R; 20 BG in PD	4 BG in R and PD	3 BG in R and Cr
Medium stretch	30 seconds in R and combined PD and Q/A	1 minute in R and combined PD and Q/A	5 BG in R and PD	4 BG in R and in combined Cr, PD, and Q/A
Slight stretch	30 seconds in R and combined Q/A and Conv	1.5 minutes in R, Q/A, and Conv	5 BG in R; 1.5 minutes in combined Q/A and Conv	2 BG in R; 30 seconds in PD
Percentage of Utterances Prolonged in Transfer				
Less exciting transfers	70–90%	50–70%	80–90%	70%–90%
More exciting transfers	20–30%	0–40%	80–90%	70%–90%
Speech Outcome				
%SS	Pre = 8.0; Post = 2.0; 7 months FU = 7.0; 19 months FU = 2.0	Pre = 11.5; Post = 2.0; 15 months FU = 5.50	Pre = 6.53[*]; Post = 1.50[†]; 4 to 5 months FU = 2.4[*]	Pre = 54.4; Post = 24.0; 3 months FU = 46.0

[*]Mean of R, Conv, and explanation.
[†]Mean of R and Conv.

BG, breath-groups; Conv, conversation; Cr, carrier; FU, follow-up; PD, picture description; Pre, pretreatment; Post, immediate post-treatment; Q/A, question/answer; R, reading; %SS, percent syllables stuttered.

the fluency-enhancing skills; however, the weighting or emphasis for some children will differ. For example, Case Patient 4's pronounced oral tension and diminished response to the fluency-evoking effects of prolongation required increased emphasis on tension modification and self-correction throughout therapy.

Fluency-enhancing skills are generally introduced in the sequence set out in **Table 8–1** using the eight training steps also described therein. For brevity, only those steps requiring elaboration (i.e., the fourth through eighth steps) are discussed next: (4) *Shape and practice skill:* The skill is established at the lowest level of utterance length and complexity necessary, and practice progresses through the hierarchies of length, complexity, cueing, and feedback; (5) *Develop self-evaluation:* Children's ability to self-monitor and self-evaluate speech production and make changes in speech patterns is developed. The criterion is 80% accuracy in self-evaluating skill production at the utterance length and complexity that is appropriate for the child. We use a 3-point rating scale that employs a basketball analogy for self-evaluation: 1 = perfect production (slam dunk); 2 = almost (rim ball: an element of the skill is missing or needs improvement); and 3 = missed (air ball). For example, if a child's production is prolonged but is not at the target rate (e.g., slow stretch), a self-rating of 2 would be the correct evaluation; (6) *Apply criterion step:* A criterion of 80% accuracy in spontaneous production (i.e., the only cue is the clinician's instruction to produce the skill) is targeted; however, the utterance length and complexity will differ for each child; (7) *Check comprehension:* A workbook is used that contains exercises that ask children to describe in their own words how each fluency skill helps speech. A formal comprehension check ends the introduction of each fluency skill and ends the introduction to the fluency-enhancing skills stage; (8) *Design and execute home practice:* Parents and children carry out daily home practice to reinforce skills learned in therapy, set the stage for generalization, and prepare the child and parent to continue with speech management during maintenance. Children are active participants in designing home practice. They choose words, sentences, readings, or discussion topics and themes that are of interest (e.g., hockey, horses). Parents learn to sequence practice activities and to manipulate the length, complexity, and spontaneity of utterances. In introducing each fluency-enhancing skill, we will further elaborate only on the "shape and practice" step to illustrate the core therapeutic procedures used in teaching each skill.

Tension Modification   Modifying a stutter by reducing tension is a foundational stuttering management skill. It is introduced first because (1) we want to establish early that stutters are not to be feared and that it is possible to modify them; and (2) it lays the foundation for subsequent self-correction skills (i.e., pull-outs and preventive rate changes; Van Riper, 1973). When tension is detected, it is released slowly and completely before continuing with phonation. A 10-point rating scale is used to shape tension modification (10 = high tension; 2 = minimal tension; 1 = normal articulatory or laryngeal tension). Various levels of tension are simulated (e.g., a 9 or a 5) and released until a tension level of 1 is achieved.

Prolongation   Fluent speech is first established at a prolongation rate of 40 to 60 syllables per minute (SPM). Vowels are prolonged and transitions through consonants are slowed but not prolonged. Natural prosody is approximated by ensuring that stressed syllables are prolonged more than unstressed syllables and that natural pitch and volume are maintained. As an introduction to prolongation, the clinician uses a rubber band analogy to explain how children will learn to "stretch" their speech to help them have smooth speech. Thereafter the term *stretch* is used throughout the program. Practice progresses from vowels to bisyllabic or trisyllabic words using word cards or work sheets and picture card stimuli.

Easy Breathing (EB)   Easy breathing (EB) develops an inspiration and expiration cycle that is appropriate for phonation and is characterized by a relaxed movement of the abdominal muscles and chest wall. The inspiration is full (but it does not exceed normal lung volume), unrushed, and has a diaphragmatic locus. Movement into expiration is smooth, and phrasing or "breath-grouping" is appropriate. The term *breath-groups* is used to help clients break their utterances into phrases or sentences that are manageable for the normal expiration cycle. As prolongation rates increase, breath-groups will comprise increasing numbers of syllables. Shaping practice progresses from producing EB without phonation (quiet breathing) to producing EB with phonation. Ideally, utterance length progresses from one breath-group to five consecutive breath-groups using monosyllabic words.

Gentle Starts   Gentle starts (GS) are used at the beginning of all breath-groups, whether consonant or vowel initiated. For children 8 years of age and older, a GS is characterized by a slow, smooth initiation of speech with a slight pre-voice expiration and a gradual increase in loudness. Full loudness is achieved within the first syllable of the breath-group. For children younger than 8 years of age, a GS is described as a slow, smooth initiation of speech. No mention is made of a pre-voice expiration for this age group because bringing attention to it can result in excessive loss of air given their lower lung volumes. Shaping begins with vowels, followed by vowel- and then consonant-initiated monosyllabic words.[2]

Smooth Blending (also called "Hooking" or "Linking")   In smooth blending (SB), airflow is continuous and there is smooth continuous movement of articulators within breath-groups. The manner or voicing characteristics of phonemes are preserved. Thus, continuous airflow does not imply voicing of unvoiced phonemes. Shaping begins with two unrelated monosyllabic words and progresses to two related monosyllabic words on one breath-group to form a phrase.

Light Touches   Lights touches (LT) are used on consonants *within* breath-groups. They prevent stutters on consonants by minimizing oral tension. In contrast, GS are used on consonants at the *beginning* of breath-groups. Articulatory contacts are lightened but remain distinct. The manner (voicing) of phoneme production is preserved. Shaping begins with bisyllabic words in one breath-group and progresses to multisyllabic words in one breath-group.

Self-Correction (Re-Breathe, Pull-Outs, and Rate Changes)   Self-correction strategies are collectively referred to as "fixes." Once all types of self-corrections have been established, children are encouraged to self-select the type of fix that they believe is necessary to modify or prevent a stutter. Although, as indicated in Table 8–1 (see Cycle Through Skills Sessions), rate changes are not introduced until the Prolongation Rate Increase and Skill Refinement stage of therapy, they are described here. Re-breathe fixes involve stopping when stuttering is detected, gradually releasing tension and breath, and re-initiating speech with an easy breath and gentle start. Pull-out fixes involve stopping when stuttering is detected, gradually releasing tension and moving smoothly to the next sound. Rate-change fixes involve reducing the rate if speech feels unstable prior to an expected stutter (preventive) or after a stutter has occurred (recovery). Shaping of re-breathe fixes progresses from simulations of stutters at the larynx (e.g., "He ate it), to velars, palatals, alveolars, and bilabials in three to four syllable phrases. Later practice incorporates the child's stuttering pattern and feared sounds and words if any. Shaping of pull-out fixes progresses from monosyllabic to multisyllabic words and then to three to four syllable phrases. Shaping of rate changes progresses from reading sentences in paragraphs to practice while talking.

3-T's (Resisting Time Pressure)   The 3-T's consolidate into a specific skill, time pressure activities that formerly had been introduced in the transfer phase (Kully & Boberg, 1991). This skill is introduced in acquisition to give clients more time to stabilize their ability to resist time pressures that disrupt ongoing speech-language production. The 3-T's skill comprises three sequential elements: **T**hink before speaking, **T**ake time to breathe, and **T**alk using fluency skills (or "smooth speech" in the later stages of therapy). During the "Think" stage children are encouraged to think about: (1) taking time to start talking; (2) what they want to say and how they will say it; and (3) what speech skills they will use. Because it is difficult for a child to actively go through the Think stage, we first encourage

---

[2]If a child has pronounced laryngeal tension on vowels and vowel initiated words and has difficulty achieving a GS, we will revert to a training progression that starts with consonant-vowel nonsense syllables or words and then fade out the consonant (e.g., da → a; or me → e; or can → an → a).

the child to silently count to 3 during this stage. This step is systematically reduced to a count of 1 to simulate a functional pause. Shaping begins in an easy question/answer task.

Prolongation Rate Increase and Skill Refinement   Slow, medium, and slight prolongation rates are outlined in **Table 8–1**. As indicated above, within each prolongation rate, increases in rate (e.g., moving from 60 to 90 SPM in medium stretch) and refinement of fluency skills are achieved through a series of Cycle Through Skills sessions ("cycle sessions"). To keep speech practice enjoyable, it is performed within the context of games and physical activities. As shown in **Table 8–1**, a cycle session consists of a sequence of fluency skill practice in which focus systematically changes from one skill to another. In the cycle sessions, children progress from focusing on stretch to EB, GS, SB, and LT to practice in which all skills are produced simultaneously (All Skills). However, an All Skills session is not introduced into the cycle until sufficient accuracy with each skill has been achieved. For some children All Skills practice will be included in the later cycle sessions in slow stretch. For others it will be introduced in the early stages of medium stretch. For each cycle session the goal for utterance length and complexity is set. Increases in length and complexity are achieved over a series of cycle sessions.

In slow stretch and the early stages of medium stretch, utterance length is increased by systematically increasing the number of consecutive breath-groups in a talking turn. Generally, when children are capable of sustaining medium stretch in an All Skills session in four or more consecutive breath-groups, utterance length is then increased by timing speech. At first, utterance length is increased in 10-second intervals until 30 seconds of sustained prolongation is achieved. Thereafter, children are often able to increase in 15- to 30-second intervals.

The complexity of talking tasks progresses from bisyllabic words or phrases (in the first cycle session in slow stretch) to carrier phrase, then to self-formulated sentences, question/answer exchanges, monologue,[3] and conversation (in slight stretch). The length and complexity goal for the *first* cycle session in slow stretch is one breath-group utterances using trisyllabic words or phrases from various stimuli. However, for children who acquire fluency skills easily, the goal may be two consecutive breath-groups. Movement up the hierarchies of length and complexity is not stringently programmed. That is, clinicians "superstep" (move up several levels quickly or skip levels if appropriate) or "substep" (return to previous levels to reestablish stability) as is appropriate for each child. For example, in the intensive program in which Case Patient 2 participated, the goal for completion of the first cycle for the group as a whole was two breath-groups in stretch in reading and two breath-groups in production of trisyllabic words and phrases. At the end of the first cycle session, Case Patient 2 had achieved two breath-groups in reading trisyllabic words, two breath-groups in EB in bisyllabic words, one breath-group in GS in bisyllabic words, and one breath-group in SB and LT in trisyllabic words.

In each intensive program group goals for length and complexity are set daily. Goals are based on: (1) the average length and complexities achieved by children in the intensive clinics over many years; and (2) the average performance of the group of children being treated. Our goal for each child is to have him or her be as stutter-free as possible in conversation at the end of the 4-week program. Each child's route to that goal, that is movement through hierarchies of length and complexity, will be different and will be influenced by stuttering severity, age, and cognitive, linguistic, and academic abilities.

Generally it takes 1.5 to 2 hours of treatment to complete the first cycle. Thereafter, a cycle session is programmed for each half-hour treatment session. That is, the focus shifts from skill to skill in the sequence described within a half-hour session. Within each session, efforts are made to move the child to the highest possible level of length and complexity. The range of cycle sessions required to complete each rate of prolongation is (1) two to three sessions for

---

[3]Monologue tasks are usually embedded within question/answer tasks that require longer answers. For example, clinicians will ask a question about a topic about which they know the child can speak at length.

slow stretch; (2) six to eight sessions for medium stretch; and (3) five to eight sessions for slight stretch.

The criterion for movement from one prolongation rate to the next is 80% accuracy in an All Skills session[4] at a rate that is: (1) near the upper limit of the range (i.e., for slow stretch the target end rate is 50–60 SPM); and (2) is at the highest possible utterance length and complexity that is appropriate for the child. The case examples illustrate the different lengths and complexities at which the criterion may be achieved. As shown in **Table 8–2**, length and complexity achieved in the criterion steps differ for each child. For example, in the criterion step for slow stretch, Case Patient 2 achieved utterance lengths of 25 and 20 consecutive breath-groups in reading and picture description, respectively. In contrast, the number of consecutive breath-groups ranged from 3 breath-groups in reading and carrier phrase for Case Patient 4, to 5 in reading and 8 in picture description for Case Patient 1. The utterance length and complexities achieved by Case Patient 1 are typical of 7-years-olds. Case Patient 2 acquired and achieved accurate production of fluency skills easily and thus was easily able to increase utterance length. The levels he achieved in slow stretch are more typical of 10- to 12-year-olds than 8- to 9-year-olds; however, the levels achieved in medium and slight stretch are typical of 8- to 12-year-olds with stuttering severities that range from mild to severe. Case Patient 3's levels in slow and medium stretch reflect the difficulty he had in acquiring fluency skills. For both Case Patients 3 and 4, timing of speech was not introduced until slight stretch, and it was not introduced in reading for either child. Case Patient 4's levels reflect the profound severity of his stuttering. His rate of prolongation remained at the lower end of slight stretch (i.e., 90–100 SPM) because he was not able to achieve stutter-free speech at higher speech rates. As a consequence, Case Patient 4 required additional therapy.

Transfer

Preparation for Transfer   Preparation for transfer begins early in the CSP-SC with strategies that are designed to promote generalization of fluency-enhancing skills beyond the clinic room. Strategies include those that target (1) use of fluency skills in "off-task" talking (see below); (2) self-correction in off-task talking; and (3) manipulation of environmental variables. Furthermore, children are transitioned from receiving feedback for use of fluency skills to receiving feedback for fluent speech achieved with or without the use of skills.

Off-task talking refers to natural exchanges between the child and clinician that are made in the course of therapy and outside of utterances that are part of the cycle sessions. For example, if, in preparation for a cycle session, the child asks "Are we going to play tic-tac-toe?" the clinician asks "Can you say that in stretch?" When the child repeats the question in stretch, he or she is praised for doing so. The concept of using stretch in off-task talking is first introduced near the end of slow stretch. Clinician reinforcement for off-task stretch progresses from continuous to intermittent and shifts from clinician to parent administered. At the same time, children self-reinforce. That is, they chart a "remember" when they have remembered to stretch in off-task talking.

The concept of using self-corrections in off-task talking is also used to promote generalization of self-correction. When children have achieved spontaneous productions in self-correction practice in cycle sessions, clinicians model stutters that are and are not corrected. Clinicians ask the children to give feedback on whether or not the stutter was self-corrected (i.e., children's feedback is "You fixed your bump" or "You forgot to fix"). Once this behavior has been established, clinicians then ask children to fix stutters that occur in the children's off-task talking ("requests for corrections"). Use of off-task stretch and self-correction is extended from the therapy room to nontherapy environments through the use of "stretch zones" (i.e., designated areas outside of the clinic room,

---

[4]For children for whom the All Skills session is not introduced until medium stretch, the criterion will be 80% accuracy in skill production with each skill individually.

in the outdoors, and in the children's homes or accommodations). After a child has the ability to "remember" to stretch or fix in a particular zone ~50% of the time, the clinician introduces "forgets," which refers to the child forgetting to stretch or forgetting to fix. Again reinforcement is clinician-, parent-, and self-administered (i.e., the child identifies a "forget" both with and without cues from the clinician).

During slight stretch practice, environmental variables are systematically manipulated. Therapy moves from the clinic room to various locations within and outside the clinic. Children make daily mini-presentations and readings to the entire group of children to prepare for return to the classroom. Siblings, friends, grandparents, and significant others in the child's life are incorporated into therapy sessions. Games and activities become more exciting, physically demanding, time pressured, and realistic (e.g., yelling to peers across the field).

Prior to 2001, a main goal in transfer was for the children to use fluency skills as much as possible. Our intention was to stabilize the continuous use of fluency skills to set the foundation for use when needed in maintenance. As shown in **Table 8–2**, the percentage of utterances prolonged during transfer across Cases 1 to 4 indicate that it is unrealistic to expect children to sustain high levels of fluency-skill use in all situations and especially in more exciting activities. Drawing from these data (obtained prior to 2001), from behavioral learning principles, from Lincoln, Onslow, Lewis, and Wilson (1996), and from our speculation that praise for naturally occurring fluent speech may serve to build children's belief in their ability to be fluent, such praise was incorporated into the CSP-SC. In the latter stages of slight stretch, after the ability to use fluency skills is well established and children are experiencing stutter-free speech with and without use of fluency skills, children are praised for having speech that is (1) naturally fluent and (2) fluent through fluency skill use (e.g., "that was really smooth"). However, in the transfer phase focused fluency skills practice is still conducted in one cycle session each day and at specific times in transfer activities. Parents are trained to identify and praise naturally occurring fluent speech while learning to model and praise fluency skills and request self-corrections.

We recognize that the contributions to treatment outcome of several elements of the CSP-SC, including the addition of praise for naturally occurring fluent speech, require empirical assessment. As Bothe (2004) indicated, "...the relative contributions of corrective feedback, reinforcement, and systematic increases in utterance length have not been definitely defined" (p. 265). In the interim, we draw on the emerging evidence base for the CSP-SC as a total treatment program.

Beyond-Clinic Transfers During beyond clinic transfers, primary feedback for fluency skill use and naturally occurring fluent speech shifts from the child's clinician to the child's parents. Children also self-reinforce for remember and forgets. As shown in **Table 8–1**, beyond-clinic transfer activities include the following: (1) *Simulated school activities*: Two half-days of therapy are conducted at a school with a certified teacher. Each day consists of lessons in math, science, and social studies. Initially, clinicians provide cues and prompts for fluency-skill use or naturally occurring fluent speech and then fade their involvement as soon as possible. Physical activities, presentations, and recess periods are also included. If a half-day simulated classroom activity is not possible in an employment setting, clinicians may wish to conduct simulated classroom activities with a group of the child's friends. School-based clinicians may work with the child in the classroom to facilitate generalization to the classroom; (2) *Field trips*: Field trips include visits to places such as the museum, zoo, and space sciences center; (3) *Shopping trips:* Shopping trips progress from those of medium excitement (e.g., the children go from store to store to find items that are within their price range and are allowed to buy one low-cost item) to those of high excitement (e.g., the children identify desired gifts for Christmas or their birthday); (4) and *Track and field*: Track and field day includes usual activities (e.g., races, broad jump) and other physical activities (e.g., shooting baskets). Parents and clinicians participate and also receive feedback from children about their use of fluency skills. Other activities include ordering food and making phone calls that are typically made by children. If, due to liability issues, such beyond-clinic transfer activities are not possible, we suggest that any usual life activity relevant to the child be used in transfer practice.

Maintenance

As indicated earlier, parents and children are being prepared for maintenance throughout acquisition and transfer. This is achieved through: (1) parent and child participation in home practice assignments; (2) parent participation in the delivery of therapy; and (3) parent training sessions. As shown in **Table 8–1**, maintenance activities include: (1) *Sit-down practice:* During these sessions children practice fluency skills in a warm-up (i.e., a 5-minute cycle session) and then in various talking and reading activities that reflect those that naturally occur in the child's life; (2) *Remembers*: Children are reinforced and self-reinforce for (a) having smooth speech and (b) remembering to self-correct or stretch. Various incentive and charting systems may be used; (3) *Planned transfers* Parents and children decide which usual daily or special (e.g., attending a wedding) talking situation will be used for a planned transfer and they decide how the parent will give the child feedback. Prior to entering the talking situation, the parent prompts the child to use fluency skills (e.g., stretch) or smooth speech; and (4) *Severity ratings*: Parents continue to make severity ratings and use them to guide adjustments in maintenance activities. In addition to parent- and child-executed home practice, maintenance sessions with the clinician may be scheduled on a performance contingent basis (i.e., decreasing in frequency as treatment gains are maintained; see Chapter 18) or at the request of the parents.

Attitudes-Emotions

The attitudinal-emotional component of the CSP-SC comprises a series of large-group, small-group, and individual discussions that target specific concepts. Before outlining the concepts addressed, we highlight the following guiding principles: (1) Children participate only in discussions that are relevant to them. Parents and clinicians discuss the concepts to be addressed and decide if they apply to the child; (2) Discussions proceed to the extent and depth to which children are prepared to go, and children are free to decide whether or how they will participate. Some children disclose freely, whereas others choose not to disclose at all or to disclose only after a period of time has elapsed; (3) Discussions begin broadly (e.g., "What might children do to hide stuttering?") and narrow to the specific child if it appears appropriate to do so. Narrowing may occur within the group discussion if the child is quite open, or it may occur in individual discussions; and (4) Clinicians watch for moments of readiness in which children indicate in some way that they are ready to discuss attitudes or emotions.

Acquisition and Transfer

The main concepts discussed in the attitude-emotional component are outlined in **Table 8–1** and are described below. Progression from one topic to the next is fluid across acquisition and transfer. Although the topic of teasing and bullying forms part of the attitude-emotional component, it will be addressed separately in this chapter. Discussions primarily take place in the large group, with the exception of sessions on self-perceptions and self-talk, which are conducted individually and only as needed. As indicated above, not all children participate in all of the attitude-emotional discussions. For example, the parents of Case Patient 1 opted not to have him participate in the discussions about feelings and acceptance of stuttering because he was a very sensitive child. They wished to keep his treatment program more objective. That is, they wanted him only to be involved in discussions of topics that related directly to managing stuttering (e.g., dealing with listener interruptions). Mentors are also invited to talk with the children. These include young teens, older teens, and adults who have undergone therapy. Clinicians and mentors work together to ensure that the discussion addresses issues that pertain to children using child-appropriate language and depth.

Feelings about Stuttering   Feelings about stuttering are explored through discussion using webs (i.e., brainstorming maps), drawings, stories, and newsletters that feature the children's stories. Different activities are used because children differ in their preferred way of expressing their feelings.

Cause of Stuttering Discussions focus on physiological features of speech and stuttering. Children learn about the muscle groups involved in speech, and they write in their own words what happens when they stutter (e.g., "I stutter because my speech muscles get jammed up"). Children often express relief after learning about the role of physiology in stuttering.

Acceptance of Stuttering Children are encouraged to speak whether or not they stutter. Also, the concept that it is brave to speak when one stutters is introduced. As an introductory exercise, children brainstorm what it means to be brave. Often they have entertaining ideas about what one does when one is being brave, and this sets the stage for a lively discussion.

Acceptance of Fluency Skills This discussion builds on the idea of speaking whether or not one stutters and introduces the idea that being brave also means that one can use fluency skills to have smoother speech. The idea that it is important to do so for oneself despite what others might think (or what one fears others might think) is introduced. Some children readily understand and embrace this concept, whereas others remain tentative about using fluency skills in public. It is our experience that most children grasp the concept cognitively; emotionally embracing it is another matter. Case 4 provides an example of the process that operates for some children in this regard. That is, the patient used his fluency skills in the classroom only when he was ready to do so. At follow-up the child's parents reported that on returning to school he at first refused to use stretch but one day decided he needed to do so and did for 4 hours (this was confirmed by the teacher). The child told his parents that "it was something I decided I needed to do."

Also, it is acknowledged that using fluency skills is not always easy. Children brainstorm the benefits of using fluency skills and finally the following take-away message is stressed: "It is important to say exactly what you want to say, when you want to say it, whether or not you stutter, and you now have skills that can help you have smoother speech."

Openness All children go through the process of preparing a formal class presentation that they give to the large group and parents in the program, and that they can give when they return to their classrooms. This is done to facilitate the development of an open objective attitude about stuttering and to give the children the opportunity to practice terminology that they might use to educate peers and teachers about stuttering. Examples from Langevin (2000) are "I stutter because my vocal folds are banging together. It is like some semi-trucks crashing together!" (p. 163), and ". . . you can help me by letting me finish saying things myself, by listening to me, especially when I'm speaking slowly, and by being my friends. When I speak smoother I feel better." (p. 158). Other topics that children may include in their presentations are: how speech is produced (e.g., "we use our breath, voice box, teeth, tongue and lips to make sounds and talk . . . we use more than 100 muscles to talk!"); how it feels to be teased (only if appropriate); what was learned in speech classes (it is suggested that children have peers try some of the speech skills); famous people who stutter (materials from the Stuttering Foundation of America and the National Stuttering Association are made available to the children and their parents); and famous people who have overcome other problems. Children may also wish to show their easy talking video, which is an accumulation of their presentations in the program. Although all children are prepared to be able to talk about stuttering openly, not all children choose to give their presentation. For example Case Patient 2 gave his presentation to a small group of supportive friends. Case Patient 3 gave his presentation to his class and received a standing ovation. In contrast, in one sentence, Case Patient 4 told his class that he had attended a speech camp over the summer.

Avoidance/Coping Strategies This discussion is tailored to deal only with avoidances that the children have identified, and it is performed in small-group or individual sessions as needed. The discussion starts with brainstorming what children might do to cope when they have trouble talking. The benefits and disadvantages of using avoidances are then discussed. That is, it is acknowledged that "tricks" (e.g., giving the wrong answer) help children be more fluent in the short term, but in the long term they are not helpful. The concepts that it is important to say what one wants to say whether or not one stutters and that they have fluency skills that can help them have smoother speech are reinforced.

Listeners Who Interrupt   Children brainstorm and role play what they might say to peers or other listeners who interrupt and finish sentences. The underlying theme of their words is always "let me finish."

Effective Communication   Although training of effective communications skills is embedded in speech practice, we believe that it is helpful to have a session that makes these skills salient. In this discussion, children brainstorm elements of effective communication that include verbal and non-verbal behaviors (e.g., voice projection, eye contact, body posture). Scenarios then are role played. Thereafter, in presentations, children are given feedback on their effective communication skills.

Self-Perceptions and Self-Talk   We address issues of negative self-perceptions and self-talk with individual children only as needed. If necessary, self-talk that is unhelpful and helpful will be identified, specific exercises will be designed to reinforce the concept of using helpful self-talk, and reinforcements will be put in place to increase the frequency of helpful self-talk. For example, Case Patient 3's parents reported that he was perfectionistic and were concerned that he would become upset if he failed to get the fluency skills right at first try. They thought that this might affect his learning process and his response to feedback. To address these concerns, we discussed the learning process with the child. We stressed that making errors or having difficulty was part of the process and that willingness to try things was important to success. Throughout therapy he was encouraged to and reinforced for willingness to try things. This discussion set the stage for his ability to cope with the difficulties he experienced in acquiring the fluency skills.

Maintenance

In maintenance, continued attention is given by parents to attitude-emotional issues as they continue to develop and as new issues arise. Parents seek help from the SLP as needed.

Parent Involvement

Acquisition and Transfer

Fundamental to our relationship with parents is an understanding and respect for the parent-child relationship and parenting style. Throughout acquisition and transfer, parents learn to make severity ratings, model and reinforce fluency skills, sequence practice activities, reinforce fluent speech that is naturally achieved, and ask for corrections. Parents become the primary agents for reinforcement of fluent speech. In addition, parents participate in a series of meetings that address parent issues, child issues, and how to create an environment that facilitates fluency. The meetings are led by a clinician and are highly interactive. Topics are introduced, information is given, and parent discussion and problem solving occur. Individual parent meetings also occur throughout therapy to deal with issues that are pertinent to the child-parent dyad. **Table 8–1** outlines the parent involvement in the program. Below we elaborate on the main topics addressed in the parent meetings.

Cause and Development of Stuttering   A summary of current research is given that encapsulates what is known or being addressed in research in terms of the cause, development ,and psychosocial impact of stuttering.

Environmental Fluency Facilitators and Disruptors   Conditions that tend to interfere with fluency and strategies to deal with these conditions are discussed. Among conditions discussed are: time pressures, emotions (e.g., positive, negative, and those associated with discipline), language demands (e.g., questions that require long, complicated answers), negative listener reactions (e.g., advice giving by adults; negative peer reactions), fatigue, and performance pressure (e.g., high self-expectations and expectations of others).

Maintenance   This discussion focuses on parental expectations and concerns about going into the maintenance period. We discuss what to expect in maintenance, when to give feedback (i.e., praise, prompts, or requests for correction), and when to just listen. It is acknowledged that: (1) it is unrealistic to expect children to use skills all of the time and especially during exciting or emotionally charged speaking situations; (2) that there will be times when children are open to praise and requests for corrections and times when they do not want any attention given to their speech; (3) that children will vary in the degree to which they want to do any sort of practice and vary in the extent to which they want their parents involved in speech practice; and (4) that variations in willingness to receive feedback and willingness to do speech practice will occur over time. In essence it is acknowledged that parents will need to perform a balancing act; that is, it will be necessary to determine when it is time to encourage speech practice, give feedback, and when it is time to just attend to the content of what is being said. At the core is the need for parents to monitor how attention to speech is affecting their parent-child relationship.

Preparing Family and Friends   Parents are encouraged to: (1) have a family meeting to discuss how the family (including grandparents, etc.) may help in the maintenance period; and (2) to be specific about what each member of the family is to do or not do. A handout is given to parents as an aid.

Educating Teachers   Parents are also encouraged to have a meeting with their child's teacher and to include or not include the child as appropriate. A handout that we have developed is given to use as a guide in the meeting and to leave with the teacher (available at http://www.istar.ualberta.ca/ content/pdf/about_stuttering.pdf). The handout includes a description of what stuttering is, how it develops and varies, underlying causes, how children can hide stuttering in the classroom, and how the teacher can help the child who stutters. Suggestions for the child's teacher are given for achieving the following four broad goals of: (1) fostering development of an objective attitude toward stuttering in the child and acceptance by classmates; (2) minimizing time pressures and stressors; (3) facilitating successful participation in classroom activities; and (4) helping children through difficult times. Clinicians also may wish to use materials from the Stuttering Foundation of America in this regard.

Parent meetings also provide a forum for parents to express and share their feelings and concerns about the welfare of their child, for example, the child's academic progress and social development. Some parent meetings also are attended by older siblings and extended family. If possible, discussions with younger siblings are conducted to help them understand stuttering and what they can do to help the child who stutters.

Maintenance

In maintenance, parents operate as independently as possible. They problem solve speech and attitudinal-emotional issues, give feedback smooth and stuttered speech as described above, participate in and monitor home practice activities, seek additional support and/or maintenance therapy for their child if needed, and liaise with teachers.

◆ Teasing and Bullying

It is well known that the school environment can be difficult for children and adolescents who stutter. It is clear that stuttering places youth at risk of being bullied (Blood & Blood, 2004; Langevin, Bortnick, Hammer, & Wiebe, 1998; Riley & Riley, 2000), being perceived negatively (Langevin and Hagler, 2004), and being less accepted than nonstuttering peers (Davis, Howell, & Cooke, 2002). It is also well known that bullying has long-term negative psychosocial consequences: low self-esteem, anxiety, depression, psychosomatic symptoms, mistrust of others, and truancy (Hawker and Bolton, 2000). In the remainder of this section we provide background information on the definition of bullying and coping strategies (limited to school-age children), and we present topics addressed in our teasing and bullying discussions.

Definition of Bullying

Bullying is generally defined as hurtful behavior by a person or group that involves an imbalance in power with the less-powerful person or group being repeatedly and unfairly attacked (see Rigby, Smith, & Pepler, 2004). Bullying behaviors include physical and verbal bullying (e.g., name calling, hurtful teasing, verbal threats). Bullying also includes relational bullying that is more indirect and social in nature and is intended to harm friendships or inclusion by the peer group (e.g., exclusion, spreading rumors) (Crick & Grotpeter, 1995). Indirect bullying can also include coercion (i.e., getting another person to do the bullying).

Coping Strategies

The relative success of different coping strategies will be affected by age, sex, social context of the school, and type, severity and frequency of bullying (Kochenderfer & Ladd, 1997; Smith, Shu, & Madsen, 2001). The child's temperament must also be considered (e.g., some may be submissive, whereas others may react with a hot temper; see Olweus, 1993). For children 12 to 13 years of age, Salmivalli, Karhunen, and Lagerspetz (1996) found preliminary evidence that the most constructive response to aggression for both boys and girls appears to be *nonchalance* (i.e., the victim stays calm, acts as if the bullying is not being taken seriously, acts as if he or she doesn't care). In interviews of victims aged 13 to 16 years, Smith, Talamelli, Cowie, Naylor, and Chauhan (2004), found that the five most frequently reported responses to aggression were "talk to someone," "ignore it," "stick up for your self (take care of myself, get more mature, sort it out with the bully)," "avoid, stay away from the bully," and "get more/different friends." However, logistic regression showed that only "talking to someone about it" and "getting more/different friends" were associated with *escape* from victimization. In a study of 10- to 14 year olds, Smith et al. (2001) found that the most frequently self-reported coping strategy was "ignored them" followed by "told them to stop," "asked an adult for help," "fought back," "cried," "asked friends for help," and "ran away." Younger children more frequently reported that they used "crying" or "running away," whereas older children more frequently reported "ignoring" the bully.

Kristensen and Smith (2003) used a modified version of the Self-Report Coping Measure (Causey & Dubow, 1992) with 10- to 15-year-olds. They found that the most used coping strategy was Self-Reliance/Problem-Solving (e.g., "Try to think of different ways to solve it," "Change something so things will work out") followed by Distancing (e.g., "Make believe nothing happened," "Tell myself it doesn't matter"), and Seeking Social Support (e.g., "Get help from a friend," "Talk to the teacher about it"). The least used strategies were Internalizing (e.g., "Become so upset that I can't talk to anyone," "Cry about it") and Externalizing (e.g., "Take it out on others because I feel sad or angry," "Curse out loud"). Girls used Seeking Social Support and Internalizing more than boys, whereas boys used Externalizing more than girls.

Taken together these studies indicate that: (1) nonchalance; (2) self-reliance/problem solving; and (3) seeking social support may be more helpful coping strategies for older children. As suggested by Kristensen and Smith (2003), "ignored the bullies" and "told them to stop" might be considered Self-Reliance/Problem Solving strategies and "talking to someone" and "asking friends for help" might be Seeking Social Support strategies. Smith et al. (2001) argue that ignoring is a socially skilled coping strategy that older children develop. However, they also address the importance of the social context. Ignoring may be relatively successful in unsupportive environments but less so in supportive environments because doing so conceals the victim's distress. In general, the implication for intervention is that victimized children need to develop successful coping strategies, and, due to the power imbalance, they need protection, support, and guidance from adults. As Pepler, Smith, and Rigby (2004) state, care must be taken to integrate and not further isolate victimized children, and it is necessary to monitor the effectiveness of interventions.

Given the saliency of having friends and the need to have quality friendships to counteract and protect against victimization (e.g., Boulton, Trueman, Chau, Whitehand & Amatya, 1999), there is some evidence that structuring supportive peer-groups for children who are at risk for bullying (Naylor & Cowie, 1999), assigning a student or students to befriend an at-risk child (Cowie & Sharp, 1996), conducting social-skills and assertiveness training for the at-risk child (e.g., Sharp and Cowie, 1994) and helping a vulnerable child to develop friendship skills (see Boulton et al., 1999) may be helpful.

Teasing and Bullying Activities in the Comprehensive Stuttering Program for School-Age Children

The teasing and bullying element comprises a series of children's discussions (**Table 8–1**),[5] a bullying seminar for parents, and individual problem solving as necessary. As with the attitude-emotion discussions, it is important to consider the individual differences of children and their readiness to disclose bullying experiences. For that reason, group discussions are kept broad, and narrow to individual experiences only when the children are ready to go to that depth.

With the guidance of a clinician, children first discuss the concept of bullying. The goal is to help children become aware of various types of bullying behaviors, and to differentiate between hurtful teasing and teasing that is fun and a part of healthy relationships. Using webs, children brainstorm what kids say or do when they bully and what they say and do when they tease. Without fail, children identify name-calling and mimicking as teasing and bullying behaviors. This provides the link to a more in-depth discussion about what constitutes teasing that is fun (i.e., the teaser and recipient are having fun; the teasing is not intended to harm the recipient) and teasing that is bullying (i.e., teasing that is intended to embarrass, hurt, taunt, or poke fun at a student with the intention of harming or putting the student down). In addition, this discussion addresses the following concepts: (1) that there is sometimes a fine line between teasing that is fun and teasing that is bullying; (2) that teasing can quickly turn into bullying (e.g., it may become upsetting to the recipient and the teaser may be insensitive to this; see Rigby 2002 for a discussion of malign and nonmalign bullying); and (3) that children who are teased may not show their distress. Children then discuss differences in addition to stuttering that make children vulnerable. This sets the stage for a later discussion that addresses respecting and celebrating differences.

Subsequent discussions address how it feels to be bullied, why a person might bully, how a person could be helped to stop bullying, coping strategies if one is being bullied, and what children can do if they witness bullying. We also discuss why children don't report bullying. We stress the importance of talking with parents about bullying: If parents do not know about it they cannot help. An exercise also addresses how children acquire power and maintain it, or get it back. Clinicians use written exercises and brainstorming throughout these discussions.

When discussing coping strategies we encourage expression of all possible response strategies and then have the children classify those that would be helpful and unhelpful. Helpful behaviors are solution oriented and do not escalate the problem. Unhelpful behaviors are those that perpetuate or escalate the problem.

The difference between tattling and responsible reporting is discussed. The following was drawn from D. Pepler (personal communication, 1999) and Langevin (2000): "Tattling is when you tell to get someone *into* trouble and you tell in front of others; telling to get help is when you tell to get someone *out* of trouble and you tell an adult in private."

Children then learn a variety of conflict resolution strategies that are helpful to all children involved: children who bully, children who are victimized, and peers who may wish to mediate

---

[5]Topics addressed in the teasing and bullying discussions are drawn from Teasing and bullying: Unacceptable behaviour [TAB] (Langevin, 2000), the large body of bullying literature, and workshops conducted in our clinic for children who did and did not stutter. Readers are also referred to others in our field who have written about teasing and bullying (e.g., see the National Stuttering Association, 2004).

conflict (Sharp & Cowie, 1994). Learning conflict strategies is particularly important in view of evidence that suggests that difficulties in managing confrontation adaptively may be associated with victimization in adolescents (Champion, Vernberg, & Shipman, 2003). Strategies are categorized into three sets and are briefly described. The first is the "I Can Speak Up—Five Finger Strategy" in which children are encouraged to tell the perpetrator of the bullying to stop. Although telling the bully to stop is a frequently suggested strategy in bullying and conflict resolution literature, its effectiveness in stopping bullying has yet to be demonstrated. Thus, its use should be judicious. The five finger component helps younger children remember how they might tell someone to stop. For example, say the person's name, tell how you feel, describe the behavior that you want stopped, be respectful, and tell what you want (i.e., "stop"). Regarding "tell how you feel," we believe that it is safer to use the term "I *don't like it* when you . . ." rather than disclosing true emotion given that the child who is bullying is not likely to be empathetic.

A second set of strategies is titled "Rules for Working It Out" (adapted with permission, Schmidt, 1994). Guidelines for working out problems effectively and "fouls" that commonly disrupt problem solving are given. Working it out rules include: (1) identify the problem; (2) attack the problem not the person; (3) treat a person's feelings with respect; and (4) take responsibility for your actions. Fouls include blaming, name-calling, threats, sneering, making excuses, getting even, and not taking responsibility. The third set of strategies includes those that encourage children to use a variety of conflict resolution strategies such as take turns, compromise, use humor, and get help.

After role playing various strategies in group discussions, children and parents carry out a home practice exercise in which the child and parent discuss bullying in general (e.g., the extent to which children in their class or school get bullied), whether or not the child has been bullied, how it felt to be bullied, and what the child might do if bullying occurs in the future or what might be done to deal with bullying that is currently occurring. Parents are encouraged to talk about their own experiences of bullying if such occurred.

Topics discussed in the parent bullying seminar are outlined in **Table 8–1**. Discussion of coping strategies includes those identified in the literature and in the children's discussion, and variables that must be considered (e.g., sex, age, social context) as described above. The following principles of intervention are discussed: (1) Each bullying event will require a different solution; (2) Each child is unique in terms of temperament and other personality characteristics, preferences, and social skills and abilities. As such, the strategies proposed for use must suit the child; (3) Children need to learn a variety of coping strategies—only being rescued may perpetuate victimization. However, given the power imbalance in bullying, victimized children need the intervention, support, and guidance of adults; (4) Role playing is fundamental for the child to be assertive and use strategies with confidence; (5) Children and parents must use judgment in responding. Different levels of intervention will be required, and the intervention or coping strategy must be appropriate for the situation. If their child is being bullied, parents are encouraged to find out as much as possible about what is happening and who is involved, consult with school personnel, and determine if adult intervention is needed or if the child will attempt to solve the problem using an agreed-on strategy. If adult intervention is necessary, parents are encouraged to work with school personnel and ideally decide on a plan of action that involves the school to ensure the safety of their child and to ensure the safety of other children who may be involved. Many schools now have bullying intervention/prevention programs in place within which the problem may be addressed; and (6) Any proposed intervention first should be discussed fully with the child, and the child should remain involved in the decision-making process.

Of the four case patients in this chapter, three were teased. Case Patient 1 had been teased by older children at school. Teachers intervened, and the problem was resolved satisfactorily. Case Patient 3 had been teased by school mates, but it stopped when his friends stood up for him. Case Patient 4 was being teased severely by older and younger children at school. At 2 months follow-up his parents reported that he was no longer being teased and that he felt more accepted and liked by peers.

♦ Case Example Treatment Outcomes

Speech outcome is reported in terms of percent syllables stuttered (%SS) and final parent report. All speech samples for Cases 1, 3, and 4 were obtained from video-recorded within clinic conversations with a stranger (in a room not associated with therapy) just prior to a refresher clinic. Audio-recorded follow-up speech samples for Case Patient 2 were obtained in his home environment. Intra-class correlations (two-way mixed model) for inter-rater reliability between the original research assistants who rated the samples and a second research assistant who rated 71% of the samples all exceeded 0.95.

Stuttering reductions for Cases 1 to 3 ranged from 52 to 75% at 6 to 19 months follow-up. At 2 months post-treatment Case Patient 4 was in relapse and needed continued maintenance therapy. Despite not maintaining speech gains, his parents reported that he was a much happier child and that his social skills had improved as a result of being in the program. Parent report at final contact for the remainder of the children indicated that: (1) at 4 years follow-up Case Patient 1 was participating freely in class and had become very open about stuttering; (2) at 15 months follow-up Case Patient 2's typical weekly severity rating was a 2 (1 = no stuttering and 10 = the worst stuttering imaginable for the child); (3) at 7 months follow-up Case Patient 3 remained highly motivated to do home practice and did so three to four times per week. He liked using GS and SB, and he was more outgoing and talkative.

The speech outcome data presented in this chapter and that of Kully and Boberg (1991) provide preliminary evidence of the effectiveness of the CSP-SC. That is, in Kully and Boberg, stuttering reductions in within-clinic conversation samples for 9 of 10 children ranged from 79 to 98% at 8 to 18 months follow-up. In covert samples obtained for 6 of the 9 children, stuttering reductions ranged 65 to 100%.

The purpose of this chapter was to provide a description of the CSP-SC and, in particular, the teasing and bullying elements of the attitude-emotional component. In so doing, the strategies and concepts addressed in each of the components were described and case examples were used to illustrate decision-making processes in programming and similarities and differences in children's treatment response. In greater detail, we reviewed the evidence base for the coping strategies discussed in the CSP-SC to help children and parents manage bullying. It is hoped that the information presented will help clinicians in their work with school-age children who stutter.

References

Blood, G. W., & Blood, I. M. (2004, Spring). Bullying in adolescents who stutter: Communicative competence and self-esteem. Contemporary Issues in Communication Science and Disorders 31, 69–79.

Bothe, A. K. (2004). Evidence-based, outcomes-focused decisions about stuttering treatment: Clinical recommendations in context. In A. K. Bothe (Ed.), Evidence-based treatment of stuttering: Empirical bases and clinical applications (pp. 261–270). Mahwah, NJ: Lawrence Erlbaum Associates.

Boulton, M. J., Trueman, M., Chau, C., Whitehand, C., & Amatya, K. (1999). Concurrent and longitudinal links between friendship and peer victimization: implications for befriending interventions. Journal of Adolescence 22, 461–466.

Causey, D. L., & Dubow, E. F. (1992). Development of a self-report coping measure for elementary school children. Journal of Clinical Child Psychology 21, 47–59.

Champion, K., Vernberg, E., & Shipman, K. (2003). Nonbullying victims of bullies: Aggression, social skills, and friendship characteristics. Applied Developmental Psychology 24, 535–551.

Conture, E. G. (2001). Stuttering: Its nature, diagnosis, and treatment. Boston: Allyn and Bacon.

Cowie, H., & Sharp, S. (1996). Peer counselling in schools: A time to listen. London: David Fulton.

Crick, N. R., & Grotpeter, J. K. (1995). Relational aggression, gender and social-psychological adjustment. Child Development 66, 710–722.

Davis, S., Howell, P., & Cooke, F. (2002). Sociodynamic relationships between children who stutter and their non-stuttering classmates. Journal of Child Psychology and Psychiatry 43, 939–947.

Hawker, D. S. J., & Bolton, M. J. (2000). Twenty years research on peer victimization and psychosocial maladjustment:

A meta-analytic review of cross-sectional studies. Journal of Child Psychology and Psychiatry 41, 441–455.

Kochenderfer, B. J., & Ladd, G. W. (1997). Victimized children's responses to peers' aggression: Behaviors associated with reduced versus continued victimization. Development and Psychopathology 9, 59–73.

Kristensen, S. M., & Smith, P. K. (2003). The use of coping strategies by Danish children classed as bullies, victims, bully/victims, and not involved, in response to different (hypothetical) types of bullying. Scandinavian Journal of Psychology 44, 479–488.

Kully, D. (2002). Venturing into telehealth: Applying interactive technologies to stuttering treatment. The ASHA Leader7(1), 6–7,15.

Kully, D., & Boberg, E. (1991). Therapy for school-age children. In W. H. Perkins (Ed.), Seminars in speech and language, 12, (pp. 291–300). New York: Thieme.

Langevin, M. (2000). Teasing and bullying: Unacceptable behaviour [TAB]: Edmonton, Alberta: Institute for Stuttering Treatment & Research.

Langevin, M., Bortnick, K., Hammer, T., & Wiebe, E. Teasing/bullying experienced by children who stutter: Toward development of a questionnaire. Contemporary Issues in Communication Science and Disorders 25, 12–24.

Langevin, M., & Hagler, P. (2004). Development of a scale to measure peer attitudes toward children who stutter. In A. K. Bothe (Ed.), Evidence-based treatment of stuttering: Empirical bases and clinical applications (pp. 139–171). Mahwah, NJ: Lawrence Erlbaum Associates.

Langevin, M., & Kully, D. (2003). Evidence-based treatment of stuttering: III. Evidence-based practice in a clinical setting. Journal of Fluency Disorders 28, 219–236.

Lincoln, M., Onslow, M., Lewis, C., & Wilson, L. (1996). A clinical trial of an operant treatment for school-age children who stutter. American Journal of Speech-Language Pathology 5, 73–85.

National Stuttering Association. (2004). Bullying and teasing: Helping children who stutter. New York: National Stuttering Association.

Naylor, P., & Cowie, H. (1999). The effectiveness of peer support systems in challenging school bullying: The perspectives and experiences of teachers and pupils. Journal of Adolescence 22, 467–479.

Olweus, D. (1993). Bullying at school: What we know and what we can do. Cambridge: Blackwell Publishers.

Pepler, D., Smith, P. K., & Rigby, K. (2004). Looking back and looking forward: implications for making interventions work effectively. In P. K. Smith, D. Pepler, & K. Rigby (Eds.), Bullying in schools: How successful can interventions be? (pp. 307–324). Cambridge: Cambridge University Press.

Rigby, K. (2002). New perspectives on bullying. London: Jessica Kinglsey Publishers Ltd.

Rigby, K., Smith, P. K., & Pepler, D. (2004). Working to prevent school bullying: key issues. In P. K. Smith, D. Pepler, & K. Rigby (Eds.), Bullying in schools: How successful can interventions be? (pp. 1–12). Cambridge: Cambridge University Press.

Riley, G., & Riley, J. (2000). A revised component model for diagnosing and treating children who stutter. Contemporary Issues in Communication Science and Disorders 27, 188–189.

Salmivalli, C., Karhunen, J., & Lagerspetz, K. M. J. (1996). How do the victims respond to bullying? Aggressive Behavior 22, 99–109.

Schmidt, F. (1994). Mediation: Getting to win win! Student handbook. Miami, FL: Grace Contrino Abrams Peace Education Foundation, Inc.

Sharp. S., & Cowie, H. (1994). Empowering pupils to take positive action against bullying. In P. K. Smith & S. Sharp (Eds.), School bullying: Insights and perspectives (pp. 108–131). London: Routledge.

Smith, P. K., Shu, S., & Madsen, K. (2001). Characteristics of victims of school bullying. In J. Juvonen & S. Graham (Eds.), Peer harassment in school (pp. 332–351). New York: The Guilford Press.

Smith, P. K., Talamelli, L., Cowie, H., Naylor, P., & Chauhan, P. (2004). Profiles of non-victims, escaped victims, continuing victims and new victims of school bullying. British Journal of Educational Psychology 74, 565–581.

Van Riper, C. (1973). The treatment of stuttering. New Jersey: Prentice-Hall.

Section III

Intervention: Children Who Stutter with Other Co-occurring Concerns

9

Language Considerations in Childhood Stuttering

Nancy E. Hall, Stacy A. Wagovich, and Nan Bernstein Ratner

The purpose of this chapter is to discuss why language is important to our understanding of childhood stuttering. We hope that the reader of this chapter will better understand that, although not likely a causal contributor to stuttering, language can be considered a potentially influential variable that is associated with fluency and stuttering. Subsequent to this consideration, we discuss ways in which assessment and treatment procedures can be improved by recognizing and taking into account the role of language.

First, from a developmental perspective, stuttering onset typically occurs between the ages of 2 and 5 years (see Bloodstein, 1995, for a review), a time of tremendous language growth. This suggests the need to acknowledge potential interactions between the development of language skills and the development of stuttering. Whether or not a causal relationship exists between language development and the progression of stuttering, it is clear that the fluent production of speech and the development of language skills interact with each other. In particular, we present research findings that can be taken to suggest that linguistic demand affects a child's ability to be fluent, an important concern in the construction of fluency therapy goals and activities.

The second reason to consider language functioning when assessing and treating developmental stuttering is the observation that some children who stutter (CWS) exhibit co-occurring language disorders (e.g., Arndt and Healy, 2001; Blood, Ridenour, Qualls, & Hammer, 2003; Yaruss, LaSalle, & Conture, 1998; see Bernstein Ratner, 2005, for reviews) requiring the identification and management of both areas of weakness. The last reason to view developmental stuttering within the scope of the child's linguistic acquisition is the broadest and perhaps most intuitive: Effective human oral communication takes place within the context of language. Thus, to overlook skills related to language use is to ignore the context in which stuttering and, indeed, oral communication, occur. Accompanying the present chapter are tables that provide a summary of studies in these areas over the past 20 years. The summary is not exhaustive; it is intended to encapsulate the most recent literature and to highlight continued efforts to understand the relation between language and fluency in CWS (see **Tables 9–1**).

Table 9–1 Summary of Studies Related to Language Skills, Effects, and Disorders in Children Who Stutter

Studies Examining Language Skills in Children Who Stutter

Author(s)	Participants	Methods	Results
St. Louis, Hinzman, & Hull (1985)	■ 24 each CWS, CWNS ■ Grades 1–6, four matched pairs at each grade level	■ Spontaneous language analysis	■ CWS produced significantly fewer verbs per utterance
Byrd & Cooper (1989)	■ 12 CWS ■ Ages 5–9 years	■ Standardized measures of language	■ Expressive language significantly delayed compared with chronological age ■ No significant difference between receptive language and chronological age
Nippold, Schwarz, & Jescheniak (1991)	■ 10 each CWS, CWNS ■ Ages 6–11 years	■ Standardized measures of language ■ Tasks of narrative skills	■ CWS did not differ from CWNS on language and narrative skills
Weiss & Zebrowski (1991)	■ 16 parent-child dyads, 8 CWS, 8 CWNS ■ Ages 4–10 years	■ Measures of assertiveness and responsiveness from conversational samples	■ Parents of two groups did not differ in assertiveness or responsiveness ratios ■ Requests more frequently produced utterance type by both parental groups
Kelly & Conture (1992)	■ 26 mother-child dyads, 13 CWS, 13 CWNS ■ Ages 3–4 years	■ Measures of speaking rates, response time latencies, interruptions in dyadic conversations with mothers	■ No differences between mothers of two groups on measures ■ Mothers of CWNS used significantly faster speech rate than children ■ Significant correlation between children's stuttering severity and duration of talking overlap
Weiss & Zebrowski (1992)	■ 8 parent-CWS pairs ■ CWS ages 4–10 years	■ Dyadic conversations ■ Identified assertive and responsive communicative acts	■ Assertions significantly more likely to be produced disfluently
Ryan (1992)	■ 20 each CWS, CWNS ■ Preschool age	■ Standardized measures of articulation and language ■ Speaking rate	■ CWS poorer on most language measures ■ No differences in articulation
Kelly (1994)	■ 11 each CWS, CWNS ■ Ages 2–10 years	■ Measures of speaking rates, response time latencies, interruptions in dyadic conversations with fathers	■ No differences between fathers or CWS and fathers of CWNS on speech and pragmatic measures ■ Higher dyadic speaking rates observed for CWS with more severe stuttering
Weiss & Zebrowski (1994)	■ 8 each CWS, CWNS ■ Ages 5–11 years	■ Narrative samples collected during story retelling	■ CWS produced nonsignificantly shorter and less complete stories
Scott, Healey, & Norris (1995)	■ 12 each CWS, CWNS ■ Ages 6–9 years	■ Narrative performance during story retelling	■ No significant differences in narratives ■ Weak relationship between stuttering and narrative complexity
Yairi, Ambrose, Paden, & Throneburg (1996)	■ 32 each, CWS, CWNS ■ Ages 2 – 5 years ■ 4 subgroups: Persistent Stuttering, Late Recovery, Early Recovery, Control	■ Spontaneous language samples analyzed for fluency, phonology, language ■ Acoustic measures ■ Genetics	■ Language behavior identified as predictive of chronicity in stuttering
Weiss & Zebrowski (1997)	■ 13 each CWS, CWNS ■ Ages 6–11 years	■ 3 conversation settings: with parent, with unfamiliar adult, with both	■ Significantly more stuttering in unstructured conversation setting in both groups

(Continued)

		• 2 conversation types: structured around goal-oriented activity, unstructured conversation	
Watkins, Yairi, & Ambrose (1999)	• 84 CWS: 62 recovered from stuttering, 22 with persistent stuttering • Ages 2–5 years	• Spontaneous language samples analyzed for lexical, morphological, syntactic characteristics	• Near or above normal expressive language skills • Similarities in language between persistent and recovered
Anderson & Conture (2000)	• 20 each CWS, CWNS • Ages 3–5 years	• Standardized measures of language and phonology • Spontaneous language samples analyzed for fluency	• Disparity between receptive/expressive language and receptive vocabulary significantly greater for CWS
Ryan (2001)	• 22 CWS • Ages 2–5 years followed longitudinally	• Standardized measures of language and articulation	• All demonstrated improvement in language and articulation • No differences in test scores between persistent and recovered CWS
Silverman & Bernstein Ratner (2002)	• 15 each CWS, CWNS • Ages 2–3 years • Within 4 months of stuttering onset	• Standardized measures of language • Spontaneous language samples analyzed for lexical diversity	• CWS scored significantly lower on measures of lexical diversity
Melnick, Conture, & Ohde (2003)	• 18 each CWS, CWNS age-and sex-matched • Ages 3–5 years	• Computer assisted picture naming in 3 conditions: no-prime, phonologically related prime, unrelated prime	• Phonological priming facilitated picture naming in both groups • Faster speech reaction times associated with articulatory mastery in CWNS only
Anderson & Conture (2004)	• 16 each CWS, CWNS • Ages 3–5 years	• Sentence structure priming task	• CWS scored significantly lower than CWNS on Test of Language Development subtests (although within normal limits) • CWS responded significantly more quickly in primed condition; no condition effect noted for CWNS • CWS produced significantly fewer accurate responses
Bajaj, Hodson, & Schommer-Aiken (2004)	• 23 each CWS, CWNS • Kindergarten, first, and second graders	• Metalinguistic tasks of phonological awareness and grammatical awareness	• CWS significantly poorer on grammatical judgement task than CWNS • No differences between groups on phonological awareness tasks
Hakim & Bernstein Ratner (2004)	• 8 each CWS, CWNS • Ages 4–8 years	• Standardized and nonstandardized measures of nonword repetition	• CWS fewer correct words and increased numbers of phoneme errors than CWNS; significantly worse for three-syllable words • CWS more errors on words with non-English stress patterns than CWNS
Anderson, Pellowski, & Conture (2005)	• 45 each CWS, CWNS matched on age, sex, race, parent socioeconomic status • Ages 3–5 years	• Profiles of scores on standardized measures of speech and language • Fluency analysis from spontaneous speech samples • Correlation-based statistical procedure for identifying dissociations among speech and language variables	• CWS more than three times as likely to demonstrate dissociations among speech and language skills • Authors argue for possible subgroup of CWS with such dissociations

(Continued)

Table 9–1   Summary of Studies Related to Language Skills, Effects, and Disorders in Children Who Stutter (*Continued*)

Author(s)	Participants	Methods	Results
Pellowski & Conture (2005)	■ 23 each CWS, CWNS age-matched ■ Ages 3–5 years	■ Computer-assisted picture naming in 3 conditions: no-prime, semantically related-prime, unrelated-prime	■ Semantically related primes associated with faster speech reaction times for CWNS compared with slower reaction times for CWS ■ Higher receptive vocabulary associated with faster speech reaction times for CWNS, not for CWS

Studies Examining Language Effects in Children Who Stutter

Author(s)	Participants	Methods	Results
Bernstein Ratner & Sih (1987)	■ 8 each CWS, CWNS ■ Ages 3–6 years	■ Sentence imitation task designed to elicit 10 different sentence types	■ Disfluency correlated more strongly with syntactic complexity than length ■ No differences between CWS and CWNS in ability to imitate a variety of sentences
Gaines, Runyan, & Meyers (1991)	■ 12 CWS ■ Ages 4–6 years	■ Spontaneous language analyzed for syntactic length and complexity	■ Stuttering associated with longer, more complex sentences
Gordon (1991)	■ 7 each CWS, CWNS ■ Ages 3–7 years	■ Sentence imitation and modeling tasks	■ Sentence modeling produced significantly more disfluencies than sentence imitation for both groups ■ Significant group x task interaction, with sentence modeling producing greater increases in disfluencies for CWS
Kadi-Hanifi & Howell (1992)	■ 17 each CWS, CWNS ■ Ages 2–12 years	■ Spontaneous language analyzed for fluency and syntax	■ Increased disfluency associated with longer, more complex sentences ■ No difference in use of different syntactic categories between the groups
Howell & Au-Yeung (1995)	■ 31 CWS, 48 CWNS ■ Age groups: 2–6 years, 6–9 years, 9–12 years	■ Spontaneous language samples analyzed for syntax	■ Stuttering occurred most frequently at clause boundaries ■ Young CWS used more simple sentence structures than young CWNS with difference between groups decreasing with age
Logan & Conture (1995)	■ 15 CWS ■ Ages 3–5 years	■ Compared fluent and stuttered spontaneous utterances for syntactic length and complexity ■ Articulatory speaking rate assessed	■ Stuttered utterances significantly longer and/or more complex than fluent utterances ■ Syllabic length for stuttered utterances significantly longer than for fluent utterances
Logan & Conture (1997)	■ 14 each CWS, CWNS ■ Ages 3–5 years	■ Compared fluent and stuttered utterances for clause and syllable structure ■ Response latency assessed	■ Stuttered utterances contained significantly more clausal constituents than fluent utterances ■ No significant difference between length-matched fluent and stuttered utterances in syllable structure
Silverman & Bernstein Ratner (1997)	■ 7 each adolescents who stutter and nonstuttering adolescents ■ Ages 10–18 years	■ Sentence imitation task designed to elicit 3 types of sentences	■ Stuttering not associated with syntactic complexity ■ Both groups showed decreases in repetition accuracy as complexity increased

(Continued)

Yaruss (1999)	■ 12 CWS ■ Ages 3–5 years	■ Spontaneous language analyzed for fluency and syntactic complexity	■ Utterance length determined to be better predictor of stuttering than sentence complexity
Melnick & Conture (2000)	■ 10 CWS with disordered phonology ■ Ages 2–6 years	■ Stuttered and fluent spontaneous utterances compared on syntactic length and complexity ■ Systematic and nonsystematic speech errors analyzed	■ Stuttering associated with grammatical length and complexity ■ Stuttering not related to presence of systematic or nonsystematic errors
Logan (2001)	■ 12 adolescent and adult persons who stutter ■ Mean age 23 years	■ Conversational and prepared sentence tasks ■ Analyses included length-matched stuttered and fluent conversational utterances	■ Significantly more disfluencies in conversational utterances than prepared sentences ■ No significant differences in fluency across syntactic complexities
Dworzynski, Howell, & Natke (2003)	■ 12 German-speaking CWS ■ Ages 7–11 years	■ Spontaneous language samples analyzed for Brown's (1945) factors and stuttering	■ Increased word length significantly associated with increased stuttering ■ Overall word difficulty not associated with stuttering
Logan (2003)	■ 15 each CWS, CWNS, age- and sex-matched ■ Ages 3–4 years	■ Language transcripts from interactive play with parent ■ Analyzed for conversational turn, conversational turn type, utterance length, and complexity	■ No significant differences between groups on disfluency rate for length-matched single-utterance or multi-utterance conversational turns ■ All subject's utterances from multi-utterance turns significantly longer and more complex than single-utterance turns
Zackheim & Conture (2003)	■ 6 each CWS, age-matched ■ Ages 3–5 years	■ Spontaneous language samples	■ Significantly more stuttering (and disfluencies) on utterances above MLU ■ Significantly more stuttering on long complex than short complex utterances
Natke, Sandreiser, van Ark, Pietrowsky, & Kalveram (2004)	■ 22 CWS ■ Ages 2–5 yeras	■ Spontaneous language samples analyzed for linguistic stress, word position, and grammatical class effects	■ Nearly 98% of all stuttering occurred on first syllable ■ Stuttering significantly associated with function words ■ Short stressed syllables and intermediate syllables more frequently stuttered than unstressed syllables

Studies Examining Concomitant Language Disorder in Children Who Stutter

St. Louis & Hinzman (1988)	■ 24 each CWS with moderate communicative deficits, CWS with severe deficits, CWNS ■ Grades 1–6	■ Compared spontaneous language samples on fluency and presence of concomitant speech and language disorder	■ CWS were likely to exhibit concomitant disorders ■ Presence of articulation disorder may be suggestive of subgroup of CWS
St. Louis, Murray, & Ashworth (1991)	■ 24 CWS from national database ■ Grades 1–12	■ Spontaneous language samples analyzed for fluency and presence of concomitant speech and language disorder	■ Considerable number of CWS exhibited concomitant disorders, specifically in articulation and voice
Arndt & Healey (2001)	■ 241 surveys on 467 CWS	■ Survey of SLPs on occurrence of concomitant speech and language disorders	■ 44% exhibited phonological and/or language disorder ■ 56% of CWS were free of concomitant disorder

Abbreviations: CWS, children who stutter; CWNS, children who do not stutter; MLK, mean length of atterance; SLP, speech-language pathologists.

♦ Stuttering Onset and Language Development

Although speculations about the role of language acquisition in stuttering onset and persistence are virtually as old as the empirical study of stuttering itself (e.g., Davis, 1939, 1940), in recent years, there has been increased interest in the relationship between language and fluency in young CWS (e.g., Anderson & Conture, 2000; Logan, 2003; Melnick & Conture, 2000; Bernstein Ratner & Silverman, 2000; Silverman & Bernstein Ratner, 2002; Yaruss, 1999; Zackheim & Conture, 2003; see also Bernstein Ratner, 1997, for a review). Interest in this area has been sparked, in part, because of the timing of the onset of stuttering and the development of major language milestones. As mentioned above, stuttering typically develops during a period of significant language growth marked by mastery of morphological and syntactic forms and dynamic vocabulary acquisition. It appears that the earliest reported onset of stuttering is 18 months (Bloodstein, 1995)—approximately the time children begin combining two words (i.e., the beginning of grammatical development). Although it is still less than clear why children experience stuttering onset when they do, there is much we do know about how stuttering and language interact in young children, information that can serve to guide assessment and treatment procedures for CWS.

Stuttering as a Function of Linguistic Demand

Some studies of normally fluent children suggest that periods of disfluency correspond to the acquisition of specific language milestones. A growing body of work, both experimental and naturalistic, has examined "trade-offs" between language demand and fluency over the course of development in children with normally fluent speech (e.g., Hall & Burgess, 2000; Rispoli, 2003; Rispoli & Hadley, 2001; Wijnen, 1990). These trade-offs include both linguistic and motor domains. For example, a CWS may have the cognitive and linguistic abilities to produce a long, grammatically complex sentence, but motorically the child may have difficulty producing such an utterance without disfluency. Thus, fluency of speech production (i.e., motor performance) is sacrificed in the face of producing complex language (i.e., linguistic performance). Recently, for example, Rispoli (2003) focused on changes in sentence production during grammatical development through a cross-sectional design including 52 normally developing children between the ages of 1 year,10 months and 4 years. Fluency of sentence production changed during the course of grammatical development, suggesting that sentence production becomes faster and more efficient in children over time, as their growing linguistic skills are more firmly mastered and habituated. Another example is the longitudinal case study by Hall and Burgess (2000), of a 2-year, 9-month-old girl with normal fluency which documented a tendency to produce more repetitions and pauses during production of advanced language forms. The percentage of disfluencies in this child's speech dramatically dropped over the course of one year as she mastered higher-level grammar.

The work of Hall and Burgess (2000), Rispoli (2003), and others provides a strong base within the literature on the *normal* development of fluency. We also have learned a great deal about the effects of linguistic demand on fluency in CWS. Both experimental and observational studies document that longer and developmentally more complex utterances are much more likely to be stuttered than shorter utterances with simpler syntax (e.g., Gaines, Runyan, & Meyers, 1991; Logan & Conture, 1995, 1997; Bernstein Ratner & Sih, 1987; Weiss & Zebrowski, 1992; Yaruss, 1999). Utterances of greater grammatical complexity, however, also tend to be longer than grammatically simpler sentences, and most studies attempting to disambiguate length from complexity present conflicting findings (e.g., Logan & Conture, 1997; Bernstein Ratner & Sih, 1987; cf. Yaruss, 1999; Yaruss, Newman, & Flora, 1999). Using a different method for examining length and complexity relative to stuttering in young CWS, Zackheim and Conture (2003) examined the rate of disfluencies in spontaneous utterances that were determined to be above the child's mean length of utterance (MLU) compared with the disfluency rate in utterances identified as shorter than the MLU. The results indicated that utterances above the MLU were more likely to be produced disfluently (with both stuttering and nonstuttering disfluencies present). In interpreting the findings, Zackheim and Conture argued that disparities in language production, such as the use of increased linguistic complexity relative to overall language proficiency (as measured by MLU), may set the stage for fluency breakdown. Thus, although it is not clear from the literature as a whole whether it is length or syntactic complexity that contributes *more* to the likelihood that an utterance will be produced with disfluency, there is evidence for trade-offs between language and fluency. That is, fluency is more likely to be compromised when children (both CWS and children who do not stutter [CWNS]) attempt to produce language that is more advanced relative to their overall linguistic proficiency.

The therapeutic ramifications of such findings are quite important. Although length of intended utterance has long been used as a guide to construct graded response hierarchies within a wide range of fluency therapy activities (e.g., Gradual Increase in Length and Complexity of Utterance [GILCU], Ryan, 1980, or Extended Length of Utterance [ELU], Costello, 1983), clinicians should be aware that the developmental difficulty of a child's utterances relative to his or her overall language development, not just utterance length, has the potential to adversely affect fluency. Because of this, targets for fluency therapy need to be chosen with care, initially to maximize the potential for fluent production and, over time, to gradually challenge the child's mastery of fluency skills through a hierarchy of successively more demanding utterances (Bernstein Ratner, 1995).

In addition to studies that demonstrate the impact of syntactic complexity on stuttering, recent work suggests that CWS may show discrepancies among language skills (Anderson & Conture, 2000; Anderson, Pellowski, & Conture, 2005). From a clinical perspective, the implication is that our assessments of CWS should include a *comprehensive* evaluation of speech and language. With the knowledge that many CWS show discrepancies in performance across language areas, we can assess the possibility of such a discrepancy in a particular CWS as part of the initial diagnostic session. Again, such information can inform our treatment procedures, particularly with respect to the language context in which we choose to embed our fluency treatment program for the child.

Thus, assessment of lexical and metalinguistic skills along with syntactic abilities will provide a clinician with an overall picture of a child's strengths and weaknesses, guiding the planning of therapeutic intervention (see Hall, 2004, for discussion of profiling language skills in treating stuttering). Fluency intervention for a young CWS should accommodate the child's level of sophistication with all components of language and allow for manipulation of linguistic contexts over time as the child experiences fluency success.

Language Proficiency and Recovery from Stuttering

Going a step further in emphasizing the clinical usefulness of early language and stuttering research, it is possible that particular associations between children's language development and stuttering may lead us in the direction of predicting the likelihood of recovery from the disorder. One basic question, therefore, would be: Do children who recover from stuttering show different patterns of stuttering (relative to those who do not recover) as they accomplish specific developmental milestones in language? In a series of insightful studies, Yairi and colleagues (e.g., Throneburg & Yairi, 2001; Watkins & Yairi, 1997; Watkins, Yairi, & Ambrose, 1999; Yairi, Ambrose, Paden, & Throneburg, 1996) addressed this question by attempting to identify factors that predict which children will persist in stuttering and which will recover. In their study of language variables as predictors of persistence, Watkins and Yairi (1997) examined three groups of children: persistent (continued stuttering for 36 months or more after onset), late recovered (recovered between 18 and 36 months after onset), and early recovered (recovered within 18 months). The researchers administered several formal tests of speech and language, and they transcribed and coded conversational language samples from the first and 1-year visits.

Results suggested that no language deficits existed for the CWS; expressive language was within or above normal limits for all subjects. However, although the *recovered* and *persistent* groups did not show language differences, the *persistent* group did display increased variability in their performances on measures of expressive language compared with those of children who recovered.

Further, the authors described "atypical patterns" of language change in the persistent group; these children either presented limited change or a loss in language growth over time. Three explanations for these findings were offered: That the persistent children likely represent a heterogeneous group (and therefore more diverse in language performance); that they begin with advanced language only to plateau later (in contrast to the language growth pattern of more typical language learners); or that their language is negatively impacted by stuttering over time as they begin to use less complex language to avoid stuttering. A second study by this group (Watkins et al., 1999) followed 84 children longitudinally for at least 48 months. Twenty-two of the children *persisted* and 62 *recovered*. Using a methodology similar to the Watkins and Yairi (1997) study, Watkins et al. found no differences between the *recovered* and *persistent* groups in expressive language; all were near or above normal at all ages on all expressive measures.

Although the longitudinal work of Watkins, Yairi and colleagues (1999) suggests that persistence of or recovery from stuttering does not appear to be systematically related to language functioning (at least in terms of whether or not children in these groups perform within the normal range on language measures), a recent report by Watkins and Johnson (2004) that followed individual children's expressive language profiles noted that children who recovered from stuttering tended to move from an above-age-level pattern on spontaneous language measures to one that was more age-appropriate as they recovered. The children who persisted in their stuttering did not show such a pattern, maintaining a more stable above-average expressive language profile. This finding is in contrast with those presented above and may be suggestive of language effects on stuttering, such that children's attempts to produce developmentally more challenging utterances have the potential to adversely affect their ability to be fluent. The finding is consistent, however, with the results of Anderson et al. (2005), and changes noted in fluency and language in the typical child case study by Hall and Burgess (2000). Findings are also consistent with those of a study by Bonelli, Dixon, Bernstein Ratner, and Onslow (2000), who found that some Lidcombe-treated children (see Chapter 4, this volume) also began therapy with above-age-level expressive language attempts, but gradually became more age-appropriate concurrent with improvements in their fluency. Although these studies did not address if and how stuttering may change as children accomplish specific language milestones over time, they do highlight that, for some CWS and typically fluent children, the processes involved in language development and mastery of fluent speech production clearly interact.

◆ Language Abilities of Children Who Stutter

Considerable research has been conducted on the nature of language skills in CWS, including investigations of syntactic, semantic, and pragmatic abilities in preschool and school-age children. Most findings indicate that CWS do not exhibit frank deficits in language skills, although subtle differences between CWS and their peers have been observed. First, we address what is known about language function in CWS not otherwise diagnosed with concomitant clinical delays in language. Second, we discuss the research related to children who exhibit concomitant language and fluency disorders.

General Patterns of Language Performance among Children Who Stutter

There has been much discussion about the ways in which CWS differ in their language skills from those who do not stutter. The question is, "If we consider only those CWS who do not display concomitant language disorders, are there subtle differences in their language performance relative to fluent peers?" This question is a particularly interesting one because if the answer is "yes" for the vast majority of CWS, then we've uncovered something about the nature of the disorder overall. In this section, we provide a brief review of the most recent literature exploring the possibility of subclinical language differences.

As discussed in the preceding section, several studies followed CWS longitudinally to investigate changes in language relative to stuttering. In addition to examining spontaneous language, some investigators assessed language skills through the use of formal test instruments (e.g., Ryan, 2001; Watkins et al., 1999; Yairi et al., 1996). Whereas Yairi and colleagues initially identified the *Preschool Language Scale-Revised* (Zimmerman, Steiner, & Pond, 1979) as predictive of chronicity (Yairi et al., 1996), Ryan (2001), who used the *Test of Language Development-Primary* (Newcomer & Hammill, 1982) as the overall language measure, found no differences in these test scores between persistent and recovered CWS. Thus, it appears that more global measures of language suggest few differences between recovered and persistent groups, whereas measures of spontaneous language reveal some differences between these groups (e.g., Watkins & Johnson, 2004).

Most recently, CWS have been shown to exhibit subtle difficulties with aspects of language beyond those of syntax and grammar. For example, in an exploratory study, Hakim and Bernstein Ratner (2004) reported that CWS, compared with CWNS, demonstrate poorer non-word repetition characterized by increased numbers of phoneme errors and more errors on words with non-English stress patterns. Likewise, Bajaj, Hodson, and Schommer-Aiken (2004) studied the metalinguistic skills of 23 early-elementary-age CWS. On a task of grammatical judgement, the CWS scored significantly more poorly than the CWNS. And finally, in their exploration of dissociations among linguistic skills in preschool-age CWS, Anderson et al. (2005) determined that discrepancies between specific linguistic domains (such as receptive and expressive vocabulary) appear more frequently in the test profiles of CWS than in those of CWNS. The findings of these studies have been interpreted as further evidence for trade-offs in the allocation of resources between language and fluency or as evidence for "a relationship between stuttering and some level of linguistic processing deficit" (Hakim & Bernstein Ratner, 2004, p. 192).

Concomitant Communication Disorders in Children Who Stutter

Language considerations are of utmost concern for those CWS who also exhibit frank language impairments. Research to date has provided some evidence to suggest stuttering and language impairment co-occur with enough regularity that such children may represent a specific subgroup of CWS (e.g., Arndt & Healy, 2001; Blood et al., 2003; Yaruss et al., 1998; cf. Nippold, 1990, 2004). For example, Yaruss et al. (1998) performed a retrospective records review of 100 diagnostic files of CWS. Among their findings were that 15% of the CWS performed below average in receptive vocabulary and 29% performed below average in expressive language. The need for the identification of a subgroup of CWS with concomitant language disorders has been questioned, however (Nippold, 1990, 2004). Nippold (2004) has argued that survey research inflates the prevalence of co-occurring language/phonological disorders with stuttering, because speech-language pathologists (SLPs) are more likely to identify CWS with concomitant impairments as needing services than CWS without concomitant impairments. We would argue, however, that logically, even if this is the case, of the children *identified* by SLPs as needing services, more of them will have concomitant language problems than the general population. In other words, the suggestion that children with concomitant problems may be referred for services more readily than children with a single area of deficit clearly indicates that this subgroup of CWS will frequently show up on SLPs caseloads. Thus, clinicians should be armed with the knowledge of appropriate treatment for these more complex cases.

Estimates of co-occurring language disorder among CWS vary. However, each of the estimates reported in the literature (e.g., Arndt and Healy, 2001; Blood et al., 2003) exceeds Leonard's (1998) estimate of 7% for the general prevalence of specific language impairment (SLI). Moreover, each value exceeds the estimate of children with learning disabilities (5 to 10%; Paul, 2001), of which *language*-learning disability is the predominant type. Thus, the prevalence of this subgroup of CWS is sufficiently large that language concerns identified through the assessment process, in addition to identified speech disfluencies, must be acknowledged and addressed in treatment. Past as well as continued objective studies of the prevalence of co-existing language disorders in CWS have extremely important ramifications for the assessment of children referred for stuttering evaluation. The evidence to date strongly suggests that best practice in all assessments of suspected or diagnosed CWS should include a full language battery as well as assessment of phonological skills in particular.

◆ Distinguishing between Stuttering and Other Forms of Disfluency

By now, the need to distinguish between *stuttered* disfluencies and other disfluencies is well-documented. This issue becomes potentially more complicated when assessing individuals with language disorder, to ascertain whether a child has two concomitant disorders (e.g., stuttering plus expressive language delay) or a primary language problem that creates atypical profiles of speech disfluency. Although some individuals with language disorder exhibit substantial linguistic disfluency (Boscolo, Bernstein Ratner, & Rescorla, 2002; Hall, Yamashita, & Aram, 1993; Thordardottir & Ellis Weismer, 2002; cf. Lees, Anderson, & Martin, 1999; Scott & Windsor, 2000), the disfluency for the most part is qualitatively different from stuttering. For example, Thordardottir and Ellis Weismer (2002) examined disfluencies produced in the narratives of children, ages 5 to 9 years, with and without specific language impairment. They found that the groups differed with respect to the number of *mazes* (a marker of linguistic disfluency in spontaneous speech), with the SLI group producing significantly more. Thus, although it appears that most studies of disfluencies in children with language impairment reveal a subgroup of individuals who are more disfluent than peers, not all studies show this pattern (see Lees et al., 2004; Scott & Windsor, 2000).

Of the studies that revealed a subgroup of children with language disorders who exhibit increased disfluency relative to peers, the disfluent subgroups demonstrated primarily disfluencies that appeared to be related to language formulation, rather than stuttering, although occasional stuttered disfluencies were noted (Boscolo et al., 2002; Hall, 1996; Hall et al., 1993; see also Bernstein Ratner, 2005; Nippold, 1990). Of interest, this pattern is not only true of children with language disorders; children with typically developing language also occasionally produce some disfluencies categorized as stuttering (e.g., Hall & Burgess, 2000; Wijnen, 1990). For example, Wijnen (1990) examined weekly language samples of a normally fluent Dutch child from ages 2 years,4 months to 2 years, 11 months, documenting sound repetitions as one type of disfluency observed. However, although the presence of *some* stutter-like disfluencies among children who are normally fluent and with typical language development has been reported, such speech disfluencies are not accompanied by struggle, tension, or awareness, nor does the child have a self-concept as a person who stutters. For these reasons, and because such disfluencies appear to be associated with general or transient problems in formulating expressive language, stuttering therapy would not be indicated in working with such children.

Perhaps a natural inclination is to infer connections, either causal or correlated, between co-occurring disorders, such as fluency and language disorders. We cannot infer such a connection. However, we know that children who have any form of communication disorder are more likely than the general population to have a co-occurring disorder (e.g., see Bernstein Ratner, 2005, for a discussion). Logically, it is possible that a third, overarching factor (such as an inherited genetic predisposition) is responsible for the development of both conditions. It is also possible that, for children with concomitant language and fluency problems, weakness in language impacts speech fluency. The observation that many children with language disorders are more apt to be disfluent (although not necessarily stuttering) than peers with normal language supports this suggestion. On the other hand, the fact that studies generally do not show a relationship between stuttering *severity* in CWS and language performance, and the finding that not all children with language disorders display increased disfluencies relative to their peers with typical language development provide evidence against this interpretation. In sum, although it is important to acknowledge the presence of a subgroup of CWS with concomitant language impairments, it is also important not to over-interpret the significance of this subgroup for yielding answers about either the overall nature of fluency disorders or the nature of language disorders.

The primary treatment implication of the work on concomitant disorders of stuttering and language is quite obvious: As noted earlier, in our assessments of children suspected of stuttering, we should explore language skills as well. And, if the child is determined to have a co-occurring language disorder, the plan for treatment should include that area (see Logan & LaSalle, 2003; Bernstein Ratner, 1995, for treatment suggestions). Comprehensively assessing the areas of communication weakness and using those observations as the basis for treatment planning is consistent with Paul's *descriptive-developmental model* (Paul, 2001, 2002; also see Miller, 1978). It takes into account the individual differences across children and the need, consequently, to develop treatments catered to the specific strengths and weaknesses observed. A second treatment implication is simply a reiteration of a central tenet in treatment theory, that is, to embed the learning of a new skill within a context with which the client is knowledgeable, familiar, and comfortable (see Paul, 2001; Slobin, 1973). In the case of fluency treatment, structuring activities to control language formulation demands is important, particularly for those children with concomitant language impairment. (The reader is directed to the Clinical Forum on child language research and the treatment of stuttering in the January 2004 issue of *Language, Speech, and Hearing Services in Schools* for assessment and treatment guidelines.)

◆ Stuttering within the Context of Language Use and the Communication of Ideas

Our final reason for considering language in the treatment of stuttering in children is that oral communication involves both language and speech, and that competence in communication is measured by an individual's ability to integrate language and speech within social contexts. In this section we discuss the literature on the communication environment of CWS and how these children respond to their environment.

The Language Environment of the Child Who Stutters

Children learn speech and language within the context of interactions with caregivers and others in their environment. Parental input can also shape the child's style of communication (Nelson, 1973). Thus, it has not been surprising to see a considerable literature that has investigated whether or not parental language models or feedback patterns may relate to the onset or persistence of stuttering symptoms in young children (see Bernstein Ratner, 2004; Yairi, 1997). Yairi (1997) provides perhaps the most comprehensive overview of historical studies that have examined parent-child variables that might potentially affect childhood stuttering. In general, the literature suggests no substantive differences between the home environments and parental interaction styles observed in CWS and their fluent peers. However, Yairi notes that the older literature can be faulted for serious design flaws and that there is much still to be learned from careful study of the home environments of CWS. In as much as the differing methodologies allow comparisons, most of the more recent studies addressing the communication patterns of parents of CWS support the belief that these parents, in fact, do not differ from those of children who are normally fluent in the language they use with their children, their communicative style, or their perceptions of the child's communicative abilities (e.g., Kloth, Janssen, Kraaimaat, & Brutten, 1995; Miles & Ratner, 2001; Yaruss & Conture, 1995; see Bernstein Ratner, 2004, and Nippold & Rudzinski, 1995, for reviews). Early work by Kelly and Conture (1992) found few differences between mothers of CWS and mothers of nonstuttering children on measures of speaking rate, response time latencies, and interrupting behavior, although a correlation was observed between stuttering frequency and the duration of mother-child overlapping speech. More recently, Miles and

Bernstein Ratner (2001) examined the language of 12 parents of CWS, close to stuttering onset, and 12 parents of normally fluent children. They found no differences between the groups in a wide range of variables including mean length of utterance and mean pre-verb length (morphosyntax), number of different words and lexical rarity (semantics), and mean length of turn (pragmatics). Similarly, parental perceptions of the children's linguistic strengths and weaknesses, important for fine-tuning language input appropriately to children, were actually likely to be more accurate in families with CWS than in those with fluent children.

Group studies that do not find generalized patterns of difference between households with stuttering and fluent children do not obviate the need to appraise individual children's environments to ascertain whether or not they appear optimal for the development of speech and language. Group studies, by design, tend to ignore individual differences among children and families. From a clinical perspective, we cannot ignore the fact that *individual* children may respond differently to particular interaction styles; this is where clinical session data are especially relevant and helpful. Both research and clinical observation support the concept that individual parental interaction styles can impact a child's fluency or expressive language strategies, particularly in terms of response to stuttered utterances (see Bernstein Ratner & Guitar, 2005, for discussion of parental feedback to fluency failure and its potential role in mediating the course of developmental stuttering). That is, it is not necessary for parents of CWS to *differ* in their interaction style from parents of fluent children for their communication to *impact* the CWS. Rather, in theory, the same parent communication style that poses no problem for a normally fluent sibling may impact the speech of a CWS.

Response of the Child Who Stutters to the Language Environment

A natural question that follows from the general observation that *parents* do not differ in their interaction styles with children, is whether *children* who stutter differ from peers in the linguistic skills necessary to make them competent communicators. We addressed general concerns about the language strengths and weaknesses of CWS in preceding sections. However, germane to more global concerns about the communicative effectiveness of CWS, Weiss (2004) reviewed the research on the pragmatic skills of CWS as a means of determining the importance of these findings for designing fluency treatment. Research examining these skills in CWS has produced little evidence for deficits in communicative competence, although some minor differences between CWS and CWNS have been observed (Nippold, Schwarz, & Jescheniak, 1991; Scott, Healey, & Norris, 1995; Weiss & Zebrowski, 1991, 1992, 1994, 1997; Wilkenfeld & Curlee, 1997). For example, in a series of studies examining a variety of pragmatic skills, Weiss and Zebrowski (1991, 1992, 1997) reported that CWS (ranging in age from 4 years to 11 years) exhibited fewer disfluencies in response to questions than when making assertions and were more disfluent during unstructured conversation than during structured conversation. Such findings stand in contrast to some conventional advisements to parents urging them to refrain from asking CWS questions as a means of creating a more fluency-enhancing communicative environment. In fact, Bernstein Ratner (2004) has argued that much of the "standard" recommended modifications to parent-child interactions for CWS have little-to-no clinical research support. Thus, a pressing need exists to empirically evaluate the effectiveness of these recommendations (as well as their potential for heightening parental guilt). And, consideration of the findings from both stuttering and child language research tells us that we should recognize that the use of reduced or simplified language will facilitate fluency at the same time as potentially dampening linguistic growth. Thus, establishing fluency may require modifications to language use in the CWS, but a *parent* does not necessarily need to overly simplify the language she or he uses with the child to achieve fluency goals. To emphasize the importance of examining the individual impact of the communication context or parental communication style on stuttering is not as provocative a suggestion as it may seem to some; careful examination of communicative context is routinely performed in the assessment of other communication impairments, as part of a comprehensive assessment. Arguably, it is no less important in the assessment of stuttering.

◆ Conclusion

This chapter presents the authors' thoughts regarding the role of language in the understanding and treatment of stuttering in children. We recognize both obvious and subtle links between key stages of language development and the onset and maintenance of stuttering, and we argue that knowledge of the research findings in this area not only enhances our understanding of childhood stuttering, but also provides the basis for making sound clinical decisions. As clinicians, we use normal language data to determine how a youngster's stuttering is impacted by changes in language development, and to inform our planning of fluency treatment—taking into account not only grammatical elements (e.g., length and complexity) but also lexical and pragmatic. We also consider the possibility that linguistic weaknesses may exacerbate a youngster's ability to produce speech fluently. In addition to careful assessment of language and contextual variables, treatment planning must include a structure whereby fluency training is provided within appropriate linguistic and environmental contexts. When assessing and/or treating CWS who exhibit a concomitant language disorder, the clinician is faced with determining therapeutic priorities. In some cases, establishing a level of fluency within a context of reduced linguistic and pragmatic expectations may be the first preference, with language and pragmatic concerns then taking precedence following mastery of basic fluency skills. In other cases, achieving a level of linguistic competence, irrespective of fluency, may be essential before targeting stuttering behavior. As always, these decisions are made on an individual basis, with the clinician documenting changes in both fluency and language. Just as stuttering has been conceptualized—etiologically as well as symptomatically—as a multifactorial disorder (e.g., Smith & Kelly, 1997), its treatment requires the consideration and integration of multiple variables, such as fluency, language, and communicative context.

References

Anderson, J. D., & Conture, E. G.(2002). Language abilities of children who stutter: A preliminary study. Journal of Fluency Disorders 25, 283–304.

Anderson, J. D., Conture, E. G. Sentence-structure priming in young children who do and do not stutter. Journal of Speech, Language, and Hearing Research 47, 552–571.

Anderson, J. D., Pellowski, M. W., & Conture, E. G. (2005). Childhood stuttering and dissociations across linguistic domains. Journal of Fluency Disorders 30, 219–253.

Arndt, J., & Healy, E. C. (2001). Concomitant disorders in school-age children who stutter. Language, Speech, and Hearing Services in Schools 32, 68–78.

Bajaj, A., Hodson, B., & Schommer-Aiken, M. (2004). Performance on phonological and grammatical awareness metalinguistic tasks by children who stutter and their fluent peers. Journal of Fluency Disorders 29, 63–77.

Bernstein Ratner, N. (1995). Treating the child who stutters with concomitant language or phonological impairment. Language Speech Hearing Service School 26, 180–186.

Bernstein Ratner, N. (1997). Stuttering: A psycholinguistic perspective. In R. F. Curlee, & G. M. Siegel (Eds.), Nature and treatment of stuttering: New directions (2nd ed.) (pp. 99–127). Boston: Allyn & Bacon.

Bernstein Ratner, N. (2004). Caregiver-child interactions and their impact on children's fluency: Implications for treatment. Language Speech Hearing Service Schoool 35, 45–56.

Bernstein Ratner, N. (2005) Treating children with concomitant problems. In R. Lees (Ed.) The treatment of stuttering in the young school aged child (pp. 161–175). London: Whurr.

Bernstein Ratner, N. & Guitar, B. Treatment of very early stuttering and parent-administered therapy: the state of the art. In N. Ratner, & J. Tetnowski (Eds.), Stuttering research and practice (pp. 99–124); Volume 2: Contemporary issues and approaches. Mahwah, NJ: Erlbaum.

Bernstein Ratner, N. B., & Sih, C. C. (1987). The effects of gradual increases in sentence length and complexity on children's dysfluency. Journal of Speech Hearing Disorders 52, 278–287.

Bernstein Ratner, N., & Silverman, S. W. (2000). Parental perceptions of children's communicative development at stuttering onset. Journal of Speech, Language, and Hearing Research 43, 1252–1263.

Blood, G. W., Ridenour, V. J. Jr., Qualls, C. D., & Hammer, C. S. (2003). Co-occurring disorders in children who stutter. Journal of Communication Disorders 36, 427–448.

Bloodstein, O. (1995). A handbook on stuttering (5th ed.). San Diego: Singular Publishing Group.

Bonelli, P., Dixon, M., Bernstein Ratner, N., & Onslow, M. (2000). Child and parent speech and language following the Lidcombe Programme of early stuttering intervention. Clinical Linguistics and Phonetics 14, 427–446.

Boscolo, B., Bernstein Ratner, N., & Rescorla, L. (2002). Fluency of school-aged children with a history of specific expressive language impairment: An exploratory study. American Journal of Speech-Language Pathology 11, 41–49.

Brown, S. F. (1945). The loci of stutterings in the speech sequence. Journal of Speech Disorders 10, 181–192.

Byrd, K., & Cooper, E. B. (1989). Expressive and receptive language skills in stuttering children. Journal of Fluency Disorders 14, 121–126.

Costello, J. (1983). Current behavioral treatments for children. In D. Prins & R. Ingham (Eds.), Treatment of stuttering in early childhood (pp. 69–112). San Diego, CA: College-Hill Press.

Davis, D. (1939). The relation of repetitions in the speech of young children to certain measures of language maturity and situational factors. Part I. Journal of Speech Disorders 4, 303–318.

Davis, D. (1940). The relation of repetitions in the speech of young children to certain measures of language maturity and situational factors. Part II and III. Journal of Speech Disorders 5, 235–246.

Dworzynski, K., Howell, P., & Natke, U. (2003). Predicting stuttering from linguistic factors for German speakers in two age groups. Journal of Fluency Disorders 28, 95–113.

Gaines, N. D., Runyan, C. M., & Meyers, S. C. (1991). A comparison of young stutterers' fluent utterances on measures of length and complexity. Journal of Speech and Hearing Research 34, 37–42.

Gordon, P. A. (1991). Language task effects: A comparison of stuttering and nonstuttering children. Journal of Fluency Disorders 16, 275–287.

Hakim, H. B., & Bernstein Ratner, N. (2004). Nonword repetition abilities of children who stutter: An exploratory study. Journal of Fluency Disorders 29, 179–199.

Hall, N. E. (1996). Language and fluency in child language disorders: Changes over time. Journal of Fluency Disorders 21, 1–32.

Hall, N. E. (2004). Lexical development and retrieval in treating children who stutter. Language, Speech, and Hearing Services in Schools 35, 57–69.

Hall, N. E., & Burgess, S. D. (2000). Exploring developmental changes in fluency related to language acquisition: A case study. Journal of Fluency Disorders 25, 119–141.

Hall, N. E., Yamashita, T. S., & Aram, D. M. The relationship between language and fluency in children with developmental language disorders. Journal of Speech and Hearing Research 36, 568–579.

Howell, P., & Au-Yeung, J. (1995). Syntactic determinants of stuttering in the spontaneous speech of normally fluent and stuttering children. Journal of Fluency Disorders 20, 317–330.

Kadi-Hanifi, K., & Howell, P. (1992). Syntactic analysis of the spontaneous speech of normally fluency and stuttering children. Journal of Fluency Disorders 17, 151–170.

Kelly, E. M. (1994). Speech rates and trun-taking behaviors of children who stutter and their fathers. Journal of Speech and Hearing Research 37, 1284–1294.

Kelly, E. M., & Conture, E. G. (1992). Speaking rates, response time latencies, and interrupting behaviors of young stutterers, nonstutterers, and their mothers. Journal of Speech and Hearing Research 35, 1256–1267.

Kloth, S., Janssen, P., Kraaimaat, F. W., & Brutten, G. J. (1995). Communicative behavior of mothers of stuttering and nonstuttering high-risk children prior to the onset of stuttering. Journal of Fluency Disorders 20, 365–377.

Lees, R., Anderson, H., & Martin, P. (1999). The influence of language disorder on fluency: A pilot study. Journal of Fluency Disorders 24, 227–238.

Leonard, L. B. (1998). Children with specific language impairment. Cambridge, MA: MIT Press.

Logan, K. J. (2001). The effect of syntactic complexity upon the speech fluency of adolescents and adults who stutter. Journal of Fluency Disorders 26, 85–106.

Logan, K. J. (2003). Language and fluency characteristics of preschoolers' multiple-utterance conversational turns. Journal of Speech, Language, and Hearing Research 46, 178–188.

Logan, K. J., & Conture, E. G. (1995). Length, grammatical complexity, and rate differences in stuttered and fluent conversational utterances of children who stutter. Journal of Fluency Disorders 20, 35–61.

Logan, K. J., & Conture, E. G. (1997). Selected temporal, grammatical, and phonological characteristics of conversational utterances produced by children who stutter. Journal of Speech, Language, and Hearing Research 40, 107–120.

Logan, K. J., & LaSalle, L. R. (2003) Developing intervention programs for children with stuttering and concomitant impairments. Seminars in Speech and Language 24, 13–19.

Melnick, K. S., & Conture, E. G. (2000). Relationship of length and grammatical complexity to the systematic and nonsystematic speech errors and stuttering of children who stutter. Journal of Fluency Disorders 25, 21–45.

Melnick, K. S., Conture, E. G., & Ohde, R. N. (2003). Phonological priming in picture naming of young children who stutter. Journal of Speech, Language, and Hearing Research 46, 1428–1443.

Miles, S., & Bernstein Ratner, N. (2001). Parental language input to children at stuttering onset. Journal of Speech, Language, and Hearing Research 44, 1116–1130.

Miller, J. F. (1978). Assessing children's language behavior: A developmental process approach. In R. L. Schiefelbusch (Ed.), The basis of language intervention (pp. 269–318). Baltimore: University Park Press.

Natke, U., Sandreiser, P., van Ark, M., Pietrowsky, R., & Kalveram, K. T. (2004). Linguistic stress, within word position, and grammatical class in relation to early childhood stuttering. Journal of Fluency Disorders 29, 109–122.

Nelson, K. (1973). Structure and strategy in learning to talk. Monographs of the Society for Research in Child Development, 38 (1–2, Serial No. 149).

Newcomer P., & Hammill, D. (1982). Test of Language Development-Primary. Austin, TX: PRO-ED.

Nippold, M. A. (1990). Concomitant speech and language disorders in stuttering children: A critique of the literature. Journal of Speech Hearing Disorders 55, 51–60.

Nippold, M. A. (2004). Phonological and language disorders in children who stutter: Impact on treatment recommendations. Clinical Linguistics and Phonetics 18, 145–159.

Nippold, M. A., & Rudzinski, M. (1995). Parents' speech and children's stuttering: A critique of the literature. Journal of Speech and Hearing Research 38, 978–989.

Nippold, M. A., Schwarz, I. E., & Jescheniak, J. D. (1991). Narrative ability in school-age stuttering boys: A preliminary investigation. Journal of Fluency Disorders 16, 289–308.

Paul, R. (2001). Language disorders from infancy through adolescence (2nd ed.). St. Louis, MO: Mosby.

Paul, R. (2002). Introduction to clinical methods in communication disorders. Baltimore: Brookes Publishing Company.

Pellowski, M. W., & Conture, E. G. (2005). Lexical priming in picture naming of young children who do and do not stutter. Journal of Speech, Language, and Hearing Research 48, 278–294.

Rispoli, M. (2003). Changes in the nature of speech production during the period of grammatical development. Journal of Speech, Language, and Hearing Research 46, 818–830.

Rispoli, M., & Hadley, P. (2001). The leading edge: The significance of sentence disruptions in the development of grammar. Journal of Speech, Language, and Hearing Research 44, 1131–1143.

Ryan, B. (1980). Programmed therapy for stuttering children and adults (3rd ed.). Springfield, IL: Charles C. Thomas.

Ryan, B. P. (1992). Articulation, language, rate and fluency characteristics of stuttering and nonstuttering preschool children. Journal of Speech and Hearing Research 35, 333–342.

Ryan, B. (2001). A longitudinal study of articulation, language, rate, and fluency of 22 preschool children who stutter. Journal of Fluency Disorders 26, 107–127.

Scott, C. M., & Windsor, J. (2000). General language performance measures in spoken and written narrative and expository discourse of school-age children with language learning disabilities. Journal of Speech, Language, and Hearing Research 43, 324–339.

Scott, L., Healey, E., & Norris J. (1995). A comparison between children who stutter and their normally fluent peers on a story retelling task. Journal of Fluency Disorders 20, 279–292.

Silverman, S., & Bernstein Ratner, N. (1997). Syntactic complexity, fluency, and accuracy of sentence imitation in adolescents. Journal of Speech, Language, and Hearing Research 40, 93–106.

Silverman, S., & Bernstein Ratner, N. (2002). Measuring lexical diversity in children who stutter: Application of vocd. Journal of Fluency Disorders 27, 289–304.

Slobin, D. (1973). Cognitive prerequisites for the development of grammar. In C. Ferguson & D. Slobin (Eds.), Studies of child language development. New York: Holt, Rinehart & Winston.

Smith, A., & Kelly, E. (1997). Stuttering: A dynamic, multifactorial model. In R. F. Curlee & G. M. Siegel (Eds.), Nature and treatment of stuttering: New directions (pp. 204–217). Boston: Allyn and Bacon.

St. Louis, K. O., & Hinzman, A. R. (1988). A descriptive study of speech, language and hearing characteristics of school-aged stutterers. Journal of Fluency Disorders 13, 331–335.

St. Louis, K. O., Hinzman, A. R., & Hull, F. M. (1985). Studies of cluttering: disfluency and language measures in young possible clutters and stutterers. Journal of Fluency Disorders 10, 151–172.

St. Louis, K. O., Murray, C. D., & Ashworth, M. S. (1991). Coexisting communication disorders in a random sample of school-aged stutterers. Journal of Fluency Disorders 16, 13–23.

Thordardottir, E. T., & Ellis Weismer, S. (2002). Content mazes and filled pauses in narrative samples of children with specific language impairment. Brain Cognitive 48, 587–592.

Throneburg, R. N., & Yairi, E. (2001). Durational, proportionate, and absolute frequency characteristics of disfluencies: A longitudinal study regarding persistence and recovery. Journal of Speech, Language, and Hearing Research 44, 38–51.

Watkins, R., & Johnson, B. (2004). Language abilities in children who stutter: Toward improved research and clinical applications. Language, Speech, & Hearing Services School 35, 82–90.

Watkins, R. V., & Yairi, E. (1997). Language production abilities of children whose stuttering persisted or recovered. Journal of Speech, Language, and Hearing Research 40, 385–399.

Watkins, R. V., Yairi, E., & Ambrose, N. G. (1999). Early childhood stuttering III: Initial status of expressive language abilities. Journal of Speech, Language, and Hearing Research 42, 1125–1135.

Weiss, A. L. (2004). Why we should consider pragmatics when planning treatment for children who stutter. Language Speech Hearing Service School 35, 34–45.

Weiss, A. L., & Zebrowski, P. (1991). Patterns of assertiveness and responsiveness in parental interactions with stuttering and fluent children. Journal of Fluency Disorders 16, 125–141.

Weiss, A. L., & Zebrowski, P. (1992). Disfluencies in the conversations of young children who stutter: Some answers about questions. Journal of Speech and Hearing Research 35, 1230–1238.

Weiss, A. L., & Zebrowski, P. (1994). The narrative productions of children who stutter: A preliminary view. Journal of Fluency Disorders 19, 39–63.

Weiss, A. L., & Zebrowski, P. (1997). Effects of conversation participation on young children who stutter. In E. Healey & H. Peters (Eds.), Proceedings of the 2nd world congress on fluency disorders (pp. 92–96). Nijmegen, The Netherlands: Nijmegen University Press.

Wijnen, F. (1990). The development of sentence planning. Journal of Child Language 17, 651–675.

Wilkenfeld, J. R., & Curlee, R. F. (1997). The relative effects of questions and comments on children's stuttering. American Journal of Speech-Language Pathology 6(3), 79–89.

Yairi, E. (1997). Home environments and parent-child interaction in childhood stuttering. In R. F. Curlee & G. M. Siegel, (Eds.), Nature and treatment of stuttering: New directions (2nd ed.) (pp. 24–48). Needham Heights, MA: Allyn and Bacon.

Yairi, E., Ambrose, N. G., Paden, E. P., & Throneburg, R. N. (1996). Predictive factors of persistence and recovery: Pathways of childhood stuttering. Journal of Communication Disorders 29, 51–77.

Yaruss, J. S. (1999). Utterance length, syntactic complexity, and childhood stuttering. Journal of Speech, Language, and Hearing Research 42, 329–344.

Yaruss, J. S., & Conture, E. G. (1995). Mother and child speaking rates and utterance lengths in adjacent fluent utterances: Preliminary observations. Journal of Fluency Disorders 20, 257–278.

Yaruss, J. S., LaSalle, L. R., & Conture, E. G. (1998). Evaluating stuttering in young children: Diagnostic data. American Journal of Speech-Language Pathology 7(4), 62–76.

Yaruss, J. S., Newman, R. M., & Flora, T. (1999). Language and disfluency in nonstuttering children's conversational speech. Journal of Fluency Disorders 24, 185–207.

Zackheim, C. T., & Conture, E. G. (2003). Childhood stuttering and speech disfluencies in relation to children's mean length of utterance: A preliminary study. Journal of Fluency Disorders 28, 115–142.

Zimmerman, I. L., Steiner, V. G., & Pond, R. E. (1979). Preschool Language Scale-revised. San Antonio, TX: Psychological.

10

Role of Phonology in Childhood Stuttering and Its Treatment

Courtney Thompson Byrd, Lesley Wolk, and Barbara Lockett Davis

The relationship between stuttering and phonology has been increasingly investigated over the past two decades (for a review, see Bloodstein, 1995, Table 18; Louko, Conture & Edwards, 1999; cf. Nippold 1990, 2002). To date, most such research has focused on clinically significant deficits in phonological development as such deficits may relate to the speech-language *production* of children who stutter (CWS), but some research (e.g., Melnick, Conture & Ohde, 2003) has also examined phonology from a *planning* perspective. Although results from the investigations that have examined the influence of phonology from a production perspective continue to indicate that disordered phonology often co-occurs with stuttering (Blood, Ridenour, Qualls, & Hammer, 2003), studies that have examined the planning perspective seem to indicate that disordered phonology does not have to be present for the child's fluency to be compromised by his or her phonological system. That is, even if CWS do not present with atypical disordered phonology, it is possible that their phonological abilities may differ, at least subtly, from those of children who do not stutter (CWNS), in ways that may either exacerbate or contribute to instances of stuttering.

The purpose of this chapter is to provide an abbreviated review of contemporary research, a review that may help to determine what role, if any, phonology has in the development of stuttering. As suggested above, this role may range from the overt perspective of an atypical degree of concomitance to the covert possibility of phonological encoding differences. Therefore, research related to the following selected areas will be reviewed: (1) the co-occurrence of stuttering and phonology; (2) the relationship between persistence of stuttering and persistence of phonological delay; (3) the phonological complexity of the stuttered word; (4) the neighborhood density of the stuttered word; (5) the phonotactic probability of the stuttered word; and (6) the phonological encoding abilities of children and adults who stutter (AWS). Following this review, the related assessment and treatment implications are explored.

♦ Review of Research on the Relationship of Stuttering and Phonology

Co-occurrence of Stuttering and Phonological Disorders

To help determine whether phonological and language disorders commonly co-occur in CWS, Arndt and Healey (2001) collected data from 241 speech-language pathologists (SLPs) from 10 states across the nation and found that of 467 CWS, 56% ($N = 205$) reportedly demonstrated a concomitant language and/or phonological disorder. Within those 205 children who presented with stuttering and a co-occurring disorder, 66 (32%) were reported to have what they referred to as a verified phonological disorder. Although this percentage does seem to concur with previous estimates (Conture, 2001), Arndt and Healey suggested that this percentage may have been positively skewed by at least one of two factors. First, the authors note that when you consider the 66 children within the total sample of CWS of 467 rather than the sample of CWS who also presented with a concomitant disorder ($N = 205$), the percentage of CWS with a concomitant phonological disorder is 14% (66/467) rather than 32% (66/205). The other potential confounding factor was the conflation of articulation disorders and language-based phonological disorders. That is, these two disorders may not have been adequately separated from each other to insure that these children did, indeed, present with phonological impairments alone. The authors further noted that the diagnostic guidelines for stuttering, language disorder, and phonological disorder varied among the 10 states surveyed. This lack of consistent diagnostic criteria limits the abilities to unambiguously assess or reliably interpret these findings.

Considering these potential confounding variables, Blood et al. (2003) followed up the Arndt and Healey (2001) study by revising the methodology in three important ways: (1) accessing SLPs nationwide (46 different states across the United States); (2) only using documented data; and (3) providing the participants (i.e., practicing SLPs) with a more comprehensive list of concomitant language, speech, and non-speech–language disorders (e.g., disorders that impact learning, attention, reading, etc.). Similar to Arndt and Healey (2001), Blood et al. (2003) employed a mail survey. This survey was completed by 1184 SLPs across the nation. Results indicated that 62.8% of the CWS had concomitant language, speech, or nonspeech disorders. Interestingly, 33.5% of these CWS presented with an articulation disorder, whereas 12.7% presented with a phonological disorder. The findings of Blood et al. (2003) are strikingly similar to those of Arndt and Healey (2001), despite the fact that the methodology was revised to take into account the aforementioned considerations. Most importantly, however, percentages reported by Arndt and Healey (2001) and Blood et al. (2003) are still at least twice as high as the 2 to 6% of children with articulation/phonological disorders reported for the general population (Beitchman, Nair, Clegg, & Patel, 1986).

A study by Nippold (2004) may provide contrasting evidence to the previously reviewed studies (i.e., Arndt & Healey, 2001; Blood et al., 2003). In her study, 127 SLPs completed a survey. When asked if they would be more likely to provide treatment to CWS with a concomitant disorder as compared with child who presents only with stuttering, 31% responded affirmatively, whereas 46% said no and 23% were unsure. The 31% who said that they would provided rationale for this, including that the child may be in more need of services and also that the child may be able to meet the guidelines more easily. To further investigate this issue Nippold (2004) asked survey participants to assess a case study of a 4-year-old male CWS. Results from this part of the survey indicated the following: (1) 71% would provide treatment if this child had no other concomitant disorder; (2) 91% would provide treatment if this child also had a phonological disorder; (3) 94% would provide treatment if this child also had a language disorder; and (4) 94% would provide treatment if the child had both a phonological and a language disorder.

Nippold (2004) interpreted her results to indicate that SLPs are more likely to provide treatment to CWS with concomitant disorders and, thus, any previous survey research (e.g., Arndt & Healey, 2001; Blood et al., 2003) may be biased by the likely increase in the amount of CWS with concomitant disorders on their caseload. However, this interpretation is significantly weakened by the fact that a nontrivial percentage (46%) of the SLPs reported that they would not be more likely to treat a CWS with a concomitant disorder as compared with a child diagnosed with stuttering alone. An additional weakness is that survey respondents were describing a relationship between what they might do without comparing it with exactly what they have done. The strength of this interpretation would have been significantly increased if SLPs surveyed had also provided a list of the children currently on their caseload. Nevertheless, Nippold's findings do raise a valuable question about whether method of data collection contributes to results. It would have been interesting if Nippold had included time since onset as a question in her survey. Perhaps it is not the concomitance of the phonological disorder but the persistence of the stuttering that results in that child with concomitant disorders being more likely to receive treatment.

Relationship between Persistence of Stuttering and Presence of a Phonological Delay

The findings of three interrelated studies on the relationship between the persistence of stuttering and the presence of a phonological delay are consistent with the possibility that stuttering and phonological difficulties are most likely to co-occur for those children whose stuttering persists. (Paden & Yairi, 1996; Paden, Yairi, & Ambrose, 1999; Yairi, Ambrose, Paden, & Throneburg, 1996). Paden and Yairi (1996) found that those CWS who continued to stutter more than 36 months post-onset exhibited significantly poorer phonological skills than age- and gender-matched CWNS. In a follow-up study with the same children Yairi et al. (1996) found that the phonological skills of each child had improved within the year after the initial measurement. This finding suggests that the presence of a phonological delay may help to predict persistence of stuttering, but the value of this predictability may decrease over time. Following their second empirical study of this issue, Paden et al. (1999) found that for those CWS who had deficient phonological skills near the time of onset of stuttering, their stuttering would be more likely to persist than resolve. Given that no one standardized measure for determination of onset of stuttering (as well as persistence) currently exists, results from these three interrelated studies should be interpreted with caution. However, taken together, these results do appear to indicate that phonology is a reasonably reliable predictor of persistence of stuttering, at least within a certain window of time (cf., Ryan, 2001).

Somewhat in contrast are the findings of Ryan (2001), who reported on the results of a longitudinal study with 14 male and eight female children who stutter. These children were formally assessed every 3 to 5 months for approximately 2 years. During each formal assessment the child's fluency (i.e., stuttered words per minute) was evaluated via an interview and the child's phonological development was evaluated via the Arizona Articulation Proficiency Scale (AAPS). Findings indicated that there were no significant differences in AAPS raw scores for those children whose stuttering persisted ($N = 7$) and those whose stuttering remitted ($N = 15$). Findings further indicated there were no significant correlations between the child's stuttering frequency and the child's AAPs score over time. However, one major confound of this study was that the age of Ryan's 22 child participants ranged from 2 years, 4 months to 5 years, 10 months, indicating that some of these children could potentially have been stuttering significantly longer than others. To that end, Pellowski and Conture (2002) found that 4-year-old, but not 3-year-old, CWS demonstrate changes in nonreiterative types of stuttering (e.g., sound prolongations) as a function of time since onset. The authors interpreted this age-dependent finding to indicate that it is possible that phonological difficulties are most apt to be associated with a stuttering problem that continues well after the time since onset, with the latter form of stuttering being associated with increasing amounts of nonreiterative types of stuttering.

Phonological Complexity of Stuttered Word

Although previous research has indicated that the phonological complexity of the word did not appear to increase the probability that the word would be stuttered (Howell & Au-Yeung, 1995; Throneburg, Yairi, & Paden, 1994), Melnick and Conture (2000) posited that this relationship might be apparent particularly in utterances that were of increased length and syntactic complexity. They analyzed the stuttered and nonstuttered utterances of 10 male CWS who also presented with disordered phonology (age range: 2 years, 10 months to 6 years, 2 months) to determine if these children produced more phonological process errors in stuttered utterances.

Using the covert repair hypothesis (see Postma & Kolk, 1993; Kolk & Postma, 1997) as their theoretical motivation, they posited that the frequency of stuttering should increase in longer and more grammatically complex utterances because of the child's detection of the increased potential of these errors and his or her attempts to covertly repair them. Prior to engaging in a conversational speech sample with his or her mother, each child completed a picture-naming task designed to identify the phonological processes used. From the conversational sample, 25 stuttered and 25 nonstuttered utterances were randomly selected for each child and then all data for the children were combined for group analyses. To determine what factors if any could systematically increase the frequency of phonological processes, a multiple regression analysis using utterance length, grammatical complexity, and utterance fluency as potential predictors was conducted. Findings indicated that phonological processes did not occur significantly more frequently in longer utterances, in more grammatically complex utterances, and/or in stuttered utterances. The authors interpreted these findings to indicate a lack of support for at least one possible prediction of the covert repair hypothesis. Perhaps this relationship cannot be seen at the larger level of the utterance; rather, it may need to be more closely examined at the smaller level of the stuttered word itself.

To that end, Wolk, Blomgren, and Smith (2000) also examined male CWS who presented with disordered phonology ($N = 7$; age range: 4 years, 5 months to 5 years, 11 months) to determine if stuttering occurred more frequently within syllables that contained phonological errors. At least 300 syllables produced by each child from within a conversational interaction with his or her mother were analyzed to determine how frequently stuttering and phonological errors co-occurred.

Although overall findings indicated that syllables produced with phonological errors were not produced with stuttering significantly more often than syllables produced without phonological errors, findings did indicate that stuttering ocurred significantly more frequently on those syllables produced with phonological errors that began with consonant clusters in comparison with those syllables that began with consonant clusters that did not contain phonological errors. One interpretation of these preliminary findings is that they lend support to the demands-capacities model (Adams, 1990) in that stuttering appears to increase within those productions requiring increased *phonological* complexity. Perhaps both the location and the nature of the consonant cluster in the syllable contributed to the increased incidence of stuttering accompanying phonological errors. Comparison of heterorganic (i.e., consonants that occur in the different places) with homorganic clusters (i.e., consonants that occur in the same place) containing stuttering moments as well as with fluently produced consonant clusters would help address this issue.

Huinck, van Lieshout, Peters, and Hulstijn (2004) used the gestural phonology model (GPM) (Browman & Goldstein, 1997) to investigate the impact of gestural overlap between two adjacent homorganic versus heterorganic consonants in clusters in coda and medial positions on speech reaction times and word durations of adults who do and do not stutter. The GPM is an articulatory-based theory of phonology that defines phonological units as coordinated gestures. Coordination of gestures enables fluid integration of sequential movements required for speech. The basic tenets of the GPM supported the authors' prediction that more time should be needed for planning and initiation of clusters of consonants that occur in the same place (i.e., homorganic), and, conversely, less time should be needed for heterorganic consonant clusters due to the overlap in time for planning these productions. Speech reaction time was also predicted to be slower in the homorganic as compared with the heterorganic condition and this difference was predicted to be greater for AWS than adults who do not stutter (AWNS). Participants were 10 AWS (mean age = 23 years, 9 months) and 12 AWNS (mean age = 24 years, 1 month) matched for age, gender, and educational level. Each participant was seated in front of a computer screen and instructed to read the target word as soon as possible upon hearing a "go-signal." Target words comprised 12 mono- and 12 bisyllabic nonwords beginning with /ba:/ presented twice in random order.

Findings indicated that both AWS and AWNS exhibited more incorrect speech productions and slower speech reaction times for homorganic than for heterorganic clusters, but there were no differences between AWS and AWNS in reaction times and word durations. However, AWS produced a greater number of speech disfluencies and demonstrated a large number of speech errors. AWS also produced longer reactions times for homorganic versus heterorganic clusters when occurring in the intersyllabic condition. The authors interpreted the findings to indicate support for the GPM in that there is a notable increase in the demands on motor planning, particularly for AWS, when producing homorganic consonants across a syllable boundary than when producing the same cluster within a syllable.

Dworzynski and Howell (2004) recently investigated how phonological complexity influences stuttering in people who stutter whose native language is not English. Participants included 50 monolingual German speakers (age range: 2–47 years) and 26 monolingual English speakers (age range: 6–18+ years). Each participant, with the exception of the youngest German age group, engaged in a spontaneous language sample with an SLP that ranged in length from 2 to 25 minutes. The German group of youngest participants engaged in a play interaction with their mothers designed to elicit a similar conversation interaction as the SLP facilitated with older children and adults. The phonetic difficulty of words produced within these samples was assessed using Jakielski's index of phonetic complexity (IPC; 1998), which scores phonetic complexity of words based on the following eight characteristics: (1) consonant by place; (2) consonant by manner; (3) singleton consonant by place; (4) rhotic vowels; (5) word shape; (6) three or more syllables; (7) contiguous consonants; and (8) cluster by place.

Findings indicated that for German function words, the frequency of stuttering was not related to phonetic complexity. By comparison, for children of at least 6 years of age and adults, results did indicate significant correlations between the frequency of stuttering and IPC score for content words. Results further indicated that the sum of the IPC mean scores for German content words was significantly higher than for English. In addition, findings indicated there was a larger difference between the IPC score for the German stuttered versus fluent words than there was for the English stuttered versus fluent words. The authors note that there are limitations to IPC with the major one being that the high degree of correlation between several of the eight scoring characteristics may have had an impact on the strength of the findings. However, overall the findings do appear to indicate that the spontaneously produced content words are more phonologically complex and that complexity may explain the higher mean IPC scores stuttered versus fluent words in German as compared with English. Perhaps this finding is not only related to content versus function categories but also to the neighborhood density of the word.

Neighborhood Density of Stuttered Word

Phonological neighbors have been defined as words that differ by one phoneme substitution, deletion, or addition and, thus, can be categorized as dense (i.e., words with many neighbors) or sparse (i.e., words with minimal neighbors) (Luce & Pisoni, 1998). Research has indicated that during perceptual tasks infants and toddlers appear to prefer phonologically dense words (Jusczyk, Luce, & Charles-Luce, 1994). By comparison, during production tasks school-age children appear to prefer sparse words (Newman & German, 2002), whereas, adults demonstrate a preference toward dense words (Vitevitch, 2002). Because sparse words have fewer neighbors, these words will not receive as much activation as dense words and, consequently, are less likely to be accurately and rapidly retrieved from the lexicon. By comparison, with increased lexical development, dense words are more easily and accurately accessed due to the simultaneous activation of multiple word forms.

Arnold, Conture, and Ohde (2005) hypothesized that preschool CWNS should demonstrate faster speech reaction time and more accurate picture-naming responses for phonologically sparse as compared with dense words, but that preschool CWS should at the least be slower and less accurate. Nine (4 females, 5 males; 3 to 5 years old) CWS and nine age- and gender-matched CWNS were presented with five phonologically dense and five phonologically sparse picture words in randomized order. Picture naming for both young CWNS and CWS was slower and less accurate for phonological dense words. In addition, there were no significant differences in the speed or the accuracy between CWNS and CWS in naming phonologically dense versus sparse words. Arnold et al. (2005) interpreted these findings to indicate that given the lack of differential influence of phonological neighborhood density on the phonological processes of CWS versus CWNS, phonological neighborhood density of words may make minimal to no contributions to the ability of a CWS to establish fluent speech-language productions. However, the influence of neighborhood variables may be more apparent when examining fluent versus stuttered words spontaneously produced by CWS in conversation.

Anderson (in press) examined the influence of phonological neighborhood variables (word frequency, neighborhood density, and neighborhood frequency) on the stuttered disfluencies of preschool CWS. Participants were 15 CWS (age range: 3 years, 0 months to 5 years, 2 months). Each participant completed a conversational interaction with his or her mother that resulted in speech sample of at least 500 words. From this 500+ word speech sample, each stuttered word was paired with the first fluent word that matched it on grammatical class, familiarity, and number of syllables/phonemes, resulting in a total of 515 useable word pairs (stuttered words and their matched controls) across all participants. These stuttered and matched fluent word pairs were then entered in the Hoosier Mental Lexicon (Luce & Pisoni, 1998) to obtain values for their word frequency, neighborhood density, and neighborhood frequency. Stuttered words were significantly lower in word frequency and neighborhood frequency than fluent words. Results further indicated that even though stuttered words appeared to be slightly more frequently composed of dense than sparse neighborhoods than fluent words were, similar to Arnold et al. (2005), neighborhood density did not significantly influence fluent speech production. In addition, results indicated that words containing part-word repetitions and sound prolongations were lower in word and neighborhood frequency than words containing single-syllable word repetitions. However, neighborhood density did not influence the type of disfluency produced. Taken together, these findings suggest that phonological neighborhood variables may influence the fluency of the production of words in running speech and that these variables may also influence the specific type of disfluency produced.

Phonotactic Probability of the Stuttered Word

Given that neighborhood density tends to be highly, positively correlated with phonotactic probability (Vitevitch, Luce, Pisoni, & Auer, 1999), recent research has also investigated the influence of phonotactic probability on the stuttered utterances of CWS. Phonotactic probability has been defined as the frequency of occurrence of different sound segments and segment sequences in the lexicon (Vitevitch, Armbrüster, & Chu, 2004). Thus, words with dense neighborhoods tend to be high in phonotactic probability, whereas words with sparse neighborhoods are more likely to be low in phonotactic probability (Vitevitch, 2002). Research with typically developing children (i.e., CWNS) has indicated that those words with high phonotactic probability, words with more common sound segments and segment sequences, are less likely to contain speech errors than those with low phonotactic probability, words containing less common sound segments and segment sequences (Storkel, 2001; Vitevitch, Luce, Charles-Luce, & Kemmerer, 1997).

Anderson and Byrd (unpublished manuscript) investigated the impact of phonotactic probability on the speech fluency of 14 CWS (age range: 3 years, 0 months to 5 years, 2 months). A conversational sample of at least 500 words was obtained for each child. Each of the children's stuttered words was randomly paired with a fluent word that was matched for the following characteristics: (1) length in syllables and phonemes; (2) grammatical class; (3) familiarity; (4) frequency;

(5) neighborhood density; and (6) neighborhood frequency. These stuttered and matched fluent words were entered into the phonotactic probability calculator (Vitevitch & Luce, 2004) to allow calculation of log-based values for the probability of co-occurrences of two adjacent sounds within a word (i.e., biphone frequency) and the probability of occurrence of a particular sound in a particular word position (i.e., positional segment frequency).

Findings revealed that stuttered disfluencies were generally not susceptible to the effects of phonotactic probability, but words containing single-syllable repetitions were significantly lower in phonotactic probability than fluent controls as well as words containing part-word repetitions. This differential impact of phonotactic probability on the type of stutter-like disfluency may be related to the underlying representation of the word, a suggestion that is in line with Anderson's (in press) neighborhood density findings. That is, those words for which the phonological segments are underspecified will not be as susceptible to the effects of phonotactic probability as those words that contain the specification for the individual segments that compose the word. In this respect, present findings point to the possibility that part-word repetitions and sound prolongations may be a consequence of difficulty at the level of the word-form, whereas single-syllable word repetitions may be due to difficulty at the lemma level. Thus, these findings suggest that CWS may lag behind their normally fluent peers in the development of fully specified phonological representations. If such underspecification is, indeed, an issue for CWS, then it would also be reasonable to suggest that the phonological encoding of these children may not be as advanced as their typically developing peers.

Phonological Encoding Abilities of Children and Adults Who Stutter

Phonological encoding has been defined as the rapid mapping of the syntactic/meaning aspects of a word (i.e., lemma) onto the phonological form of a word (i.e., lexeme) (Levelt, 1989). Recent research (Weber-Fox, Spencer, Spruill, & Smith, 2004) investigated the phonological encoding of AWS in comparison with AWNS through the analysis of event-related brain potentials (ERPs), judgment accuracy, and reaction times during the completion of a rhyme judgment task of visually presented primes and targets (i.e., word pairs). These word pairs were separated into two categories: (1) congruent and (2) incongruent. In the congruent category, the word pairs were phonologically and orthographically congruent across words. Thus, in this category the words either looked similar and rhymed or did not look similar and did not rhyme. For the incongruent category the words either looked similar but did not rhyme or did not look similar but rhymed.

Overall, AWS demonstrated phonological encoding similar to AWNS. However, AWS demonstrated longer reaction times than AWNS during the incongruent category tasks. Weber-Fox et al. (2004) interpreted this slowness in reaction time to indicate that AWS are more sensitive to increases in cognitive load. Additionally, unlike AWNS, AWS demonstrated right-hemisphere asymmetry in the rhyme judgment task. Although these investigators concluded that an integrated view of these findings do not lend support to the theories of stuttering that suggest difficulties with phonological encoding as a major contributor to the development of stuttering, the investigators did acknowledge that these findings need to be explored with CWS and in overt speech production rather than nonspeech tasks.

Consistent with this suggestion, Hakim and Bernstein Ratner (2004) investigated the phonological encoding of young CWS (age range: 4 years, 3 months to 8 years, 4 months; mean age: 5 years, 10 months) in comparison with age- and gender-matched CWNS during a nonword repetition task. This task included 40 nonsense words consisting of 10 words comprising 2 syllables, 10 comprising 3 syllables, 10 comprising 4 syllables and 10 comprising 5 syllables. The set of ten 4-syllable words were repeated a second time but with an altered stress pattern atypical of English. Results indicated CWS performed more poorly than CWNS on measures of number of words correct and number of phoneme errors at all nonword lengths; however, the only significant difference was observed for the repetition of the 3-syllable nonwords. In addition, although both CWNS and CWS demonstrated more errors when repeating the nonword set that was composed of the altered stress pattern, the CWS made more errors. Findings were taken to suggest that CWS may have a deficiency in their ability to hold novel phonological sequences in memory and, subsequently, in their ability to adequately repro-duce those novel sequences. Perhaps this deficiency impacts the speed with which CWS are able to phonological encode words.

To investigate such a possibility, Melnick et al. (2003) employed a picture-naming task. Partici-pants were 18 CWS (mean age: 50.67 months) and 18 age- and gender-matched CWNS (mean age: 49.44 months). For this task, immediately prior to picture presentation the participants were: (1) not presented with an auditory prime (no prime condition); (2) presented auditorily with a word onset related prime that comprised the consonant onset plus the formant transitions and most of the vowel of the name of the target picture (related prime condition); or (3) presented auditorily with a word onset unrelated prime that comprised a consonant onset plus formant transitions and most of the vowel target of a word that did not correspond with the target picture (unrelated prime condition).

Findings indicated that CWNS exhibited a greater (though not significantly greater) phonological priming effect (i.e., speech reaction time [SRT] faster in related than neutral condition) than CWS. However, CWNS did exhibit a significant correlation between articulatory mastery scores (based on the Goldman-Fristoe test of articulation) and SRTs during each of the three priming conditions. By comparison, CWS did not exhibit a significant correlation between SRT and any of the priming con-ditions. The authors interpreted this finding to indicate that the articulatory production system of CWS is not as well organized and/or developed as that of their normally fluent peers. Although not surprising, it is important to note that results of this study indicated across all conditions that the SRT of both CWS and CWNS became faster with age, indicating that cognitive processing speed in-creases with development.

One additional interesting aspect of the Melnick et al. (2003) data that was not examined or re-ported was differences seen for SRT in the related prime condition between 3- versus 5-year-old CWNS that were not apparent for 3- versus 5-year-old CWS. In essence, for the related prime con-dition, 5-year-old CWNS demonstrated a faster speech reaction time than 3-year-old CWNS, but no such age-related differences in SRT were apparent for CWS. This perhaps suggests that CWS may continue to use a more immature form of phonological encoding (i.e., holistic processing) at a later age in development than is typically expected.

Holistic processing has been defined as the processing of a unit of speech of at least syllable size (see Charles-Luce & Luce, 1990; Walley, 1988). By comparison, incremental processing has been defined as the processing of the word as individual sounds from the beginning to the end. Typically, developing young children's phonological representations are more holistic than older children and adults (Walley, 1988, 1993; Walley, Smith, & Jusczyk, 1986) due to young children's tendency to "employ more global recognition strategies because words are more discriminable in memory" (Charles-Luce & Luce, 1990, p.205). A relatively consistent finding in childhood stuttering research is that the mean onset of stutter-ing typically occurs between 30 and 36 months of age (e.g., Mansson, 2000; Yairi & Ambrose, 1999; Yaruss, LaSalle, & Conture, 1998), an age range during which the shift from holistic to incremental pro-cessing is thought to occur in typically developing children (i.e., CWNS) (Charles-Luce & Luce, 1990; Walley, 1988). Although the putative shift from holistic to incremental processing is but one of several changes that may occur with 30- to 36-month-old children, childhood stuttering may be more likely to begin during the developmental period when changes from holistic to incremental processing are most apt to occur and/or begin in typically developing children (i.e., CWNS).

To examine this possible developmental difference between CWS and CWNS, Byrd, Conture, and Ohde (in press) studied 3- (N = 13) and 5-year-old (N = 13) female and male CWS and an identical number of age- and gender-matched CWNS during a picture-naming task (e.g., Glaser, 1992). This priming task required the participants to name computer-presented line drawings of common age-appropriate items during three auditory priming conditions: (1) *neutral prime*; (2) *incremental prime*; and (3) *holistic prime*. In the *neutral prime* condition, 600 ms prior to picture presentation participants were presented with a cue consisting of a 100-ms, 1-kHz "beep" presented 45 dB(SPL) free-field from a pair of standard computer speakers. In the *incremental prime* condition, partici-pants were presented with the target word's initial consonant(s) and two to six glottal pulses of the transition into the following vowel. In the *holistic prime* condition, participants were presented with a prime that contained all of the acoustic information of the target word except for the initial consonant(s) and two to six glottal pulses of the transition to vowel.

Byrd et al. (in press) reported that 3-year-old CWNS exhibited significantly faster SRT than 5-year-olds in the holistic condition; however, for the incremental condition, 5-year-old CWNS were significantly faster than 3-year-old CWNS. Within the group of 3-year-old CWNS, there was no significant difference in SRT between the priming conditions, but within the group of 5-year-old CWNS, SRT was faster in the incremental than holistic conditions. By comparison, although 5-year-old CWS exhibited significantly faster SRT than 3-year-old CWS in the incremental condition, there was no significant difference in SRT for the holistic condition between 3- and 5-year-old CWS. Furthermore, both 3- and 5-year-old CWS exhibited faster speech reaction time in the holistic than the incremental condition. Findings lend support to the hypothesis that CWS are delayed in making the developmental shift from holistic to incremental processing of phonological representations and that this delay may contribute to their difficulties initiating and/or maintaining fluent speech.

Summary

The previous review of contemporary research indicates that phonological disorders continue to co-occur with stuttering and that the persistence of this disorder may contribute to the persistence of stuttering. In addition, for those CWS who do not present with phonological disorders the review suggests that there may subtle phonological differences that contribute to their inability to produce and/or maintain fluent speech. This review further indicates that the underlying representation of the stuttered word may provide valuable information regarding the factors contributing to fluency breakdown. It is hoped that this abbreviated review will serve to ignite additional interest in this area of research that will ultimately lead to a better understanding of the phonological piece of the stuttering puzzle.

♦ Assessment and Treatment

Since we do not yet have definitive information on the exact symptomatological differences of CWS who present with phonological disorders, we need to extrapolate from what we know about each disorder in isolation. Our suggestions for assessment and treatment are based on clinical experience and limited data drawn from small subject pools.

Assessment

With regard to stuttering assessment, the following dimensions are useful: (1) mean frequency, and range of all speech disfluencies based on a 300-word sample; (2) mean frequency of each disfluency type; (3) mean duration (in milliseconds) from onset to offset of 10 randomly selected speech disfluencies; (4) mean number of iterations per sound syllable repetition for 10 randomly selected disfluencies; (5) a stuttering severity index (e.g., SSI-3; Riley, 1994); and (6) mean rate of speech in words or syllables per minute (see Wolk, Edwards, & Conture, 1993). Phonological assessment should include the following: (1) the development of a phonetic inventory for each child; (2) percentage consonants correct (Shriberg & Kwiatkowski, 1982); and (3) phonological process analysis (there are multiple published procedures that can be used for such analysis). More research is needed to develop and refine clinical assessments appropriate for this specific dually disordered population. For example, future study might suggest closer analysis of the actual instance of co-occurrence of stuttering and disordered phonology (e.g., Wolk et al., 2000). In the interim, application of individual assessment tools as described here represents the most effective assessment methods available.

Treatment

As we have seen, approximately one-third of children who exhibit fluency disorders also have a concomitant phonological impairment. This amount is a sufficiently large proportion to justify clinicians' concern for and attention to specific treatment strategies for this population. To date, we have limited data on treatment outcome using various techniques for children with these co-existing disorders. Therefore, the following section includes clinical suggestions drawn from clinical experience and adapted and modified from treatments for each individual disorder. Clearly, it is a simpler task to treat childhood stuttering as a single disorder than it is to manage two co-existing disorders in a given child. When fluency and phonological disorders co-exist, clinicians face a double challenge. The first challenge is to decide whether to treat the two disorders sequentially or simultaneously at a given time in therapy. The second challenge is to decide which disorder to treat first in the case of sequential treatment.

Some findings do support the value of simultaneous treatment. Conture, Louko, and Edwards (1993) compared the changes in stuttering behavior from the simultaneous treatment of children who exhibited both stuttering and disordered phonology, with changes in stuttering observed in the treatment of children who exhibited only stuttering. They evaluated eight children: (1) four children with stuttering (S) and disordered phonology (DP) who participated in a "stuttering-phonology" treatment group and (2) four children with stuttering alone who participated in a "stuttering" treatment group. The goal for the S+DP group was to decrease disordered phonology without increasing stuttering. Stuttering behavior changed appreciably for two of the children in the stuttering-phonology treatment group, and for three children in the stuttering group. In addition, three of the children in the stuttering-phonology group made appreciable improvements in their phonology. These findings provide some degree of support for a simultaneous treatment approach to childhood stuttering and disordered phonology when they co-exist in young children.

Empirical data evaluating a sequential treatment model are not available. Clinical observations seem to suggest that parents are often more anxious about their child's disfluency and its interruption of the overall communication process than about their child's articulatory disruption. Consequently, clinical intuitions suggest that it may be most beneficial to first target the disfluency, and once fluency begins to improve, attention could be given to the phonological impairment. This clinical intuition is in need of empirical validation. Obviously, before we can be more certain regarding the most appropriate treatment programs for CWS, more treatment outcomes on larger sample-size studies are needed.

The choice of a sequential approach to treatment presents both pros and cons that must be considered by the clinician. On the plus side, if a child's disfluency was initially ignored and the treatment focused on disordered phonology, phonology is likely to improve. On the negative side, however, the disfluency may begin to worsen. This is not optimal for overall prognosis. A second negative factor is that there are obvious ethical considerations for the clinician when deciding to leave a diagnosed problem (i.e., stuttering) untreated for a period of time. On the other hand, if the phonological disorder is ignored initially, it may not necessarily worsen, but articulatory disorder may limit a child's ability to be understood. This affects all of his or her interpersonal interactions, which is a significant negative consequence.

Whether simultaneous or sequential treatment approaches are chosen, basic principles of childhood stuttering intervention are still applicable for the child who exhibits stuttering and disordered phonology. However, an inherent problem exists in the application of traditional phonological treatment where sounds are directly and repeatedly modified to achieve accurate places and manner of articulation. If we consider the phonological encoding component as possibly integral to the stuttering complex itself, it is possible that any conscious attention to the articulatory precision may exacerbate the disfluency. Hence, one basic principle in the treatment of these children with co-existing disorders may need to involve a modification of the traditional approach. Most importantly, phonological changes have to be targeted in a manner that does not exacerbate the stuttering issues for the child.

Wolk (1998), together with Conture et al. (1993), have proposed a novel approach to treatment with this group of children. This perspective involves an indirect approach to the treatment of phonological errors rather than a more direct traditional approach to sound modification. The conceptual framework behind this is that these children have special needs. Direct articulation therapy may exert too much pressure on their conscious attempt to program articulatory sequences and produce articulatory accuracy, thereby exacerbating disfluency. Wolk (1998) outlines six clinical principles guided by this conceptual approach for phonology-fluency therapy for children ages 4 to 7 years. These are as follows: (1) indirect approach to the treatment of phonological errors; (2) use of a phonological process approach; (3) use of direct fluency modification techniques; (4) concurrent application of phonology and fluency intervention strategies; (5) parental involvement; and (6) use of a group rather than individual treatment setting whenever possible. A detailed review of the basic principles for treatment of children who exhibit stuttering and disordered phonology can be found in Wolk (1998).

The overarching framework is an indirect approach to the modification of phonological errors but a direct modification of disfluency. Hence, principles 1 to 4 are all essential. Principles 1 and 2 involve an indirect approach to the phonological approach using processes, and principle 3 involves direct fluency modification techniques. Principle 4 involves the attention to both disorders concurrently. Principle 5 is also essential for a positive outcome but will have differing levels of possible application depending on the clinical setting. For example, in the school setting, it is more difficult to engage in direct parent contact, whereas in a private or other setting, regular parent contact may be more feasible. Parent/caregiver involvement, however, is critical to overall outcome. Finally, principle 6 is nonessential, and its utility depends on the type of clinical setting. Group work with children may help to facilitate games and "fun," thereby reducing pressure on "speech focus." Group work with parents can be very supportive because of shared experiences.

Principle 1: Indirect Approach to the Treatment of Phonological Errors

This approach refers to any method that does not explicitly or directly try to change the child's speech sound production. Focus is placed on creating a relatively relaxed, enjoyable communication rather than pressuring/encouraging the child to speak accurately, clearly, and quickly. This involves a lot of modeling on the part of the clinician and emphasizing slow, physically relaxed speech production. Phonological targets are modeled and introduced indirectly via play. No expectation is placed on the child for accurate production of specific sounds, although closer approximations are rewarded positively. The child is not told directly about the speech goal; rather the clinician incorporates it through play. The following is a concrete example:

The goal of a session might be to determine how accurately he or she can produce the "shh" sound. The child is not directly told about the speech goal, rather the clinician may tell the child, *"Today we are going to have fun shooting basketballs through the hoop."* The clinician provides the child with several model productions of "shh." Each time the child hears the sound, he or she is allowed to shoot the basketball. The rationale for this listening activity is an assumption that the child's auditory awareness of that sound is enhanced. In the next step, the clinician encourages the child to say "shh" each time to help *shoot* the basketball correctly. The following step encourages the child, not only to use the singleton "shh," but to move toward the goal, on the word level, of producing *"shoot."* Approximations toward the target sound are accepted and rewarded rather than expecting 100% sound accuracy. In summary, the main focus of the approach is on the activity that includes the phonological target, but the target is not directly highlighted to the child. Any speaking pressure placed on the child to achieve accurate articulation is reduced as much as possible.

Principle 2: Use of a Phonological Process Approach

This approach implies a systematic organization of the child's sound changes that may involve entire classes of sounds. It involves sensitization to the phonological system and rules that operate to define the use of particular features rather than drill work on a single sound. During each therapy session one or more phonological processes may be targeted. If the child makes a consistent error on more than one sound in a phonemic group, a particular session may not necessarily involve targeting each and every sound. This is done deliberately so as to reduce the communicative demand on the child. Thus, one sound, or several sounds are not the focus of every therapy session. Treatment sessions provide general speech practice for the child.

In the phonological process approach the clinician needs to: (1) select target processes and sounds and (2) select a treatment paradigm for the phonological concerns. Any phonological treatment approach used must involve the gradualness principle, that is, selecting stimulus items that increase in linguistic complexity (e.g., stimuli should progress from consonant vowel consonant (CVC) words, to consonant consonant vowel consonant (CCVC) words, to sentences, to conversational speech). To minimize a disfluent child's attention to articulatory errors, all productions (accurate/inaccurate) should be accepted. Accurate productions specifically should be rewarded verbally. (See Wolk, 1998, for further detail of selection and treatment paradigm).

Principle 3: Use of Direct Fluency Modification Techniques

Many researchers have highlighted the benefits of speech rate reduction in fluency modification (e.g., Bloodstein, 1995; Conture, 2001). In the case of children who exhibit co-existing stuttering and disordered phonology, there is an additional benefit in reducing the child's speech rate. Slowing the rate of speech affords the child more time to plan semantic and pragmatic elements. It also allows time to select, sequence, and execute speech sound output. In particular, when the phonological target is complex (e.g., consonant clusters, multisyllabic words), there is a presumed increased demand on the phonological and motor plan. Thus, providing the child more time for phonological organization and execution can reduce disfluency in children with both stuttering and disordered phonology (Wolk, 1998).

In addition to rate reduction, prolonged speech also allows a child more time for phonological planning and execution. Other methods used to achieve fluency include the use of soft/light articulatory contacts and slight vowel elongation, which help to decrease the chances that the child would be unable to pronounce a specific sound.

Principle 4: The Concurrent Application of Phonology and Fluency Intervention Strategies

It can be challenging to treat children who exhibit both stuttering and disordered phonology as both components co-exist in successful communication. If you treat the stuttering first and facilitate fluency, the phonological errors will probably become more salient to the listener. Clinically, we have found that, as fluency increases, parents pay greater attention to articulatory disruptions and become more concerned with how they affect overall communication. However, if the phonological component is treated first, disfluency may be exacerbated. The disorders may be directly linked, which would further indicate that a combined therapy approach is needed to achieve optimum results.

Results of Conture et al. (1993) suggest that clinicians can concurrently introduce phonological targets with fluency facilitation techniques. Specifically, slower, physically relaxed speech should be modeled and encouraged while indirectly working on phonological targets in therapy. A key feature of this form of therapy is to not draw attention to the child's speech errors. The clinician should not provide direct feedback but rather should allow the child to remain involved in the fun of the activity. We feel this is the optimum method in spite of the possibility that progress could be slowed slightly.

Let us consider for a moment how the use of contrasts may applicable in both phonology and fluency therapy. In phonological therapy, the child is sensitized to contrasting visual, auditory, and tactile features (e.g., contrasting stop versus fricative or oral versus nasal sounds). In fluency therapy, some of the modification techniques also involve contrasts (e.g., tension versus relaxation, soft versus hard contact). Contrasts can also be effective in demonstrating a slow versus fast speaking rate. A specific clinical application could be to contrast "turtle speech" versus "rabbit speech." It is implied that stuttering may result from the demand of a "low" capacity speech production system. Thus, for children with concomitant disorders, the demands may be significantly larger and the capacities may be weaker for a given time (Starkweather & Gottwald, 1990).

Principle 5: Parental Involvement

It is beneficial for parents to become involved with their children's therapy program (see Chapters 4 and 5, this volume). It allows the parents to observe their child and to learn the optimum methods to use in facilitating the child's communicative behavior. Several suggestions that have been made to include parents are:

1. Parents should reduce their own normal speaking rate to slow to make it easier for the child to process as well as respond to parents' oral communication.

2. Parents should reduce the time urgency for speech by increasing the pause-time between conversational exchanges with their child.

3. Parents should casually correct or restate the child's error, rather than expecting the child to repeat accurate productions after the parents' model.

4. Parents should not directly drill and/or expect articulation accuracy.

5. Parents should make an effort to communicatively interact with their child while applying these techniques for at least 10 minutes every day.

6. Parents should listen and demonstrably show support of their child and commitment to their child.

Principle 6: The Use of a Group Setting

Ideally, a combination of individual and group therapy could maximize treatment outcome. A group setting provides an opportunity for a wide variety of communication interactions between clinician and child, and child and his or her peers. In particular, peer groups provide natural conversational communication, thus facilitating a seemingly ecologically appropriate form in therapy. Furthermore, a group setting reduces the focus and stress on an individual child to achieve accurate phonological targets. Although group settings are appropriate and enjoyable for most children, some children simply appear unable to modify their speech in a group setting. In such situations, the child should be placed in individual therapy. When selecting children for a group, differences in speech intelligibility and severity in disordered phonology should be kept to a minimum. Obviously, other behavioral issues such as hyperactivity, impulsivity, extreme sensitivity, perfectionist traits, and attention span should all be taken into account when selecting group members.

Summary

In summary, the suggestions made regarding assessment and treatment are based on the available literature as well as clinical intuition. To review, the suggestions for assessment consist of general guidelines that are widely supported by stuttering specialists. The suggestions for treatment involve facilitating the emergence of new sound patterns through the indirect treatment of phonological processes. Simultaneously, attention is given to the child's fluency difficulties by reducing the clinician's speech rateand not interrupting or speaking for the child and/or requiring the child to initiate and maintain overly rapid speech-language production. In general, this approach tries to capitalize on parental modeling of appropriate pragmatics as well as group dynamics of communication. All of these perspectives on therapeutic intervention require empirical validation that meets the guidelines for establishing evidence-based practice that are becoming the gold standard in the field of communication sciences and disorders.

♦ Conclusion

Much knowledge has been gained during the past two decades in the understanding of the potential relationships between stuttering and phonology in young children. Future research is needed to explore the exact nature and interactions of these two disorders when they co-occur in children. Differentiating the stuttering symptomatology of children who exhibit stuttering in isolation versus children with co-existing disorders has important implications for diagnosis, treatment, and, ultimately, for further understanding of stuttering etiology and possible subgrouping of CWS. Deeper implications for the very essence of the stuttering complex may, in part, be rooted in the phonological components of speech planning and production.

From a clinical prospective, we have outlined suggestions for the assessment treatment of children with co-existing disorders. We have encouraged a simultaneous intervention approach, including stuttering modification techniques suited to young children, combined parental involvement, and an indirect approach to the modification of phonological errors. Such intervention techniques need to be applied on larger samples of children with co-existing disorders before generalizations about the benefits of such therapy can be made. Long-term treatment outcome studies following evidence-based practice guidelines would be useful in the evaluation of overall results of therapy.

References

Adams, M. R. (1990). The demands and capacities model I: Theoretical elaborations. Journal of Fluency Disorders 15, 135–142.

Anderson, J. (in press). Phonological neighborhood and word frequency effects in the speech disfluencies of children who stutter. Journal of Speech Language, and Hearing Reserach.

Arnd, t. J, & Healey, E. C. (2001). Concomitant disorders in school-age children who stutter. Language, Speech, and Hearing Services in Schools 32, 68–78.

Arnold, H. S., Conture, E. G., & Ohde, R. N. (2005). Phonological neighborhood density in the picture naming of young children who stutter: Preliminary study. Journal of Fluency Disorders 30, 125–148.

Beitchman, J. H., Nair, R., Clegg, M., & Patel, P. G. (1986). Prevalence of speech and language disorders in 5-year-old kindergarten children in the Ottawa–Carleton region. Journal of Speech and Hearing Disorders 51, 98–110.

Blood, G. W., Ridenour, V. J., Qualls, C. D., & Hammer, C. S. (2003). Co-occurring disorders in children who stutter. Journal of Communication Disorders 36, 427–448.

Bloodstein, O. (1995). Handbook on stuttering (5th ed.). San Diego, CA: Singular.

Browman, C. P., & Goldstein, L. (1997). The gestural phonology model. In W. Hulstijn, H. F. M. Peters, & P. H. H. M. van Lieshout, (Eds.), Speech production: Motor control, brain research and fluency disorders (pp. 57–71). Amsterdam, The Netherlands: Elsevier.

Byrd, C. T., Conture, E. G., & Ohde, R. N. (2006). Phonological priming in young children who stutter: Holistic versus incremental processing. American Journal of Speech–Language Pathology.

Charles-Luce, J., & Luce, P. A. (1990). Similarity neighborhoods of words in young children's lexicon. Journal of Child Language 17, 205–215.

Conture, E. G. (2001). Stuttering: Its nature, diagnosis, and treatment. Boston: Allyn & Bacon.

Conture, E. G., Louko, L. J., & Edwards, M. L. (1993). Simultaneously treating stuttering and disordered phonology in children: Experimental treatment, preliminary findings. American Journal of Speech-Language Pathology 2, 72–81.

Dworzynski ,K., & Howell, P. (2004). Predicting stuttering from phonetic complexity in German. Journal of Fluency Disorders 29, 149–173.

Glaser, W. (1992). Picture naming. In W. J. M. Levelt (Ed.), Lexical access in speech production (pp. 61–105). Cambridge, MA: Blackwell Publishers.

Hakim, H. B., & Bernstein Ratner, N. (2004). Nonword repetition abilities of children who stutter: an exploratory study. Journal of Fluency Disorders 29, 179–199.

Howell, P., & Au-Yeung, J. (1995). The association between stuttering, Brown's factors, and phonological categories in child stutterers ranging in age between 2 and 12 years. Journal of Fluency Disorders 20, 331–344.

Huinck, W. I., van Lieshout, P. H. H. M., Peters, H. F. M., & Hulstijn, W. (2004). Gestural overlap in consonant clusters: Effects on the fluent speech of stuttering and nonstuttering subjects. Journal of Fluency Disorders 29, 3–24.

Jakielski, K. J. (1998). Motor organization in the acquisition of consonant clusters. Doctoral dissertation, , University of Texas, Austin.

Jusczyk, P. W., Luce, P. A., & Charles-Luce, J. (1994). Infants' sensitivity to phonotactic patterns in the native language. Journal of Memory and Language 33, 630–645.

Kolk, H., & Postma, A. (1997). Stuttering as a covert repair phenomenon. In R. F. Curlee, & Siegel, G. M. (Eds.), Nature and treatment of stuttering: New directions (2nd ed.) (182–203). Boston: Allyn & Bacon.

Levelt, W. (1989). Speaking: From intention to articulation. Cambridge, MA: Bradford Books/The MIT Press.

Louko, L. J., Conture, E. G., & Edwards, M. L. (1999). Treating children who exhibit co-occurring stuttering and disordered phonology. In R. F. Curlee (Ed.), Stuttering and related disorders of fluency (2nd ed.) (pp. 124–138). New York: Thieme Medical Publishers.

Luce, P. A., & Pisoni, D. B. (1998). Recognizing spoken words: the Neighborhood Activation Model. Ear and Hearing 19, 1–36.

Mansson, H. (2000). Childhood stuttering: Incidence and development. Journal of Fluency Disorders 25, 47–57.

Melnick, K. S., & Conture, E. G. (2000). Relationship of length and grammatical complexity to the systematic and nonsystematic speech errors and stuttering of children who stutter. Journal of Fluency Disorders 20, 331–344.

Melnick, K. S., Conture, E. G., & Ohde, R. N. (2003). Phonological priming in picture-naming of young children who stutter. Journal of Speech, Language, and Hearing Research 46, 1428–1444.

Newman, R. S., & German, D. J. (2002). Effects of lexical factors or lexical access among typical language-learning children and children with word-finding difficulties. Language and Speech 45, 285–317.

Nippold, M. A. (1990). Concomitant speech and language disorders in stuttering children: A critiqe of the literature. Journal of Speech and Hearing Disorders 55, 51–60.

Nippold, M. A. (2001). Phonological disorders and stuttering in children: What is the frequency of co-occurrence? Clinical and Linguistic Phonetics 15, 219–228.

Nippold, M. A. (2002). Stuttering and phonology: Is there an interaction? American Journal of Speech-Language Pathology 11, 99–110.

Nippold, M. A. (2004). Phonological and language disorders in children who stutter: Impact on treatment recommendations. Clinical Linguistics and Phonetics 18, 145–159.

Paden, E. P., & Yairi, E. (1996). Phonological characteristics of children whose stuttering persisted or recovered. Journal of Speech and Hearing Research 39, 981–990.

Paden, E. P., Yairi, E., & Ambrose, N. G. (1999). Early childhood stuttering: II. Initial status of phonological abilities. Journal of Speech, Language, and Hearing Research 42, 1113–1124.

Pellowski, M. W., & Conture, E. G. (2002). Characteristics of speech disfluency and stuttering behaviors in 3- and 4-year-old children. Journal of Speech, Language, and Hearing Research 45, 20–35.

Postma, A., & Kolk, H. H. J. (1993). The covert repair hypothesis: Prearticulatory repair processes in normal and stuttered disfluencies. Journal of Speech and Hearing Research 36, 472–487.

Riley, G. D. (1994). Stuttering severity instrument for children and adults-3 (SSI-3) (3rd ed.). Austin, TX: PRO-ED.

Ryan, B. P. (2001). A longitudinal study of articulation, language, rate, and fluency of 22 preschool children who stutter. Journal of Fluency Disorders 26, 107–127.

Shriberg, L. D., & Kwiatkowski, J. (1982). Phonological disorders: I. A diagnostic classification system. Journal of Speech and Hearing Disorders 47, 226–241.

Starkweather, C. W., & Gottwald, S. R. (1990). The Demands and capacities model: II. Clinical applications. Journal of Fluency Disorders 15, 143–157.

Storkel, H. L. (2001). Learning new words: Phonotactic probability in language development. Journal of Speech, Language, and Hearing Research 44:1321–1337.

Throneburg, R. N., Yairi, E., & Paden, E. P. (1994). Relation between phonologic difficulty and the occurrence of disfluencies in the early stage of stuttering. Journal of Speech and Hearing Research 37, 504–509.

Vitevitch, M. S. (2002). The influence of phonological similarity neighborhoods on speech production. Journal of Experimental Psychology: Learning, Memory, and Cognition 28, 735–747.

Vitevitch, M. S., Armbrüster, J., & Chu, S. (2004). Sublexical and lexical representations in speech production: effects of phonotactic probability and onset density. Journal of Experimental Psychology: Learning, Memory, and Cognition 30, 514–529.

Vitevitch, M. S, & Luce, P. A. (2004). A web-based interface to calculate phonotactic probability for words and non-words in English. Behavior Research Methods, Instruments, & Computers 36, 481–487.

Vitevitch, M. S., Luce, P. A., Charles-Luce, J., & Kemmerer, D. (1997). Phonotactics and syllable stress: Implications for the processing of spoken nonsense words. Language and Speech 40, 47–62.

Vitevitch, M. S., Luce, P. A., Pisoni, D. B., & Auer, E. T. (1999). Phonotactics, neighborhood activation and lexical access for spoken words. Brain and Language 68, 306–311.

Walley, A. C. (1988). Spoken word recognition by young children and adults. Cognitive Development 3, 137–165.

Walley, A. C. (1993). The role of vocabulary development in children's spoken word recognition and segmentation ability. Developmental Review 13, 286–350.

Walley, A. C., Smith, L. B., & Jusczyk, P. W. (1986). The role of phonemes and syllables in the perceived similarity of speech sounds for children. Memory and Cognition 14, 220–229.

Weber-Fox, C., Spencer, R. M. C., Spruill, J. E., & Smith, A. (2004). Phonological processing in adults who stutter: Electrophysiological and behavioral evidence. Journal of Speech, Language, and Hearing Research 47, 1244–1258.

Wolk, L. (1998). Intervention strategies for children who exhibit coexisting phonological and fluency disorders: A clinical note. Child Language Teaching and Therapy 14, 69–82.

Wolk, L., Blomgren, M., & Smith, A. B. (2000). The frequency of simultaneous disfluency and phonological errors in children: A preliminary investigation. Journal of Fluency Disorders 25, 269–281.

Wolk, L., Edwards, M. L., & Conture, E. G. (1993). Coexistence of stuttering and disordered phonology in young children. Journal of Speech and Hearing Research 36, 906–917.

Yairi, E., & Ambrose, N. (1999). Early childhood stuttering: I. Persistency and recovery rates. Journal of Speech, Language, and Hearing Research 42, 1097–1112.

Yairi, E., Ambrose, N. G., Paden, E. P., & Throneburg, R. N. (1996). Predictive factors of persistence and recovery: Pathways of childhood stuttering. Journal of Communication Disorders 29, 51–77.

Yaruss, J. S., LaSalle, L. R., & Conture, E. G. (1998). Evaluating stuttering in young children: Diagnostic data. American Journal of Speech-Language Pathology 7(4), 62–76.

11

Assessment and Treatment of Stuttering in Bilingual Speakers

Patricia M. Roberts and Rosalee C. Shenker

Millions of people speak two or more languages. Yet, there is little research on the symptoms, assessment, or treatment of stuttering in bilingual speakers. This chapter provides the reader with some key concepts about bilingualism and then reviews many of the studies done to date on bilingual stuttering. Based on the existing literature and on their own extensive clinical experience with bilingual children and adults, the authors provide concrete suggestions for the assessment and treatment of bilingual children and adults who stutter. The reader will also gain an understanding of the need for data from well-controlled studies to address the many unanswered questions concerning assessment and treatment of bilingual individuals who stutter.

Throughout the chapter we use the terms *bilingual* and *bilingualism* to refer to bilingual and to multilingual (or polyglot) speakers. This is a convenient shorthand because there is not yet sufficient data on whether there are clinically relevant differences between bilingual speakers (knowing/using two languages) and polyglot or multilingual speakers (knowing/using more than two languages). We begin by discussing the nature of bilingualism to provide the reader with the necessary framework to then consider assessment and treatment of bilingual speakers who stutter (BWS).

◆ Bilingualism: Myths and Definitions

Although there is a limited literature on stuttering in bilingual speakers, there is a large body of research on bilingualism. Because most speech-language pathologists (SLPs) are not familiar with this literature, this chapter begins by reviewing some of the popular myths about bilingualism and bilingual stuttering, contrasting each myth with the known facts, and pointing out the main clinical implications of these facts.

Some readers may think that bilingual people who stutter will be seen by bilingual clinicians, allowing unilingual clinicians to say to themselves "if I am not bilingual, I don't need to know anything about bilingual stuttering." This is not the case. There is a serious mismatch between the languages spoken in many countries, including the United States, Canada, Australia, and South

Africa, and the number of clinicians able to serve clients in these languages. In the United States and Canada, few clinicians speak languages other than English compared with the number of languages spoken by residents. For example, according to US Census data (United States Census, 2000), there are 2 million Chinese speakers, yet the American Speech Language and Hearing Association records show only 14 Chinese/Cantonese-speaking SLPs. Similar situations exist in other countries where immigration brings people from many different parts of the world. Countries with many indigenous languages also report a mismatch between the languages spoken in the country and the languages of training programs and professionals in many fields (Bortz, Jardine, & Tschule, 1996; Extra & Maatens, 1998). Thus, clinicians should expect to see clients with different language backgrounds, whether or not they themselves are bilingual (at least until there are many more bilingual and multilingual clinicians!).

Myth 1: Bilingualism Is Rare

Reality   Exact figures on the incidence of bilingualism worldwide are not available and would depend on one's definition of bilingualism, but bilingualism may be more common than unilingualism (Harris & Nelson, 1992; Tucker, 1998).

Clinical Impact of Myth 1   Speech-language pathology training programs need to prepare clinicians to assess and treat bilingual clients, and the field needs much more research on which to base our clinical service to this very large segment of the population.

Myth 2: Bilingualism Means "Speaking Two Languages Perfectly"

Reality   This level of proficiency is extremely rare, if it exists at all. Many experts think it is impossible to attain native-like and equal competence in two languages (Grosjean, 1989). This is, in part, because the languages in a person's brain modify each other, with interference going from the native language (or first language: L1) to the second language (L2) and also from L2 to L1 (Cenoz, Hufeisen, & Jessner, 2001; Cook, 2003; Pavlenko, 2000; Pavlenko & Jarvis, 2002).

Clinical Impact of Myth 2   Even in a client who claims to be "perfectly bilingual," clinicians should expect gaps in knowledge of vocabulary and syntax and also cross-language interference in pronunciation, vocabulary, and syntax. There is no predictable level of proficiency associated with "learned both languages from age 2" because so much depends on the total exposure to each language and patterns of use of each language over time. In presenting written and verbal instructions and in assigning conversation and transfer tasks, clinicians need to keep in mind that individual abilities in each language vary across each language modality, across domains of use, and across language registers.

Myth 3: One Is Either Bilingual or Unilingual

Reality   Bilingualism is a continuum, not a dichotomy (Hakuta, 1986; Macnamara, 1967). Furthermore, competence in each language varies across the four modalities of auditory and written comprehension and verbal and written expression. Some people who routinely speak two or more languages in their daily lives cannot read or write at all, or can read and/or write in only one language. So, a bilingual speaker's level of proficiency is not a unitary thing; it must be defined in relation to each modality.

The fact that bilingualism and unilingualism are end points of a continuum means that the tendency to think of people as either second language learners or as "true bilingual speakers" is problematic. Some authors use "second language speaker/learner" to mean someone in the process of learning a new language, in many cases the language spoken by the majority of people in the country to which the person has recently moved, or a student formally studying a new language. But there is no dividing line that separates so-called second language students from so-called bilingual speakers in how many words they know or how many grammatical errors they make. Each individual can be placed at some point along a continuum of proficiency for each of the four language modalities. Furthermore, there is no consensus as to the definition of the so-called true bilingual. One study proposes that babies whose exposure to a second language begins after 1 month of age are L2 learners, not true bilinguals (Håkansson, Salameh, & Nettelbladt, 2003). Other studies put the hypothetical cutoff point for "true bilinguals" at many different points ranging up to puberty (e.g., Flege, Yeni-Komshian, & Liu, 1999; Harley & Wang, 1997; Johnson & Newport, 1989). Language acquisition research demonstrates that there is no defensible cutoff point at which the age of first exposure to each language determines the ultimate level of proficiency attained (Hakuta, Bialystok, & Wiley, 2003; Piske, Flege, & MacKay, 2001).

Another argument against the label "true bilingual" is that, unlike some attributes such as eye color, bilingualism is not a permanent, stable characteristic. Children growing up in a bilingual home often have a high level of ability in each language, then drift into a pattern of using one of their two languages more than the other due to the influence of school, clubs, and friends. This causes attrition (gradual forgetting) of the less often-used language, resulting in a stronger language (Ls) and a weaker language (Lw), and making these speakers impossible to distinguish from people who began learning their L2 later in childhood.

Clinical Impact of Myth 3 It is important to understand what clients means when they describe themselves or their child as "bilingual" or "not bilingual." Each client may mean something different when using these terms. Avoid the use of labels, including "L2 learner," "L2 speaker," "bilingual," and "true bilingual" because there is no agreement on the definitions for these often-misleading labels. Focus instead on the person's level of proficiency for each language modality, and for different types of communication.

Myth 4: Bilingualism Increases the Risk of Stuttering

Reality There is no credible research to either support or refute this often-repeated statement. In support of his statement that "a child who is bilingual appears to be more likely to stutter than one who is unilingual," Silverman (1996, p.108) cites two very flawed studies. In one of these studies (Travis, Johnson, & Shover, 1937), people with no training in communication disorders such as priests and steel company personnel directors identified children as stuttering. In the other study (Stern, 1948), no information is given about the basis for judging a child to be stuttering or not. The author "interviewed" children identified by their parents as stuttering, but there is no information about the sample length, language(s) of the interview, topics, or how stuttering was defined. In both of these early studies, and in the more recent study by Dale (1977) that claimed more disfluency in four Cuban-American adolescents because of their bilingualism, the authors fail to distinguish between normal speech disfluencies and disfluencies that are part of clinical stuttering. This methodological flaw makes it impossible to interpret their results. (see the section Possible Threats to the Validity and Reliability of Stuttering Assessments, pages 189 to 190, regarding normal disfluencies across different languages, and in one's Lw).

Is there any more recent research showing a link between stuttering and bilingualism? A recent on-line survey by Howell and colleagues reported that bilingualism may be a risk factor for some children, depending on their genetic vulnerability and the pattern and age of language acquisition. However, this survey was abandoned, due, in part, to the biased sample of people who chose to respond (Howell, personal communication, January 5, 2006). The accuracy of some of the respondents' replies was also doubtful. For example, the average reported age of onset of stuttering was 7 years old. Empirical studies of children place the mean age of onset of stuttering much younger than this, at around 3 years of age (e.g., Mansson, 2000; Yairi & Ambrose, 2005; Yaruss, LaSalle, & Conture, 1998).

Karniol's (1992) often-quoted case description reports anecdotally on one boy who was exposed to English and Hebrew from birth, with frequent periods of exposure to Hungarian as well (maternal grandparents). The boy began to stutter, suddenly and quite severely, in both languages, at approximately age 2 years, 1 month. Three months later, his parents began using only Hebrew when speaking to him, and they allowed him to speak only Hebrew to them. The stutter soon disappeared. When he resumed using English at age 3 years, 2 months, it is not clear from the diary descriptions given in the article whether he still stuttered. He may have been one of the majority of children who recover naturally from stuttering with no formal help. The anecdotal form of all the data (in a diary kept by parents with no training in stuttering or the identification of disfluencies), the fact that the boy continued to be exposed to English in the home, and in other places throughout the period described in the diary, and the lack of experimental control all mean that Karniol's narrative cannot be interpreted as showing why this boy stopped stuttering. The study raises several interesting questions that need to be tested, but it fails to demonstrate any relationship between bilingualism and the risk for stuttering or between bilingualism and the prognosis for recovery in children. Stahl and Totten (1995) suggest that if a child has both a history of persistent stuttering and other speech and language problems, it may be reasonable to limit the child's environment to one language; however, there is (still) no clinical research to support this opinion and recent reviews no longer recommend creating an artificially monolingual environment for stuttering children (Bernstein Ratner, 2004; Van Borsel, Maes, & Foulon, 2001).

If bilingualism were a significant risk factor causing stuttering or preventing spontaneous recovery in children, then countries or regions with high levels of bilingualism would have higher incidences of stuttering than countries or regions with low levels of bilingualism. This does not appear to be the case (see Bloodstein, 1995, p. 106–107). In a recent and very rigorous study by Mansson (2000), the incidence and recovery rates for stuttering are approximately the same in Denmark as for unilingual groups in the United States. Comparisons of the incidence of stuttering in countries such as Japan, where low immigration rates and cultural factors combine to create a homogeneous and largely unilingual population, with countries such as the Netherlands, where bilingualism is widespread, will be helpful in determining whether bilingualism contributes to the risk for stuttering.

On the other hand, evidence is mounting that children who stutter have a higher incidence of phonological and language delays and have motor speech differences compared with children who do not stutter (e.g., Blood, Ridenour, Qualls, & Hammer, 2003; Gagnon & Wolk, 2006; Hakim & Bernstein Ratner, 2004; Huinck, Van Lieshout, Peters, & Hulstijn, 2004; Ingham et al., 2004; Yaruss et al., 1998). These findings may raise questions that have implications for bilingual children with family histories of stuttering. Does learning two languages tax a vulnerable system in a bilingual child or not? Does learning a larger number of articulatory and motor patterns to produce the phonemes of two languages stress a bilingual child's developing motor control abilities or not? Until research is done on these and other related questions, we need to keep an open mind.

Clinical Impact of Myth 4   When parents ask "Does my child stutter because he is bilingual?" or "Should we stop using Language X?" the only defensible answer is "I don't know. There is too little research on this." The research to date on bilingual stuttering and bilingual language acquisition does not provide evidence that would justify asking a child to "become monolingual" in a community and family where two or more languages are spoken by those around him or her and both languages are part of his or her daily routine. We return to this question later in this chapter.

Myth 5: Some BWS Stutter in Only One Language

Reality   There is no adequately documented case of this occurring. Van Riper (1971) cites second- and third-hand reports of two individuals reported to stutter in only one of their two languages, but the author offers no data. Given the roles of genetics and motor processes in stuttering, it is highly unlikely that someone would stutter in only one of his or her languages.

Clinical Impact of Myth 5   Clinicians should thoroughly test each language and be aware of ways in which a BWS might "hide" his or her stuttering. Speaking a new language might act in the same way as acting a part in a play, and (temporarily?) facilitate fluency. A BWS may use language switching to

Table 11–1   Is Stuttering Possible in Only One Language?

To convincingly demonstrate that a bilingual individual stutters in only one of his or her languages, the speech samples must be long enough and on topics the speaker is used to discussing in that language. In addition, future reports will need to include:

1. The level of proficiency of each language estimated by self-assessment and also the clinician's judgment

2. Patterns of use of each language, that is, how often does the speaker use each of his or her languages, and for what kinds of topics and situations?

3. Analysis of more than one speech sample in each language, with each sample being long enough to reduce the chance of false negatives (i.e., failing to find stuttering because the sample is too short)

4. Analysis of the samples by people who are proficient speakers of each language

5. Appropriate levels of inter- and intra-rater reliability in transcriptions and in disfluency counts

6. A clear statement of the definition of stuttering used either to classify each disfluency as stuttering or not, or to classify a particular sample as displaying symptoms of stuttering or not

avoid anticipated stutters in one language, resulting in a speech sample that has no overt stutters in that language. **Table 11–1** presents the information that will be needed to convincingly document a case of a bilingual speaker stuttering in only one language.

But, until there is evidence to the contrary, clinicians should expect to find stuttering in all the languages spoken. Future reports of BWS who stutter in only one language must provide data that are sufficiently valid and reliable to be convincing. It will be particularly important to provide readers with the operational definition of stuttering used because this is important in separating stutters from disfluencies due to limited proficiency in one or more of the languages tested.

Cultural Factors

In recent years, there has been a growing interest in what are called "multicultural issues" or "culturally and linguistically diverse" populations (CLD). Research into how cultural factors can influence clinical work has repeatedly demonstrated two things. First, verbal and nonverbal communication are both influenced by culture, to some degree. Second, misunderstandings can occur if clients or clinicians misread some of the culturally influenced features of communication. There are several encyclopedia-like guides to various cultural groups that may be useful to clinicians (e.g., Brislin, 1994; Galens, Sheets, & Young, 1995; Lynch & Hanson, 1992) (**Table 11–2**).

While reading these cultural summaries, however, it is critical to avoid cultural stereotypes, as several authors have pointed out (Cooper & Cooper, 1993; Finn & Cordes, 1997; Kayser, 1998; Leith, 1986; Tellis & Tellis, 2003). The danger of very short descriptions of various groups is that they make it easy to forget that people from a given country or background are *not* all the same. This is especially true of immigrants, who may have left their native country because they reject aspects of its prevailing culture. In addition to overall cultural background (African American, Chinese, German, Guatemalan, etc.), one must expect influences from microcultures, which are determined by factors such as age, education, occupation, sex, religion, and whether one comes from an urban or rural setting (Gollnick & Chin, 1990). Thus "a 55-year-old lawyer from Hong Kong may have more in common with a 52-year-old Anglo architect from Chicago than he does with a 22-year-old Hong Kong street vendor" (Roberts, 2001, p. 209). In dealing with clients who come from cultures different from our own, we need to see the client not the culture.

One example of individuals' beliefs going against cultural stereotypes: Some Caucasian, English-speaking, Canadian and American adults believe stuttering is a form of divine punishment, yet a study currently underway found that almost all Africans surveyed in Cameroon believe stuttering is caused by genetic factors (St. Louis, Roberts, Lukong, & Meese, 2006). Tellis and Tellis (2003) provide similar examples. With experience, clinicians learn to explore and probe; they learn not to assume or stereotype.

Table 11–2 Aspects of Communication Most Likely To Vary across Cultures

- How the client views time: Is being punctual important? Is lateness seen as rude? Does the client understand the clinician's tight pattern of time slots for each session?

- Who speaks for the family: It could be a father, mother, grandfather, grandmother, oldest surviving male, or oldest surviving female member.

- Gender roles: Some decisions such as discipline may be the role of one parent, making it inappropriate to ask the other parent to take on this responsibility. Who decides to begin or end therapy? Who deals with the child's school? For adult clients, especially younger adults, to what extent does the client defer to someone else in the family for certain issues?

- Taboo topics: family dynamics, arguments; failures. Is disability (or the stuttering itself) seen as a taboo topic? In some cultures, clients will feel it is polite to ask about the clinician's family and children. In other cultures, this is inappropriate for a professional relationship.

- Whether or not and how children should be praised.

- Rules for children speaking or not speaking to adults, both inside and outside the family circle. In some cultures, well-behaved children may be reluctant to speak to the clinician (older, opposite sex, position of authority), especially when their parents are present.

- Being alone with strangers—especially a female client or parent with a male clinician.

- Touching the client: for reinforcement, greetings, tapping rhythm. The head and the left hand have special status in some cultures. Shaking hands is not always appropriate.

- Eye contact: In some cultures, making eye contact shows respect, honesty. In others, especially across age and sex differences, it is disrespectful.

- Distance and height relationships when speaking: Each culture defines personal space differently. So, what may seem "too close" or threatening to some, can be normal and collaborative to others.

- Loudness of the voice: Appropriate levels can vary with age and status.

- Giving and receiving gifts: Who gives to whom? What is an appropriate cost for a gift? Whether to open a gift in front of the giver or not. Whether to ask or not ask how much the gift cost. These are all aspects of polite gift giving that vary across cultures.

- Use of first names versus more formal titles such as Mr. or Mrs. The American informality and use of given names is seen as disrespectful in some other cultures.

Note: Some items taken from Leith, W. R. (1986) Treating the stutterer with atypical cultural influences. In K. O. St. Louis (Ed.), The atypical stutterer (pp. 9–34). London: Academic Press.

Several publications recommend that clinicians "ask about cultural factors in the assessment." Watson and Kayser (1994) recommend using the initial interview to learn about the client's view of stuttering and people who stutter. Relating these issues to Latino culture, Bernstein Ratner (2004) suggests that it is important to discuss the cultural and specific concerns related to interpretations of clinical information. However, questions about culture can easily trigger resentment in the client. So, the clinician must walk a fine line: on the one hand being aware of the potential impact of macro- and microcultural factors, while on the other hand remembering that each client comes to us with his or her own individual values and views, not as a representative of any particular group.

Also, it is important not to overstate the importance of cultural factors. We ask all clients/parents what they think caused the stuttering, what strategies they have tried so far to reduce or manage it, and, once sufficient rapport has been developed, we ask what feelings the stuttering elicits in the child and/or in the family. These same questions are appropriate for the so-called CLD clients. Their answers (and, for children, our own observations of the parent-child interactions) will tell us much of what we need to know, without ever mentioning "culture" or asking potentially offensive or perplexing questions such as, "How is stuttering seen in your culture?"

Other culturally influenced behaviors such as child-rearing and discipline practices, and views about school and professional success, can be explored as the need arises in the assessment and intervention. Again, this is true of all clients, not just those labeled CLD. It is appropriate to explain the rationale for activities and to negotiate treatment goals and priorities with all clients

(Leahy & Wright, 1994). The experienced clinician never assumes that clients share his or her views or values, or therapy goals, no matter what their background.

Having addressed some of the key concepts relevant to bilingualism and with these cultural caveats in mind, we now turn to more concrete questions of how to assess and how to treat bilingual children who stutter and bilingual adults and adolescents who stutter.

♦ Assessment of Bilinguals Who Stutter

Most textbooks on stuttering, including the present volume, present one chapter or more on assessment procedures (e.g., Conture, 2001; Ham, 1990; Manning, 2001). Clinicians working with bilingual clients need to be familiar with these procedures. However, there are some unique twists and extra steps involved in assessing a BWS. The purpose of this section is to make the reader aware of these.

Components of Stuttering Assessment

An assessment of a BWS should include: (1) a complete language history; (2) speech samples in each language spoken, using tasks for each client's domains of use for each language; and (3) reliable analyses of these speech samples to allow the clinician to make some judgment about rate of speech, normal speech disfluencies, disfluencies related to level of proficiency in each language, and moments of stuttering.

Language History

There are three parts to an adequate language history. First, find out the age of first exposure to each language and the course of language acquisition for each. This is particularly important for children, where part of the assessment involves screening for language and articulation problems. Second, identify the recent and current domains of use for each language (e.g., school, work, family, and sports or other hobbies). **Table 11–3** provides a list of domains of use. This information allows

Table 11–3   Domains of Language Use

Depending upon each client's age and circumstances, some of these may not apply.

- ♦ At home with family
- ♦ With extended family (out of town, other countries)
- ♦ School:
  - ♦ Language of instruction in classes
  - ♦ Language of most required reading
- ♦ At home with roommate(s)
- ♦ For main hobbies and sports activities
- ♦ Reading newspapers, books, magazines (outside work and/or outside school)
- ♦ Religious community activities
- ♦ Watching TV/movies
- ♦ Internet and computer use
- ♦ Listening to the radio
- ♦ Social life: friends, family friends, relatives
- ♦ Shopping

clinicians to interpret performance on assessment tasks and to consider appropriate topics and difficulty levels for tasks and assignments in therapy. The form provided in **Appendix 11.1** provides appropriate interview questions to cover these first two areas.

The third component of a client's language history is an estimate of his or her proficiency in each language. To estimate a person's level of bilingualism (LOB), ask the person to rate his or her own ability, on a 7-point scale, for each of the four language modalities: auditory comprehension, verbal expression, reading comprehension, and written expression. For young children, parents' ratings should be used. For clients who cannot read or write, skip these modalities in the ratings (young children, illiterate adults). Depending on a speaker's need to use each of these modalities, exposure to each, and several other factors, each speaker will have a higher or lower level of expertise in each modality, which may vary with the language register (formal or informal) and with the topic (see Grosjean, 1998, for excellent arguments on this point). Some adolescents and adults may be able to read in only one language, especially when their two languages use different scripts. The form in Appendix 11.1 also contains a section for proficiency rating. This self-rating may seem technical. However, most clients (and parents and research participants) easily come up with numbers that appear to have reasonable validity (i.e., they seem to match, roughly, proficiency on various assessment tasks).

The accuracy of self-assessments of language ability is still being investigated (e.g., Oscarson, 1989). However, self-assessment is widely used in studies of bilingualism. Language histories and self-ratings of level of proficiency are used to create groups as homogeneous as possible in their linguistic background or to match people who stutter with nonstuttering control cases. Language histories and information about proficiency are essential to allow comparisons between studies. However, as with any measurement tool, it is important to recognize its limitations. Self-assessments of language proficiency should be used as rough indicators, and they should never be taken as precise "scores."

The word *fluent* is often used in describing how well someone masters a given language. Clinicians who work with stuttering use the word *fluent* to describe a construct that includes disfluencies, speech rate, and the smoothness of the flow of speech. Written reports and conversations quickly become confusing when the word *fluent* is used in both these senses. Therefore, we recommend not using *fluent* to describe a level of knowledge of a given language. It quickly becomes impossible to know what is meant by things like "he speaks Mandarin fluently." Does this mean with few stutters? Few normal disfluencies? With a good command of the grammar and vocabulary? With a rapid rate of speech?

Speech Sample Analyses

After obtaining the language history and the normal background information that is part of all stuttering assessments, the next step is to obtain speech samples for all tasks that are appropriate to the client's age and severity of stuttering. We do not yet have norms for normal disfluencies or for normal rates of speaking or reading aloud for speakers of a range of languages although there are several studies on English-speaking American children of different ages (e.g., Guitar, 2006; Yairi & Ambrose, 2005; Yaruss et al., 1998) which may or may not have accidentally included some bilingual children. Even if there were perfect studies of unilingual speakers of many of the world's languages, there is scant evidence on whether these results would apply to bilingual speakers, given the often-quoted axiom that the bilingual is "not two monolinguals in one person" (Grosjean, 1989) and the more recent evidence cited above about how the two languages influence and modify each other. Therefore, one purpose of the assessment is to compare one language with the other, for each client, in terms of the rate of speech, number and type of disfluencies, and type and duration of moments of stuttering.

In addition to obtaining these ratings of LOB, clinicians should explore the client's and/or parents' view of the severity of stuttering in each language and reasons for the perceived patterns. Some clients make self-assessments that agree with the data from objective analysis of their speech, whereas others do not (Bernstein Ratner & Benitez, 1985; Jankelowitz & Bortz, 1996;

Table 11–4   Six Steps in Assessing Bilinguals Who Stutter

To maximize the chances that your assessment will allow you to draw valid conclusions about the client's stuttering:

1. Obtain a sufficiently detailed language history, including age of first exposure, patterns of use (what language was used for school, home life, social life, work, etc., in childhood and as an adult), and current domains of use for each language (see **Appendix 11.1**).

2. Ask the parents of young children and adolescents and ask adolescent and adult clients for ratings of level of bilingualism (see **Appendix 11.1**). These ratings must be done separately for each language modality. An overall, global rating is impossible to interpret.

3. Obtain speech samples for all relevant and age-appropriate tasks (300 syllables for each sample). In each language, obtain two samples for each task (three if possible). This will allow you to compare within-language variability to between-language variability. It is impossible to accurately judge the severity of stuttering in each language based on a single, short sample in each language. Tasks may include conversation, a monologue, story retelling, telephone calls (typically shorter samples), and reading aloud.

4. Analyze each sample, identifying all disfluencies and/or unambiguous moments of stuttering. For languages that you do not speak, ask the client, a parent, a colleague, or an interpreter to help with this task. Accuracy will be higher if you limit the scope of this analysis for languages you do not speak. Untrained raters may do better identifying moments of stuttering than identifying normal speech disfluencies. Obtain appropriate consent before involving outsiders in the assessment. Accept that these analyses will *not* be as accurate as your own analysis in your native language(s), and draw your conclusions taking this into account.

5. Interpret the observed patterns of disfluency in light of: (a) the client's level of bilingualism; a slower speaking rate, frequent interjections, revisions, pauses, and single word repetitions may be part of the stuttering and avoidance/postponement strategies, but they can also be caused by less than perfect proficiency in the language being assessed; and (b) the phonological and prosodic features of the language being spoken, including rhythm, prosody, appropriate loudness levels, and phonemes that you are unfamiliar with, such as clicks and glottal stops.

6. Ask the parent's and/or the client's opinion about the severity of stuttering in each language and compare this with your objective data. If their opinion and your data disagree, consider possible reasons including confusion between stuttering and language proficiency issues (and resulting normal disfluencies), day-to-day variability, influence of domains of use for each language, and the accuracy of your analysis in your non-native language.

Roberts, 2002). They may confuse disfluencies caused by weak language skills with stuttering and report that they "stutter more" in their Lw, when, in fact, they simply speak with a higher rate of normal disfluencies. Clinicians and researchers should ask the client or the child's parents for their view, but they should also objectively assess normal disfluencies and stuttering patterns in each language (**Table 11–4**).

Possible Threats to the Validity and Reliability of Stuttering Assessments

There are several challenges in assessing the stuttering of a bilingual client. These include adaptation effects, test-retest reliability issues, the impact of domains of use for each language, the possibility of a role-playing effect, and the lack of published data on the range of normal disfluency rates and types in different languages and on the rate of speech. (see also **Appendix 11.2** for a checklist of criteria for valid assessments and descriptions of stuttering in published studies.)

Adaptation or Practice Effects   It is well known that people who stutter become more fluent on repeated readings of the same passage (see Bloodstein, 1995, for an overview). In assessing bilingual speakers, they must do each task at least twice. Roberts (2002) speculated that the second time a client is asked to provide a monologue, answer questions about his or her work, or read a text aloud, the client's speech could be different (faster rate and/or fewer disfluencies). An unpublished study found little evidence of cross-language adaptation effects in disfluencies or in speaking rate, using the tasks commonly used in clinical assessments (Mazzocca, Tarte, & Roberts, 2001).

A study of two adult bilingual men found different patterns of adaptation within and across languages on a reading aloud task (Hall & Evans, 2004). Hall and Evans used multiple readings, whereas Mazzocca et al. used only two, to simulate real clinical procedures. Still, the possibility of an adaptation effect influencing results in the L2 assessed cannot be ruled out. Taking more than one speech sample in each language (see below) and counter-balancing the order of these samples may help to reduce any potential adaptation effect in assessments, for both clinical and research purposes.

Test-Retest Reliability   It is well known that stuttering behavior changes from one day to the next, especially in children. Therefore, clinicians (and researchers) need to be cautious in making judgments about the relative severity of the stuttering in each language based on one sample in each language. For example, if a client displays 5% SS (percent of syllables stuttered) in one language and 10% SS in the other language, this might or might not mean stuttering is more severe in the latter. This is especially true given that inter- and intra-rater tallies of %SS are rarely identical.

Ideally, judgments about the severity of stuttering in a particular language should be made only on the basis of multiple speech samples in each language. Using the model of three pretreatment baseline scores for single-subject treatment studies, and based on the authors' clinical experience, we recommend obtaining three samples for each task, ideally (thus, three monologues, three texts read aloud, etc.). Analysis of these samples should take into account not just %SS, but also factors such as visible and audible physical tension, the number of iterations, and the number and severity of any observed secondary behaviors. In a clinical context, there may not be time to do this repeated sampling, and two samples for each task may be a more realistic protocol. Using a button-press or computer-based counting device will greatly shorten the time needed to analyze each sample. In collecting multiple samples of speech across languages, varying the order of languages will reduce the chances of the adaptation effect mentioned above.

Domains of Use of Each Language   Bilingual speakers often use one language for some areas of their lives, such as work, and their other language for other areas of their lives, such as speaking with friends and family. In the language they are unaccustomed to using for a particular topic or activity, speakers may do one or more of the following: speak more slowly; produce interjections, pauses, and revisions due to word finding and syntax planning problems; use shorter sentences; or switch back and forth between languages using their task-specific, preferred language to fill in the gaps in vocabulary or syntax. All of these behaviors could mistakenly be attributed to their stuttering, when in fact, they are simply normal, bilingual coping strategies.

Non-Native Language as Role Playing   Does speaking in one's non-native language have a fluency-enhancing effect similar to playing a role onstage? Perhaps. Some bilingual adult clients report things like "it's easier to speak because I don't have all those old fears" or "it's like it's not really me talking when I speak in English." (Maillet & Roberts, 1997). No published research has addressed this question.

Limited Proficiency Can Cause Disfluencies   When a speaker has limited proficiency in a language, coping strategies often include frequent pauses, changing to the other language to fill in a word or phrase, normal speech disfluencies, including interjections, revisions (because of a syntactic or pronunciation error or anticipated error), and word and phrase repetitions. In some languages, sound prolongations are also used for some instances where interjections might be used in English (Nwokah, 1988; Roberts & Meltzer, 2004).

Characteristics of Stuttering in Different Languages

One way to assess the severity of stuttering is to compare the speaker's rate and overall disfluency level with appropriate norms. The further outside the normal range the speaker falls, the more severe the problem is. What do we know so far about the characteristics of stuttering in different languages? Several studies have documented the kinds of disfluencies present in both stuttering and nonstuttering speakers in a small range of languages and conditions (Van Borsel, Sunaert, & Engelen, 2005, including Spanish (Au-Yeung, Vallejo Gomez, & Howell, 2003; Carlo & Watson, 2003), German (Dworzynski, Howell, & Natke, 2003; Howell et al., 2004; Sandrieser, Natke, Van Ark, Pietrowsky, & Kalveram, 2004), Kannada (Jayaram, 1983), Portuguese (De Andrade, Sassi, & Zackiewcz, 2004; Juste & de Andrade, 2004), and French (Grosjean & Deschamps, 1975; Roberts & Hébert, 2001; Roberts & Meltzer, 2004).

In all of these languages, the same types of disfluencies found in English occur. However, there are differences in their distribution in various languages on dimensions such as content versus function words, the influence of consonant clusters, and the number of what are called stutter-like disfluencies (SLDs) in English-speaking children (Yairi & Ambrose, 2005).

Disfluencies that are rarely produced by non-stuttering English speakers—such as prolongations—are more frequent in some other languages. In French, Roberts and Meltzer (2004) found that non-stuttering, French-speaking men produced twice as many SLDs as unilingual, English-speaking men of similar age and education. This was true regardless of the level of English proficiency in the French-speaking group. The French speakers produced higher numbers of prolongations and one-syllable word repetitions. Also, the overall mean number of disfluencies per 100 syllables across three different speaking tasks was 13 for the French-speaking group compared with 6 for the English-speaking group. This study demonstrates that we cannot assume that other languages fall within the documented normal range for English speakers. For many languages there are little or no data about the expected range for normal disfluencies. Clinicians must rely on perceptual judgments about the number of iterations, the length and types of the disfluencies, and the level of visible and audible tension during disfluencies to make a judgment about the severity of the stuttering.

Rate of Speech in Different Languages

There are several studies of rate of speech in different languages, but they reveal far less than one might hope, mainly because there is no consistent methodology. Some studies use single sentences, others use connected speech; some include disfluent syllables, whereas others do not; some exclude pauses as short as one-quarter of a second, whereas other studies include pauses of up to 3 seconds. Finally, most studies fail to report the language background of their speakers (to exclude bilingual speakers), and most fail to provide inter-and intra-rater reliability data. Therefore, the search for data on rate of speech in different languages is, ultimately, a frustrating one. It is important for readers to critique what they read and to discard studies that fail to meet appropriate standards.

For example, a paper by Verheoven, De Paux, and Kloots (2004) provides a list of rates of speech in several languages taken from different studies but all calculated in syllables per second. British English was much slower than Spanish: 3.2 versus 7.8 syllables per second. But, the British study (Tauroza & Allison, 1990) used samples of connected speech that included pauses of up to 3 seconds, whereas the Spanish study (Rebello Couto, 1997) used single, isolated utterances, with all pauses excluded. Thus, the very different mean rates of speech, presented without commentary or explanation, reflect the different methodologies of the studies more than they reveal rates of speech across different languages.

Accurate Judgments of Stuttering Severity

One of the skills needed to assess and treat people who stutter is the ability to accurately identify disfluencies. Depending on the approach used, this may mean identifying moments of stuttering or identifying all disfluencies. Can clinicians accurately identify disfluencies in a language they do not speak? Humphrey (2004) compared the mean disfluency rates identified by a group of six unilingual English students with those of a group of six English-Spanish bilingual students. There was no significant difference in the mean number of disfluencies reported by the two groups. However, both groups failed to identify large numbers of disfluencies, there is little information on the level of bilingual proficiency of the bilingual judges, and the study involved a single speech sample in each language. Therefore, it is difficult to know how to interpret these results. Van Borsel and de Britto Pereira (2005) asked native speakers to watch videotaped samples of adult speakers and to decide whether or not each one stuttered, and they found that judges' decisions were significantly more accurate for speech samples in their native language than in a language they had little or no knowledge of. These findings are consistent with the present authors' impression based on years of working with bilingual students and bilingual new clinicians: They are less accurate and require more training identifying disfluencies in their non-native language (English or French), even when they speak it quite well. On a related topic, Schwab and Grosjean (2004) have found that bilingual adults' ability to judge speech rate is correlated with their own level of proficiency in each language.

Because of the uncertainty around accurate identification of disfluencies and accurate judgments of speaking rate, clinicians should be aware that their own accuracy in analyzing speech in a language other than their own L1 may be less than adequate. When reporting their findings, authors must pay particular attention to demonstrating adequate levels of reliability in their fluency counts in studies of bilingual speakers and in studies of languages other than their native language. Some published studies have failed to demonstrate adequate reliability in fluency counts (e.g., Nwokah, 1988), thus seriously undermining the credibility of their findings.

Another tool for assessing both stuttering severity and treatment outcomes is a naturalness rating scale. There is evidence that naturalness ratings can be affected by the presence of foreign or regional accents (Mackey, Finn, & Ingham, 1997). This might or might not make naturalness ratings unsuitable for use with clients who speak one or more of their languages with an accent. Replications of this initial study, using speakers of different languages as both speakers and judges, are needed.

Deciding if a given disfluency is stuttered or not is problematic at the best of times. Stutters that last for one or more seconds and stutters that are accompanied by tension and nonspeech secondary behaviors are relatively easy to identify. Briefer, more subtle stutters of shorter duration with no accompanying secondary behaviors are much harder to accurately identify, as are word substitutions and inappropriate use of interjections, yet these are common behaviors particularly in adolescents and adults who stutter. Clinicians need to know something about the normal rhythm and prosody of a language and have a basic knowledge of the phonemes in the language being assessed. Two examples illustrate this point. To a clinician hearing them for the first time, the clicks in some African languages could sound like nonspeech sounds inserted before word-initial vowels or they could sound like laryngeal or glottal blocks. In standard Japanese, high vowels can be voiceless when they occur between two voiceless consonants (Fujimoto, Murano, Niimi, & Kiritani, 2002). Adolescent and adult clients and parents can often provide helpful information, contrasting the sounds in their L1 with those in English, especially if they have formally studied English.

◆ Treatment for Bilinguals Who Stutter

In planning treatment for bilingual clients, clinicians must make decisions about several issues. Given the very limited number of published studies with sound and clinically relevant data, the available literature provides little guidance for clinicians who want to base their actions on empirical evidence. The next section presents a review of some of what is known about how cultural factors might affect therapy outcomes, and whether to treat both/all languages spoken by the client.

Cultural Factors in the Treatment of Bilingual Children Who Stutter

Most authors who write about CLD issues stress the importance of considering a CLD client's culture and beliefs and providing "culturally appropriate" intervention. (e.g., Bernstein Ratner, 2004). Too often, however, recommendations are based on opinion, with little or no data supporting them. It seems appropriate to modify one's style of interviewing to some degree, based not only on cultural factors but on education level, anxiety levels, and other factors, and it makes sense to be aware of how culture can affect the pragmatic aspects of communication (e.g., interpreting eye contact). But many recommendations such as playing "music consistent with the African American culture" in the waiting room to improve "clinical results" (Terrell, Battle, & Grantham, 1998, p. 37) have not been tested and need to be.

One study in stuttering has tested the impact of cultural factors on therapy outcomes. At the Hospital for Sick Children in Toronto, Waheed-Kahn (1998) found that only 20% of the non-native English-speaking (NNE) children reached the target fluency levels, as compared with 85% of the native English speakers. The NNE group was made up primarily of school-age children of very recent immigrants to Canada, coming primarily from India, southeast Asia, Ethiopia, and Somalia. Attendance was also much poorer for the NNE group. Waheed-Kahn changed her approach to require that a family member attend all sessions with the child, to learn the fluency-shaping targets and to develop suitable practice vocabulary, homework, and transfer tasks in the child's home language. She observed the family member practicing with the child in the clinic, offering correction and encouragement. With this increased family involvement, 75% of the NNE children achieved the fluency criteria, and attendance improved from 73 to 97%. Homework completion also improved. Fluency improved in English and in the children's home language. This study provides data to support the often-made recommendation to use culturally appropriate stimuli (for in-clinic practice and for homework), and to ensure that clients have opportunities to apply fluency skills in contexts that are relevant to their cultural circumstances (Kathard, 1998; Bernstein Ratner, 2004; Watson & Bernstein Ratner, 2005).

In other studies, however, bilingual clients receiving treatment in their non-native language, with no adjustments made to the therapy program, reached and maintained the same levels of fluency as those of native speakers in the same therapy group (Druce, Debney, & Byrt, 1997; Euler, personal communication, June 9, 2005). The contradictory—and preliminary—results from these studies highlight the urgent need for studies of how or if cultural factors influence treatment participation and outcomes. It seems likely that different levels of cultural accommodation may be needed depending on the client's home culture and how different it is from that of the new country, how long the client has been in the new country before starting therapy (if the client is an immigrant), the client's age, and the client's LOB. Socioeconomic status, level of education, and reasons for immigration may also be relevant factors and probably interact with the cultural factors to influence clients' willingness to seek treatment, their compliance, and the treatment outcomes.

Do Treatment Methods Developed in One Language Work in Other Languages?

Clinical experience and published studies agree that the most popular treatment methods developed in English can produce similar results in various languages whether they are based on: (1) fluency-shaping principles (Franken, Boves, Peters, & Webster, 1992; Euler & Wolff von Gudenberg, 2002; Jehle, 1995; Frokjaer-Jensen, 1995); (2) stuttering modification methods (Eichstadt, Watt, & Girson, 1998; Hansen, 1995); or (3) use a blend of methods (Forne-Wästlund, 2004). Readers able to access and read the clinical literature in other languages will no doubt find many more examples.

The literature search for this chapter failed to find any outcome studies designed to compare bilingual with unilingual speakers. The only available evidence is serendipitous. In a study of the treatment outcomes for children 6 to 8 years old, Druce et al. (1997) found that the outcomes for a group of 6 bilingual children (LOB and language histories not described) were not significantly different from those of the nine unilingual English-speaking participants. The low power and low external validity that inevitably obtain with such small numbers of participants and the lack of data on whether or not the family practiced with the child in their home language make this report very incomplete and its results difficult to interpret. In a study with larger numbers, Euler found that 32 adults who were non-native speakers of German showed improvement in a fluency-shaping program administered entirely in German that did not differ from the improvement shown by native German speakers (H. Euler, personal communication, June 9, 2005). Once again, clients may or may not have practiced outside the clinic in their L1. In studies that assess treatment outcomes, logs of practice time may be helpful in tracking whether and to what degree clients are doing practice in the language(s) other than the language of the therapy in the clinic. This information will be critical in measuring between-language generalization of progress and in establishing protocol validity (i.e., in studies measuring the effects of treatment given in only one language, demonstrating to what extent treatment really was administered in only one language).

Do Clients Need Therapy in All Languages That They Speak? (Table 11–5)

Ideally, all BWS should be seen by clinicians who speak all of the client's languages with near-native-level proficiency. Ideally, treatment would continue for as long as needed, moving seamlessly from one language to another. Unfortunately, this is rarely—if ever—the clinical reality. It is very time-consuming and therefore costly to recruit, train, and then conduct treatment working through interpreters. Schools and clinics often cannot refer clients to other districts or agencies to gain access to an appropriately bilingual clinician. Even in large cities, there is a shortage of clinicians with expertise in stuttering who speak the many languages of the BWS living there. Therefore, the question "do clients need therapy in all languages they speak?" is an important one, both ethically and financially.

Table 11–5 Treatment Studies of Bilingual Stuttering

Study	Subjects	Description of Treatment	Findings
Humphrey, Al Natour & Amayreh (2001)	11-year-old identical twin girls L1: Arabic L2: English	Aspects of stuttering modification and fluency shaping; treatment was only for reading. Language of treatment: Arabic. 21 treatment sessions.	S1: Pretreatment: 27%SS (Arabic); 29%SS (English). Posttreatment: 2%SS (Arabic); 3%SS (English). S2: Pretreatment: 18%SS (Arabic); 23%SS (English). Posttreatment: 3%SS (Arabic); 1%SS (English). Fluency increased in Arabic reading and generalized to English reading in both girls.
Shenker, Conte, Gingras, Courcy, & Polomeno (1998)	3-year-old girl; exposed to English/French from birth	The Lidcombe Program began after 16 weeks of indirect therapy. Language of treatment: began in English in the clinic with French added starting at week 23. Both English and French continued to be spoken at home. 30 clinic visits.	Pretreatment: 13%SS (English); 9.9%SS (French). Post-reatment: 2.8%SS (English); 4.4%SS (French).
Rousseau, Packman, & Onslow (2005)	7-year-old boy L1: French L2: English, was introduced at 5.5 years	The Lidcombe Program. Language of treatment: French. 41 clinic visits over a period of 51 weeks.	Pretreatment: stuttering ranged from 2%SS to 6% SS (English); and from 2.5%SS to 5.5%SS (French) for samples taken both within and beyond the clinic. Posttreatment: <1%SS for both English and French samples taken both in the clinic and outside, and averaged per week. A simultaneous decrease of stuttering rate in both English/French.
Harrison, Kingston, & Shenker (in press)	5-year-old boy exposed to English/French from birth	The Lidcombe Program. Both parents attended treatment and feedback was provided in English and French both in and beyond the clinic. 8 clinic visits over a period of 12 weeks.	Pretreatment: English and French ranged from 3.8%SS to 12%SS, in and beyond the clinic. Posttreatment: English and French ranged from 0.4%SS to 1.4%SS, in samples in-clinic and outside. Fluency stable at <1%SS on 1-year follow-up visit in both English and French.

(Continued)

Humphrey (1999)	Adult female exposed to English and Spanish from birth (English Ls)	Fluency-shaping and counseling. Language of treatment: English. Treatment given by a succession of graduate students. 10 hours treatment with a 2-month break after 5 treatment hours.	Pretreatment: 10.5%SS (English); 17.4%SS (Spanish). Posttreatment: 3.1%SS (English); 10.4%SS (Spanish).
Humphrey (2003)	S1: Adult female exposed to Spanish and English from birth (English Ls) S2: Adult male. L1: Arabic L2: French L3: English from age 20. S3: Adult male exposed to English and Spanish from birth; more English. S4: Adolescent male exposed to English and Spanish from birth	Method: not specified. Weekly treatment sessions. Language of treatment: English. Treatment time: not specified.	S1: Pretreatment: 10.5%SS (English); 17.4%SS (Spanish). Posttreatment: 3.1%SS (English); 10.4%SS (Spanish). S2: Pretreatment: 27.1%SS (English); 14.7%SS (French). Posttreatment: 11.5%SS (English); 6%SS (French). S3: Pretreatment: 31%SS (English); 51.9%SS (Spanish). Posttreatment: 2.4%SS (English); 9.1%SS (Spanish). S4: Pretreatment: 22.6%SS (English); 15.4%SS (Spanish). Posttreatment: 11.3%SS (English); 6.6%SS (Spanish).
Lim, Lincoln & Onslow (2005)	S1: Adult male exposed to English/Mandarin (English Ls) S2: Adult male exposed to English/Mandarin; balanced bilingual	3-day intensive utilizing speech restructuring technique (Block et al., 2004).	S1: Pretreatment: 13.9%SS (English); 20.7%SS (Mandarin) in clinic. 14.3%SS (English); 18.6%SS (Mandarin) beyond clinic. Posttreatment: 0.2%SS (English); 0.6%SS (Mandarin) in clinic. 0.6%SS (English); 2.5%SS (Mandarin) beyond clinic. S2: Pretreatment: 3.7%SS(English); 4.7%SS (Mandarin) in clinic. 4.2%SS (English); 4%SS (Mandarin) beyond clinic. Posttreatment: 0.3%SS (English); 0.4%SS (Mandarin) in clinic. 1.4%SS (English); 1.4%SS (Mandarin) beyond clinic.

S, subject; %SS, percent of syllables stuttered; L1, Native language, first language learned; Ls, stronger language.

Based on the authors' clinical experience and the few studies done to date, it seems that BWS often, but not always, need treatment in both languages. Studies that provide data on the generalization of treatment gains across languages are listed in **Table 11–5**.

In some cases, gains made in therapy given in one language generalize to an untreated language (Harrison, Kingston, & Shenker, in press; Humphrey, 2003; Humphrey, Al Natour, & Amayreh, 2001; Lim, Lincoln, & Onslow, 2005; Rousseau, Packman, & Onslow, 2005; Shenker, Conte, Gingras, Courcy, & Polomeno, 1998). In other cases, there is some improvement in the untreated language, but less than in the treated language (Humphrey, 1999). Clinically, the authors have seen bilingual adults who stutter where there is no improvement in an untreated language. Interestingly, this is the same range of outcomes found in therapy for bilingual adults with aphasia. We do not yet understand what factors explain these widely different results.

Given what is known about bilingualism, and about cross-language generalization of treatment effects in other disorders such as aphasia, and child language disorders (Edmonds & Kiran, 2006; Gutierrez-Clennen, 1999; Holm & Dodd, 2001; Paradis & Crago, 2000) the following factors merit investigation: the client's age; level of proficiency in each language; age of acquisition of each language; current and recent patterns of use of each language; level of similarity between the two languages (e.g., Russian/English BWS compared with French/Italian BWS). Some authors speculate that this linguistic distance is an important factor in the ease of transfer of new skills across languages. The frequency and intensity of treatment and the length of treatment are also variables that should be studied. A child or adult with no cross-language generalization after a short period of treatment might generalize gains to an untreated language if given a longer period of treatment.

The Lidcombe Program of early stuttering intervention is a parent-administered program (Chapter 4, this volume; Onslow, Packman, & Harrison, 2003), in which a parent attends weekly clinic visits to learn how to provide the treatment in the child's everyday environment. This approach is particularly easy to use with families where the clinician does not speak the language spoken by the family at home. In the studies to date, the preschool children treated with the Lidcombe Program have all transferred the gains in fluency in the language of treatment to an untreated language, but to varying degrees (Harrison et al., in press; Rousseau et al., 2005; Shenker et al., 1998). In one case (Shenker et al., 1998), the child's %SS after treatment was higher in French (L2) than in English, perhaps because he received fewer hours of treatment in French, or perhaps because it was his less proficient language. In another case study using the Lidcombe Program with a preschool-age child (Harrison et al., in press), treatment was provided both in the clinic and at home in English by the father and in French by the mother. The criteria for maintenance (<1%SS and severity ratings of 1–2) were reached in eight clinic visits over 12 weeks. Fluency stabilized at these levels 8 weeks into Stage 2, and the child's speech remained stutter-free at 1 year posttreatment. The successful outcome in both languages is due, perhaps, to the treatment being administered in the child's home, or perhaps it occurred because of the young age of children suitable for this method and their neural plasticity and high chance for natural recovery. Perhaps better results are obtained for the Lidcombe Program (or, indeed, for any treatment method) if both languages are treated. These initial case reports do not answer these questions. We need studies of preschool-age bilingual children using the Lidcombe Program and other therapy methods, with a range of pairs of languages and LOBs, comparing outcomes when children of various ages are treated in just one language or in two languages.

Until these studies are available, each clinician will need to collect data as therapy progresses to determine if treatment is needed in a second or third language. Generalization of gains in treatment from one language to another should be measured. In BWS who are school-age and older, and therefore less likely (perhaps?) to spontaneously generalize across languages, generalization should be facilitated by providing home assignments and some in-clinic practice for each language. Ratings of stuttering severity and speech naturalness done by the parents and/or the client can be used to monitor changes over time in languages the clinician does not speak. Accuracy of these ratings is often better if the client and clinician do some joint ratings of in-clinic speech. The authors have found that it is not necessary for a clinician to understand the client's language to hear things like speech rate, gentle onsets, or laryngeal tension. However, clinicians should recognize, as most intuitively do, that their discrimination may be less than accurate in languages they do not speak well.

In Treatment, which Languages(s) to Work in?

In considering which language(s) to work in, the clinician should look at the language(s) the BWS needs to use in daily activities, and provide treatment in these languages, if generalization does not spontaneously occur. These "other-language sessions" can be done by conducting treatment and demonstration sessions in the language that the client and clinician have in common, and then relying on the client and/or family to devise parallel exercises and ways of practicing in the client's other language(s). The case studies of M.K. and O.D. at the end of this chapter provide examples of treatment using this approach.

Clinical experience suggests that most bilingual adolescents and adults who stutter spontaneously generalize skills like slower speaking rates, gentle onsets, or cancellation to their different languages after learning them in one language. However, the degree of spontaneous generalization varies from one person to another, perhaps due to language proficiency, similarity between languages, patterns of language use, learning styles, and, no doubt, other factors. Most adolescent and adult BWS seem to need some structured practice in all languages spoken to reach a high level of proficiency and confidence in using the techniques in their various languages. It is not a question of repeating the entire therapy process in each language. It seems sufficient for most clients to have them do some practice at home as they are taught each new skill, and then help them to build the different languages spoken into the transfer hierarchies. Clients must take responsibility for the languages not spoken by the clinician, playing a more active role earlier in the therapy than they normally would to assist in devising ways to practice relevant words, content, and tasks in each of their languages. To assist the BWS practice in a language the clinician does not speak, it is often possible for the clinician to identify the most obvious stutters if the client speaks slowly. Similarly, the clinician can provide feedback on gentle onsets without understanding what is being said. The problem is, of course, that the clinician's ability to perceive subtle stutters, word substitutions, or avoidances, and to provide accurate feedback will be limited, to an unknown extent, when listening to speech in a language the clinician does not understand. It is important to recognize these limitations. It appears beneficial to start these "other language" exercises early in the therapy process so that the therapy techniques are associated with both languages. A caveat: These recommendations are based on the authors' clinical experience and have not been empirically tested.

For many methods, part of the therapy process consists of working through tasks of progressively greater difficulty. Each list of tasks is constructed based on feedback from each client on what factors increases his or her difficulty speaking in a particular situation (telephone; number of listeners, etc.). As noted above, it is important to consider cultural factors when designing hierarchies of difficulty. Factors that have little importance in one culture, such as the age and marital status of the person spoken to, can be very important in other cultures. Therefore, the hierarchies need to reflect these factors, as well as patterns of use and levels of proficiency for each language.

The case reports cited in **Table 11–5** are encouraging in that they document what clinicians working with BWS see in their daily practice: Treatment in one language often results in gains in the client's other language(s), with no practice or minimal practice in the latter. However, we need to move beyond such case reports (which constitute a very weak level of evidence) and conduct well-controlled treatment studies using both single-subject designs and group designs (Hoyle, 1999; Jones, Gebski, Onslow, & Packman, 2001; Kazdin, 1998) with speakers of various pairs of languages for clients of different ages, using a wider range of treatment methods.

Case Examples

Simultaneous English/French Bilingual Preschool Child

P.S. was 3 years, 11 months of age when treatment with The Lidcombe Program of early stuttering intervention began. The reported onset of stuttering was at 2 years of age. P.S. was exposed to both English and French in the home from birth. His pretreatment stuttering rates ranged from 5.6%SS to 9.8%SS in English and French conversation samples taken in both in-clinic and out-of-clinic settings. Overall, he averaged 7.0%SS in English and 7.3%SS in French. Pretreatment severity ratings were 8 in English and 6 in French (1 = no stuttering; 2 = mild stuttering; 10 = severe stuttering).

Treatment began 1 month following assessment. The language of therapy was English because that was the common language between P.S. and his mother, who would be providing the verbal feedback that is essential to the Lidcombe Program. The %SS in the clinic at the first treatment session was 18%SS (English) and 10%SS (French). Note that although the pretreatment data suggest roughly equal %SS in the two languages, the two samples on the day the client began therapy differ

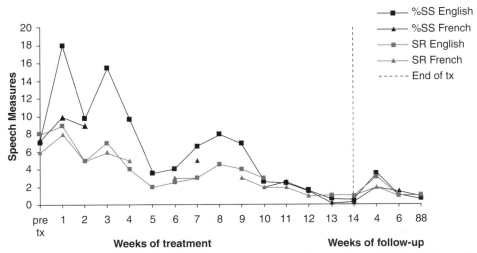

Figure 11–1 Treatment of stuttering both in English and French in a male aged 3 years, 11 months. *SR*, severity rating; *tx*, treatment.

by 8%. This kind of variability is not unusual in young children. No other speech and language concerns were present.

English was the language of treatment for the first six sessions. French was introduced at week 7 with the father now participating in therapy. This change resulted in an initial increase in the %SS (**Fig. 11–1**). After 15 sessions (23 weeks), P.S. met criteria for Stage 2 (Maintenance), and visits to the clinic tapered off, with his mother continuing to provide appropriate reinforcements in his day-to-day speech. Follow-up at 88 weeks after discharge from Stage 2 indicated that P.S. had met the criteria for successful maintenance of fluency at 0.6%SS in English and 0.9%SS in French, and a severity rating of 1 in both languages. The %SS for measures taken in the clinic as well as the parent's average severity rating for each week are shown in **Fig. 11–1.**

School-Age Arabic/English Bilingual Child, English Introduced At Age 4

O.D., age 6 years, lives with his parents and 3-year-old brother in the Middle East. O.D. speaks Arabic at home and was introduced to English at age 4 years, 6 months when he started attending a school where English was the language of instruction. English is O.D's father's L1. He began stuttering at age 3, and his parents report some improvement but still variable severity day to day. There is a history of recovered stuttering in one paternal uncle.

On assessment, O.D. displayed 5.0%SS in English and 7.8%SS in Arabic. Stuttering was characterized as syllable and part-word repetitions, audible and inaudible sound prolongations, and associated blinking and facial grimaces when trying to speak. O.D.'s parents confirmed that this was typical of his stuttering. He shows some frustration when trying to speak and has stopped talking on occasion when confronted with severe stuttering. No developmental, learning, or behavioral concerns were raised, and his parents described him as engaging easily with other children. At the time of assessment, O.D.'s parents rated the severity of his stuttering as 6 (1 = no stuttering; 10 = extremely severe stuttering). A pretreatment videotaped conversation sample showed the frequency of stuttering to be 5.8%SS in English and 8%SS in Arabic. Stuttering moments in Arabic were reviewed from the video samples with O.D.'s parents to confirm accurate identification by the parents of unambiguous moments of stuttering.

This family spent 1 month at the Montreal Fluency Centre, to start treatment for stuttering that could be continued by distance. Although he was a little older than is ideal, the Lidcombe Program of early stuttering intervention was administered. Treatment was provided in English by the clinician

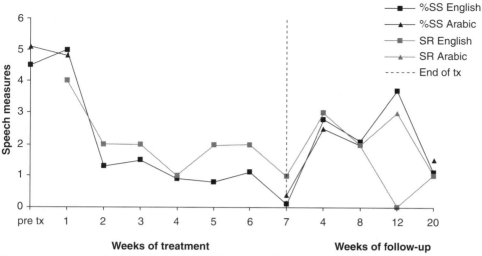

Figure 11–2 Treatment of stuttering both in English and Arabic in a 6-year-old male. SR, severity rating; *tx*, treatment.

and equally in the daily treatment sessions in English and Arabic by both parents. Over the course of treatment, O.D.'s stuttering frequency decreased to 2.4%SS in English and 1.4%SS in Arabic. Severity ratings were provided on a daily basis by both parents for beyond-clinic conversations. Severity ratings made by parents in-clinic were found to be a reliable rating of O.D..'s severity when rated jointly by both clinician and parents. Severity was rated at 2 for both English and Arabic at the final session.

After the final session, his parents have continued to provide the feedback required to maintain stutter free speech and have followed treatment with weekly exchange of severity ratings, videotapes, stutter counts, and telephone calls from their home. Fluency fluctuated initially after the family returned home and then stabilized at 1.1%SS (English) and 0.9% SS (Arabic) with a severity rating of 1 for the last shared video sample, taken at 4 months posttreatment. The severity ratings and %SS for O.D. are shown in **Fig. 11–2**.

Arabic/English/French Adolescent, English as a Second Language/French Introduced at Age 3

M.K., a 13-year-old trilingual (English/Arabic/French) speaker, was exposed to both English and Arabic from birth. French was introduced in school at age 5. Stuttering was first observed at age 3.5, and it varied in severity across situations, but it never disappeared. Previous treatments at age 6 and 8 for a period of 1 year each focused on "talking slower," with no lasting changes in stuttering noted as a result. No stuttering modification or fluency-shaping skills were included in these early treatments. M.K. was aware of and concerned about his stuttering and was motivated to try treatment again. He changed words to avoid stuttering and avoided situations in which he anticipated stuttering such as talking on the phone and in front of audiences. There were no reports of teasing or bullying.

M.K. was treated in an intensive therapy program that consisted of speech restructuring using prolonged speech (PS): the Camperdown Program (O'Brian, Onslow, Cream, & Packman, 2003). Treatment data for M.K. are provided in **Fig. 11–3**. In this program, PS is taught without reference to traditional speech targets. Development of stutter-free speech involves no programmed instruction or speech rate targets. Clients are encouraged to use whatever features of the PS pattern they require to control their stuttering, and they are free to individualize their speech pattern. There is no structured or hierarchical transfer phase. Clients evaluate their stuttering severity using a 9-point rating scale. Over the course of treatment, PS is shaped into natural-sounding speech and generalized to "real-world" settings.

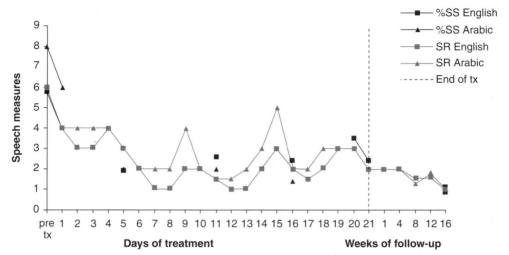

Figure 11–3 Treatment of stuttering both in English and Arabic in a male aged 13 years, 4 months. *SR*, severity rating; *tx*, treatment.

Pretreatment evaluation 1 year prior to starting treatment indicated a range of 3.9 to 5.1%SS in English on a variety of speaking/reading tasks (average 4.5%SS) and 5.1%SS for a conversation sample in Arabic. Stuttering severity was mild to moderate with the majority of stutters including audible sound prolongations and multisyllabic unit repetitions, with some nonverbal behaviors such as head movements accompanying moments of stuttering. On the first day of treatment, stuttering in English ranged from 2.7 to 6.7%SS in a variety of speaking situations that included reading (average 5%SS), and stuttering was 4.8%SS in spontaneous conversation with his mother in Arabic. During treatment the clinician provided therapy in English and the mother in both English and Arabic. At the end of the intensive program, stuttering was reduced to less than 1%SS in both English and Arabic.

Follow-up has been done through a distance monitored protocol comprising regular telephone contact, and continued data collection. Severity ratings are ranging from 1 to 2 (mild stuttering on a 10-point scale), and M.K. has increased his willingness to speak to teachers, order in restaurants, and read in front of the class. At the fourth follow-up session, 4 months following the intensive treatment, stuttering frequency was 1.1%SS on the telephone talking with the therapist, and 1.5%SS in conversation in Arabic with his mother. Severity ratings by his mother were 1 in both languages for the week prior to the follow-up session.

♦ Conclusion

This chapter contains a brief glimpse of the information about bilingualism that is relevant to stuttering. There are initial studies touching on several topics, including disfluencies and speaking rates in different languages, and a discussion of issues relating to the reliability and validity of assessments. We have presented some initial studies of the treatment of BWS. Because there are so many clinically important issues for which there is little or no research, this chapter has also included some impressions based on the authors' clinical experience. In addition to the reviews of research, the chapter provides some practical guidelines for assessing bilingual clients and some insights stemming from our experiences in providing treatment for BWS.

It is clear that much remains to be done. The existing studies serve to identify questions more than to provide answers. Replications and studies with more rigorous methodologies and larger numbers of participants will constitute the next steps on the road to understanding bilingual stuttering and how best to assess and then help BWS. International collaboration will allow researchers to gather larger numbers of cases, and design better studies.

The literature presented here reflects, to some degree, our own linguistic limitations and the difficulty in finding studies published in languages other than English. We welcome correspondence from readers pointing out studies we may have missed, in all languages.

It is our hope that future research on stuttering in bilinguals will avoid the pitfalls that have marked the development of knowledge about stuttering. Research on bilingual stuttering will need to take into account the new findings about stuttering, the importance of demonstrating the reliability of data, and the need to obtain representative participants (BWS and nonstuttering bilinguals) and to adequately describe their linguistic backgrounds and abilities. If authors report the findings of published studies without considering the quality of the study—and therefore the likely accuracy of the findings—progress will be slowed. As the now classic incident around "the Indians have no word for it" demonstrates, it is important not to turn rumors, second-hand reports, or erroneous findings into "facts" by (uncritically) repeating them (see Finn & Cordes, 1997, for a recent summary of this incident).

By comparing the performance of bilingual and unilingual speakers, it will be possible to study stuttering from new and potentially valuable perspectives. More than 20 years ago, Bernstein Ratner and Benitez (1985) pointed out that researchers will be able to use studies of BWS to separate motor from language phenomena to a greater degree than is possible in unilingual speakers. Sadly, this avenue of research has remained untapped. Given the large number of bilingual speakers in all parts of the world, there is a great need for studies on all aspects of the nature, assessment, and treatment of stuttering in bilinguals of all ages, and from all linguistic and cultural backgrounds.

References

Au-Yeung, J., Vallejo Gomez, I., & Howell, P. (2003). Exchange of disfluency from function words to content words with age in Spanish speakers who stutter. Journal of Speech, Language, and Hearing Research 46, 754–765.

Bernstein Ratner, N. (2004). Fluency and stuttering in bilingual children. In B.Goldstein (Ed.), Bilingual language development and disorders in Spanish-English speakers (pp. 287–308). Baltimore: Paul H. Brookes.

Bernstein Ratner, N., & Benitez, M. (1985). Linguistic analysis of a bilingual stutterer. Journal of Fluency Disorders 10, 211–219.

Block, S., Onslow, M., Roberts, R., White, S. (2004). Control of stuttering with EMG feedback. Advances in Speech Language Pathology 6, 100–106.

Blood, G. W., Ridenour, V. J., Qualls, C. D., & Hammer, C. S. (2003). Co-occurring disorders in children who stutter. Journal of Communication Disorders 36, 427–448.

Bloodstein, O. (1995). A handbook on stuttering (5th ed.). San Diego, CA: Singular.

Bortz, M. A., Jardine, C. A., & Tschule, M. (1996). Training to meet the needs of the communicatively impaired population of South Africa: A project of the University of the Witwatersrand. European Journal of Disorders of Communication 31, 465–476.

Brislin, R. W. (1994). Intercultural training: An introduction. Thousand Oaks, CA: Sage Publications.

Carlo, E. J., & Watson, J. B. (2003). Disfluencies of 3- and 5-year old Spanish-speaking children. Journal of Fluency Disorders 28, 37–53.

Cenoz, J., Hufeisen, B., & Jessner, U. (Eds). (2001). Cross-linguistic influence in third language acquisition: Psycholinguistic perspectives. Clevendon, UK: Multilingual Matters.

Conture, E. G. (2001). Stuttering: its nature, diagnosis and treatment. Boston: Allyn and Bacon.

Cook, V. (Ed.). (2003). Effects of the second language on the first. Clevendon, UK: Multilingual Matters.

Cooper, E. B., & Cooper, C. S. (1993). Fluency disorders. In Battle, D.E. (Ed.), Communication disorders in multicultural populations (pp.189–211). Boston: Andover Medical Publishers.

Dale, P. (1997). Factors relating to disfluent speech in bilingual Cuban-American adolescents. Journal of Fluency Disorders 2, 311–314.

De Andrade, C. R. F., Sassi, F. C., & Zackiewcz, D. V. (2004). Aspects of normally fluent speech in Brazilian adults. In A. Packman, A. Meltzer, & H. F. M. Peters (Eds.), Theory, research and therapy in fluency disorders: Proceedings of the 4th World Congress on Fluency Disorders (pp. 376–381). Nijmegen: Nijmegen University Press.

Druce, T., Debney, S., & Byrt, T. (1997). Evaluation of an intensive treatment program for stuttering in young children. Journal of Fluency Disorders 22, 169–186.

Dworzynski, K., Howell, P., & Natke, U. (2003). Predicting stuttering from linguistic factors for German speakers in two age groups. Journal of Fluency Disorders 28, 95–113.

Edmonds, L. A. & Kiran, S. (2006). Effect of semantic naming treatment on cross-linguistic generalization in bilingual aphasia. Journal of Speech, Language, and Hearing Reserach 49, 729–748.

Eichstadt, A., Watt, N., & Girson J. (1998). Evaluation of the efficacy of a stutter modification program with particular reference to two new measures of secondary behaviors and control of stuttering. Journal of Fluency Disorders 23, 231–246.

Euler, H. A., & Wolff von Gudenberg, A. (2002, November). Stuttering therapy with a relapse prevention program: 3-year follow-up data. Poster presented at the Annual Convention of the American Speech-Language-Hearing Association. Atlanta, GA.

Extra, G., & Maatens, J. (1998). Multilingualism in a multicultural context: Case studies on South Africa and Western Europe. In (Series Eds.) R. Appel, G. Extra, K. Jaspaert, & L. Verhoeven. Vol. 10 of Studies in multilingualism. Tilburg: Tilburg University Press.

Finn, P., & Cordes, A. K. (1997). Multicultural identification and treatment of stuttering: a continuing need for research. Journal of Fluency Disorders 22, 219–236.

Flege, J. E., Yeni-Komshian, G., & Liu, S. (1999). Age constraints on second-language acquisition. Journal of Memory and Language 41, 78–104.

Forne-Wästlund, H. (2004). Swedish comprehensive stuttering program-evaluation two to four years after treatment. In A. Packman, A. Meltzer, & H. F. M. Peters (Eds.), Theory, research and therapy in fluency disorders: Proceedings of the 4th WorldCongress on Fluency Disorders (pp. 189–194). Nijmegen: Nijmegen University Press.

Franken, M. C., Boves, L., Peters, H. F. M., & Webster, R. L. (1992). Perceptual evaluation of the speech before and after fluency shaping stuttering therapy. Journal of Fluency Disorders 17, 223–241.

Frokjaer-Jensen, B. (1995). Evaluation of results obtained after one year in a physiological stutter treatment. In C. W. Starkweather & H. F. M. Peters (Eds.), Stuttering: Proceedings of the 1st World Congress on Fluency Disorders (pp. 213–214). The International Fluency Association.

Fujimoto, M., Murano, E., Niimi, S., & Kiritani, S. (2002). Differences in glottal opening pattern between Tokyo and Osaka dialect speakers: factors contributing to vowel devoicing. Folia Phoniatrica et Logopedica 54, 133–143.

Gagnon, B., & Wolk, L. (2006, November). Coexistence of dysfluency and phonological impairment in two bilinguals. Poster presented at the annual conference of the American Speech-Language-Hearing Association. Miami, FL.

Galens, J., Sheets, A., & Young, R. V. (1995). Gale Encyclopedia of multicultural America. New York: Gale Research.

Gollnick, D., & Chin, P. (1990). Multicultural education in a pluralistic society. Columbus, OH: Merrill Publishers.

Grosjean, F. (1989). Neurolinguists beware—The bilingual is not two monolinguals in one person. Brain and Language 36, 3–15.

Grosjean, F. (1998). Studying bilinguals: methodological and conceptual issues. Bilingualism, Language and Cognition 1, 131–149.

Grosjean, F. & Deschamps, A. (1975). Analyse contrastive des variables temporelles de l'anglais et du français: Vitesse de parole et variables composantes, phénomènes d'hésitation. Phonetica 31, 144–184.

Guitar, B. (2006). Stuttering: an integrated approach to its nature and treatment 3rd ed. Baltimore: Lippincott, Williams & Wilkins.

Gutierrez-Clennen, V. F. (1999). Language choice in intervention with bilingual children. American Journal of Speech-Language Pathology 8, 291–302.

Håkansson, G., Salameh, E. K., & Nettelbladt, U. (2003). Measuring language development in bilingual children: Swedish-Arabic children with and without language impairment. Linguistics 41, 255–288.

Hakim, H. B., & Bernstein Ratner, N. (2004). Nonword repetition abilities of children who stutter: An exploratory study. Journal of Fluency Disorders 29, 179–199.

Hakuta, K. (1986). Mirror of language: The debate on bilingualism. New York: Basic Books.

Hakuta, K., Bialystok, E., & Wiley, E. (2003). Critical evidence: a test of the critical-period hypothesis for second-language acquisition. Psychological Science 14, 31–38.

Hall, N. E., & Evans, D. L. (2004). Examining adaptation and bilingualism in stuttering. In A. Packman, A. Meltzer, & H. F. M. Peters (Eds.), Theory, research and therapy in fluency disorders: Proceedings of the 4th World Congress on Fluency Disorders (pp. 410–413). Nijmegen: Nijmegen University Press.

Ham, R. E. (1990). Therapy of stuttering: preschool through adolescence. Inglewood Cliffs, NJ: Prentice-Hall.

Hansen, D. (1995). Treatment of school-aged stutterers. In C. W. Starkweather & H. F. M. Peters (Eds.), Stuttering: Proceedings of the 1st World Congress on Fluency Disorders (pp. 213–214). The International Fluency Association.

Harley, B., & Wang, W. (1997). The critical period hypothesis: Where are we now? In A. M. B. de Groot & J. F. Kroll (Eds.), Tutorials in bilingualism (pp. 19–52). Mahwah, NJ: Lawrence Erlbaum Associates.

Harris, R. J., Nelson, E. M. (1992). Bilingualism: Not the exception any more. In R. J. Harris (Ed.), Cognitive processing in bilinguals (pp. 3–14). New York: Elsevier.

Harrison, E., Kingston, M., & Shenker, R. (in press). Case studies in evidence-based management of stuttering preschoolers. In M. Onslow (Ed.), Evidence based clinical management of stuttering. Austin, TX: PRO-ED.

Holm, A., & Dodd, B. (2001). Comparison of cross-language generalisation following speech therapy. Folia Phoniatrica et Logopedica 53, 166–172.

Howell, P., Ruffle, L., Fernandez-Zuniga, A., Guitierrez, R., Fernandez, A. H., O'Brien, M. I., et al. (2004). Comparison of exchange patterns of stuttering in Spanish and English monolingual speakers and a bilingual Spanish-English speaker. In A. Packman, A. Meltzer, & H. F. M. Peters (Eds.), Theory, research and therapy in fluency disorders. Proceedings of the 4th World Congress on Fluency Disorders (pp. 415–422). Nijmegen: University of Nijmegen Press.

Hoyle, R. H., (Ed.) (1999). Statistical strategies for small sample research. Thousand Oaks, CA: Sage Publications.

Huinck, W. J., Van Lieshout, P., Peters, H. F. M., & Hulstijn, W. (2004). Gestural overlap in consonant clusters: Effects on the fluent speech of stuttering and non-stuttering subjects. Journal of Fluency Disorders 29, 3–25.

Humphrey, B. D. (1999, November). Bilingual stuttering: can treating one language improve fluency in both? Poster presented at the annual conference of the

American Speech-Language-Hearing Association, San Francisco, CA.

Humphrey, B. D. (2003). Bilingual stuttering: Transfer of treatment effects across languages. Poster presented to the annual convention of the American Speech-Language-Hearing Association, San Francisco, CA.

Humphrey, B. D. (2004). Judgments of disfluency in a familiar vs. an unfamiliar language. In A. Packman, A. Meltzer, & H. M. F. Peters (Eds.), Theory, research and therapy in fluency disorders: Proceedings of the 4th World Congress of Fluency Disorders (pp. 423–427). Nijmegen: Nijmegen University Press.

Humphrey, B. D., Al Natour, Y., & Amayreh, M. (2001, May). Does treatment of stuttering in language 1 generalize to language 2: A case study. Paper presented at the Florida Speech and Hearing Assocation conference (FLASHA), Orlando.

Ingham, R. J., Fox, P. T., Ingham, J. C., Xiong, J., Zamarripa, F., Hardies, L. J., et al. (2004). Brain correlates of stuttering and syllable production: Gender comparison and replication. Journal of Speech, Language, and Hearing Research 47, 321–341.

Jankelowitz, D. L., & Bortz, M. A. The interaction of bilingualism and stuttering in an adult. Journal of Communication Disorders 29, 223–234.

Jayaram, M. Phonetic influences on stuttering in monolingual and bilingual stutterers. Journal of Communication Disorders 16, 287–297.

Jehle, P. (1995). Results of the evaluation of a German version of the "Comprehensive Stuttering Program" by Boberg and Kully. In C. W. Starkweather & H. F. M. Peters (Eds.), Stuttering: Proceedings of the 1st World Congress on Fluency Disorders (pp. 442–444). The International Fluency Association.

Johnson, J. S., & Newport, E. L. Critical period effects in second language learning: the influence of maturational state on the acquisition of English as a second language. Cognitive Psychology 21, 60–99.

Jones, M., Gebski, V., Onslow, M., & Packman, A. (2001). Design of randomized controlled trials: Principles and methods applied to a treatment for early stuttering. Journal of Fluency Disorders 26, 247–267.

Juste, F., de Andrade, C. R. F. (2004). Distribution of disfluencies according to word class categorization in Brazilian Portuguese. In A. Packman, A. Meltzer, & H. F. M. Peters (Eds.), Theory, research and therapy in fluency disorders: Proceedings of the 4th World Congress on Fluency Disorders (pp. 369–375). Nijmegen: Nijmegen University Press.

Kathard, H. (1998). Issues of culture and stuttering: A South African perspective. Paper published for the First International Stuttering Awareness Day online conference. Available at http://www.mnsu.edu/comdis/isad/papers/kathard.html. Accessed February 22, 2007.

Karniol, R. (1992). Stuttering out of bilingualism. First Language 12, 255–283.

Kayser, H. (1998). Assessment and intervention resources for Hispanic children. San Diego, CA: Singular Publishers.

Kazdin, A. E. (1998). Research design in clinical psychology (4th ed.). Boston: Allyn & Bacon.

Leahy, M., & Wright, L. (1994). Therapy for stuttering facilitating working with people from different ethnic backgrounds. In C.W. Starkweather & H. F. M. Peters (Eds.), Stuttering: Proceedings of the 1st World Congress on Fluency Disorders (pp. 355–360). International Fluency Association.

Leith, W. R. (1986). Treating the stutterer with atypical cultural influences. In K.O. St. Louis (Ed.), The atypical stutterer (pp. 9–34). London: Academic Press.

Lim, V. P. C., Lincoln, M., & Onslow, M. (2005). Generalization effects to the non-treated language in English-Mandarin bilinguals who stutter. Paper presented at the 6th Oxford Disfluency Conference, Oxford, UK.

Lynch, E, W., & Hansonm J. (1992). Developing cross-cultural competence: A guide for working with young children and their families. Baltimore: Brookes.

Mackey, L. S., Finn, P., & Ingham, R. J. (1997). The effect of speech dialect on speech naturalness ratings: A systematic replication of Martin, Haroldson, and Triden (1984). Journal of Speech, Language, and Hearing Research 40, 349–360.

Macnamara, J. (1967). The bilingual's linguistic performance. In F. Cordasco (Ed.), Bilingualism and the Bilingual Child. New York: Arno Press.

Maillet, L., & Roberts, P. M. (1997). Perceptions de disfluidité chez les bègues bilingues. Unpublished manuscript, University of Ottawa.

Manning, W. H. (2001). Clinical decision making in fluency disorders (2nd ed.). San Diego: Singular-Thomson Learning.

Mansson, H. (2000). Childhood stuttering: Incidence and development. Journal of Fluency Disorders 25, 47–57.

Mazzocca, P., Tarte, C., & Roberts, P. M. (2001). Effets d'adaptation en lecture pour adultes francophones. Unpublished manuscript, University of Ottawa.

Nwokah, E. E. (1988). The imbalance of stuttering behavior in bilingual speakers. Journal of Fluency Disorders 13, 357–373.

O'Brian, S., Onslow, M., Cream, A., & Packman, A. (2003). The Camperdown Program: Outcomes of a new prolonged-speech treatment model. Journal of Speech, Language, and Hearing Research 46, 933–946.

Onslow, M., Packman, A., & Harrison, E. (2003). The Lidcombe Program of early stuttering intervention: A clinician's guide. Austin, TX: PRO-ED.

Oscarson, M. (1989). Self-assessment of language proficiency: rationale and applications. Language Testing 6, 1–13.

Paradis, J., & Crago, M. (2000). Tense and temporality: Commonalities and differences in French-speaking children with specific language impairment and French second language speakers. Journal of Speech, Language, and Hearing Research 43, 834–848.

Pavlenko, A. (2000). L2 influence on L1 in late bilingualism. Issues in Applied Linguistics 11, 175–205.

Pavlenko, A., & Jarvis, S. (2002). Bidirectional transfer. Applied Linguistics 23, 190–214.

Piske, T., Flege, J. E., & MacKay, I. R. A. (2001). Factors affecting degree of foreign accent in an L2: A review. Journal of Phonetics 29, 191–215.

Rebello Couto, L. (1997). Le rythme en espagnol et en portugais. Travaux de l'institut de phonétique de Strasbourg, 27, 3–90.

Roberts, P. M. (2002). Disfluency patterns in four bilingual adults who stutter. Journal of Speech-Language Pathology and Audiology 26, 5–19.

Roberts, P. M. (2001). Aphasia assessment and treatment for bilingual and culturally diverse patients. In R. Chapey (Ed.), Language intervention strategies in aphasia and related neurogenic communication disorders. (4th ed.) (pp. 208–232). Baltimore: Lippincott, Williams & Wilkins.

Roberts, P. M., & Hébert, T. (2001, August). Le débit et les disfluidités chez des enfants francophones bilingues (Rate of speech and disfluencies in bilingual Francophone children). Paper presented at the 25th world congress of the International Association of Logopedics and Phoniatrics, Montreal.

Roberts, P. M., & Meltzer, A. (2004). Normal rates and disfluencies in French and English. In A. Packman, A. Meltzer, & H. F. M. Peters (Eds.). Theory, research and therapy in fluency disorders: Proceedings of the 4th World Congress of Fluency Disorders (pp. 389–395). Nijmegen:Nijmegen University Press.

Rousseau, I., Packman, A., & Onslow, M. (2005). Treatment of early stuttering in a bilingual child. Paper presented at the 26th World Congress of the International Association of Logopedics and Phoniatrics. Brisbane, Australia.

Sandrieser, P., Natke, U., Van Ark, M., Pietrowsky, R., & Kalveram, K. T. (2004). A temporal analysis of disfluencies in children who stutter close to onset and controls. In A. Packman, A. Meltzer, & H. F. M. Peters (Eds.), Theory, research and therapy in fluency disorders: Proceedings of the 4th World Congress on Fluency Disorders (pp, 257–264). Nijmegen: Nijmegen University Press.

Schwab, S., & Grosjean, F. (2004). La perception du débit en langue seconde [The perception of speech rate in a second language]. Phonetica 61(2–3), 84–94.

Shenker, R. C., Conte, A., Gingras, A., Courcy, A., & Polomeno, L. (1998). The impact of bilingualism on developing fluency in a preschool child. In E. C. Healy & H. F. M. Peters (Eds.), Proceedings of the 2nd World Congress on Fluency Disorders (pp. 200–204). Nijmegen: Nijmegen University Press.

Silverman, F. H. (1996). Stuttering and other fluency disorders. (2nd ed.). Needham Heights, MA: Allyn and Bacon.

St. Louis, K., Roberts, P. M., Lukong, J., & Meese, M. (2006, July). Linguistic, cultural, and geographic influences on public attitudes toward stuttering: Cameroon, Canada, USA. Paper presented at the 5th World Congress on Fluency Disorders, Dublin, Ireland.

Stahl, V., & Totten, G. (1995). Bilingualism in young disfluent children. In C. W. Starkweather & H. F. M. Peters (Eds.), Stuttering: Proceedings of the 1st World Congress on Fluency Disorders (pp. 213–214). The International Fluency Association.

Stern, E. (1948). A preliminary study of bilingualism and stuttering in four Johannesburg schools. Journal of Logopaedics 1, 15–25.

Tauroza, S., & Allison, D. (1990). Speech rates in British English. Applied Linguistics 11, 90–105.

Tellis, G., & Tellis, C. (2003). Multicultural issues in school settings. Seminars in Speech and Language 24, 21–26.

Terrell, S. L., Battle, D. E., & Grantham, R B. (1998). African American cultures. In D.E. Battle (Ed.), Communication disorders in multicultural populations (2nd ed.) (pp. 31–71). London: Butterworth-Heinemann Medical.

Travis, L. E., Johnson, W., & Shover, J. (1937). The relation of bilingualism to stuttering: a survey in the east Chicago, Indiana, Schools. Journal of Speech Disorders 12, 185–189.

Tucker, G. R. (1998). A global perspective on multilingualism and multilingual education. In J. Cenoz & F. Genesee (Eds.), Beyond bilingualism: multilingualism and multilingual education (pp. 3–15). Clevendon, UK: Multilingual Matters.

United States Census. 2000. Available at: http:// www.census.gov/prod/2003pubs/c2kbr-29.pdf. Accessed June 2, 2005.

Van Borsel, J., & de Britto Pereira, M. (2005). Assessment of stuttering in a familiar versus an unfamiliar language. Journal of Fluency Disorders 30, 109–124.

Van Borsel, J., Maes, E., & Foulon, S. (2001). Stuttering and bilingualism: A review. Journal of Fluency Disorders 26, 179–205.

Van Borsel, J., Sunaert, R., & Engelen, S. (2005). Speech disruption under delayed auditory feedback in multilingual speakers. Journal of Fluency Disorders 30, 201–217.

Van Riper, C. (1971). The nature of stuttering. Englewood Cliffs, NJ: Prentice-Hall.

Verhoeven, J., De Paux, G., & Kloots, H. (2004). Speech rate in a pluricentric language: a comparison between Dutch in Belgium and the Netherlands. Language and Speech 47, 297–308.

Waheed-Kahn, N. (1998). Fluency therapy with multilingual clients. In E. C. Healey & H. F. M. Peters (Eds.), Proceedings of the 2nd World Congress on Fluency Disorders (pp.195–199). Nijmegen: University of Nijmegen Press.

Watson, J. B., & Kayser, H. (1994). Assessment of bilingual/bicultural children and adults who stutter. Seminars in Speech and Language 15, 149–164.

Yairi, E., & Ambrose, N. G. (2005). Early childhood stuttering. In (Series Eds.) D. Vogel & M. P. Cannito. Vol. 14 of For clinicians by clinicians. Austin, TX: PRO-ED.

Yaruss, J. S., LaSalle, L. R., & Conture, E. G. (1998). Evaluating stuttering in young children: diagnostic data. American Journal of Speech-Language Pathology 7, 62–76.

Appendix 11.1   Bilingual Language History and Proficiency Form

Ask as many questions as needed to find out the information for each item.

Name / Case Number: _____

Sex: F   M   Age: _____   Date assessed: _____

What languages have you/has your child learned and still remember?

1 _____   2 _____   3 _____   4 _____

Native language(s) (languages exposed to before age 2 or 3). Circle one or more than one of the languages listed above:

Numbers refer to the languages identified above.

	1	2	3	4
How learned each language:				
One column per language:	_____	_____	_____	_____
At home, starting at age:	_____	_____	_____	_____
At school, starting at age:	_____	_____	_____	_____
From TV or radio, from age:	_____	_____	_____	_____
From friends, starting at age:	_____	_____	_____	_____
From books or taught as a subject in school:	_____	_____	_____	_____

Encourage client/parent to think about all possible influences, talking to relatives in other countries, access to books, friends in different periods of client's life, etc.

Language of instruction at school (*Add details if needed, for example, if went to two different high schools.*) *Label each column with the appropriate language.*

Elementary school: age ___ to ___	1	2	3	4	NA
Senior elementary or middle school: age ___ to ___	1	2	3	4	NA
High school: age ___ to ___	1	2	3	4	NA
Community college: age ___ to ___	1	2	3	4	NA
University: age ___ to ___	1	2	3	4	NA
Other _____: age ___ to _____	1	2	3	4	NA
Other _____: age _____ to _____	1	2	3	4	NA

If more than one school in each age range, use the *Other* lines.

Language used in different domains:

(*Some of these domains apply more to adults than children. To use as needed.*)

	1	2	3	4	NA
In work, for all activities combined	_____	_____	_____	_____	NA
i.e., whatever you do in a typical week at work, how much of it is in _____ ?					
or, what percent of your total time doing work do you spend using _____ ?					
At home with your family	_____	_____	_____	_____	NA
At home with your roommate(s)	_____	_____	_____	_____	NA
For your main hobbies and sports activities	_____	_____	_____	_____	NA
Reading newspapers, books, magazines (outside work and/or outside school)	_____	_____	_____	_____	NA
Religious community activities	_____	_____	_____	_____	NA
TV/movies	_____	_____	_____	_____	NA
Internet and computer use	_____	_____	_____	_____	NA

(Continued)

Appendix 11.1 Bilingual Language History and Proficiency Form *(Continued)*

	1	2	3	4	
Listening to the radio	_____	_____	_____	_____	NA
Social life: your friends, family friends, your relatives	_____	_____	_____	_____	NA
Shopping	_____	_____	_____	_____	NA

For all above items, indicate what percentage of time each language is used. If the client has had more than one job recently, or changes in the home or hobbies, ask for a combined rating for the past several years, or ask the client to rate each period separately. The purpose of this section is to start to understand the mix of languages in the client's daily life, including percentage of use in oral and written language(s). The figures will not be exact, but they will give you a general idea of overall patterns.

Where did you / your child live from age:

0–5 _____ 6–10 _____ 11–15 _____

Since age 15 _____

Ask what was the dominant language spoken around client for each period. Some cities have neighborhoods that expose people to one or more languages other than the dominant language of that country or region; it is surprising how many people forget to mention exposure to various languages. This question aims at uncovering these omissions.

Assessment of Level of Bilingualism (LOB)

Instructions to read verbatim. **READ EXACTLY WHAT IS WRITTEN HERE.**

"Now I want you to rate your abilities on a scale that goes from 0 to 7

On this scale, 0 means you can't do it at all.

A rating of 1 means you can understand just a few words, not enough to understand sentences or make up sentences.

A rating of 7 means like an average native speaker of that language (at the same age, for children).

Your rating should reflect ability for all topics, in all situations.

Note that 7 does not mean perfect or ideal ability, but the level of a typical person who only speaks that language.

So a higher number means a higher level of ability.

How would you rate your ability/your child's ability to":

Label each column with appropriate language.

	L1	L2	L3	L4
Understand what people say in:	_____	_____	_____	_____
Express ideas in:	_____	_____	_____	_____
Understand what is read in:	_____	_____	_____	_____
Write:	_____	_____	_____	_____

If the client says things like: "in Spanish I'd give myself 7, but for some topics it is harder," explore this with the client. A normal unilingual speaker can discuss all aspects of his or her life. So, the client who says this does not qualify for a 7. However, if the client gives ratings that you disagree with, and says nothing to indicate uncertainty or equivocation, do not try to correct the client's ratings. You will form your own opinion, separate from these ratings, based on the client's performance during the assessment.

Appendix 11.2   Checklist for the Evaluation of Articles about Bilingual Speakers and Bilingual Stuttering

Published studies and conference presentations vary widely in quality. Some studies have such poor methodology, low reliability, and low validity that we should not accept their results. It is impossible to list all the relevant factors. However, for each study you read, ask the following questions, as a minimum. The more "yes" answers, the more likely it is that the results presented in the article are accurate.

◆ Have the authors described the participants adequately? This means have they told the reader: (1) the age of the participant(s); (2) their native language(s); (3) the age when exposure to each language began; (4) some indication of proficiency in each language, broken down by modality (auditory comprehension, verbal expression [syntax and vocabulary], reading, written expression); (5) some information about domains of use of each language; and (6) some information about screening for language and articulation disorders, especially in studies of children.

◆ Have the authors clearly stated what types of disfluencies they counted, and have they defined each of these types? Is this a complete analysis or have they omitted some types of disfluencies?

◆ If they say they have calculated %SS, did they define how they decided which syllables are stuttered? If they fail to do this, it is impossible to interpret their findings or compare them with other studies.

◆ Have the authors done inter-rater and intra-rater reliability checks? That is, (1) did someone else count disfluencies and check the transcription to see if their results agree with those of the authors. The second rater should be unaware of the purpose of the study, whether the tape they are analyzing is pre-therapy or post, etc.; and (2) did the person who did the original counts redo 10 to 20% of them to see if he or she obtained the same totals the second time?

◆ Are the inter-rater and intra-rater levels of agreement acceptable?

Section IV

Intervention: Adolescents and Adults Who Stutter

12

Intensive Treatment of Stuttering in Adolescents and Adults

Deborah A. Kully, Marilyn Langevin, and Holly Lomheim

The purpose of this chapter is to describe the ISTAR-Comprehensive Stuttering Program[1] (CSP) for adolescents and adults. Before describing the goals, clinical strategies, and components of the CSP, we begin with a brief overview of the development of the program, its various treatment formats, and the similarities and differences in treating adolescents and adults. Case examples are provided to illustrate the program for a typical adult and an adolescent client. We conclude with a brief discussion of the outcomes of the program.

The CSP, first published by Boberg and Kully in 1985, has been developed over a 30-year period of research and experience. In addition to our own clinical experience and client feedback, we have drawn from the work of many clinicians and researchers (see Langevin & Kully, 2003[2]). The present chapter provides an update of the CSP for teens and adults described in Kully and Langevin (1999). Because of space constraints, only the treatment program will be discussed in this chapter. Readers are referred to Kully and Langevin (1999) for a discussion of assessment issues and case selection decisions.

The CSP addresses both overt and covert aspects of stuttering. Treatment procedures include: (1) fluency-enhancing techniques (fluency skills and stuttering modification skills), which deal with core stuttering and learned struggle behaviors; and (2) cognitive-behavioral methods, which deal with the emotional and attitudinal aspects of stuttering. Family participation in therapy is encouraged with the degree of participation being determined by the developmental level of the client and the nature of the client-family relationship. Inherent in the process of treatment is the ongoing collection of behavioral and self-report data to evaluate clients' progress and make needed adjustments.

---

[1]ISTAR, the Institute for Stuttering Treatment and Research, is a nonprofit center located in Edmonton, Alberta, Canada. The ISTAR Comprehensive Stuttering Program is not related to the Swedish Comprehensive Stuttering Program (Forne-Wastlund, 2004) and is distinguished by specifying that it is the ISTAR program.

[2]Owing to space limitations, readers are referred to Langevin and Kully (2003) for references to publications that have influenced the development of the CSP. The authors again acknowledge these clinicians and researchers for their valued contributions.

◆ Treatment Formats and Schedules

Depending on the needs and goals of the client, treatment in the CSP is provided in group and individual formats and in intensive, semi-intensive, or extended schedules. More recently, we have also provided treatment through a combination of in-clinic and telehealth sessions (i.e., using videoconferencing systems to provide distance delivery of assessment, treatment, and consultative services; see Bashshur, Reardon & Shannon, 2000). For example, the client may attend the clinic for 1 week of intensive individual therapy to establish basic proficiency with the fluency skills and then return home where treatment is continued through the use of videoconferencing systems accessed though the client's community health center (Kully, 2000, 2002). The treatment format is selected in consultation with clients, with consideration of such factors as severity of overt and covert stuttering, presence of co-existing problems, and the client's ability to attend the clinic.

A 3-week intensive group-therapy approach is the preferred format for the majority of clients. We believe that intensive schedules offer several advantages. First, they provide opportunities for concentrated practice, which accelerates acquisition of fluency skills and provides impetus for transfer of skills to nonclinic environments. Second, intensive schedules reduce interference from other life activities and provide the opportunity to invest fully in the treatment process. Thus, dropout rates tend to be very low. Third, the group format allows for much practice to be accomplished in interactive speaking situations and provides a context for practice of demanding speaking tasks (e.g., debates and impromptu speeches), thus promoting generalization. Fourth, groups enable discussion and sharing of experiences among clients. Through both informal and clinician-led exchanges and exercises, clients discuss their feelings, thoughts, and experiences relating to stuttering (Boberg & Kully, 1985).

Despite their potential advantages, group intensive clinics are not suitable for all clients. Some clients simply will not be able to attend at times when intensive group clinics take place. Others who have pronounced cognitive, social, or physical problems will be unlikely to participate successfully in a group context. Still others who have mild overt and covert stuttering may not require the quantity of therapy that an intensive clinic provides. In such cases, we have conducted the CSP in individual intensive, semi-intensive, or extended formats, with the amount of therapy provided being dependent on individual needs. Based on empirical data obtained from 17 teen and adult clients, we have found that most clients who have been suitable for individual intensive or nonintensive formats have required 10 to 30 hours of therapy, with the median number of hours being 18, to complete acquisition and transfer phases.

If, after assessment (see Kully & Langevin, 1999), intensive group treatment is recommended, we determine the most suitable age group for the client. Our center offers intensive programs for three age groups: (1) children (7–12; see Chapter 8, this volume); (2) young teens (12–14); and (3) older teens and adults (15+). Several factors are considered in a placement, including chronological age, social-emotional maturity, and cognitive skills. For example, a 12-year-old with attention, language, or social-emotional difficulties may be placed in the children's clinic, which has more structure, greater parental involvement, and shorter therapy sessions (3 hours a day). A 14-year-old with good linguistic, academic, and social skills may be placed with older teens and adults, who are able to work more independently.

Group intensive clinics provide 83 hours (12–14-year-olds) to 90 hours (15+ years) of therapy each week day plus an additional hour of home practice each evening. Family meetings involve an average of 4 or 8 hours in adult and young teen clinics, respectively. In the intensive group clinics, therapy consists of a combination of individual, small-group, and large-group activities. Total group size ranges from 2 to 12 clients. In all clinics, the clinician-client ratio varies from 1:1 to 1:3, depending on the needs of the client and the demands of the activity. In most cases, client-clinician and client-client pairings are rotated daily to facilitate generalization.

◆ Similarities and Differences in Treatment for Adolescents and Adults

By early adolescence, the typical client will have been stuttering for several years and will have well-established motoric, behavioral, emotional, and cognitive aspects of stuttering. Thus, the general goals, clinical strategies, and components of treatment in the CSP are common to teens and adults. However, quite obviously, these two age groups are at very different stages socially, cognitively, and experientially. Accordingly, the *delivery* of treatment must be adjusted for adolescents to take into account their interests, ability to attend, emotional awareness, cognitive development, motivation, social skills, interaction styles, and so on (i.e., treatment must be age-adjusted and experientially adjusted to meet the developmental levels of the two age groups).

◆ Treatment Goals and Components

In addition to speech and attitudinal-emotional goals, the CSP includes self-management and environment-related goals as described below:

1. *Speech-related goals* These include: (1) the ability to sustain controlled fluency in all speaking environments with prosody and rate approximating normal and; (2) ability to manage residual stuttering (i.e., instances of stuttering that remain after treatment).

2. *Attitudinal-emotional goals* These include: (1) positive attitudes toward communication; (2) openness about stuttering and fluency-enhancing techniques; (3) reduced avoidance behavior; (4) ability to manage general and situationally related fear and anxiety; (5) ability to deal with teasing and negative listener reactions; and (6) improved communication and social skills.

3. *Self-management goals* These include: (1) self-monitoring, self-evaluation, and problem-solving skills; (2) ability to manipulate the environment to support needs; (3) ability to sequence practice activities; and (4) ability to handle regression and recognize when relapse is occurring.

4. *Environmental goals* These include: (1) increased family understanding of the etiology and development of stuttering and the long-term process of change and (2) family ability to support the client during and after therapy.

◆ Treatment Procedures

Clinical Strategies

Prior to discussing specific treatment procedures, we discuss several clinical strategies that appear to facilitate client success.

Maintaining Client Individuality

Because treatment programs may sometimes be viewed as unalterable, it is important to emphasize that we focus on each individual with whom we work. In all respects we strive to make our treatment responsive to the needs of each client. Client individuality is maintained through constant tailoring of every phase, step, and activity to meet individual needs. Fluency skill emphasis, target speech rates, speaking tasks, task sequences or hierarchies (tasks that progress from easier to more difficult), feedback, transfer exercises, maintenance plans, and family education and counseling are all adjusted—to the extent possible—according to each client's particular responses and needs.

Modeling

The tenet of observational learning (Bandura, 1997) suggests that modeling can facilitate the acquisition of concepts and new behavior patterns. Accordingly, clinicians continuously model cognitive-behavioral skills (e.g., effective "self-talk") and fluency skills (within and outside the clinic). Former clients also act as role models. We incorporate former clients into discussions of attitudinal-emotional issues and in transfer activities. In sessions that do not include clinicians, former clients share with present clients their experiences regarding anxiety management, avoidance reduction, and challenges in maintaining speech and attitudinal gains.

Self-Management Strategies Incorporated into All Therapy Activities

Self-management refers to a set of cognitive-behavioral processes that promote generalization and help clients extend new behaviors into their home and daily lives, under their own direction and control (Rehm & Rokke, 1988; Chapter 18, this volume). Self-management strategies are incorporated into both speech and attitudinal-emotional components of therapy. We view clinicians as facilitators who strive to help clients become their own clinicians.

Speech Practice in Non-English Languages

For bilingual or English-as-a-second-language clients, speech practice in their primary language is incorporated as soon as they achieve proficiency with fluency skills in English. In our experience, it is not necessary for clinicians to understand the other language to conduct such practice. To ensure that the integrity of stress patterns and word meanings are preserved, however, we involve clients and families in evaluating these aspects when fluency skills are practiced in other languages. Homework and transfers are also completed in the other languages.

Phases of Treatment: Acquisition, Transfer, and Maintenance

The CSP has three interrelated *phases: acquisition, transfer,* and *maintenance.* Acquisition and transfer occur during the 3-week program, whereas maintenance occurs in the posttreatment period. In acquisition, which occurs during the first half of the intensive program, clients learn the fluency-enhancing and cognitive-behavioral skills. In transfer, clients apply the skills in everyday life and increasingly challenging beyond-clinic situations. In maintenance, clients carry out daily fluency skill practice and self-directed transfers and work to integrate cognitive-behavioral skills.

Movement from one phase to the next is fluid, with strategies to promote generalization and maintenance integrated into acquisition but becoming more concentrated during the transfer phase. Although fluency skills and cognitive-behavioral treatment techniques are discussed separately here, they are delivered in an integrated way throughout treatment.

Fluency-Enhancing Techniques during the Acquisition Phase

This phase consists of three general stages.

Identification and Introduction to Self-Rating

In this first stage of the acquisition phase, clients learn to identify stutters and are introduced to the concepts of tension modification and self-rating. Clients learn that overt stuttering is a result

Table 12–1   Progression of Stages in Acquisition

Identification
Introduction to fluency skills

- Prolongation
- Easy breathing (EB)
- Gentle starts (GS)
- Smooth blending (SB)
- Light touches (LT)
- Refining prosody/naturalness
- Preparation for sustained prolongation

Rate increase and fluency skill refinement

- Slow stretch: EB, GS, SB, LT, all skills, Self-correction (SC), 3T's Self-assessment (SA)
- Medium stretch: EB, GS, SB, LT, all skills, SC, Rate Change session, SA
- Slight stretch: as for medium
- Control rate: as for medium

3T's, Think, Take a breath, Talk using skills.

of what they do physically to interfere with the smooth flow of speech. Following a brief description of the speech production process, they discuss how stuttering interrupts the speech flow at various levels in the vocal tract and identify where and how this occurs in their own speech. Physical tension modification exercises are then introduced in which clients practice simulating and releasing tension, first at various levels in the speech system without voice, and gradually, while emulating their own stuttering patterns. Clients use a 10-point scale to self-evaluate their physical tension levels as they simulate and release varying degrees of tension.[3] Clients are encouraged to focus on the kinesthetic feeling of releasing the tension. This tension modification practice lays the foundation for later self-correction (SC) training. Clients are also introduced to the process of making daily ratings of the severity of their stuttering as well as an emotional-attitudinal variable they wish to change[3] (e.g., situational anxiety). These daily ratings of stuttering severity and attitudinal-emotional variables are an aspect of self-management training that continue into maintenance. They also provide valuable information for both the client and clinician when problem-solving (e.g., if the client's ratings increase or plateau) and in tracking progress.

Introduction to Fluency-Enhancing Skills

In this second stage of the acquisition phase, the fluency-enhancing skills are introduced and shaped in a series of structured practice tasks, and self-evaluation training of the accuracy of fluency skill production is introduced. Practice generally proceeds in the order listed in **Table 12–1.** Although this order is used with most clients, it may be varied to fit the needs of differing stuttering patterns and abilities to acquire fluency-enhancing skills. **Table 12–2** provides a brief description of these fluency skills. Fluency skill practice begins with single syllables and progresses to longer utterances. Throughout the acquisition phase of treatment, clients are encouraged to focus on the kinesthetic feeling of each skill.

After clients achieve 80% accuracy in producing skills with clinician feedback, they learn to evaluate their own productions. This is done by having clients use a gesture or a +/− tally after each production to indicate whether or not a target skill (e.g., gentle start [GS]) was accurately produced. Clinicians indicate whether they agree with the client's self-evaluation, and if they do not, they indicate how their evaluation differs from the client's (Ingham, 1982). This self-evaluation practice continues throughout treatment and is fundamental to self-management training.

---

[3]All ratings are based on 10-point scales where 1 = nonexistent and 10 = very pronounced.

Table 12–2   Fluency-Enhancing Skills

Fluency Skills	Brief Description
Prolongation	Vowels are prolonged; transitions through consonants are slowed but not prolonged; stressed syllables receive more prolongation than unstressed syllables; natural prosody is maintained
Easy breathing	Full, unrushed diaphragmatic inspiration; smooth movement into expiration; appropriate breath grouping
Gentle starts	Slow, smooth initiation of speech with a slight pre-voice expiration and a gradual increase in loudness; full loudness achieved on the first syllable
Smooth blending*	Continuous air flow and smooth continuous movement of articulators within breath groups; manner and voicing characteristics of phonemes are preserved
Light touches*	Lightened but distinct articulatory contacts; manner and voicing characteristics of phonemes are preserved
3T's	Think, Take a breath, Talk using skills; used to consolidate skills and resist time pressure

Stuttering Management Skills	Brief Description
Self-correction	"Re-breathe": gradual release of tension and breath; re-initiation of speech with easy breath and gentle start
	"Pull-out": gradual release of tension; continuous smooth movement to next sound

*It is important to note that in producing smooth blending and light touches, manner and voicing characteristics of phonemes are preserved. Stops are not fricated, voiceless phonemes are not voiced, and consonants are not slurred.

Before progressing to the next skill, clients complete a self-evaluation task. The criterion is 80 to 90% accuracy in self-evaluating at least 10 productions of short phrases, usually four syllables long. Clients rate their skill proficiency immediately after each production, using a +/− tally system while clinicians covertly make their own tally. After five utterances, the clinician and client compare their ratings. In most cases the self-evaluation criterion is easily achieved; however, a few clients experience great difficulty with self-monitoring, a behavioral observation that is consistent with brain-imaging research which shows deactivation of regions involved in self-monitoring speech and voice in adults who stutter (see Ingham, Ingham, Finn & Fox, 2003). For these clients, extra self-monitoring training is provided.

A session devoted to refining speech naturalness (see Schiavetti & Metz, 1997; Chapter 18, this volume) concludes the introduction to fluency skills. Clients review the features of natural prosody and practice various stress patterns in words and sentences. Voice and resonance characteristics are evaluated to ensure that clients are using their natural pitch and resonance. A naturalness rating scale[4] is also introduced as a means of providing feedback, encouraging client self-evaluation, and appraising progress. Naturalness is an ongoing goal in all speech practice throughout the program.

Rate Increase of Speech with Fluency Skill Refinement

In this third stage of acquisition, fluency skills are practiced within the context of systematically increasing rates of speech. Speech rates increase from "slow" (40–60 syllables per minute [SPM]), to

---

[4]On this naturalness scale, 1 = highly natural and 10 = highly unnatural.

Table 12–3   Variables Manipulated in Sequencing Tasks

Variable	Hierarchy
Length	From single syllables to connected speech
Complexity	From linguistically and conceptually simple to complex and abstract (clients generally progress from reading to answering and asking questions to monologue and then conversation)
Cuing	From strong to minimal cuing
Feedback	From continuous to intermittent feedback
Emotionality	From low to high emotion
Interest level	From low to high interest
Spontaneity	From structured to natural exchanges
Time pressure	From low to high time pressures
Environmental variables such as physical setting, audience, and distracters*	From easier to more challenging

*One distracter that is incorporated into later rating sessions for teens—which senior clinicians find challenging and clients thoroughly enjoy—is the inclusion of popular background music.

"medium" (60–90 SPM) to "slight" prolongation (90–120 SPM) and, finally, to a "controlled rate" (120–210 SPM). At each prolongation rate, clients find an optimal rate that allows them to use the fluency skills well and maintain a feeling of stability. By the end of this stage, most clients are speaking at a rate of 150 to 190 SPM, which is on the lower end of the normal range (estimated at 162–230 SPM; see Andrews & Ingham, 1971).

At each prolongation rate, fluency skills are practiced in a series of 5-minute rating sessions. Each skill is practiced individually at first, then all skills are practiced together. The progression of rating sessions is outlined in the lower portion of **Table 12–1**. Rating sessions are carefully sequenced, moving from easier to more challenging speaking tasks by manipulating the variables listed (e.g., length, complexity) in **Table 12–3**, although task sequences are individualized for each client. Practice for teens incorporates age-appropriate games to foster motivation and interest. To promote generalization and active use of fluency skills to resist time pressure, physical activities are also incorporated into practice, particularly with teens. The last minute of each rating session is devoted to client self-evaluation using the gestures or written tallies described earlier.

To meet criteria for completing each rating session, clients must: (1) be within the SPM range for the target rate; (2) have less than 1% stuttering; and (3) have no more than five fluency skill errors, except in the "All Skills" sessions, in which errors must not exceed 10. Clients typically have 0% stuttering; however, a few may exhibit mild stuttering during prolongation. In such cases, SC is practiced extensively and stutters that are self-corrected are not counted.

After completing the All Skills sessions, clients practice SC, which incorporate aspects of Van Riper's (1973) cancellations and pull-outs. The first level of SC is called a "re-breathe" in which clients stop when they begin to stutter, slowly release physical tension and remaining air, re-breathe, and begin the word again using exaggerated fluency skills. Once proficiency with the re-breathe skill has been achieved, clients progress to using a pull-out. This involves stopping when physical tension is detected, gradually releasing tension, and making a smooth transition through the next syllable using exaggerated fluency skills. In both methods, clients are to use slight prolongation until their fluency stabilizes (i.e., speech is stutter-free and client feels stable). Practice of SC begins on day 3 of the program with simulated stutters, and in a series of steps, progresses to correction of true stutters. Modification of true stutters also progresses gradually, from structured tasks with clinician support to self-managed corrections during transfer tasks.

Rate Change sessions are introduced at the slight stretch rate. Clients learn to reduce their rate of speech as both a preventative and recovery strategy. As a preventative strategy, rate changes incorporate aspects of Van Riper's (1973) preparatory sets. This is done by having clients reduce their rate slightly and exaggerate fluency skills when they approach a feared or avoided word or are feeling a loss of control or increased anxiety. As a recovery strategy, clients reduce their rate and exaggerate fluency skills to regain stability after a stutter. In both cases, clients are to reduce their speaking rate until stability has been reestablished.

To progress from one rate to the next, clients complete a formal self-assessment (SA) task. The purposes of SA are, first, to ensure that clients can produce fluency skills accurately before moving to a faster rate and, second, to ensure that self-evaluation skills are accurate. Clients evaluate their fluency skill proficiency, rate of speech, number of stutters identified and self-corrected, naturalness, stability, and loudness. To meet criteria they must: (1) achieve 80% accuracy in fluency skill production and self-evaluation; (2) have an SPM that is within the target rate range; (3) identify and self-correct 80% of any stutters; (4) achieve acceptable naturalness; (5) have adequate levels of loudness; and (6) have a feeling of stable fluency.

Beginning on the third day of therapy, rating sessions are preceded by a fluency skill "warm-up" wherein clients briefly review tension modification, fluency skills and SC at various speech rates. To foster self-management, responsibility for conducting the morning warm-up is shifted to the clients at the beginning of the second week. Clients design and lead warm-up practice, first in the clinic room, then in large groups within and outside the clinic.

As mentioned earlier, movement between the acquisition and transfer phases is fluid, with self-management procedures incorporated into acquisition to promote generalization of behavior change. In addition to the sequenced practice activities and self-evaluation training described earlier, other strategies to promote generalization include:

1. *Prolongation in off-task comments* As soon as clients are able to use fluency skills in sustained prolongation in question-and-answer activities during rating sessions, they are required to use prolongation in off-task comments within the therapy room, then in all talking within the clinic with clinical and support staff. This generally occurs when clients are nearing the end of slow prolongation (e.g., 60 SPM) rating sessions.

2. *Peer and self monitoring outside of clinic* During lunch and other breaks outside the clinic, clients monitor each other and provide cues and feedback. They record the percentage of time they used prolongation during breaks and the number of times they used SC.

3. *Structured home practice* Each evening, beginning on the third day of the program, clients complete structured home practice in pairs and groups. Tasks are always at a level at which clients can be expected to achieve 70 to 80% accuracy. Clients self-evaluate their tape-recorded practice and bring their recording and evaluation for review by the clinician the following day. Family members are often involved in completing home practice activities with teens and may also support or facilitate group evening practice.

Fluency Enhancing Techniques during the Transfer Phase

The goal of transfer is for clients to generalize speech and cognitive changes established in the clinic to everyday life and challenging situations. Accordingly, progressively more time is spent outside the clinic during this phase. However, morning rating sessions continue to be conducted to help clients refine fluency skills and naturalness.

The transfer phase begins with preliminary activities that are designed to prepare clients for transfer. These activities, which we call *pre-transfers,* incorporate situational elements or antecedents (see Chapter 18, this volume) that tend to be associated with stuttering (e.g., the telephone and talking to strangers) but still provide some structure associated with the clinic. These pre-transfers include: (1) conversations with staff and volunteers within and outside the clinic; (2) "walk-'n-talk" tasks that are tape-recorded conversations while walking outside in pairs or groups; (3) telephone calls made to and received from clinical staff and volunteers; (4) large-group activities incorporating humorous situations so that clients can practice using skills while laughing and having fun; and (5) time-pressured tasks such as running to answer the phone and, for teens, scavenger hunts that require them to make as many contacts as possible with staff and volunteers within and outside the clinic. Pre-transfers are completed first in slight stretch, then in controlled rate.

Once clients complete the pre-transfer activities, they move to actual *transfer activities,* which involve beyond-clinic situations. In these transfer activities, clients: (1) engage in conversations with strangers on campus; (2) make telephone calls to businesses and to volunteers they have not met. Clients also leave messages on answering machines as well as make long-distance calls to family and friends; (3) conduct opinion surveys that involve approaching people on campus and asking a series of questions about stuttering; (4) engage in shopping activities in which shopkeepers are asked for items and items of interest are discussed; (5) give presentations on various aspects of stuttering and subjects of special interest to each client. Teens practice a "classroom education presentation," which also promotes openness about stuttering and fluency skills, whereas adults give work- or school-related presentations and (6) give a speech in a lecture theater on campus to an audience of family, friends, and other guests. In addition, older teens and adults participate in a simulated job interview conducted by personnel at a career and placement center on campus, and young teens go on field trips to museums and local attractions. A classroom simulation is also arranged for young teens. The classroom simulation attempts to mirror a usual school day with a real teacher from a local school following a schedule that includes core subjects such as math, language arts, science, and physical education activities.

In addition to these activities, clients complete special transfers that are particularly relevant to their personal interests and goals. For example, actual job interviews or meetings at workplaces will be arranged. Transfers are completed ordinarily in a controlled rate and are repeated several times at each level of difficulty to ensure that clients develop stability. To further develop self-management abilities, clients learn how to sequence transfer tasks.

As in the acquisition phase, treatment in transfer is individualized. Skill and rate goals, the specific sequence of transfer activities and types of transfers are tailored to individual needs.

Prior to beginning each transfer task, clients specify their skill and rate goals. They also examine and, if necessary, change their self-talk (described below). To meet criteria for completing a transfer task, clients must achieve 80% accuracy in: (1) fluency skill production; (2) maintaining the target rate; (3) self-evaluation of fluency skills; and (4) identifying and self-correcting stutters. Clients must also identify areas of strength and areas for improvement. If criteria are not met, then clients redo the transfer.

The majority of the pre-transfer and transfer activities are tape-recorded so that clients may subsequently analyze their performance. This analysis further develops clients' self-evaluation skills. However, some transfer activities are not tape-recorded. For instance, the simulated classroom activity and brief exchanges (e.g., asking for the time) are not recorded. This is done to preserve the naturalness of the exchange and to ensure that clients can use the fluency skills independent of the tape recorder, which can become a cue for fluency. These unrecorded transfers are evaluated using the same parameters as recorded transfers; however, clients estimate their percentages of accuracy in achieving fluency skill and target rate goals.

Fluency Enhancing Techniques during Maintenance Phase

The goal of maintenance is for clients to continue the behavioral and cognitive changes achieved in the clinic. Preparation for maintenance is a focus throughout the program. Discussions regarding the need for, requirements of, and challenges of maintenance begin during assessment and are included in client and family discussions throughout the program. In addition, the self-management strategies incorporated in acquisition and transfer prepare the clients to plan and carry out maintenance activities.

In-Clinic Preparation for Maintenance

In their final week of therapy, clients attend special maintenance seminars and learn about the speech-related and attitudinal components of a maintenance plan. The speech-related components are as follows:

1. *Warm-up* Warm-up consists of fluency skill practice in the morning and for short periods throughout the day. In the morning, clients focus on specific skills while prolonging at various rates and end with a conversation in slight prolongation with a family member. They are encouraged to vary the practice material and location daily to counteract boredom. Practice can include reading from magazines, reviewing school work, and discussing daily activities, news items, or anything else of interest to the client. Parents of young teens are urged to be involved in warm-up practice as much as possible so that warm-up becomes part of the family's routine.

2. *Ongoing practice* Ongoing practice can be completed using any daily talking activity and is both pre-planned and spontaneous. In pre-planned exercises, clients use fluency skills in routine activities such as talking during dinner and nonroutine activities such as requesting a book at the library. In spontaneous activities, they take advantage of unexpected situations that occur and are encouraged to keep a record of their performance in these ongoing activities.

3. *Transfers* Any daily or special talking activity can be used, but a transfer differs from ongoing practice in that it is formally evaluated and specifically related to clients' long- and short-term goals (see below). Transfers should include both easy and more difficult speaking situations as well as those speaking situations that have been avoided in the past. Clients are encouraged to tape-record at least one transfer per week and to keep a record of their transfers. They are also encouraged to be creative, seek out talking situations, and take risks.

Clients then identify short- and long-term goals, learn how to sequence practice activities, and plan specific practice activities for the first 3 days posttreatment. Long-term goals are those that clients want to achieve within 1 year posttreatment. Most often these goals are related to increasing the client's comfort in talking in avoided or feared situations, such as presentations or on the telephone. They may also be attitude-based. For instance, some clients want to be more open about stuttering (e.g., tell their listeners that they stutter) and more comfortable using fluency skills with friends. Short-term goals are those that clients want to achieve by the end of the first month after treatment. They often are substeps used to achieve long-term goals. An example for students might be giving a presentation to a group of three friends in the classroom after school as a substep toward giving a presentation to the whole class during the school day.

Daily and weekly transfers are designed around short- and long-term goals. Clients plan and write a hierarchy of transfers for each month. This gives the transfers purpose and promotes goal-directed transfer activities. In planning practice activities for the first 3 days posttreatment, clients identify what they will be doing in the course of the day, decide where and when they will do their warm-up, and write out a warm-up plan. They think about the usual or special talking events that will occur in the day and decide which ones can be used for ongoing practice or transfers. They also think about how to create talking situations that will help them achieve short-term goals for the month. As a final step in preparing for maintenance, they identify barriers to carrying out speech practice and brainstorm solutions for dealing with them.

Post treatment Maintenance Activities

Maintenance activities in the post treatment period consist of daily home practice with fluency skills, transfers, and attention to attitudinal issues, and one or more maintenance therapy options including: (1) follow-up sessions with a local speech-language pathologist; (2) participation in regularly scheduled refresher clinics as needed; and/or (3) participation in a long-distance maintenance program via the telephone or teleconferencing systems. Clients are also encouraged to maintain contact with fellow clients for speech practice and support and to participate in self-help groups.

Cognitive-Behavioral Skills

We believe that clients' positive attitudes (cognitions, emotions, and behaviors) toward communication and their speaking abilities contribute to maintenance of improved fluency. The use of cognitive-behavioral techniques to help clients achieve these goals is grounded in theoretical tenets and research on the efficacy of cognitive-behavioral therapies.

According to Ivey, Ivey, & Simek-Downing (1987) cognitive-behavioral theory integrates thought and action. The task of therapy is twofold: "(1) to examine how one thinks and if necessary, to change thinking and cognition; and (2) ensure that clients act on those cognitions through behavior in their daily life" (p. 302). A third dimension is the process of decision-making in which "one must *decide* how one will act" (p. 303). In several meta-analytic studies (Cartwright-Hatton, Roberts, Chitsabesan, Fothergill, & Harrington, 2004; Leichsenring & Leibing, 2003; Taylor, 1996), cognitive-behavioral therapies have reportedly been found to be effective in treating a variety of disorders. Although not necessarily superior to other forms of treatment, it has been postulated that cognitive-behavioral therapies may be one of the best modes of therapy for some disorders. Preliminary studies of the effectiveness of cognitive-behavioral methods in stuttering treatment have yielded encouraging results (e.g., Klein & Amster, 2003; McColl, Onslow, Packman, & Menzies, 2001). However, more research is needed to investigate applications of these methods to the treatment of stuttering.

In our program, applications of cognitive-behavioral strategies are highly individualized. Although clients have many attitudinal-emotional issues in common, each individual has a unique constellation of concerns. Each client's stage of cognitive and emotional development, state of readiness to discuss emotional issues, and desire to make changes is considered in designing group and individual discussions and exercises. Because the analytical and reflective abilities of many young adolescents may not be as developed as those of older teens and adults, the cognitive-behavioral component of therapy for young adolescents tends to be more concrete or action oriented and less abstract or analytically based than that for adults.

We introduce cognitive-behavioral concepts and strategies in a series of seminars that are supported by readings **(Table 12–4)**. Readings for young teens are drawn from *Do You Stutter: A Guide*

Table 12–4   Cognitive-Behavioral Therapy Components

Component	Purpose
Psychoeducation	*Purpose is to develop understanding of:*
Etiology and development of stuttering	Factors contributing to onset, development, and exacerbation of stuttering
Process of change	Long-term and variable nature of change
Link between thoughts, feelings, and behaviors	Reciprocal relationship between thoughts, feelings, and behaviors
Attitude modification	*Purpose is to facilitate development of:*
Effective self-talk	Self-talk that supports talking and use of fluency skills
Cognitive-emotional issues	*Purpose is to facilitate:*
Feelings	Awareness of and acceptance of feelings
Acceptance and openness	Acceptance of stuttering and comfort with speech-management skills
Listener reactions	Adaptive responses to perceived listener reactions
Confronting avoidances	Systematic confrontation of feared situations
Confidence	Understanding that confidence is built through success in managing stuttering and facing challenges
Expectations for fluency	Realistic vs perfectionist expectations
Regression, relapse	Understanding of how to manage regression and relapse
Teasing and bullying	Understanding of how to identify and manage bullying
Communication and social-skills training	*Purpose is to facilitate improved social skills*

for Teens (Fraser, 2004) and strategies are incorporated from *Facilitating Fluency*[5] (Webster & Poulos, 1989). The *Facilitating Fluency* manual is the primary source of readings and strategies for older teens and adults. Discussions are supported by behavioral exercises in communicative situations that follow hierarchies of difficulty progressing from contrived to natural, simple to more complex, and easier to harder tasks. Cognitive-behavioral skills training is introduced during the acquisition stage and continues through the transfer stage.

Our discussion of cognitive-behavioral skills is organized into four inter-related areas: (1) psychoeducation; (2) attitude modification; (3) cognitive-emotional issues; and (4) skills training.

Psychoeducation Although psychoeducation is interwoven throughout all aspects of treatment, we believe it important to highlight the following three areas.

Etiology and Development of Stuttering Clients acquire an understanding of the neurophysiological, genetic, environmental factors, and internal reactions that are presumed to contribute to the development of stuttering. Acquiring such an understanding, in our experience, helps: (1) relieve guilt (that they did not try hard enough to stop stuttering) and shame (about being different); (2) facilitate acceptance and openness about stuttering; and (3) develop understanding of the overall process of treatment and change.

Process of Change Discussing the process of change helps clients develop realistic expectations and prepares them to deal with difficulties and keep difficulties in perspective (see Manning, 2001). Discussions include the following concepts: (1) change takes time and requires patience (i.e., there will be no "quick fixes"); (2) there are ups and downs; (3) it is important to be pleased with small successes; and (4) therapy initiates a long-term process.

Linkage between Thoughts, Feelings, and Behavior Clients learn about the reciprocal relationship between thoughts, behavior, and emotions—that is, how what one feels and does is intimately related to what one thinks. They learn that experience influences attitudes, and that attitudes, in turn, influence experience (Grant, Mills, Mulhern, & Short, 2004). This discussion lays the foundation for the attitude modification strategies described below.

Attitude Modification The tripartite definition of attitude (Rosenberg & Hovland, 1960) proposes that attitudes have affective, cognitive, and behavioral components. Common to each of these components are verbal evaluative statements. Examining and changing verbal evaluative thoughts, or self-talk, about one's cognitions, emotions, or behavioral responses is one way to change attitudes. We believe that attitude change is facilitated and maintained through a combination of effective self-talk that we call "helpful thoughts," and success in using fluency skills, confronting avoidances, dealing with listeners, and managing feelings.

Clients learn that thoughts affect how feelings and reactions are handled. They identify helpful and unhelpful thoughts. Drawing from Webster and Poulos (1989) and our own clinical experience, we describe helpful self-talk as that which: (1) reminds clients of the fluency skills they have acquired to manage or modify stuttering; (2) tells clients exactly what they can do to manage speech (e.g., "slow my rate" or "use a gentle start"); (3) puts feelings into perspective (e.g., "it's okay to feel anxious. This will be a chance for me to practice"); (4) is encouraging and positive; (5) is realistic (allows mistakes); and (6) is reality-based (e.g., "I don't *really* know what she thinks about my speech"). Unhelpful self-talk or thoughts are maladaptive in that they: (1) make it harder to use skills; (2) are negative and show helplessness; (3) continually expect perfect fluency (i.e., zero tolerance for mistakes); (4) make it harder to enter feared situations; (5) make it harder to talk in social and other speaking situations; and (6) focus on what listeners might think, do, and say.

---

[5]Available from the Institute for Stuttering Treatment and Research.

In a series of preparatory written exercises, clients identify unhelpful self-talk they have previously used before and after difficult situations as well as brainstorm effective self-talk that they could use now and in the future in place of these unhelpful thoughts. They then practice identifying and changing self-talk before and after each transfer. They are also encouraged to keep a record of their self-talk in maintenance. This process of examining self-talk is integral to all our discussions of attitudinal-emotional issues, including those described below.

Cognitive-Emotional Issues   The following discussion of cognitive-emotional issues addressed in therapy is not exhaustive. Only the main concepts are presented. Always, there is a myriad of other social and emotional issues that are interrelated, client-specific, and of great concern to clients.

Feelings   Feelings refer to both emotions and somatic sensations. Discussions of feelings are conducted in both group and individual sessions throughout the program, and we strive to foster an environment in which clients are comfortable and willing to discuss their feelings. Most clients talk readily about the fear and anxiety felt before, during, and after communicating in different situations; however, many are reluctant to talk about such feelings as shame, guilt, or humiliation. Indeed, it is often difficult for some clients to separate and identify different feelings. We respect a client's stage of readiness to acknowledge and discuss feelings, and we ensure that contributions in group discussions are always voluntary. These discussions focus on several interrelated issues.

1. Identifying and acknowledging feelings rather than denying them

2. Understanding the role that fear and anxiety play in perpetuating avoidances and interfering with the use of fluency skills

3. Understanding normal levels of speech-related anxiety, managing feelings through effective self-talk, scanning for tension and using relaxation techniques

4. Systematically confronting feared situations

Like Luterman (2001), we believe that "feelings just *are* and should never be judged" (p. 123). We try to help clients move toward a stage of being comfortable with normal levels of speech-related anxiety. Too often, clients unrealistically desire and expect to have no anxiety after improved fluency has been achieved. They are helped by the knowledge that all speakers, regardless of level of fluency, experience such feelings from time to time.

Acceptance and Openness   We encourage an attitude wherein clients are accepting of themselves, of their stuttering, and of the speech management techniques. We believe that being open about stuttering (also described as "self-disclosure"; Van Riper, 1973) and about speech management techniques facilitates anxiety- and avoidance-reduction, use of fluency skills, and ultimately, self-acceptance. It is imperative that clients do not use fluency skills as a way to hide stuttering. We focus discussions on acceptance of stuttering; acceptance of the sound and feel of fluency skills; being open about stuttering and using fluency skills—how, when, and who to be open with; and perceptions of listener reactions to stuttering and fluency skills. Clients are encouraged to discuss their stuttering and therapy with family, friends, and coworkers.

As part of the process of encouraging openness, teens are asked to prepare a presentation that can be given to their class when they return home. In it they discuss, in their own words, why people stutter, how they have learned to manage stuttering, and how listeners can help people who stutter. The presentation they have prepared is also delivered to an audience during the treatment program. Although many teens do not deliver their presentations to classes when they return home, they often proudly report being open with listeners and family in individual or small-group situations. Teens are also encouraged to take the lead in carrying out meetings with teachers to discuss what they learned in treatment and how teachers can help in the classroom. During the transfer phase, teens carry out openness exercises with family members who have accompanied them to the clinic and with family members at home, by telephone. These exercises are taped and analyzed. Clients are also encouraged to use voluntary stuttering (also referred to as psuedostuttering; Van Riper, 1973) as a way of being open and desensitizing themselves to the fear of stuttering. In our experience, voluntary stuttering is one of the more challenging techniques for clients to embrace and apply. Consequently, some transfers specifically incorporate voluntary stuttering.

Listener Reactions   Clients need to develop an awareness of the potential difference between what they perceived to be a listener's reactions and what are, in reality, the listener's true reactions. Thus, we have our clients discuss why listeners' seemingly negative reactions may relate to uncertainties in knowing how to respond. They also discuss reactions that have been unmistakably negative and brainstorm and role-play different ways of responding to such reactions and educating listeners.

Confronting Avoidances   A fundamental goal of treatment is for clients to decrease avoidance and increase approach to situations (for discussion of avoidance, see Sheehan, 1975). Accordingly, clients learn how avoidances develop, how they are reinforced and perpetuated, and why it is important to confront them. They also learn how to sequence anti-avoidance activities, beginning with easier and moving to more challenging situations to increase the likelihood of approaching situations and successfully managing speech. Transfer exercises always include avoided situations.

Building Confidence   Improved confidence is built by experiencing success in managing stuttering in a variety of situations, by coping successfully with challenges and setbacks, and through discussing how one builds self-confidence. Beginning in the first week of therapy, clients record their successes in a Success Diary and are encouraged to continue doing so during maintenance.

Expectations for Fluency   Clients need to understand that a realistic long-term goal is maintaining the ability to manage stuttering rather than expecting to have 100% fluency.

Handling Regression and Recognizing Relapse   We distinguish between regression and relapse. Regression is defined as some slippage in fluency that includes variations in stuttering across time and situations, variations in the ability to monitor and use fluency skills, and temporary setbacks. In contrast, *relapse* is defined as a pronounced and persistent return to pretreatment levels of stuttering. Like Craig (1998), we believe that relapse should not be viewed as final, or as a sign of failure, but as a time to identify problems and to take action to correct them, thus building confidence and making change more robust. Discussions include the antecedents and cues for stuttering; adaptive ways of dealing with stuttering, which include use of effective self-talk and self-correction techniques; adopting a problem solving approach; dealing with related feelings of fear, anxiety, and disappointment; identifying internal and external factors that contribute to relapse; and getting back on track after a setback.

Teasing and Bullying   Generally, bullying occurs less often in adolescence than in elementary school; however, the topic often arises in discussions with teens. Readers are referred to Chapter 8, this volume for a more detailed discussion of coping strategies that teens report using and that have been found to be associated with escape from victimization.

Communication and Social Skills Training   Clients vary in the degree to which stuttering has affected their development of communication and social skills. For those with limited social and communication skills, intervention is both direct and indirect. Indirect interventions occur when clients practice fluency skills in various speaking situations within the clinic and in transfer. *Direct* instruction includes learning how to: (1) initiate, sustain, and end conversations; (2) appropriately and effectively present ideas; (3) include the listener by asking questions; (4) interrupt or get one's turn when necessary; and (5) take turns.

Role-plays and scripts are incorporated in clients' fluency skill practice. Clients also attend a seminar in which they define effective communication and brainstorm qualities, both nonverbal and verbal, of effective communicators. After appraising their areas of relative strength and weakness, clients identify goals for improvement (e.g., eye contact, initiating conversation, active listening, etc.). They then have the opportunity to work on these goals during conversation practice in the transfer phase.

Family Involvement in Therapy

We encourage family involvement in both adult and teen clinics (Boberg & Kully, 1997). As would be expected given the difference between the two age groups in terms of degree of independence and self-responsibility, family involvement is greater with young teens than with older clients. Whereas the adult program offers two meetings of 1.5 to 2 hours each, the young teen program includes weekly family meetings for a total of ~8 hours of meeting time. When necessary, individual family-client discussions are also held to help families and clients come to an understanding and resolution of issues. We encourage clients and family to engage in discussions in which clients are free to share information, beliefs, and feelings without judgment or penalty. Likewise, family members are encouraged to share their feelings and experiences with the client.

Topics typically addressed in family meetings with both teen and adult groups include:

1. *Etiology and development of stuttering and impact of stuttering on client and family;*

2. *Treatment components, strategies and process* Fluency skills are demonstrated, and family members are introduced to cognitive-behavioral strategies (particularly self-talk) and learn about common client responses to the discussion topics. Of course, the confidentiality of particular clients' responses is always preserved;

3. *What family members can expect during and after treatment* This includes family expectations for fluency and maintenance. It is important that family understand that continual monitoring is challenging, that variations in fluency and the ability to use fluency skills will occur, that there likely will be residual stuttering, and that some regression can be expected; and

4. *How family members can support clients during therapy and in maintenance.*

In addition, parents of teens learn: (1) how to produce the fluency skills and monitor their child's skill production; (2) about fluency disruptors and strategies for facilitating the use of fluency skills and cognitive-behavioral skills; (3) about components of the maintenance plan; (4) about when and how to remind clients and avoid constant reminding; (5) how to reinforce the use of techniques and cognitive-behavioral strategies; (6) how to help their child get back on track after a relapse; and (7) how to facilitate and support their child's meetings with teachers.

Family members of teen clients are also given opportunities to observe speech practice sessions and participate in home practice and transfer exercises, with extent of involvement depending on the needs of the client and the dynamics of the relationship. The aims of family members' participation in treatment sessions are to foster the teens' comfort in using the new speech pattern with parents and other family members. Parents are also instructed how to appropriately model the controlled speech pattern and how to encourage open and ongoing discussion of stuttering and the therapy process.

♦ Case Examples

The following case composites are intended to illustrate the process of treatment in the CSP with a "typical" adult and young teen. These cases highlight selected aspects of the program to demonstrate how treatment may be tailored to client's needs and to provide examples of individual responses to treatment.

Case 1: Adult male   Craig, age 28, presented with moderate stuttering characterized by silent prolongations, part-word repetitions, and pressurized articulatory contacts. Accessory behaviors included eye closure, head nodding, lip and neck tension, and use of "uh" and "um." Attitude and self-perception scale scores (see Kully & Langevin, 1999) were moderate to severe, and Craig reported many word and situational avoidances. Craig worked as a bush pilot and was an active church member, giving readings to the congregation and participating in Bible studies. Situations of particular difficulty were the telephone, reading and speaking to groups, and relaying information via radio to air traffic controllers. Craig's goals were to improve his fluency control at work and to feel more confident when speaking to new people and socializing at church.

In treatment, Craig readily was able to identify locus of tension, core stuttering, and accessory behaviors. Likewise, Craig performed well in tension modification exercises introduced here and continued throughout therapy. On the 10-point severity rating scale, introduced as a means of facilitating self-evaluation and problem-solving as well as tracking progress, Craig rated his stuttering severity as an 8 and his avoidances as a 6.[3]

The fluency-enhancing skills **(Table 12–2)** were then introduced and practiced in the typical sequence **(Table 12–1)**. Because laryngeal stoppages (silent prolongations) were predominant, special focus was given to GS and smooth blending (SB). Craig had mild difficulty acquiring GS, demonstrating slight tension evidenced by mild pitch elevation. This was addressed by conducting brief relaxation exercises prior to GS practice, encouraging focus on sensations of ease and "looseness" while voicing, periodically having Craig contrast spontaneous with prolonged productions, and striving to retain the voice quality of spontaneous productions while initiating speech with GS.

Subsequent sessions focused on developing proficient use of fluency skills at gradually increasing rates of speech. Practice followed the general sequence of: reading sentences, using carrier phrases, answering short questions, describing pictures, reading paragraphs, speaking in monologue (short to long topics) and conversation (low to high interest), impromptu speeches, and debating. Because Craig's first language was German, practice in German was integrated into these sessions in a graded way. Craig's difficult sounds and words (e.g., name, address, city names) were incorporated into tension modification, self-correction, and fluency skill practice, first in warm-ups and then in rating sessions. Having strong self-evaluation skills, Craig progressed through evaluation tasks quickly.

Cognitive-behavioral skills training was initiated with a seminar in which Craig began identifying his physical, emotional, and avoidance reactions as well as the consequences of avoidance and cues associated with his stuttering. Craig was then introduced to the concept of self-talk as a means of changing negative attitudes associated with stuttering, and he was encouraged to begin "tuning in" to his self-talk, that is, thoughts relating to himself, others, and his circumstances. In a series of exercises, Craig identified feelings of anxiety, embarrassment, and incompetence associated with specific events, and he examined thoughts and beliefs underlying these feelings. He also began examining the links between his thoughts, feelings, and behavior, identifying how thoughts like "*I can't do this*" and "*They'll think I'm incompetent if I stutter*" heightened his anxiety and tension and led to avoidance. Craig then practiced developing more effective self-talk statements that would help him to manage his anxiety, use fluency skills, and talk whether or not he stuttered. For instance, statements he generated for managing anxiety were: "*I can handle this. I'll focus on easy breathing and releasing tension.*" As Craig continued to self-reflect, he was able to identify beliefs that underlay his reactions to stuttering. Some of these beliefs were: "*Stuttering is bad and I must hide it.*" "*Others think less of me because I stutter,*" and "*When I stutter I am seen as less competent.*" Craig recognized how these beliefs contributed to apprehension but was initially unable to see how he might be able to change them. Nonetheless, he agreed that he had a choice in how he reacted to his thoughts and feelings, and he began considering how he might view his stuttering and the need for managing it in a more accepting way. As Craig continued to gain experience with the fluency skills and with confronting his stuttering and avoidances, a shift in his perspective about stuttering became evident. He began taking steps to talk about his stuttering, first with family and then with strangers while conducting surveys about stuttering. He conducted these exercises with a view to objectively examining others' reactions and discovered his tendency to "mind read" his listeners and to assume they evaluated him and his stuttering negatively. Although Craig at first felt very uncomfortable, he began using voluntary stuttering followed by a self-correction as a way to reduce sensitivity about stuttering and to keep it in the open. Craig then began to reflect on his many competencies and to recognize that his tendency to equate competence with fluency was limiting. The shift in perspective also became evident in his self-talk statements, as follows: "*I might talk different* [sic] *than most people but that doesn't make me inadequate.*" As Craig progressed into the transfer phase, he continued to check his thinking before, during, and after situations, and he worked to develop more effective self-talk that encouraged skill use and reframed situations as opportunities rather than threats.

In addition to the standard transfer assignments, Craig had conversations with German-speaking volunteers, gave bible readings to groups of volunteers, and role played leading a bible study and speaking to an air traffic controller over a walkie talkie.

Post treatment testing revealed marked improvements in speech and questionnaire measures as well as in self-ratings of severity (from 8 to 2).[3] Having no local support, Craig enrolled in a distance follow-up program involving bimonthly phone sessions. Follow-up recommendations included continued focus on: refining use of GS and SB in spontaneous speech, scanning and releasing tension, noting speech and other successes in a daily journal, and systematically confronting feared words and situations.

Case 2: Adolescent Female   Sarah, age 13, presented with mild-to-moderate stuttering characterized by audible prolongations and part- and whole-word repetitions. Accessory behaviors included blinking, gaze aversion, lip tension, and use of "well" and "um." Attitude and self-perception scale scores (see Kully & Langevin, 1999) were mildly severe, and Sarah reported that she sometimes substituted words but rarely avoided situations. Sarah was active in her drama class and had performed in many school plays. She often took airline flights independently as her parents were divorced and lived in different cities. Difficult situations were using the telephone and asking for directions or instructions when traveling. Sarah's presenting goal was to "get rid of" her stuttering.

In treatment, Sarah was able to identify locus of tension, core stuttering, and accessory behaviors only with assistance after viewing herself on videotape. She performed well in initial tension modification exercises but required considerable graded practice in transfer to improve her ability to identify and release tension in spontaneous speaking situations. Sarah rated her physical tension during stuttering and her stuttering severity as 5. Later, she began tracking "comfort with controlled speech," giving this aspect an initial rating of 6.[3]

The fluency skills **(Table 12–2)** were then introduced and practiced in the typical sequence **(Table 12–1).** Because consonant prolongations were predominant, special focus was given to light touches (LT) as a means of reducing articulatory tension. Sarah acquired the skills with relative ease but as is typical of many teens, she did not readily apply them to spontaneous speech. Praise, gestural and verbal cues and incentive systems were used to encourage Sarah to use the skills, first in off-task comments in the clinic room and later in outside clinic sessions.

Subsequent sessions focused on developing proficient use of fluency skills at gradually increasing rates of speech with practice following a similar sequence as for adults. Games such as Hangman, 20 Questions, and Taboo, personal items like photo albums, scrapbooks and magazines, scripts from plays, and Sarah's difficult words and sounds ("hello", "Wh" questions, b/p-initial words) were incorporated into practice in a graded way. Sessions were often conducted in informal settings (e.g., picnic table outside) and in physical games like Frisbee tossing. To further facilitate generalization and interest, games involving the entire group were integrated into practice, many of which incorporated competition or time pressure to enable practice of the 3T's (Think, Take a breath, Talk using skills; e.g., Family Feud game). Self-evaluation training was a special focus for Sarah. By the end of acquisition she was able to self-evaluate her skills with ~70% accuracy.

Cognitive-behavioral seminars were adjusted in content and complexity to accommodate to Sarah's developmental level and awareness. Sarah identified feelings of embarrassment, fear of being different, and discomfort with controlled speech. She examined the link between thoughts, feelings, and actions, noting how thoughts like *"They'll think I'm weird"* heightened her discomfort and physical tension and interfered with her use of her skills. In discussions regarding consequences of word avoidance, Sarah was first able to identify only the immediate feelings of relief; however, her later self-talk reflected increased awareness of the negative longer-term consequences of avoidance (e.g., increased fear, decreased confidence) and the importance of facing feared words. Sarah also became increasingly aware of her tendency to hold back when meeting new people and to sometimes use gestures to minimize talking.

During transfer, Sarah worked to develop more accepting attitudes toward her managed speech. She made a notable shift after speaking with a former teen client who shared his experiences in treatment, commenting that she no longer felt she was the only one with this problem and that she could overcome it. Further progress was apparent after transfer assignments in which she discussed her therapy and demonstrated exaggerated fluency skills with her family and a friend. Sarah continued to work on developing more supportive self-talk statements before and after transfers, developing statements such as *"I'm talking slow for myself and not for them and if I keep doing this it will make me stronger and help me overcome bigger things"* or *"If I use my skills, I can achieve my goals."*

In addition to the usual transfer assignments for teens, Sarah taught a friend a new card game, performed skits in front of people, role played speaking to airport employees, ordered fast food through an intercom, and asked for tickets and information at local attractions. Sarah was not willing to use voluntary stuttering outside the clinic. Although she cognitively understood the concept, she was not ready to use the technique.

Post treatment testing revealed marked improvement on all speech and nonspeech measures and on self-ratings of severity (from 5 to 2). Sarah scheduled follow-up sessions with her local speech-language pathologist to begin on her return home. Follow-up recommendations included continued focus on: consistent use of LT and rate control in spontaneous situations, openness about stuttering and managed speech, self-evaluation training (verifying accuracy using a tape recorder), ongoing use of difficult words, and initiating conversation with new people.

◆ Treatment Outcomes

Since 1986, ~650 teens and adults have completed intensive clinics at our center. They came from all parts of North America and around the world, ranged in age from 10 to 78, and in severity from mild to profound. Several clients had co-existing speech, language, cognitive, neurological and/or learning problems. Treatment programming for many of these clients was highly modified and individualized, and referrals were made to other specialists, such as neurologists and psychologists, in some cases.

We routinely obtain several measures of clients' speech, self-perceptions, and attitudes before and after therapy. With few exceptions, our adolescent and adult clients have shown marked improvements on all objective and self-report measures immediately after treatment. Of far greater interest, however, is the extent to which treatment gains are sustained across time. We have conducted several investigations of the effects of therapy on teens and adults in the longer term. Two studies that examined outcomes 1 and 2 years posttreatment found that between 76% (Boberg & Kully, 1994) and 80% (Langevin & Boberg, 1993) of clients were maintaining satisfactory (<3% stuttering) or marginally satisfactory (3.1–6%) outcomes, and 80% rated their speech as satisfactory. Langevin and Boberg (1993) also reported that improvements in attitudes and self-perceptions of performance were being maintained. An investigation of the cross-cultural effectiveness of the CSP delivered in Holland has been conducted (Langevin, Huinck, Kully, et al. 2006). Further, a preliminary report of a 5-year outcome investigation provided a longitudinal illustration of trends in speech and nonspeech performance in the posttreatment period (Langevin & Kully, 2004). Finally, a study that evaluated the effectiveness of the program with adults who stutter and clutter (Langevin & Boberg, 1996) showed positive results.

◆ Conclusion

The CSP arises out of our conceptualization of persistent stuttering as a disorder of speech that has environmental consequences and results in maladaptive cognitions, emotions, and behaviors. Accordingly, treatment integrates speech skills to enhance fluency and manage stuttering with cognitive-behavioral techniques to deal with the attitudinal-emotional consequences of stuttering. Self-management skills are interwoven throughout therapy to promote generalization and maintenance of speech and attitudinal changes. Results of several long-term outcome studies suggest that the program is effective in producing durable improvements in both stuttering frequency and associated negative reactions; however, to ultimately improve treatment efficiency and effectiveness, further research is needed to determine how and why the components and procedures work. Notwithstanding, clinical outcomes have been encouraging and provide support for the effectiveness of the program as a whole.

References

Andrews, G., & Ingham, R. J. (1971). Stuttering: Considerations in the evaluation of treatment. British Journal of Disorders of Communication 6, 129–138.

Bandura, A. (1997). Self-efficacy: The exercise of control. New York: W.H. Freeman and Company.

Bashshur, R. L., Reardon, T. G., & Shannon, G. W. (2000). Telemedicine: a new health care delivery system. Annual Review of Public Health 21, 613–637.

Boberg, E., & Kully, D. (1985). Comprehensive stuttering program. San Diego, CA: College-Hill Press.

Boberg, E., & Kully, D. (1994). Long-term results of an intensive treatment program for adults and adolescents who stutter. Journal of Speech and Hearing Research 37, 1050–1059.

Boberg, J., & Kully, D. (1997). Spouses as adjuncts in fluency therapy. Seminars in Speech and Language 18, 357–369.

Cartwright-Hatton, S., Roberts, C., Chitsabesan, P., Fothergill, C., & Harrington, R. (2004). Systematic review of the efficacy of cognitive behaviour therapies for childhood and adolescent anxiety disorders. British Journal of Clinical Psychology 43, 421–436.

Craig, A. (1998). Relapse following treatment for stuttering: A critical review and correlative data. Journal of Fluency Disorders 23, 1–30.

Finn, P. (2007). Self-control and the treatment of stuttering. In: R. F. Curlee (Ed.). Stuttering and related disorders of fluency (pp. 342–355). New York: Thieme.

Forne-Wastlund, H. (2004). Swedish comprehensive stuttering program-evaluation two to four years after treatment. In A. Packman, A. Meltzer, & H. F. M. Peters (Eds.), Theory, research and therapy in fluency disorders: Proceedings of the fourth world congress on fluency disorders (pp. 189–194). Nijmegen, The Netherlands: Nijmegen University Press.

Fraser, J. (2004). Do you stutter: A guide for teens. Memphis, TN: Stuttering Foundation of America.

Grant, A., Mills, J., Mulhern, R., & Short, N. (2004). Cognitive behavioral therapy in mental health care. London: Sage Publications.

Ingham, R. J. (1982). The effects of self-evaluation training on maintenance and generalization during stuttering treatment. Journal of Speech and Hearing Disorders 47, 271–280.

Ingham, R. J., Ingham, J. C., Finn, P., & Fox, P. T. (2003). Towards a functional neural systems model of developmental stuttering. Journal of Fluency Disorders 28, 297–318.

Ivey, A. E., Ivey, M. B., & Simek-Downing, L. (1987). Counseling and psychotherapy, (2nd ed.). Englewood Cliffs, NJ: Prentice-Hall, Inc.

Klein, E. R., & Amster, J. (2004). The effects of cognitive behavioral therapy with people who stutter. In A. Packman, A. Meltzer, & H. F. M. Peters (Eds.), Theory, research and therapy in fluency disorders: Proceedings of the fourth world congress on fluency disorders (pp. 195–203). Nijmegen, The Netherlands: Nijmegen University Press.

Kully, D. (2000). Telehealth in speech pathology: Applications to the treatment of stuttering. Journal of Telemedicine and Telecare, 6, S2:39–S2:41.

Kully, D. (2002). Venturing into telehealth: Applying interactive technologies to stuttering treatment. The ASHA Leader, 7, 1, 6–7, 15.

Kully, D., & Langevin, M. (1999). Intensive treatment for stuttering adolescents. In R. F. Curlee (Ed.), Stuttering and related disorders of fluency (pp. 139–159). New York: Thieme.

Langevin, M., & Boberg, E. (1993). Results of an intensive stuttering therapy program. Journal of Speech-Language Pathology and Audiology 17, 158–166.

Langevin, M., & Boberg, E. (1996). Results of intensive stuttering therapy with adults who clutter and stutter. Journal of Fluency Disorders 21, 315–327.

Langevin, M., Kully, D., & Ross-Harold, B. A comprehensive stuttering progarm with strategies for managing teasing and bullying for school age children. In: R. F. Curlee (Ed.) Stuttering and related disorders of fluency. (pp. 129–147). New York: Thieme.

Langevin, M., Huinck, W., Kully, D., Peters, P., Lomheim, H., & Tellers, M. (2006). A cross-cultural, long-term outcome evaluation of the ISTAR Comprehensive Stuttering Program across Dutch and Canadian adults who stutter. Journal of Fluency Disorders 31, 229–256.

Langevin, M., & Kully, D. (2003). Evidence-based treatment of stuttering: III. Evidence-based practice in a clinical setting. Journal of Fluency Disorders 28, 219–236.

Langevin, M., & Kully, D. (2004). Longitudinal treatment outcome: Four case studies. In A. Packman, A. Meltzer, & H. F. M. Peters (Eds.), Theory, research and therapy in fluency disorders: Proceedings of the fourth world congress on fluency disorders (pp. 195–203). Nijmegen, The Netherlands: Nijmegen University Press.

Leichsenring, F., & Leibing, E. (2003). The effectiveness of psychodynamic therapy and cognitive behavior therapy in the treatment of personality disorders: A meta-analysis. American Journal of Psychiatry 160, 1223–1232.

Luterman, D. (2001) Counseling persons with communication disorders and their families. Austin, TX: Pro-Ed.

Manning, W. H. (2001). Clinical decision making in fluency disorders. San Diego, CA: Singular.

McColl, T., Onslow, M., Packman, A., & Menzies, R. (2001). A cognitive behavioural intervention for social anxiety in adults who stutter. Speech Pathology Australia National Conference Proceedings, Melbourne, Australia, pp. 93–98.

Rehm, L. P., & Rokke P. (1988). Self-management therapies. In K. S. Dobson (Ed.), Handbook of cognitive-behavioral therapies. New York: The Guilford Press.

Rosenberg, M. J., & Hovland, C. I. (1960). Cognitive, affective and behavioral components of attitudes. In M. J. Rosenberg, C. I. Hovland, W. J. McGuire, R. P. Abelson, & J. W. Brehm (Eds.), Attitude organization and change: An analysis of consistency among attitude components. New Haven, CT: Yale University Press.

Schiavetti, N., & Metz, D. (1997). Stuttering and the measurement of speech naturalness. In: R. F. Curlee & G. M. Siegel (Eds.), Nature and treatment of stuttering: New directions (2nd ed.) (pp. 398–412). Needham Heights, MA: Allyn & Bacon.

Sheehan, J. G. (1975). Conflict theory and avoidance-reduction therapy. In J. Eisenson (Ed.), Stuttering: A second symposium (pp 97–198). New York: Harper & Row.

Taylor, S. (1996). Meta-analysis of cognitive-behavioral treatments for social phobia. Journal of Behavior Therapy and Experimental Psychiatry 27, 1–9.

Van Riper, C. (1973). The treatment of stuttering. Englewood Cliffs, NJ: Prentice-Hall.

Webster, W. G., & Poulos, M. G. (1989). Facilitating fluency: Transfer strategies for adult stuttering treatment programs. Edmonton, AB: Institute for Stuttering Treatment and Research.

13

Traditional Approaches to Treatment of Stuttering in Adolescents and Adults

Walter H. Manning and Anthony DiLollo

The purpose of this chapter is to describe principles that clinicians can utilize when helping adults and adolescents who stutter. The chapter begins with a discussion of how individuals who stutter are likely to instinctively cope with their situation. We discuss the important connection between the more obvious overt aspects of stuttering and the more subtle cognitive features of how stuttering impacts the speakers. After briefly discussing some of the unique characteristics of adolescents who stutter we describe several important characteristics of the treatment process, describe some refinements of the more common treatment strategies, and comment on the importance of several treatment techniques for promoting long-term change. We conclude the chapter with a discussion of one way to conceptualize and facilitate the process of long-term therapeutic change. We hope that the reader will gain insight about the exciting and rewarding process of helping older speakers who have stuttered for many years to learn to successfully manage their stuttering and become effective communicators.

◆ Finding a Direction for Therapy and Developing a Roadmap for Change

Coping with the Experience of Stuttering

After years of adjusting to the experience of stuttering, adolescents and adults often develop creative and habituated strategies for coping with the requirements of everyday conversation. To the extent that adult speakers have been successful and their coping strategies meet their needs, they are not likely to seek help from clinicians. For others, assistance is necessary to change what has become an unacceptable way of living and communicating. In general, because adult speakers have accumulated years of experience with their coping or survival strategies, the behavioral, cognitive, and affective adjustments that they make typically require more time and effort than is generally the case for younger preschool and school-age children. Although adolescents have had fewer years to develop coping strategies and may be less entrenched in the role of a speaker who stutters, they present their own unique challenges to the adults who are attempting to provide help. For both adults and adolescents the clinician must consider the extent to which stuttering will increase the *difficulty* the person will face when performing a wide range of tasks (the disability) and the extent to which stuttering is likely to result in a range of *disadvantages* to be faced in achieving life goals (the handicap).

Because these older speakers have experienced the socialization and learning process provided by years of various school, social, and work environments, their problems in achieving successful communication more than likely requires a multivariate solution. In essence, these older individuals who stutter have become adept at negotiating their way through our typically fluent culture. The fact that they stutter often becomes a major theme in their self-concept. Beginning in early adolescence, the person is likely to have made many choices, sometimes important life decisions, based on the fact that they are a person who stutters (e.g., the vocation they will pursue may be strongly influenced by how much spoken speech-language it will require). Much learning and adaptation has taken place and often, because of the shame and stigma associated with stuttering earlier in life (Chmela & Reardon, 1997; Murphy, 1999), they have learned subtle ways to hide and avoid disclosing themselves and/or their speaking difficulties. It is not unusual for the original disruptions in speech fluency to be so well disguised that overt stuttering behavior is subtle or not apparent, particularly to the unsophisticated listener. Instead of disclosing themselves as someone who stutters, they may appear—to the casual observer—as if they are nervous, shy, unintelligent, or a little strange (See Jezer, 1997; Rabinowitz, 2001).

To Back Away from the Problem or Ask for Help?

Because adults who stutter have lived for many years with the possibility as well as the reality of stuttering, the problem can and often does evolve far beyond the issue of fluently communicating a message. Often the adult who stutters takes great care to arrange his or her academic, social, or vocational life by dismissing or narrowing options. Certainly, this is also true of some adults with typically fluent speech. Few of us take as many risks as life offers or push the envelopes of our lives as much as possible. Every so often we realize how much we live, as Maslow (1968) suggests, in the "psychopathology of the average"; however, people who stutter are usually more likely to step back from the edge of the speaking situations that life has to offer. There are important exceptions to this, of course, and many people who stutter successfully forge ahead with their lives despite numerous and nontrivial challenges. However, we see relatively few of these "risk-taking" people who stutter in our clinics and research centers. Many such individuals do not seek help, and the professional community seldom has the opportunity to study their response to the problem (Finn, 1996; Manning, 2001). Although we have no empirical data to suggest what percentage of people who stutter in the general population seek formal assistance, the proportion may be similar to what is known about similar problems. Prochaska, DiClemente, and Norcross (1992) indicate that relatively few people having a chronic or long-standing problem are ready to take action. For example, data obtained on smoking cessation illustrates this point. They noted that 50 to 60% of smokers are in a pre-contemplation stage where they have no intention of seeking help and 30 to 40% are in a contemplation stage where they are in the early stages of obtaining information about assistance. Only 10 to 14% of all smokers were categorized as being ready to actively seek professional help.

The Strong Connection among the Overt and Covert Features of Stuttering

The strong linkage of the overt and covert features of stuttering has many critical implications for moving people forward to achieve success in the therapeutic process. It is not unreasonable to suggest that helping people change the overt features of stuttering that are readily observable is usually not difficult. At least this is the case as long as the client attends to basic techniques of fluency and stuttering modification practices with some responsibility; however, changing surface behaviors, as important as that may be for an adult, is only a portion of the process. The more covert features of the problem that lie under the surface must also shift and move off a well-established and often comfortable center. These less observable but nonetheless salient features of stuttering are often referred to as cognitive or cognitive-affective features of the problem. Obviously, such behaviors as sound/syllable repetitions, sound prolongations, and facial and body movement contribute to the inability to effectively communicate; however, it is the person who stutters decision not to pursue certain social, educational, and vocational opportunities because of his or her speaking difficulties that often has the greatest handicapping impact on the person's life. Therefore, it is understandable that these changes in the person's quality of life—due to his or her reactions/attempts to cope with stuttering—are often one of the main sources of the client's complaints when the client asks for help.

The Clinician as a Counselor, Helping Those Who Stutter to Approach the Problem

The majority of research on stuttering has focused on overt or surface behavior, particularly the frequency of stuttering events. Relatively little effort has been devoted to the nature of the intrinsic features of stuttering. These features may not be assessed during diagnosis, they often go unattended during treatment, and they may not be used as indicators of progress during or following treatment. One of the reasons for this, undoubtedly, is the relative lack of measurement procedures and techniques that allow identification and quantification of the cognitive and attitudinal features of stuttering. In addition, dealing with these features may be intimidating for some clinicians. It requires an understanding of the nature of stuttering, in general, and of the psychodynamics of the older person who stutters, in particular; this is not necessarily an easy task for the typically fluent clinician (see Manning, 2004). Such understanding allows the use of counseling techniques and that can be threatening to some clinicians, especially those who have not had such training. That is unfortunate because counseling is an exciting and rewarding part of the therapeutic experience. Basic counseling responses are an integral part of any good therapeutic relationship, a relationship that begins as the clinician demonstrates an authentic understanding of the phenomena of stuttering as it manifests itself for each person. This is most easily accomplished by the clinician demonstrating an authentic interest and curiosity in the client's story. The clinician listens with an emphatic (indicating understanding without judgment) rather than a sympathetic (indicating agreement) perspective. The clinician appreciates that each person will require varying degrees of support, modeling, challenge, and encouragement. Even though the client may show some distress as he or she attempts new and sometimes threatening speaking experiences, the clinician is comfortable as they accompany the client and encourage experimentation with new speaking roles.

When counseling individuals who stutter it is important to understand that many of the choices that adults and adolescents make in response to the experience of stuttering are normal coping strategies. The most basic and intuitive of these are likely to be in the form of avoidance and escape behaviors in an effort to minimize the effect of stuttering (or potential stuttering). For the most part, they are typical or normal responses to a chronic but unpredictable problem, similar in many ways to the reactions that most everyone has when they are asked to enter a feared speaking situation. Student clinicians, for example, when asked to take on the role of a person who stutters, report anxiety, fear, avoidance, shame, and embarrassment as well as the wide variety of physiological attributes associated with the experience. Of course these student clinicians—who are generally normally fluent speakers—know that they are able to escape from the experience when the threat becomes too great. Nevertheless, even prior to entering speaking situations, many of these student clinicians recognize the threatening nature of the experience. They rapidly adopt coping strategies to hide or lessen the effect of their unusual speech by carefully selecting their speaking situations, listeners, topics of conversation, and words. Were they required to stay in the role of a person who stutters for many weeks or months, the reactions of their listeners would eventually result in a narrowing of their communicative options and possibly an altered quality of life.

◆ The Special Case of Therapy for Adolescents Who Stutter

It's easy to stereotype teenagers, and, of course, there are reasons for such stereotypes. As with all stereotypes, there are many exceptions. Adolescents (teenagers essentially) have often been identified as some of our more difficult clients by such people as Van Riper (1971), Daly, Simon, and Burnett-Stolnack (1995), Blood (1995), Brisk, Healey, and Hux (1997), Conture (2001), and Manning (2001; 2003). The literature suggests that adolescents can be (select one or more from the following menu): noncompliant, difficult, complex, uncooperative, resistive, rebellious, sensitive, contentious, argumentative. Of course, we might say the same about some of our adult clients; however, in this portion of our chapter, we are focusing on adolescents and what experienced clinicians have observed about them.

Although we cannot fix adolescence, we can appreciate some of the characteristics and particularly how they may impact stuttering and the response to the possibility of therapy. For example, it is often difficult to convince teenagers to enter into speech-language therapy. Despite the likelihood that the socialization processes and demands of school are likely to increase both the disability and the handicap of stuttering, formal treatment is not the response of choice for most junior and senior high school students (Silverman & Zimmer, 1982). Parents and teachers can drag them to us, but unless we are able to intellectually, emotionally, and/or socially connect with them, the requirements of therapy are not likely to be attractive. One basic coping response of most people who stutter is to hide the problem (even if it means hiding themselves). Another common response is to deny the problem, not so much the fact that stuttering occurs, but that it is of any real significance. A prime directive for many teenagers is to avoid anything that will distinguish them from their peers. Of course, stuttering generally causes them to stand out in a negative fashion; however, they appear to believe that attending speech-language therapy—especially if they are pulled out of a daily scheduled class—will spotlight their distinctiveness, making it all the more apparent to their peers.

Therapy involves several issues that are likely to be unappealing to anyone, especially a teenager. Therapy requires, to varying degrees, a mind-set for taking responsibility, self-analysis, introspection, confrontation of emotions, considerable practice of new or modified old behavior, self-discipline, and a reduction of avoidance behaviors. Particularly aversive for some adolescents is the fact that successful therapy requires the involvement of their family. Parental/family involvement may be an anathema to teenagers, who are characteristically striving on many levels to become independent of adults (often with limited success). In addition, teenagers are typically involved in a variety of academic, social, and athletic activities. Taking time out from these activities to deal with their speaking difficulties on a daily or weekly basis is not something that often rates a high priority.

Another characteristic of therapy that can get in the way is that it requires entering into a trusting relationship with an adult clinician. Dependence on an adult may be especially difficult for a teenager who already feels vulnerable in the midst of these aliens from the older generation who "don't understand." Adolescents are known to be resistant to engaging in treatment, especially if they feel they are being talked down to (Haig, 1986). This may be exacerbated somewhat if the clinician is not someone who is able to communicate that he or she truly understands the experience of stuttering.

Teenagers as well as adults may also be resistant to therapy if one or more of their previous therapy experiences were unsuccessful. Another rarely mentioned dynamic that may inhibit the therapeutic relationship is the possibility that the client will be male and the clinician will be female, which is frequently the case. Asking a teenage male to be forthright and honest about his stuttering behavior and feelings of helplessness, loss of control, and shame with a female clinician is not something that some teenage males who stutter find easy to do, at least at first.

Finally, it has often been reported by adults that, as teenagers, they always harbored the thought that they would eventually grow out of the stuttering. This hope may prevent many teenagers from entering treatment until later in life when they realize that the problem is not going to simply go away and that they must take action. All of these factors may contribute to the resistance we encounter when we encourage teenagers to seek or stay with treatment. And, of course, if we push too hard we are likely to encounter even greater resistance. Still, our appreciation of the teenage experience can guide our clinical decisions about how to proceed with the process of treatment. When we do have the opportunity to meet with a teenager who stutters, it is important to demonstrate more than our understanding of the stuttering experience. We also need to show that we have some "street smarts" about how stuttering is likely to be impacting this young person's life on many levels.

◆ Treatment Decisions and Objectives

Recent Revisions of the International Classification of Functioning, Disability, and Health by the World Health Organization

The World Health Organization's (WHO) most recent revision of a framework for describing the consequences of disorders resulted in the *International Classification of Functioning, Disability, and Health* (ICF; WHO, 2001). Yaruss and Quesal (2004) have interpreted this revision and its implications for the experience of stuttering. The new ICF framework acknowledges that all disabilities involve more than overt or observable behaviors. Within this new (2001) ICF framework, no distinction is made between the idea of the "disability" (the difficulty performing tasks) and the "handicap" (disadvantages experienced in the ability to achieve life goals). Furthermore, the revision construes both environmental and personal factors as central to the disorder. That is, beyond the observable features of the problem of stuttering (e.g., repetitions, prolongations, blocking of airflow and voicing), this framework permits consideration of less apparent or overt, sometimes even covert, environmental influences (e.g., support from others, attitudes of society, communication services, support organizations, educational services) and the individual's response to their ability to participate across many aspects of life (e.g., social, education, employment, civic involvement).

And what does all this mean to speech-language pathologists researching, studying, or treating stuttering? In essence, this framework provides clinicians and researchers with a much broader, and seemingly more ecologically valid, interpretation of the stuttering experience. It means a greater appreciation that individuals who stutter are likely to respond in unique ways according to the internal and external factors that influence their experience. It means that a basic goal of assessment is to attempt to measure, observe, and understand the wide variety of external and internal factors that uniquely impact the disability and handicap of each individual. It means the goals of treatment involve helping the person to not only change the obvious, relatively overt behaviors of stuttering but to also improve the quality of his or her life with increased involvement at all levels of interaction relative to the person's environment. It means that, as clinicians, we pay attention to the many (and many times less apparent) cognitive and affective features of the stuttering experience and that we include this information in our interpretation of treatment efficacy.

Decisions at the Outset of Treatment

As with many things in life, timing is crucial. For example, if a person has been more or less successful in dealing with the problems presented by stuttering for many years, what has made the person ask for help now? One possibility is that a person may feel "stuck" and, despite years of trying, finally realize that he or she cannot change this situation without some form of outside assistance (Egan, 1994). There are, however, several reports of success by individuals who stutter who have achieved significant and successful changes without the help of professionals (Anderson & Felsenfeld, 2003; Finn, 1996; 1997; Plexico, Manning, & DiLollo, 2005)

Of course, as Peck (1978) points out, choosing formal treatment from a professional is often the more difficult path, and many clients drop out of treatment long before they have reached the goals the clinician has in mind. This can be the case even in programs that demonstrate a high rate of success for those who continue with treatment (O'Brian, Onslow, Cream, & Packman, 2003; Quesal, 2003). Long-term change usually requires long-term commitment and is more likely to occur during significant periods in the life cycle of most people. Such moments occur throughout life but seem to occur with greater frequency while a person is in his or her early 20s (Plexico et al., 2005). During this decade, people are likely to complete formal schooling, change their living status and location, enter and leave military service, initiate careers, get married, have children, and sometimes, go through a divorce. It is at such "nodes" in a person's life when self-awareness and introspection may be heightened and consequently when significant decision-making and restructuring take place (Kimmel, 1974; Sheehy, 1974; Valiant, 1977). During these periods, people are more likely to assume increased responsibility for their lives and begin the new and often necessary journeys.

The timing of the therapeutic alliance between a client and clinician may also be crucial to the success of treatment. The matching of client and clinician is not a simple one and undoubtedly is an area in need of considerably more study than it has received (Wampold, 2001). There are several investigations in the area of counseling and psychotherapy that indicate the importance of congruence between the client's and clinician's conceptualization of the problem and the best way for the clinician to approach treatment (Lyddon, 1989; 1991; Simons, Lustman, Wetzel, & Murphy, 1985; Wampold, 2001). Choosing an effective clinician involves more than locating someone with experience and a good reputation or finding a clinician who has specialized in working with people who stutter, although that can be an excellent first step (See www.stutteringspecialist.org for clinicians who are board recognized in fluency disorders). Beyond these basic competencies, the clinician should be experienced enough to be congruent with the treatment and the techniques that are employed (Luterman, 1991). As Luterman points out, the strategy and associated techniques of treatment must be "congruent" with the personality of the clinician. Ideally the techniques used by the clinician should seamlessly blend into the interaction and dialogue taking place during the session. If not, such techniques are likely to be discontinuous with the process and even have the possibility of undermining the authenticity and development of the clinical relationship. This would be unfortunate, for often, it is this therapeutic alliance (Wampold, 2001) that is at the core of the change process for many treatments, including that of adolescents and adults who stutter (Cooper & Cooper, 1985).

Some Observations and Measures of the Subtle, Intrinsic Features of the Stuttering Experience

The clinician must acquire and process a considerable amount information during the initial treatment sessions. Not only is it important to appraise the nature of the nonverbal behaviors associated with stuttering but it is also important to learn about the person in a more general sense. What does this person sound and look like when not stuttering? What are the linguistic and acoustic qualities of his or her nonstuttered speech; is it truly flowing and easy or does it sound unstable, irregular, rapid, or unnatural? Does it appear that stuttering is about to "break through" to the surface or become overt to the listener? Does the person's body language provide clues that stuttering nearly occurred or is about to take place? In what ways does the speaker signal the possibility of avoidance or word substitution? Are there clues that the individual would be taciturn, reticent to socially interact, even if he or she did not stutter? Many of these clues are likely contained in a speaker's body language, choice of vocabulary, speaking rate, and syntax. Obviously, with all this information to process, it may take many meetings for the clinician to become calibrated to a new client.

Many formal assessment procedures and techniques may be used to assign severity ratings and to measure change in stuttering as a function of intervention. The majority of these procedures tend to address overt or observable features of stuttering, particularly the percentage of syllables (%SS) or words (%WS) stuttered and struggle or escape behaviors. However, some examples stress self-evaluation by the speaker (Ingham & Cordes, 1997), particularly for measuring the more covert, subtle, intrinsic features of the stuttering experience. As an example of these nonspeech and language but nonetheless important means of assessing people who stutter, the present writers would like to discuss the following tests that have been shown to be of assistance to a comprehensive assessment of stuttering.

The *Locus of Control of Behavior (LCB)* (Craig, Franklin, & Andrews, (1984) is a 17-item, Likert-type scale designed to indicate the degree to which a person perceives occurrences as a consequence of his or her own behavior. The scale was initially developed based on a sample of 100 nonstuttering university students. The 17-item scale has an acceptable internal consistency (α of 0.79). One-week test-retest reliability with 25 nonstuttering adults resulted in a Pearson correlation of 0.90. A 6-month test-retest reliability of 0.73 was found for 25 adults who stuttered and were awaiting treatment. Clients record their agreement or disagreement to the 17 statements using a 6-point bipolar Likert-type scale. Items 1, 5, 7, 8, 13, and 16 are reverse scored before item scores are summed to obtain a total score. Lower scores indicate greater internal control (which is desirable), and higher scores indicate greater perceived external control over the person's actions. Administration of the LCB by Craig et al. (1984) to two groups of nonstuttering adults, 123 university students (mean score 28.3) and 53 nurses (mean score of 27.9), resulted in significantly lower scores ($p < .05$) compared with a group of 70 adults who were awaiting treatment for stuttering (mean score of 31.0). Craig et al. (1984) also noted that a reduced LCB score (greater internality) during treatment predicted maintenance of fluency, whereas an increase (or no change) in the LCB score was predictive of relapse 10 months after treatment. Craig and Andrews (1985) found that changes in LCB scores successfully predicted the outcome in 15 of 17 participants 10 months following treatment. However, De Nil and Kroll, (1995) found that LCB scores do not seem to be related to a person's fluency and may be influenced by whether or not increased assertiveness and responsibility are a focus of the treatment program (Ladouceur, Caron, & Caron, 1989).

The *Self Efficacy for Adults Who Stutter Scale (SESAS)* (Ornstein & Manning, 1985) is based on the work of Bandura (1977) on perceptual self-efficacy scaling and is intended to measure the confidence with which an adult who stutters can approach and maintain fluent speech in a wide variety of extra-treatment speaking situations. Ornstein and Manning (1985) found that 20 adults (mean age 26.11 years; range of 18–44 years) who stutter scored significantly lower ($p < .05$) on both the approach (66.2) and performance (55.8) portions of the SESAS than did a matched group of nonstuttering speakers. The latter speakers scored 94.2 and 98.0 for the approach and performance portions, respectively. Several investigators have reported increases in SESAS scores as a result of treatment (Blood, 1995; Hillis, 1993; Manning, Perkins, Winn, & Cole, 1984), and in some cases, adults who consider themselves recovered from stuttering have recorded SESAS scores that exceed those of nonstuttering adults (Hillis & Manning, 1996).

The *Self Efficacy for Adolescents Scale (SEA-Scale)* (Manning, 1994) is designed for older school-age children and adolescents. The 100-item scale allows clients and clinicians to map a client's predicted performance in 13 categories (Watson, 1988) of beyond-therapy speaking situations appropriate for these younger speakers. Clients use a scale of 1 through 10 to rate their confidence in their ability to enter into and speak in each of the 100 progressively more difficult speaking situations (higher scores indicate greater confidence). The SEA-Scale was normed on 40 adolescent children who stuttered and a matched group of nonstuttering children. The children who stuttered scored significantly ($p < .001$) higher (mean of 8.65, SD = 1.2) than the nonstuttering children (mean of 7.21, SD = 1.8). The overall α level of the entire scale was 0.98 with the 13 subscale α ranging from 0.74 to 0.94.

The *Subjective Screening of Stuttering Severity (SSS)* (Riley, Riley, & McGuire, 2004) was developed because of the potential disparity between listener-determined ratings and the speaker's self-perceptions of the communication experience. The authors' state their belief that the most important opinion concerning communication ability and satisfaction with the experience is that of the speaker.

Four years of clinical trials resulted in eight items across three subtests that provide screening information about the speaker's perceived stuttering severity (two items), level of internal/external locus of control (three items), and word or situation avoidance (three items). Each item is rated on a 9-point semantic differential format where 1 represents a normal speaking experience (target level) and 9 the most severe. All items are self-rated for three audiences: a close friend (ratings used for comparison but not included in the scoring), an authority figure, and use of the telephone. Test-retest agreement was obtained with 16 adults. Pearson product correlations for the three subtests were 0.90 (severity), 0.93 (locus of control), and 0.79 (avoidance). Individual subtests correlated well with the total SSS scores (0.92 for perceived severity, 0.92 for locus of control, 0.95 for avoidance). The SSS appears to provide an efficient way to determine desirable change in three important intrinsic factors known to be associated with successful therapeutic intervention.

A recently published tool is the Overall Assessment of the Speaker's Experience of Stuttering (OASES) (Yaruss & Quesal, 2006). The OASES is designed to obtain information about the totality of the stuttering experience as described by WHO's ICF (WHO, 2001) as described earlier. Following the development and testing of several preliminary versions ($N = 173$ adults ages 18 to 70) to establish validity and reliability, test-retest reliability of the final version was provided by 14 adults (mean age 45.4, SD $= 9.26$ years). Participants' scores on individual items were identical for 77.7% of the 1399 responses and within ± 1 for 98.5% of all responses. Pearson product-moment correlations for two administrations of the test were 0.90 to 0.97.

The OASES contains four main sections. Section I (*General Information*) contains 20 items that provide information about the speaker's self-assessment of impairment as well as the speaker's knowledge about stuttering and stuttering therapy. Section II (*Reactions to Stuttering*) contains 30 items that provide information about the speaker's affective, behavioral, and cognitive reactions to stuttering. Section III (*Communication in Daily Situations*) contains 25 items that provide information about the *difficulty* speakers experience when communicating in key situations. Section IV (*Quality of Life*) contains 25 items that provide information about the overall impact of stuttering on the speaker's quality of life. Items assess such factors as how much stuttering interferes with the speaker's communication, relationships, and sense of confidence and well-being. To control for items that may not apply to all participants, a ratio of the total points selected by the respondents divided by the total possible points for each section was used, resulting in an "impact score." Although not a direct indication of stuttering severity, the scores provide an indication of the impact of stuttering on the speaker's life. Impact scores in each section range from a minimum of 20 to a maximum of 100, with higher scores indicating a greater degree of negative impact. Numerical scores from the OASES can be translated to ratings used to reflect the degree of impact stuttering has on a speaker's life (mild, mild-to-moderate, moderate, moderate-to-severe, severe). Psychometric testing to date indicates that this measure appears to have good reliability and validity.

One final comment about the assessment process: Although perhaps obvious, the initial meeting with a new client can be crucial. It is our first, and possibly only, opportunity to indicate our understanding about the experience of stuttering (indeed, the initial diagnostic is as much about orienting the client to who we are and what we believe and know as it about assessing his or her concerns). Based on our interactions and our realistic presentation about the demands of treatment we can often get a sense about the client's motivation. It is our first opportunity to show the potential client that we are: unafraid of stuttering; are highly interested in the client and his or her problem; have both empathy and insight about the process of change for someone who stutters; have a variety of treatment options as well as a sense of direction about the treatment process; and are willing to accompany the client in his or her quest.

The goals of treatment for stuttering are as multidimensional as the problem. Beyond the obvious objective of helping the speaker to reduce the frequency with which he or she stutters, we also want these individuals to be able to become not only better but also more willing communicators. As much as anything, change is indicated by the speaker's ability to alter his or her habitual, reflexive, and struggled stuttering and to produce stuttering that is both emotionally and physically easier. Similarly, success is also indicated by speakers' ability to improve the quantity and quality (e.g., rate, resonance, intelligibility, intensity) of their nonstuttered speech. Improvement in the person's ability to problem solve unexpected and difficult speaking experiences is also an indicator of success. There are often important lifestyle changes that indicate that persons are increasing their ability to live an unrestricted and satisfying life, even if they occasionally stutter. We are especially interested in the ability of people to incorporate the successes they are able to achieve with their speech into other aspects of their lives. We would like them to reconstruct the view of themselves and their lives that may have been dominated by the theme of stuttering (See DiLollo, Neimeyer, & Manning, 2002) and characterized by themes of failure, helplessness, and shame (See Corcoran & Stewart, 1998; Plexico et al. 2005).

The Nonlinear Process of Change

It is common to think of processes such as learning, change, and adaptation as a linear process. In some cases, particularly if the issues are relatively uncomplicated, the process may, indeed, be linear or a straight, smooth trajectory from beginning to end. For example, linear models of human adaptation to the loss of a loved one (e.g., Kubler-Ross, 1969) imply that people work through the various stages of grief, eventually reaching a stage called "acceptance." However, most anyone who has ever worked through the arduous and complicated process of mastering a complicated athletic activity, obtaining an advanced degree, or adjusting to the issues associated with moving to a new city or the loss of a relationship or a job knows that the process is rarely linear. The experience requires revisiting the various stages of the process, stages that one thought were finished. Things are never quite "back to normal" and, in some ways, a person may do this for the rest of his or her life. This cyclical view of the change or adaptation process corresponds to consistent findings by authors who have studied the counseling process (Neimeyer, 2000; Prochaska & DiClemente, 1992; & Prochaska et al., 1992).

The process of changing complex human problems such as stuttering could hardly be expected to be linear. For an assortment of reasons, there are peaks and valleys along the way. Motivation for change fluctuates. Schedules and priorities must be adjusted (one's own and often others) to set aside the time to spend on the task. So, it should not be surprising if changing something as complex as stuttering will be a circular and rigorous process. It is necessary for the client, as well as the clinician, to understand this at the outset of treatment so that no one gets overly frustrated and quits whenever there is a dip in energy or achievement. It is essential for all involved, including family members and friends, to appreciate the larger pattern of change. Both the clinician and the client must keep their eyes on the prize and not become discouraged by temporary cycles and setbacks because such nonlinearities, starts and stops, are the norm rather than the exception when dealing with human change and learning.

Whatever overall treatment strategy and associated techniques are used, the clinician as well as the client should be in relatively close agreement concerning the nature and direction of treatment. Research in counseling and psychotherapy (See Wampold, 2001) has demonstrated that there is no single treatment strategy that is best for all clients, and this is likely to be the true for adults who stutter (Huinck & Peters, 2004; Franken, Van der Schalk, & Boelens, 2005).

Client motivation typically is high at the outset of treatment. The person has accepted the fact that a problem exists, at least at some level, and has initiated the process of change by contacting a professional who can provide helpful information and begin to demystify the problem. Thus begins the process of clients becoming more objective about their predicament. At the outset, some clients appear to be highly motivated, saying all the right things; however, it is never what one *says* but rather, what one *does*, that indicates one's true level of motivation. Thus, we must distinguish between our client's verbiage and their actions in attempts to discern each client's true level motivation. One way to help with this assessment is to clearly describe to the client the nature of the treatment process. The clinician can provide examples of the tasks that will have to be done, making it clear that although the clinician is the coach, it is the client who "runs the laps." Clinicians can provide specific examples and give concrete assignments to be completed by the following treatment session. To be sure, at times clinicians will demonstrate or model desired behavior changes and perform some of the tasks that are asked of the clients. In the final analysis, however, it is the client's journey, and it is his or her responsibility to take action, problem solve, and, on occasion, lead the way.

Distinguishing Treatment from Techniques

An important observation concerning treatment techniques is that the procedures themselves are not the treatment. Of course, the mastery of techniques is important, sometimes critical, to learning and change. In much the same way that the specific techniques required of an athlete during a competition reveal relatively little about the overall nature of the competitive experience, the particular techniques used in the treatment of stuttering tell us little about the essence of therapeutic change.

DiClemente (1993) argues that successful treatment is not the result of using techniques, but of using the right techniques at the right time. This has also been pointed out in the area of fluency disorders (Culatta & Goldberg, 1995; Manning, 2001; Max & Caruso, 1997). As Culatta and Goldberg (1995) insightfully suggest, failure of a client to make effective use of a technique is more often due to the inappropriate selection of the technique by the clinician rather than the characteristics of the technique. The many techniques associated with rate control, fluency shaping, and stuttering modification strategies have an important, even critical, place in the repertoire of an experienced clinician. Experienced clinicians, just as experienced coaches and teachers, need to have many options available to them, applying them judiciously and at the right points in time during the therapy process.

Technical and Professional Approaches: Rule-Based versus Principle-Based

Rules are created and serve as specific prescriptions for whether or not something was achieved, and how well something was done (Levitt, Neimeyer & Williams, 2004). A *rule-based* approach tends to be mechanistic, algorithmic, and often quantitative. An individual using this approach would follow a structured set of formalized guidelines that are unequivocally applied. A *principle-based* approach tends to be less structured, clear-cut, and specific. An individual using this approach would likely be guided by his or her professional and personal experience. The determination of whether or not behavior as well as internal changes (e.g., attitudes about talking) are accomplished would be qualitative and contextual.

In the case of a treatment intervention, a rule-governed approach is generally associated with a particular treatment methodology and specifically prescribed techniques. The treatment protocol is predetermined (or programmed) and session activities are rigorously maintained. Accordingly, manuals are typically developed to ensure that the rules are followed and that the treatment protocol is consistent both within and across clients. Behavioral change relative to stuttering is often determined in a quantitative manner, commonly % SS (percentage of syllables stuttered) and rate of speech. On the other hand, a principled approach to treatment allows the clinician the option of selecting from various methodologies and associated techniques from a variety of therapeutic approaches. Both the clinician and the client are able to respond creatively and "on-the-fly" to the dynamic nature of the change process. Change is often determined in a qualitative and contextual manner.

Braithwaite (2002) suggested that the application of explicit standards without regard to the context of the situation or action works best when the type of action to be regulated is relatively straightforward, simple, and stable. He suggests that in such cases, rules tend to regulate with greater certainty than principles. One example would be the rules for driving a car (e.g., what speed to maintain, when to turn on red, when to pass another vehicle) in regular, everyday, "dry pavement" conditions. However, Braithwaite makes a convincing case that when the type of action to be regulated is complex and dynamic (such as driving with ice or snow on the road or negotiating traffic during an emergency), principles tend to regulate with greater certainty than rules. Or, when predicting the outcome of say, a two-person political contest, one could not use the simple odds of heads or tails to predict the winner; rather, one's predictions would need to be based on much more complex, principle-informed decisions, and they would need to allow for the dynamic changes of public opinion inherent in such contests. Clearly in such a cases, when dynamically changing and challenging circumstances and events present themselves, the rules need to be adjusted. Braithwaite proposes that using rules to regulate complex procedures results in lower consistency and validity when determining outcome.

◆ Refinement of Some Common Treatment Techniques

Stuttering Modification

Having argued that treatment is more than technique, we now discuss aspects of some of the techniques that are commonly used. The goal of *stuttering modification* techniques are also referred to as traditional, Van Riparian (Van Riper, 1973) nonavoidance, or stutter-more-fluently (Gregory, 1973) approaches. The primary goal when using techniques associated with the stuttering modification approach is to change the form of a person's stuttering to an open, flowing, and easy (although not necessarily normally fluent) form of speaking. The goals of stuttering modification have been described in detail in several sources (Van Riper, 1973; 1989; Van Riper & Erickson, 1996). There are, however, key elements that can easily be overlooked.

Because primary emphasis of this approach to treatment is on decreasing avoidance behavior, desensitizing a speaker to his or her own fluency breaks, and modifying instances of stuttering, some presume that fluency is neither a major nor long-term goal. Because stuttering has to be out in the open and exposed to be identified and altered, there can be an *increase* in the client's frequency of stuttering, particularly early in treatment. As the client increases the frequency and duration of his or her everyday, social communications, it is not unusual to observe more frequent fluency breaks. However, even as breaks in speech fluency increase, this approach encourages and helps the client to make better decisions and use less avoidance behavior. Indeed, in spite of this temporary increase in stuttering, a realistic long-term goal of the stuttering modification approach is spontaneously fluent speech.

A primary principle of stuttering modification techniques is to monitor and change old automatic, reflexive, and struggled fluency breaks into physically easier and smoother forms of stuttering. Clients initially learn to do this following (cancellation or post-event), then during (pull-out or para-event), and finally, prior to (preparatory set or pre-event) instances of stuttering (see Van Riper, 1973, for details). Modification proceeds in this order (from after to before) to give clients the opportunity to overcome their emotional discomfort and/or anxious reaction to this experience and make it easier for them to detect and modify their fluency breaks during ongoing conversational speech.

A goal throughout each stage of stuttering modification is not to become immediately fluent but rather to "take charge" of the stuttering event and selectively modify the speech pattern. When first attempting the cancellation technique—typically one of the first steps with this approach—it is common for clients to simply say the stuttered word again but fluently. Instead, the goal is to repeat the word using a form of "easy stuttering." Although not spoken in a normally fluent manner, their speech is slightly stretched, open, and flowing. At this point, fluency-enhancing techniques (e.g., full breath, light articulatory contact, blending of sound and syllable transitions) are helpful. Once the cancellation technique is mastered in a variety of speaking situations, most clients quite naturally begin using para- (e.g., pull-outs) or even pre-event (e.g., preparatory sets) modifications. Again, however, the key aspect of this technique is to take charge of the instance of stuttering, rather than helplessly fighting through it.

As these modification techniques become (over)learned, a client achieves more success in progressively more difficult speaking situations beyond the treatment settings. Pre-stuttering modifications are, of course, preferred. If this is not possible, then the client has a second opportunity to modify stuttering by using the para-event or pull-out technique. Finally, if unsuccessful in taking charge of the stuttering moment using these techniques, the client's final opportunity is a post-event or cancellation technique. Although this may take several attempts, clients should not move forward with the sentence until they have taken charge of the word. This is often difficult for clients to do, especially at the outset of treatment. They may even feel that it is an impossible task, particularly during more difficult speaking situations. If a speaker is unable to modify his or her stuttering, it is often because he or she has not yet become sufficiently desensitized to the stuttering experience. But once a person begins to think of stuttering moments as an opportunity for victory, he or she can begin to "score some runs."

If clients are focused on fluency rather than control when using any of the stuttering modification techniques, they will not be as effective. Thus, many clients have to become more comfortable with stuttering, to be able to "stay in the stuttering moment" rather than trying so hard to escape from the experience. They have to stay with the moment of stuttering, to vary it, and to allow themselves to experience it fully. Although it will seem contradictory to clients, only by getting to "know" and accept stuttering by experiencing it is it possible to achieve some distance from the fear and helplessness of that experience.

There is often a delicate balance between the desire to effectively modify the stuttering into a smooth form of disfluency and an overstriving for fluency (or the urge not to stutter). The extent to which the speaker is trying excessively hard to successfully modify the stuttering is the extent to which more physical tension and possibly blocking may result. The speaker may do better to find a balance between successful smoothing of the old form of stuttering and an attitude of "giving oneself permission to stutter." Letting go of the urge not to stutter is often liberating. There is a reason why the newsletter of the National Stuttering Association is titled *Letting Go* (http://www.nsastutter.org.)

The client's decision to substitute or avoid sounds, words, people, or situations is one of the more insidious features of stuttering and therefore one of the most difficult to alter. This decision can be so subtle that the client may not even be aware of it. It is a form of stuttering that never becomes overt and thus observable to listeners. The decision not to speak will not be identified as stuttering but is, in fact, a profound stuttering event. Along with the changes in surface behaviors of the problem, the choices that a client makes because of the *possibility* of stuttering must also begin to change. Stuttering modification strategies require a good deal of introspection, self-awareness, self-monitoring, motivation, and courage on the part of the client as well as perceptive leadership and support on the part of the clinician.

We have a few final comments concerning stuttering modification approaches. Because the cancellation technique requires so much desensitization, discipline, and resistance to the possibility of negative listener response, many clients report that they rarely use this technique beyond the safety of the clinic setting. Still, to the degree that it is possible, this technique provides a litmus test of the determination to successfully replace the old pattern of effortful stuttering with a new elegant and smooth behavior. All of the stuttering modification techniques require diligent self-monitoring of the status of the speech production system including the respiratory, phonatory, and articulatory systems. Consistent progress requires kinesthetic monitoring of one's speech system for tension and hesitations in air flow, voicing, and contact of the articulators to achieve smooth and effortless production. For most adolescents and adults who are accustomed to (anticipating and in fact) struggling with their speech on a daily basis, change requires a long process of openness and disclosure of their stuttering and a diligent and persistent effort to systematically alter their approach to producing speech. In many ways, this is also true with the other generic approach to treatment that focuses on the enhancement of fluency.

Fluency Modification

Fluency modification strategies (also called fluency-shaping or speak-more-fluently approaches) are closely related to the rate control and rate reduction/prolonged speech therapies that became popular beginning in the 1960s/1970s. These approaches focused almost exclusively on reducing the frequency of the stuttering behavior, often using behavioral modification techniques to decrease stuttering. (e.g., Brutten & Shoemaker, 1967; Ingham, 1993; Ingham, Martin, & Kuhl, 1974; Ryan, 1971). Rate reduction remains a popular approach for modifying stuttering (O'Brian et al., 2003; St. Louis & Westbrook, 1987) and has been shown to significantly reduce the frequency of stuttering, particularly in a clinical setting. As Max and Caruso (1997) point out, a reduction of speaking rate is often a treatment goal in and of itself, a temporary goal to promote fluency before the client's rate is gradually increased, or a technique for smoothing an anticipated stuttering event.

In any case, the emphasis of treatment with a fluency-shaping approach is not on modifying instances of stuttering but rather on changing the client's overall speech pattern (Andrews, Guitar, & Howie, 1980; Howie & Andrews, 1984; Ingham, 1993). Rate reduction often emphasizes the use of prolonged speech in which the duration of articulatory movements is increased and smooth articulatory transitions between sounds and syllables are accentuated. Such slowing and smoothing of speech promotes the coordination and integration of respiratory, phonatory, and articulatory movements. Once such movements are well learned and integrated, the client is able to gradually increase speed of performance, often without fluency breaks. In addition, a reduction in the length of phrases, even as short as two to five syllables (Perkins, 1984), with pauses at natural syntactic junctures (Neilsen & Andrews, 1993) promotes an open vocal tract and provides clients the opportunity to achieve a full breath. Continuous phonation (Shames & Florence, 1980) or constant vocalization (Max & Caruso, 1997) of both voiced and unvoiced sounds is recommended to promote continuous airflow and articulatory movement. Boberg and Kully (1995) suggest blending the sounds, syllables, and words of an utterance together as if saying one continuous word. Although earlier fluency modification approaches focused almost exclusively on surface features of stuttering, more recent versions (Boberg & Kully, 1995; Langevin & Kully, 2007, Chapter 8 this volume) are more comprehensive in nature and often incorporate procedures for facilitating cognitive and affective change.

Fluency-shaping procedures can be beneficial for any speaker (fluent or not) as they increase understanding of speech physiology, and speakers learn to use techniques that make the most efficient use of the speech production mechanism. Mastery of these techniques can lead to smooth, flowing, easy respiratory, vocal and articulatory adjustments that may result in more efficient as well as more fluent speech. If done well and practiced diligently, speakers become considerably easier to listen to even if some (easy) fluency breaks continue to be present.

Stuttering Modification Melded with Fluency Modification

Based on these writers' experience, it is often effective to begin treatment using a stuttering modification approach. As a client is able to identify and become desensitized and knowledgeable about stuttering in general and his or her own stuttering in particular, the various fluency modification techniques provide a natural way to successfully modify the old forms of effortful stuttering. On other occasions, when clients' are having difficulty producing any fluent speech and are demonstrating profound struggle behavior, it is helpful to begin with fluency facilitating techniques for the speakers to achieve some immediate fluency. Once they have experienced success, they can learn to identify, become desensitized to, and modify specific features of their stuttering. Most adolescents and adults who stutter need both sides of this therapeutic "coin." The speaker benefits from learning how to produce speech in a way that promotes fluency. The physiological characteristics of dynamically changing speech production and the increased awareness of the distinctive features of sound production provide the speakers with information that is essential for analyzing and monitoring their speech. But most speakers also need to know what to do when they are producing and feel they are unable to release from an instance of stuttering. As they develop confidence in using techniques for "moving through and out of" the stuttered moment, many clients find that the helplessness that accompanies their stuttering begins to subside.

Both fluency and stuttering modification approaches tend to heighten a speaker's monitoring and self-evaluation abilities and development of the critical ability to self-monitor speech.[1] As clients are able to take charge of their stuttering moments and achieve higher levels of fluency there are fewer stuttering events left to modify. Voluntary stuttering in an easy, open manner is often useful at this point. It provides a good test of whether or not a client still possesses the strong desire to avoid and/or escape his or her stuttering. As treatment progresses and there are fewer stuttering moments available to modify, fluency modification techniques, quite naturally, take precedence. These procedures can sometimes be used to smooth out (i.e., to make more continuous and flowing) any remaining unstable speech. And finally, fluency modification techniques provide clients with helpful techniques for smoothly modifying stuttering moments, particularly during later stages of stuttering modification programs when pre-event or preparatory sets are being mastered.

◆ Procedures for Promoting Long-Term Change

The Importance of Practice

Anyone who has attempted to learn a complex physical or mental activity begins to realize that it will be necessary to practice to the point where the activity is overlearned and habitual. Only when such a level of performance is achieved will a person be able rely on a technique under stress or time pressure (or a threat to a person's physical or psychological well-being). Although people who stutter do not necessarily need to attain an extreme level of expertise to produce fluent speech, the importance of persistence and practice can hardly be over-emphasized. As a point of reference, the work of Ericsson and Smith (1991) may be helpful. These authors found that a minimum of 10,000 to 20,000 hours of practice are required to perform an activity appropriately and effortlessly. Once a technique has been habituated and integrated it becomes far more than a sequence of behaviors; the technique becomes part of who a person is, and the person uses it with little or no thought. Smith (1999), Guitar (1998), and others have reported data indicating that what we do when we practice is to reform or "reformat" our central nervous system. There is increasing support for the notion that this is occurring for adults who have been able to change their pattern of stuttering (DeNil & Kroll, 2001; Neumann Preibisch & Euler et al., 2005).

In addition, for people who stutter the issue isn't only one of developing the many features necessary for producing fluent speech. Adolescents or adults who have stuttered for many years have accumulated an untold number of hours practicing how they stutter as well as how they cognitively process their communicative as well as social experiences. They will likely have to "unlearn" many of the behaviors they have habituated and reconstrue how they think about themselves and their ability to communicate (DiLollo, Manning & Neimeyer, 2003; Plexico et al. 2005).

The Value of Group Treatment

One effect of a group treatment situation that brings together stuttering clients and nonstuttering clinicians is that both clinicians and clients soon understand the common nature of most

---

[1]The recent meta-analysis of functional neuroimaging studies by Brown, Ingham, Ingham, Laird, and Fox (2005) provides some intriguing results that may relate to the ability of speakers to monitor their speech output. A comparison of neural signatures of fluent and stuttering speakers indicate that one most distinctive markers for individual who stutterer is "the absence of activation in auditory areas bilaterally" (p. 112). This inhibition of auditory activity appears to be positively related to the frequency of stuttering and clinical determination of severity. It also seems lessened by fluency-enhancing activities. The authors describe a phenomenon of "efference copy" to explain the lack of speech-associated auditory activation in people who stutter.

anxiety-producing situations. Many people who stutter are often surprised to learn that some people who don't stutter may also be intensely afraid of public speaking experiences and go to great lengths to avoid speaking in front of a group. Although the threshold of avoidance may be reached sooner if a person stutters, everyone shares the anxiety associated with many speaking situations (e.g., public speaking, making introductions, speaking on the telephone to members of the opposite sex, speaking with a superior at work). As the group discusses the nature of negative and positive "self-talk" and takes both speech and nonspeech risks during therapy, clinicians often express the idea that they feel as if they are also undergoing treatment. Together, group members experience the excitement and challenge of pushing the envelope of their speech and communication, and of their lives.

Group treatment can be especially helpful for student clinicians because the group setting provides them an opportunity to learn about other clients and to see their own client in a somewhat more typical communication situation. The diversity of a group setting provides a wide variety of communicative opportunities (e.g., introductions, role playing, public speaking). It also enables clients to realize that they are not alone with their problem (Stewart & Richardson, 2004). Perhaps most important, others in the group can provide support for clients during the process of change at a time when they can benefit from helping relationships (Prochaska & DiClemente, 1986).

Expected Outcomes

An ideal outcome of treatment would have clients speaking with normal fluency that sounds natural in all situations, particularly outside the confines of the clinic. This is possible, of course, and it happens, but it is the exception. It may not even be desirable for all persons. Following treatment, some people are speaking with what may be termed "technical" fluency. Their speech is, in a technical sense, free from repetitions, prolongations, and obvious struggle behavior that can certainly be interpreted as progress; however, on occasion, some of these individuals are controlling their speech so carefully, and working so hard to maintain fluency, that they are speaking with strain and effort. Oral expression of their thoughts, their communication, is for them is neither truly spontaneous nor effortless. In essence, they are not communicating with ease, even the ease that is possible for a person whose speech contains easy, tension-free fluency breaks. Being in continuous, conscious, if not grim, pursuit of fluency can result in overcontrolled speech and, even in the absence of stuttering, result in less than natural, desirable communication.

Speaking carefully is not a preferred outcome. Like writing carefully, it is not likely to be spontaneous or creative or enjoyable for listeners. Speaking carefully is far from a functional way of communicating. As Perkins (1979, 1984) has commented, clients will not likely use techniques that feel or sound to them at least as abnormal as their stuttering. However, even traditional techniques of stuttering modification may result in adverse listener reactions (Manning, Thaxton, & Ells, 1997). Clients not only must work against the inertia of their own long-standing responses to the stuttering experience but also the expectations and reactions of others. To reduce the possibility of post-treatment relapse, clinicians may need to assist clients in preparing for such negative responses and inform those in clients' environments about appreciating and reinforcing their use of modification techniques.

Maintenance of Success

Many clients leave treatment with relatively high levels of fluency; however, the maintenance of that fluency will continue to take considerable effort, at least during the period immediately following the end of formal treatment. Consistent effort and practice can usually lead to high levels of fluency that, in turn, may result in less practice when the problem is no longer prominent. Of course, what usually follows decreased practice is an increase in stuttering. This sequence of events is not unusual and should not be surprising, and both client and clinician should be prepared for this possibility. In addition, there will be many speaking situations when maintenance of fluency will not have the highest priority. This is apt to be the case in high stimulus social situations such as weddings, receptions, or parties where there are many things to concentrate on other than fluency. For some speakers, it may not be worth the effort to monitor and modify all moments of stuttering in every communicative situation. It may be more important on such occasions not to work so hard on speech and simply enjoy the situation. Of course, the "ideal" client would use such speaking situations as an opportunity to practice. However, if this was not the choice, clients should not berate themselves for such decisions are natural and to be expected. Positive self-talk following either success or failure to maintain fluency is an important feature of clients' continued progress (Emerick, 1988; Maxwell, 1982).

Just as with the completion of an academic degree, the completion of formal treatment is the initial stage for years of further growth. Usually, it takes a long time for changes in the affective and cognitive features of stuttering to catch up to the behavioral changes, changes that may occur rather quickly over the course of a few weeks or months. Even though clients may be able to demonstrate high levels of fluent speech in several speaking situations, it will take some time before they no longer think or feel about themselves primarily as persons who stutters. (Manning, 1991; Plexico et al., 2005).

Of course, a principal goal of treatment is to reduce the disability and handicap associated with stuttering. As indicated by the revisions of the ICF by the WHO (2001), this requires our focus on the observable as well as the less observable features of the problem. Accordingly, it is often far less important to achieve a complete absence of stuttering as it is to significantly decrease the influence of the problem during most aspects of daily living. It may be that complete fluency is neither necessary nor sufficient for the achievement of high levels of successful stuttering management (Plexico et al. 2005). Daily goals are accomplished within the context of important personal and environmental influences such as the client's ability to demonstrate more open decision-making, expanded risk-taking behavior, and the achievement of greater freedom in speaking to anyone, anywhere, at anytime about anything. In short, with successful therapy, the quality of the client's life should improve across all communication and many noncommunication situations.

Self-Help, Support Groups

Throughout treatment, and especially following treatment, client involvement with a support group can be extremely important (Reeves, 2005; Chapter 14, this volume). DiClemente (1993) indicates that support groups often play a critical role for eliciting change and especially for maintaining it. There are several organizations that promote such groups for children and adults (See: The Stuttering Home Page at http://www.mnsu.edu/comdis/kuster/stutter.html), with the National Stuttering Association being the most prominent in the United States. The value of such support to people with similar challenges can hardly be underestimated. The nurturing provided by a well-run and active support group can facilitate continued growth during the maintenance stage of change. The support and information that support meetings can provide to spouses, parents, and other interested family members can be critical for validating successes and promoting continued progress both during and following treatment. Support group experiences and professional treatment can be complementary and should be thought of as enhancing one another. The Stuttering Home Page on the Internet is the most comprehensive source and provides many links to support networks throughout the world.

◆ Future Directions

Our discussion of treatment for adults who stutter has, so far, focused on the traditional approaches of stuttering modification and fluency shaping, and the ways in which these two approaches might be used, either individually or in combination, to provide the individual with the most effective and satisfying treatment options and outcomes. In combination, these approaches can effectively address various components of the stuttering problem, including the speech and accessory behaviors, avoidances, fears, and emotional reactions to stuttering. One component that these approaches fail to address, however, is a consideration of the "meaningfulness" of the changes that occur in the treatment process. As an illustration of what we mean by this, consider the following quote from the late Marty Jezer, author, and a person who stuttered:

> My hands were trembling as I began. . . . I felt very much alone. So great was my fear that I seemed to go into a trance. It was a kind of out-of-body experience: a fluent person seemed to be speaking out of my mouth. I heard his words, but they did not come from me. When I was finished, the teacher complimented me for my fluency and for my courage. I think the class may even have applauded – not in sarcasm but in appreciation for my triumph and also, I imagine, in relief. My feeling of success was fleeting, however, as at my Bar Mitzvah, I had somehow been fluent. But my fluency mystified me. There was no way to remember how I felt being fluent, because my fluency did not seem to come from me. I was beginning to fear fluency. I knew myself when I was stuttering. But I felt estranged from myself when I was fluent.
> (Jezer, 1997, p.108).

As this example dramatically illustrates, some persons who stutter, as they begin to experience increases in fluent speech, also start to feel increased anxiety, fear, and even guilt and depression as a response to the therapeutic changes in their speech (Manning, 2001). Experiences such as these suggest that some clients struggle to relate the changes being made in their speech behaviors to their understanding of themselves as speakers and communicators; they end up feeling "estranged" from themselves when they are fluent.

In the following section of this chapter, we look at some past and recent research indicating that an additional, counseling-based component to treatment, perhaps used in conjunction with traditional treatment approaches, may facilitate more complete and favorable long-term outcomes for adult persons who stutter.

Fransella's Personal Construct Theory of Stuttering

Based on Kelly's (1955) Theory of Personal Constructs, Fransella (1972) hypothesized that a person stutters "because it is in this way that he can anticipate the greatest number of events; it is by behaving in this way that life is most meaningful to him" (p.58). In Kelly's Theory of Personal Construct, *meaning* is the key to behavior, as individuals extract (in Kelly's terminology, "construe") only what is meaningful to them from the unending stream of experience that constitutes the world. They then use these "constructions" to relate themselves to their environment by being able to predict events and outcomes. For example, Jason is a person who stutters. He can confidently predict how events will unfold if he stutters when he attends an office party, allowing him to prepare for and deal with the situation. If, however, Jason is to be fluent in that situation, he can no longer predict the myriad of possible outcomes. He begins to feel anxious and afraid, perhaps even guilty that he will be "deceiving" people into thinking he is a "fluent speaker." The likely outcome, if he has a choice, is that Jason will "choose" to stutter, not because he prefers it in the usual sense, but because it is what is familiar; it is how he understands the world (Dalton, 1983).

Fransella (1972) demonstrated some support for her theory in an uncontrolled study in which she found that by using personal construct counseling to increase the meaningfulness of being a "fluent speaker" she was able to improve the fluency of 16 adults who stuttered. More recently, DiLollo et al. (2002; 2003) found support for Fransella's theory in two studies that examined the meaningfulness of speaker roles for persons who stutter. DiLollo et al. found a relative lack of meaningfulness of the "fluent speaker role" for individuals who stuttered that was mirrored by a lack of meaningfulness of the "stutterer role" for fluent speakers. These findings suggested that this lack of a meaningful fluent speaker role for persons who stutter may be the result of a natural process of construing only the events from their communication experiences that supported their self-concept (i.e., stuttered events for the persons who stutter; fluent events for the fluent speakers).

Clinical Implications of Fransella's Theory

According to this Theory of Personal Construct of stuttering, then, people continue to stutter because that is the most meaningful way for them to behave. If that is the case, then at least some aspects of therapy need to be directed toward making *fluency* a more meaningful way to behave (Fransella, 1972, 2003).

In her initial study, Fransella (1972) primarily used a technique called "controlled elaboration" to increase the meaningfulness of the fluent speaker role for her persons who stuttered. Kelly (1955) described controlled elaboration as a method by which the counselor can help clients to examine one part of their construct system through verbal and other behavioral experiments to make it possible to contrast its validity. In Fransella's case, this meant guiding the persons who stutter to focus on any occasions in which fluency was experienced and questioning them about the experience, thereby *elaborating* the experience of fluency. DiLollo et al. (2003) demonstrated that persons who stutter tend to "protect" their "stutterer" self-image by ignoring or discounting episodes of fluent speech, referring to them as "lucky" or "a fluke," and always predicting a return to stuttering. The effect of controlled elaboration of fluency, then, is to require the person who stutters to pay attention to his or her fluent speech, to examine it, experiment with it, see what it feels like, and see how other people react to it. Fransella (2003) suggests that the "crucial question" in this method is, "Did you predict you would be fluent?" As clients learn to be more aware of their fluent speech, predictions of fluency become more frequent, and they are able to attribute their fluency to themselves rather than some "fluke" or external source. In essence, their fluency becomes more *meaningful* to them.

Questioning about occurrences of fluent speech is not the only method that might lead to a reconstruing of the meaningfulness of fluency. As Kelly (1955) described, controlled elaboration can also take nonverbal forms. For example, in traditional stuttering therapy, we often have clients make up "hierarchies" of situations in which they may have trouble speaking more or less fluently. As part of therapy, we often ask clients to practice their fluency-enhancing skills in some of these situations. Such exercises can be used as part of a controlled elaboration approach by asking clients *before* going into the situation to examine their thoughts and feelings about the action: How will this turn out? How will you feel? How will the others in the situation react? Do you predict being fluent? After considering the activity carefully, and noting their predictions, clients then carry out the "experiment." Finally, clients report back to the clinician and discuss the outcome of the experiment, carefully comparing their predictions with the actual outcomes. Elaboration of the fluent speaker role tends to begin in early stages of therapy through the contrasting of clients' predictions of stuttering with demonstrations of successful fluency. Later, with increasing predictions of fluency that are then confirmed by the experiment, the fluent speaker role may even replace the stutterer role as the dominant speaker role used by the client.

Other Personal Construct Theory-based methods have also been used with persons who stutter. Botterill and Cook (1987), for example, discuss the use of a "problem solving" exercise based on Kelly's (1955) "circumspection, pre-emption, and control" cycle, and a role-playing method based on Kelly's "fixed-role" therapy.

Narrative Therapy

In addition to specific Personal Construct Theory methods, DiLollo et al. (2002) suggested a *narrative therapy* approach to the treatment of stuttering (in conjunction with traditional speech therapy) as a way of facilitating fundamental changes in the ways in which individuals who stutter construe themselves as speakers and communicators. As with personal construct methods, this approach aims to facilitate elaboration of spontaneous or treatment-induced episodes of fluency and to start to consolidate a preferred story of the self as capable of fluency. An added aspect of a narrative approach is that it also takes into account the social aspect of behavior, looking to secure social validation for the achievements made in treatment. We view this approach as more complementary than competitive with both Fransella's (1972) controlled elaboration approach and traditional speech therapy for stuttering.

Based on the work of White and Epston (1990), the narrative approach described by DiLollo et al. (2002) makes use of "externalizing" language to encourage persons who stutter to move from feeling like a "problem person" (i.e., "I'm a stutterer") to a "person with a problem" (i.e., "I am a person who stutters"). Although this suggestion seems to be at odds with findings by St. Louis (1999) regarding the lack of an effect of "person-first" terminology, St. Louis's research was conducted to assess the effect of the terminology on the *listener* and not on the *speaker* as is being suggested here. The act of referring to "Stuttering" as an external "entity" can often help in recruiting the client to be an active participant in the treatment process, as opposed to feeling like a problem person who requires "fixing" by the clinician.

The narrative approach is based on repeated telling and retelling of the individual's story, initially mapping out the influence of Stuttering on the life of the person (i.e., How does the problem affect the person's life?), followed by an investigation of the influence of the *person* on the life of Stuttering (i.e., How does the person affect the course of the problem?). Similar to Kelly's (1955) controlled elaboration, the investigation of the influence of the *person* on the life of "Stuttering" may be facilitated by the use of questions that help the individual identify "sparkling moments" (Winslade & Monk, 1999), or times when the individual's experiences have been contradictory to the problem story (e.g., getting the client to "elaborate" on times when he or she was fluent). Such questions might then be followed by questions that further focus on the sparkling moments and begin to invite clients to make sense of these exceptions to their dominant narrative of disfluency that may not have previously registered as significant and to retain them as part of an emerging coherent narrative. Further questions may be used to facilitate individuals' re-describing themselves and projecting forward to speculate about various personal and relational alternatives that derive from their emerging alternative narrative. As a new story that is focused on fluency rather than stuttering begins to emerge, the story is told and retold many times and with many different audiences, strengthening the meaningfulness of the fluent speaker role for the client and establishing predictions of fluency, not only on the part of the client, but also on the part of significant others in his or her social environment.

The Problem of Relapse

As described earlier in this chapter, under the right circumstances, traditional approaches to the treatment of adult persons who stutter can be highly successful. Despite this, "relapse" following successful treatment has been a major cause for concern for both consumers and professionals working with persons who stutter, even being called the "Achilles' heel" of stuttering intervention (Kuhr & Rustin, 1985). Authors (Silverman, 1992; Craig & Hancock, 1995) have suggested that between 50% to 70% of adults relapse following successful treatment prompting Cooper (1977) to suggest that relapse may actually be "part of the human condition." As evidence, Cooper cited the high rate of occurrence of relapse in other areas of clinical intervention such as addiction problems, weight loss, and marital problems. Craig (Craig & Andrews, 1985), in a review of the relapse literature, indicated that relapse rates in the treatment of addictive disorders are reported to be in the range of 40 to 60%, uncomfortably similar to those reported for stuttering treatment.

Understanding the problem of relapse, however, takes on new meaning when viewed from the perspective of Kelly's (1955) Theory of Personal Construct. Earlier in this section, we described how Fransella (1972) suggested that individuals will continue to stutter because that is what is most meaningful to them. We also described some of the emotional reactions some persons who stutter can have to successful treatment for stuttering. Perkins (1979) summarized how these issues might relate to relapse when, in reference to lapses by clients who appeared to have mastered behavioral techniques to control their speech, he stated that, "these lapses seem to have more to do with the person's sense of identity as a stutterer, and his misgivings about relinquishing that identity, than with inability to maintain the skills of normal sounding speech" (p. 109).

A personal construct view of relapse, therefore, relates back to the lack of meaningfulness of the fluent speaker role for persons who stutter—even once they have learned to produce consistently fluent speech. The clear implication of this view of relapse, then, is to take a more holistic approach to the treatment of adult stuttering and to incorporate personal construct (e.g., Botterill & Cook, 1987; Fransella, 1972, 2003) or narrative therapy (DiLollo et al. 2002) components into our traditional speech-language pathology stuttering treatments.

◆ Conclusion

It can be a demanding task to help an adolescent or adult who has had many years to develop what can be less than ideal strategies for negotiating communication situations. Because stuttering, especially in teens and adults, is a dynamically changing, multidimensional problem strongly influenced by fear and feelings of helplessness, it may take several cycles of treatment, sometimes with different clinicians, before things begin to come together and the client begins to achieve lasting success. It is important for clinicians, especially those who are just beginning in the field, to understand that success is possible and some speakers are able to achieve spontaneous fluency that is indistinguishable from the speech of nonstuttering speakers. There are adults who have stuttered (and some who still do) who are more confident about communicating than adults who have never stuttered (Hillis & Manning, 1996). Even with some residual stuttering, they can be extremely successful communicators.

Successful treatment does not appear to depend so much on the overall treatment strategy and its associated clinical techniques. It has been suggested in our field (Van Riper, 1975; Manning, 2001; 2006) and demonstrated in related fields (Wampold, 2001) that the quality of the clinician is a critical variable in the process of therapeutic change. The more influential factors appear to be clinician allegiance to the treatment protocol, the quality of the therapeutic alliance of the client and the clinician, and the expertise of the clinician. As the speaker is able to predict and become gradually more accepting and comfortable with the successes related to the achievement of fluency, he or she typically begins to develop an agentic lifestyle.

In constructivist literature, agency is thought of as "the extent to which individuals can act for themselves and speak on their own behalf" (Monk, Winslade, Crocket, & Epston, 1997, p. 301). Agency is created in spite of an undesired but dominant discourse and associated themes, and success involves a deliberate break from the influence of such themes (Monk et al., 1997). As Drewery, Winslade, & Monk (2000) state: "Health, in our view, has much to do with the capacity for agency and less to do with the absence of disease" (p. 256). In our clinical pursuit of the client's fluency it is important to appreciate that agency, or the ability of the person to live his or her life and achieve a voice in a literal as well as a metaphorical sense, is not dependent on total fluency. It's more profound and considerably more exciting than that.

References

Anderson, T. K. & Felsenfeld, S. (2003) A thematic analysis of late recovery from stuttering. American Journal of Speech-Language Pathology, 12, 243–253.

Andrews, G., Guitar, B., & Howie. P. (1980). Meta-analysis of the effects of stuttering treatment. Journal of Speech and Hearing Disorders 45, 287–307.

Bandura, A. (1977). Self-Efficacy: Toward a unifying theory of behavioral change. Psychological Review 84, 191–215.

Blood, G. (1995). POWER²: Relapse management with adolescents who stutter. Language, Speech, and Hearing Services in Schools 26, 169–179.

Boberg, E., & Kully, D. (1995). The comprehensive stuttering program. In C. W. Starkweather & H. F. M. Peters (Eds.), Stuttering: Proceedings of the 1st World Congress on Fluency Disorders (pp 305–308). Munich: International Fluency Association.

Botterill, W., & Cook. F. (1987). Personal construct theory and the treatment of adolescent dysfluency. In: L. Rustin, H. Purser, & D. Rowley (Eds.), Progress in the treatment of fluency disorders (pp. 147–165). London: Taylor Francis.

Braithwaite, J. (2002). Rules and principles: A theory of legal certainty. Australian Journal of Legal Philosophy 27, 47–82.

Brown, S., Ingham, R. J., Ingham, J. C., Laird, A. R., & Fox, P. T. (2005). Stuttered and fluent speech production: An ALE meta-analysis of functional neuroimaging studies. Human Brain Mapping 25, 105–117.

Brisk, D. J., Healey, E. C., & Hux, K. A. (1997). Clinicians' training and confidence associated with treating school-age children who stutter: A national survey. Language, Speech, and Hearing Services in Schools 28, 164–176.

Brutten, G. J., & Shoemaker, D. J. (1967). The modification of stuttering. Englewood Cliffs, NJ: Prentice-Hall.

Chmela, K., & Reardon, N. (1997). The emotions of stuttering. Presentation to the annual Conference on Stuttering Therapy: Practical Ideas for the School Clinician, Memphis, TN.

Conture, E. (2001) Stuttering, Its nature, diagnosis, and treatment. Boston: Allyn & Bacon.

Cooper, E. B. (1977) Controversies about stuttering therapy. Journal of Fluency Disorders 2, 75–86

Cooper, E. B, & Cooper, C. S. (1985).The effective clinician. In E. B. Cooper & C. S. Cooper (Eds.), Personalized fluency control therapy - revised. Allen, TX: DLM 21-31.

Corcoran, J. A., & Stewart, M.(1998). Stories of stuttering: A qualitative analysis of interview narratives. Journal of Fluency Disorders 23, 247–264.

Craig, A., & Andrews, G. (1985). The prediction and prevention of relapse in stuttering. The value of self-control techniques and locus of control measures. Behav Modif 9, 427–442.

Craig, A., & Hancock, K. (1995). Self-reported factors related to relapse following treatment for stuttering. Australian Journal of Human Communication Disorders 23, 48–60.

Craig, A. R., Franklin, J. A., & Andrews, G. (1984). A scale to measure locus of control behavior. Br J Med Psychol 57, 173–180.

Culatta, R., & Goldberg, S. A. (1995). Stuttering therapy: An integrated approach to theory and practice. Boston: Allyn & Bacon.

Dalton, P. (1983). Psychological approaches to the treatment of stuttering. In P. Dalton (Ed.), Approaches to the Treatment of Stuttering. London: Croom Helm.

Daly, D., Simon, C., & Burnett-Stolnack, M. (1995). Helping adolescents who stutter focus on fluency. Language, Speech, and Hearing Services in Schools 26, 162–168.

De Nil, L. F., & Kroll, R. M. (1995). The relationship between locus of control and long-term stuttering treatment outcome in adult stutterers. Journal of Fluency Disorders 20, 345–364.

De Nil, L. F., & Kroll, R. M. (2001). Searching for the neural basis of stuttering treatment outcome: recent neuroimaging studies. Clin Linguist Phon 15, 163–168.

DiClemente, C. C. (1993). Changing addictive behaviors: a process perspective. Curr Dir Psychol Sci 2, 101–106.

DiLollo, A., Manning, W., & Neimeyer, R. (2003). Cognitive anxiety as a function of speaker role for fluent speakers and persons who stutter. Journal of Fluency Disorders 28(3), 167–186.

DiLollo, A., Neimeyer, R., & Manning, W. (2002). A personal construct psychology view of relapse: indications for a narrative therapy component to stuttering treatment. Journal of Fluency Disorders 27(1), 19–42.

Drewery, W., Winslade, J., & Monk, G. (2000). Resisting the dominating story: Toward a deeper understanding of narrative therapy. In R. Neimeyer & J. D. Raskin (Eds.), Constructions of disorder (pp. 253–263). Washington, DC: American Psychological Association.

Egan, G. (1994). The skilled helper: A problem-management approach to helping. Pacific Grove, CA: Brooks/Cole Publishing.

Emerick, L. (1988). Counseling adults who stutter: A cognitive approach. Seminars in Speech and Language 9(3), 257–267.

Ericsson, A. K., & Smith, J. (1991). Prospects and limits of the empirical study of expertise: an introduction. In A. K. Ericsson & J. Smith (Eds.), Toward a general theory of expertise: prospects and limits. Cambridge: Cambridge University Press. 1–38.

Finn P. (1996). Establishing the validity of recovery from stuttering without formal treatment. Journal of Speech and Hearing Research 39(6), 1171–1181.

Finn, P. (1997). Adults recovered from stuttering without formal treatment: Perceptual assessment of speech normalcy. Journal of Speech, Language, and Hearing Research 40, 821–831.

Franken, M. C., Van der Schalk, K., & Boelens, H. H. (2005). Experimental treatment of early stuttering: A preliminary study. Journal of Fluency Disorders 30, 189–19.

Fransella, F. (1972). Personal Change and Reconstruction: Research on a treatment of stuttering. London: Academic Press.

Fransella, F. (1992). Personal change and reconstruction. London: Academic Press.

Guitar B. (1998). Stuttering: An integrated approach to its nature and treatment. Baltimore: Williams & Wilkins.

Gregory, H. H. (1973). Stuttering: Differential evaluation and therapy. Indianapolis, IL: Bobbs-Merrill.

Haig, R. A. (1986). Therapeutic uses of humor. American Journal of Psychotherapy 40(4), 543–553.

Hillis, J. W. (1993). Ongoing assessment in the management of stuttering: A clinical perspective. American Journal of Speech-Language Pathology 2(1), 24–37.

Hillis, J., & Manning, W. (1996). Extraclinical generalization of speech fluency: A social cognitive approach. Presentation to the annual meeting of the American Speech-Language-Hearing Association, Seattle, WA.

Howie, P., & Andrews, G. (1984). Treatment of adult stutterers: Managing fluency. In R. Curlee & W. Perkins (Eds.), Nature and treatment of stuttering (pp. 424–445). Austin, TX: PRO-ED.

Huinck, W. J., & Peters, H. F. M. (2004). Effect of speech therapy on stuttering: Evaluating three therapy programs. Paper presented at the IALP Congress, Brisbane.

Ingham, J. C. (1993). Current status of stuttering and behavior modification-I: Recent trends in the application of behavior modification in children and adults. Journal of Fluency Disorders 18, 27–55.

Ingham, R. J., & Cordes, A. K. (1997). Self-measurement and evaluating stuttering treatment efficacy. In R. F. Curlee & G. M. Siegel (Eds.), Nature and Treatment of Stuttering, New Directions (2nd ed.) (pp 413–437). Allyn & Bacon, Boston.

Ingham, R. J., Martin, R. R., & Kuhl, P. (1974). Modification and control of rate of speaking by stutterers. Journal of Speech and Hearing Research 17, 489–496.

Jezer, M. (1997). Stuttering: a life bound up in words. Basic Books: New York.

Kimmel, D. C. (1974). Adulthood and aging. New York: John Wiley and Sons.

Kelly. G. A. (1955). The psychology of personal constructs. Vol. 1. New York: Norton.

Kubler Ross, E. (1969). On death and dying. New York: Simon and Schuster.

Kuhr, A., & Rustin, L. (1985). The maintenance of fluency after intensive inpatient therapy: Long-term follow-up. Journal of Fluency Disorders 10, 229–236.

Ladouceur, R., Caron, C., & Caron, G. (1989). Stuttering severity and treatment outcome. Journal of Behavior Therapy and Experimental Psychiatry 20, 49–56.

Langevin, M., & Kully, D. (2003). Evidenced-based treatment of stuttering: III. Evidence-based practice in a clinical setting. Journal of Fluency Disorders 28, 219–236.

Levitt, H. M., Neimeyer, R. A., & Williams, D. (2004). Rules vs. principles in psychotherapy: Implications of the quest for universal guidelines in the movement for empirically supported treatments. Journal of Contemporary Psychotherapy 35(1), 117–129.

Luterman, D. M. (1991). Counseling the communicatively disordered and their families (2nd ed.). Austin, TX: PRO-ED.

Lyddon, W. J. (1989). Personal epistemology and preference for counseling. Journal of Counseling Psychology 36, 423–429.

Lyddon, W. J. (1991). Epistemic style: Implications for cognitive psychotherapy. Psychotherapy 28, 588–597.

Manning, W. (2001). Clinical decision making in fluency disorders (2nd ed.). San Diego, CA: Singular Publishing.

Manning, W. (2003). Counseling adolescents who stutter. Perspectives in Fluency and Fluency Disorders 13, 11–14.

Manning, W. H. (1991). Making progress during and after treatment. In: W. H. Perkins (Ed.) Seminars in speech and language (12, pp. 349–354). New York: Thieme.

Manning, W. H. (1994). The SEA-Scale: Self-efficacy scaling for adolescents who stutter. Presented at the annual meeting of the American Speech-Language-Hearing Association, New Orleans.

Manning, W. H. (2004). How can you understand? You don't stutter! Contemporary Issues in Communication Science and Disorders 31, 58–68.

Manning, W. H. (2006). Therapeutic change and the nature of our evidence: Improving our ability to help. In N. Bernstein Ratner & J. Tetnowski (Eds.),Current issues in stuttering research and practice (pp. 125–158). Mahwah, NJ: Lawrence Earlbaum, Inc.

Manning, W., Perkins, D., Winn, S., & Cole, D. (1984). Self-efficacy changes during treatment and maintenance for adult stutterers. Paper presented to the annual meeting of the American Speech-Language-Hearing Association, San Francisco.

Manning, W., Thaxton, D., & Ells, A. (1997). Listener response to stuttering versus modification techniques. Paper presented at the 2nd World Congress on Fluency Disorders, San Francisco.

Maslow, A. (1968). Towards a psychology of being (2nd ed.). Princeton: Van Nostrand.

Max, L., & Caruso, A. (1997). Contemporary techniques for establishing fluency in the treatment of adults who stutter. Contemporary Issues in Communication Science and Disorders 24, 45–52.

Maxwell, D. (1982). Cognitive and behavioral self-control strategies: Applications for the clinical management of adult stutterers. Journal of Fluency Disorders 7, 403–432.

Monk, G., Winslade, J., Crocket, K., & Epston, D. (1997). Narrative therapy in practice. San Francisco: Jossey-Bass Publishers.

Murphy, B. (1999). A preliminary look at shame, guilt, and stuttering. In N.B. Ratner & E. C. Healey (Eds.), Stuttering research and practice: Bridging the gap (pp.131–143). Mahwah, NJ: Lawrence Erlbaum.

Neilsen, M., & Andrews, G. (1993). Intensive fluency training of chronic stutters. In. R. F. Curlee (Ed.), Stuttering

and related disorders of fluency (pp. 139–165). New York: Thieme.

Neimeyer, R. A. (2000). Lessons of loss: A guide to coping. Keystone, FL: PsychoEducational Resources, Inc.

Neumann, K., Preibisch, C., Euler, H. A, et al. (2005). Cortical plasticity associated with stuttering therapy. Journal of Fluency Disorders 30, 1, 23–39.

O'Brian, S., Onslow, M., Cream, A., & Packman, A. (2003). The Camperdown Program: Outcomes of a new prolonged-speech treatment model. Journal of Speech, Language, and Hearing Research 46, 933–946.

Ornstein, A. F., & Manning, W. H. (1985). Self-efficacy scaling by adult stutterers. Journal of Communication Disorders 18, 313–320.

Peck, M. S. (1978). The road less traveled. New York: Simon and Schuster.

Perkins, W. H. (1979). From psychoanalysis to discoordination. In H. H. Gregory (Ed.), Controversies about stuttering therapy (pp. 97–127). Baltimore: University Park Press.

Perkins, W. H. (1984). Techniques for establishing fluency. In W. H. Perkins (Ed.), Stuttering disorders (pp.173–181). New York: Thieme-Stratton.

Plexico, L., Manning, W., & DiLollo, A. (2005). A phenomenological understanding of successful stuttering management. Journal of Fluency Disorders 30(1), 1–22.

Prochaska ,J. O., & DiClemente, C. C. (1986). Toward a comprehensive model of change. In R. W. Miller & N. Heather (Eds.), treating addictive behaviors, process of change (pp. 3–28). New York: Plenum.

Prochaska, J. O., & DiClemente, C. C. (1992). Stages of change in the modification of problem behaviors. In M. Herson, R. Eisler, & R. Miller (Eds.), Progress in behavior modification (pp 184–218). Sycamore, IL: Sycamore Publishing Company.

Prochaska. J. O., DiClemente, C. C., & Norcross, J. C. (1992). In search of how people change: applications to addictive behaviors. Am Psychol 47(9), 1102–1114.

Quesal, R. (2003). Evidenced-based practice in stuttering: Current controversies and considerations. The Newsletter of the Illinois Speech-Language-Hearing Association 29(2), 10–11.

Rabinowitz, A. (2001) Beyond the last village. Washington: Island Press, Shearwater.

Reeves, L. (2005). The role of self help/mutual aid in addressing the needs of individuals who stutter. In N. Bernstein Ratner & J. Tetnowski, (Eds.), Stuttering research and practice: Contemporary issues and approaches (pp. xx–xx). Mahwah, NJ: Lawrence Earlbaum, Inc. 255–278.

Riley, J., Riley, G., & McGuire, G. (2004). Subjective screening of stuttering severity, locus of control and avoidance: research edition. Journal of Fluency Disorders 29, 51–62.

Ryan, B. P. (1971). Operant procedures applied to stuttering therapy for children. Journal of Speech and Hearing Disorders 36, 264–280.

Shames, G.H., & Florence, CL. (1980). Stutter free speech: A goal for therapy. Columbus: Merrill.

Sheehy, G. (1974). Passages: Predictable crises of adult life. New York: Bantam

Silverman, F. H. (1992). Stuttering and other fluency disorders. Englewood Cliffs, NJ: Prentice-Hall.

Silverman, E. M., & Zimmer, C. H. (1982). Demographic characteristics and treatment experiences of women and men who stutter. Journal of Fluency Disorders 7, 273–185.

Simons, A. D., Lustman, P. J., Wetzel, R. D., & Murphy, G. E. (1985). Predicting response to cognitive therapy of depression: The role of learned resourcefulness. Cognitive Therapy and Research 9, 79–89.

Smith, A. (1999). Stuttering: A unified approach to a multi-factorial, dynamic disorder. In N. B. Ratner & E. C. Healey (Eds.), Stuttering research and practice: Bridging the gap (pp. 27–44). Mahwah, NJ: Lawrence Erlbaum.

Stewart. T., & Richardson, G. (2004). A qualitative study of therapeutic effect from a user's perspective. Journal of Fluency Disorders 29, 95–108.

St. Louis, K. O. (1999). Person-first labeling and stuttering. Journal of Fluency Disorders 24, 1–24.

St. Louis, K. O., & Westbrook, J. B. (1987). The effectiveness of treatment for stuttering. In L. Rustin, H. Purser, & D. Rowley, (Eds.), Progress in the treatment of fluency disorders (pp 235–257). London: Taylor & Francis.

Valiant, G. E. (1977). Adaptation to life. Boston: Little, Brown, and Co.

Van Riper, C. (1971). The nature of stuttering. Englewood Cliffs, NJ: Prentice-Hall.

Van Riper, C. (1973). The treatment of stuttering. Englewood Cliffs, NJ: Prentice-Hall.

Van Riper, C. (1975). The stutterer's clinician. In Jon Eisenson (Ed.), Stuttering, a second symposium (pp. 453–492). New York: Harper & Row.

Van Riper, C. (1989). Modifying the stuttering. In C. W. Starkweather (Ed.), Therapy for stutterers (pp 61–73). Memphis, TN: Stuttering Foundation of America.

Van Riper, C., & Erickson, R. L. (1996) Speech correction: An Introduction to speech pathology and audiology (9th ed.). Needham Heights: Allyn & Bacon.

Wampold, B. E. (2001). The great psychotherapy debate: Models, methods, and findings. Mahwah, NJ: Lawrence Erlbaum Associates.

Watson, J. B. (1998). A comparison of stutterers and nonstutterers affective, cognitive, and behavioral self reports. Journal of Speech and Hearing Research 31, 377–385.

White, M., & Epston, D. (1990). Narrative means to therapeutic ends. New York: Norton.

Winslade, J. & Monk, G. (1999). Narrative counseling in Schools: Powerful & brief. Thousand Oaks, CA: Corwin Press, Inc.

World Health Organization. (2001). International classification of functioning, disability, and health. Geneva: World Health Organization.

Yaruss, J. S., & Quesal, R. W. (2004). Stuttering and the International Classification of Functioning, Disability, and Health (ICF): An update. Journal of Communication Disorders 37, 35–52.

Yaruss, J. S., & Quesal, R. W. (2006). Overall Assessment of the Speaker's Experience of Stuttering (OASES): Documenting multiple outcomes in stuttering treatment. Journal of Fluency Disorders 31(2), 90–115.

14

Self-Help and Mutual Aid Groups as an Adjunct to Stuttering Therapy

J. Scott Yaruss, Robert W. Quesal, and Lee Reeves

The purpose of this chapter is to discuss several ways that self-help groups can serve as an adjunct to stuttering therapy. Specifically, the chapter describes how self-help or mutual aid groups can help people who stutter to receive greater benefits from the therapy they receive, achieve gains in communication even if they are not successful in therapy, or find ways of helping themselves if they decide not to participate in formal therapy. The chapter begins with a brief review of the history of self-help groups for people who stutter, including an overview of currently available self-help groups and other supportive resources for individuals who stutter and their families. The chapter continues with an exploration of the potential benefits of self-help group participation, including a summary of presently available research data pertaining to stuttering support groups. Finally, the chapter concludes with a discussion of service models that incorporate self-help groups as an adjunct to speech therapy to enhance treatment outcomes for children and adults who stutter.

Considerable evidence indicates that people who stutter can achieve substantive improvements in speech fluency, reductions in negative reactions to stuttering, and improvements in overall communication skills through therapeutic intervention (see reviews in Andrews, Guitar, & Howie, 1980; Blood, 1993; Bloodstein, 1995; Conture, 1996; Cordes, 1998; Thomas & Howell, 2001). Several methods for achieving these and other clinical goals are described in this book, and it is clear that many people who stutter have experienced success through a variety of commonly used treatment approaches. Still, not all people who stutter experience the same degree of success in treatment, even though they may have participated in speech therapy on several occasions (Yaruss, Quesal, Reeves, et al, 2002). In addition, even those individuals who are successful in treatment may have difficulty transferring gains in speech fluency or communication attitudes to "real-world" settings (see reviews in Hillis & McHugh, 1998; Ingham & Onslow, 1987). They may also face challenges in maintaining changes over time, as evidenced by the high relapse rates reported for some treatment approaches (Boberg, 1981; Craig, 1998).

There are many reasons that people who stutter may not attain or maintain optimal treatment outcomes. Some individuals may find that goals of a particular treatment are not consistent with their own needs and goals, or they may not be comfortable using speaking techniques during everyday, conversational speech. Others may feel that treatment strategies, such as fluency shaping or stuttering modification, are too difficult to be used consistently in different speaking situations, or they may not prefer the quality or naturalness of their speech when they use the modifications learned in therapy. Still others may not have participated fully in their treatment program or they may not have followed their clinician's recommendations for practice or generalization. Regardless of the specific reasons for some individuals' lack of success, it is clear that speech therapy—just like any form of therapeutic intervention—does not provide the same benefits for all people. This appears to be true no matter what the specific nature of the treatment program may be, for as reported in the reviews cited above, there does not appear to be any single approach to therapy that works for all people at all times or in all situations.

Helping individuals who do not achieve either short- or long-term success in speech therapy presents a significant challenge to people who are interested in improving the lives of those who stutter. If clinicians and researchers are to develop treatment strategies that are effective for a broader range of people who stutter, various means of enhancing the outcomes of stuttering treatment should be considered. This chapter explores one such enhancement to stuttering treatment by describing some of the ways that participating in *self-help* or *mutual aid* groups can help people who stutter and their families achieve and maintain greater success, both in and out of therapy.

♦ A Brief History of Self-Help Groups for People Who Stutter and Their Families

Self-help groups have been defined as "voluntary, small group structures for mutual aid and the accomplishment of a special purpose...usually formed by peers who have come together for mutual assistance in satisfying a common need, overcoming a common handicap or life-disrupting problem and bringing about desired social and/or personal change" (Katz & Bender, 1976, p. 141). Self-help groups have been known by various names over the years, including "support groups" and, more recently "mutual aid groups." Some authors (e.g., Borkman, 1999) have differentiated between groups that are managed by professionals (i.e., support groups) and groups that primarily involve individuals experiencing difficulty, without direct management by a professional (i.e., self-help or mutual aid groups). To reduce confusion about the names for various types of groups, and in an attempt to adopt newer terminology, this chapter refers to all such groups as "self-help" or "mutual aid" groups without a distinguishing between those groups that involve professionals and those that do not. (Note that this does not apply to groups that were *originated* by professionals, such as therapy groups or maintenance groups associated with a particular method of treatment.)

The first self-help groups are said to have begun among ethnic communities in the United States in the mid-1800s, when immigrants joined together to help each other adjust to their new lives (Katz & Bender, 1976). In 1935, the concept of self-help was formalized with the creation of Alcoholics Anonymous, a structured meeting group based on the now widely used "twelve steps" and "twelve traditions." Since then, the number of self-help groups in the United States has grown to 500,000 (Adamsen & Rasmussen, 2001), and today, it is estimated that self-help groups exist for every condition identified by the World Health Organization (Banks, 2000). Indeed, a Google search for the term, "self-help," yielded more than 19 million Web sites at the time of the present writing.

Self-help groups for people who stutter had their formal beginning in the United States in the mid-1960s, although people who stutter had come together in small groups for mutual aid and support much earlier than that (e.g., the "Kingsley Clubs" described in an undated pamphlet on the history of the Stuttering Foundation of America). The first nationally recognized self-help group for stuttering, the *Council of Adult Stutterers*, was formed at Catholic University in Washington, DC, in 1965, with the assistance of speech-language pathologist Eugene Walle. According to Michael Heffron, one of the founders of that group, the purpose of the Council was to provide an opportunity for people who stutter "to help themselves and to help other people who stutter" (cited in Van Riper, 1973, p. 169). Before long, independent but related groups of adults who stutter were formed in other states, and the organization came to be known as the *National Council on Stuttering* (NCOS). A detailed description of the early days of stuttering self-help groups can be found in Borkman (1999).

Subsequently, in 1977, two other stuttering self-help organizations were created: *Speak Easy International*, founded in New Jersey by Bob Gathman, and the *National Stuttering Project* (NSP), founded in California by Michael Sugarman and Bob Goldman. These groups differed from the original NCOS, in that they sought to develop a network of related self-help groups under the umbrella of a broader regional or national organization (Reeves, 2006). In addition, the formation of Speak Easy and the NSP was generally driven by the efforts of people who stutter, rather than through partnerships with speech-language pathologists, as was originally true for the NCOS. Both of these newer groups were intended to help individuals who stutter provide mutual aid and support for one another, while raising awareness about stuttering and simultaneously advocating for the needs of people who stutter (Reeves, in press).

Over the years, the NSP, in particular, began to develop a national presence, with numerous local chapters across the nation, a national office, and annual conferences that brought together people who stutter from around the country. In 1997, these organizations were joined by *Friends: the National Association for Young People Who Stutter* (Friends), which was founded in New York by John Ahlbach and Lee Caggiano. Friends also hosts annual conferences and workshops, though it focuses exclusively on children who stutter and their families. All three of these groups, Speak Easy International, Friends, and the NSP, which is now known as the *National Stuttering Association* (or NSA), continue to operate, and it appears that the number of individuals participating in these and other stuttering groups is still growing worldwide (Krall, 2001; Ramig, 1993; Yaruss et al., 2002). Contact information for currently active self-help groups in the United States for people who stutter is included in **Table 14–1**.

Of course, the United States is not the only country that has seen a growth in the establishment of self-help and mutual aid groups for people who stutter. Canada, for example, is home to the *Canadian Association for People Who Stutter* (CAPS), the *Canadian Speak Easy*, the *British Canadian Association of*

Table 14–1   Self-Help/Mutual Aid and Related Groups for People Who Stutter in the United States

Friends: National Association of Young People Who Stutter
c/o Lee Caggiano
38 South Oyster Bay Rd.
Syosset, NY 11791
Phone: (866) 866–8335
Email: lcaggiano@aol.com
Web site: www.friendswhostutter.org

National Stuttering Association (NSA)
119 W. 40th St., 14th Floor
New York, NY 10018
Phone: (800) We Stutter (937–8888)
Email: info@WeStutter.org
Web site: www.WeStutter.org

Speak Easy International
c/o Bob Gathman
233 Concord Dr.
Paramus, NJ 07652
Phone: (201) 262–0895
Email: speakezusa@juno.com

Stuttering Foundation of America (SFA)
P.O. Box 11749
3100 Walnut Grove Road #603
Memphis, TN 38111
Phone: (800) 992–9392
Email: stutter@stutteringhelp.org
Web site: www.stutteringhelp.org

For a more complete list of self-help/mutual aid groups for people who stutter around the world, visit the Stuttering Home Page at www.stutteringhomepage.com.

People Who Stutter, and other similar groups. The *International Stuttering Association*, an umbrella organization linking stuttering self-help and mutual aid groups around the world, has member organizations in 35 countries, and many of these countries host more than one group. In fact, at the time of this writing, the Stuttering Home Page, an information clearinghouse developed by Judy Kuster of the Minnesota State University in Mankato, lists more than 60 distinct self-help groups for people around the world who stutter. (http://www.mnsu.edu/comdis/kuster/support.html). It is apparent that the number of people participating in self-help for stuttering (as well as the number of self-help organizations) continues to grow rapidly. Furthermore, there also appears to have been an increase in the number of speech-language pathologists who refer their clients to self-help groups (Cooper, 1987; Diggs, 1990; Ramig, 1993; Starkweather & Givens-Ackerman, 1997).

It is also worth noting that self-help and mutual aid groups are not the only types of organizations dedicated to helping people who stutter. Perhaps the most widely known stuttering organization in the United States—and around the world—is the *Stuttering Foundation of America* (SFA), which was founded by Malcolm Fraser in 1947. Although it is not a self-help or mutual aid organization, SFA provides many helpful resources for people who stutter and clinicians, and especially for the families of children who stutter. Most notable among these are the SFA's popular booklets, videos, and DVDs for parents of children who stutter and clinicians, which are mentioned throughout this chapter. A complete list of SFA materials is available at the Stuttering Foundation Web site, http://www.StutteringHelp.org, and various SFA materials are discussed in this chapter together with materials from self-help and mutual aid groups.

There are also many other, less formal groups for people who stutter, including Internet listservs (e.g., Stutt-L, founded by Woody Starkweather in 1985 (Starkweather, 1995) and chat rooms (e.g., the *stutteringchat* Yahoo group, founded in 2000 and having more than 2700 members registered at the time of this writing). Some speech-language pathologists also maintain "practice" therapy groups or discussion groups for their clients (e.g., Yaruss & Soifer, 1998). Such groups give clients the opportunity to practice the skills learned in therapy, either during therapy as a formal part of a treatment program, or following therapy to support long-term maintenance of therapy gains. In many cases, these practice groups may be viewed as a type of self-help group, for they provide people who stutter with the chance to help one another achieve success both in and out of treatment. Regardless of the specific structure of a group, it is clear that, throughout the world, there are numerous opportunities for people who stutter to interact with one another, to share experiences, and to provide each other with needed support in overcoming the challenges associated with their stuttering. The next section examines some of the specific benefits people who stutter indicate that they gain through participation in stuttering self-help groups.

◆ Self-Help Groups for People Who Stutter

Benefits Reported by Participants

The benefits of participating in self-help groups have been reported for a wide variety of conditions (e.g., Borkman, 1999; Katz, 1993; Katz & Bender, 1976, 1987), and research on the benefits of self-help and mutual aid groups has been ongoing in many fields for decades. An annotated bibliography prepared by Kyrouz and Humphries (2002) lists numerous peer-reviewed studies on the effectiveness of self-help groups in assisting people with a variety of conditions, including addiction, bereavement, cancer, chronic illness, diabetes, mental health concerns, and other difficulties. Such studies have also examined the benefits of self-help groups for caregivers, the elderly, and those seeking to lose weight. As Kyrouz and Humphries report, research in these and other fields has included interviews, questionnaire- and observation-based studies, and experimental designs, as well as large-scale record reviews, direct group comparison, randomized control trials, and meta-analyses. Results have demonstrated that the benefits of self-help group participation can include: better short-term and long-term success with treatment goals, both in and out of treatment; enhanced ability to maintain goals across environments; increases in social attachment and interpersonal skills; benefits in general health, emotional well-being, adjustment, and self-confidence; enhanced understanding of the condition faced by self-help participants; and improvements in several other variables directly related to treatment outcomes and quality of life. Thus, it appears that people can benefit from support group participation, regardless of the specific nature of the concerns they are facing. Particularly relevant to self-help groups for stuttering was the finding that the benefits of self-help were not limited to the psychological realm; they also included positive changes in behavior management and long-term maintenance of treatment outcomes.

Within the field of stuttering, relatively few empirical studies (including primarily questionnaire-based research) have sought to determine why people who stutter participate in self-help groups or to evaluate the benefits group members may receive. It is worth noting that all of the studies conducted thus far have examined self-help groups for *adults* who stutter. Although there are a growing number of services available for young children who stutter and their families, as well as for school-age children and teens who stutter, there is, thus far, no empirical research that has examined self-help for these populations. Further research is clearly needed.

In the early days of stuttering self-help groups, it was suggested that many members participated because they felt that traditional treatment had failed to help them achieve or maintain their goals (Bradberry, 1997; Cooper, 1987; Ramig, 1993). Empirical investigations, however, highlighted several other reasons that people participate in stuttering self-help. For example, in a questionnaire-based survey of members of the NSP (now the NSA), Krauss-Lehrman and Reeves (1989) found that participants reported benefits from group activities such as "sharing feelings, thoughts, and experiences," and "speaking in a non-threatening place." In another survey, Ramig (1993) found that self-help participants believed that their attendance at meetings and their interactions with others who stutter had helped them feel better about themselves and had improved their confidence. Similarly, Yaruss et al. (2002) found that the majority of respondents in a survey of 71 NSA members felt that group participation had improved their self-image. Positive findings about support group participation are not limited to groups found in the United States. In a survey by Hunt (1987), adults in Britain's Association for Stammerers (AFS) reported that participation facilitated not only attitudinal changes, but also their ability to maintain speech fluency gains over time. Thus, just as was reported in the broad review of self-help research presented by Kyrouz & Humphries (2002) described above, people who stutter indicate that they experience a wide range of benefits from participation in self-help groups. In addition to these findings, there is a considerable amount of less formal evidence highlighting benefits people receive from stuttering self-help groups. As Yaruss et al. (2002) summarized, many people have described their experiences with self-help groups in memoirs (e.g., Jezer, 1997), collections of personal stories (e.g., Ahlbach & Benson, 1994; Hood, 1998; St. Louis, 2001), and online discussion groups (e.g., Starkweather, 1995).

Through these studies and anecdotal reports, people who stutter have indicated that their participation in self-help groups helped them to focus on aspects of their stuttering disorder that were not addressed to the same degree, or at all, in traditional treatment. Still, it does not appear that people who stutter participate in self-help groups solely because they feel that their treatment was unsuccessful. For example, 75% of the respondents in the Krauss-Lehrman and Reeves (1989) study reported that their treatment was successful to varying degrees. A similar finding was reported by Yaruss et al. (2002). It seems, therefore, that at least some people who stutter seek out self-help groups as a way of *supplementing* their speech therapy experiences. This finding will be considered in more detail later, in our discussion of ways that speech therapy and self-help may be combined to help people who stutter achieve improved treatment outcomes. First, several other potential benefits of self-help groups will be reviewed to provide a more complete picture of the services provided by current self-help groups.

Other Benefits and Outreach Programs

In addition to offering opportunities for people to engage in personal interaction through local chapters and online connections, self-help groups also serve several other functions for people who stutter and their families, as well as for clinicians and researchers interested in stuttering. Specific examples of the benefits offered by stuttering self-help groups can be categorized in terms of "meetings and conferences," "published material," and "other services." (Note: although it is not a self-help group, the SFA also provides numerous resources that can be used by individuals who stutter, their families, and their clinicians. Therefore, SFA materials are included throughout the following review to ensure that readers are aware of helpful information from a variety of sources.)

Meetings and Conferences

A particularly important aspect of the self-help experience involves personal interactions. As described above, this can be accomplished through regular meetings of local chapters, which may bring together as few as two or three people, or as many as a dozen or more. Such interactions can also be facilitated on a much larger scale through regional or national conferences and workshops that may involve several hundred people. Examples of the types of meetings and conferences hosted by current self-help and related organizations include:

- *Annual conferences* gather people who stutter, their families, speech-language pathologists, and researchers from around the country. In 2005, for example, more than 600 people gathered in Chicago for the NSA's 22nd annual conference. That same year, Friends held its 8th annual conference and drew participants from around the country, and at the time of this writing, Speak Easy International was planning its 25th annual symposium in 2006.

- *Youth and family day* programs focus specifically on the needs of children who stutter and their families, as well as the clinicians who serve them in school settings. These workshops provide advanced clinical training for speech-language pathologists as well as support and self-help for children and their families.

- *Regional conferences* and *continuing education (CE) workshops* provide education for speech-language pathologists concerning the diagnosis and treatment of stuttering. The most well-known and widely attended CE conferences are those hosted by the SFA around the country each year. Because CE activities help to educate the professionals who directly interact with people who stutter, both the NSA and Friends also host CE workshops as part of their broader mission to improve clinical services for children and adults who stutter and their families.

Published Materials

Personal contact is a primary means of providing support for self-help groups. Still, published materials offer another meaningful way for organizations to communicate with individuals who stutter and their families. Following are several examples of the publications provided by stuttering self-help groups, such as Friends, the NSA, and the SFA. For a more complete list of resources, readers should visit the Web sites listed below.

- *Newsletters* provide background information about stuttering and speech therapy, share news about individuals in the stuttering community, and inform members about upcoming events. Newsletters also provide opportunities for members (including adults who stutter, teens and school-age children who stutter, and family members) to share their personal stories of success in dealing with stuttering. Examples of newsletters, which are typically available primarily to subscribing members, include the *NSA's Letting Go* for adults, *Our Voice* for teens, *Stutter Buddies* for school-age children, and *CARE: Connections, Advocacy, Resources, and Empowerment* for parents of children who stutter. Friends publishes *Reaching Out*, which is particularly geared for children. The SFA publishes a newsletter that focuses on the efforts of that organization, including information about stuttering research and other events of interest to people who stutter and speech-language pathologists.

- *Web sites* provide information for individuals interested in stuttering. In recent years there has been a growing emphasis on informative Web sites, including those of the NSA (www.WeStutter.org),

Friends (www.FriendsWhoStutter.org), and the SFA (www.StutteringHelp.org). Through their Web sites, each of these organizations provides information not only about the organization itself, but also about stuttering and stuttering treatment in general. Another notable website that provides online support for people who stutter is the Stuttering Homepage mentioned previously (www.Stuttering Homepage.com).

- *Brochures and pamphlets* educate members, clinicians, and the public about the nature of stuttering, treatment options for people who stutter, strategies for handling challenging situations, and other issues related to the daily experiences of those who stutter and their families. Examples of brochures and pamphlets produced by the SFA include: *If You Think Your Child Is Stuttering* for parents, and *Using the Telephone* for adults who stutter. Examples from the self-help groups include the *Stuttering Presentation Guide,* which is available on the Friends Web site, and the *NSA's Notes to Listeners* and *Information for Educators.* Some of these materials can be downloaded for free from the Web sites listed above, whereas others can be purchased for a nominal fee.

- *Booklets* address key topics for people who stutter or their families. The SFA has produced many excellent booklets for many years, including *Stuttering and Your Child: Questions and Answers,* for parents and *Sometimes I Just Stutter,* for children ages 7 to 12. Recently, the NSA has created booklets that address specific issues raised by the stuttering community. Examples include *Young Children Who Stutter*, which provides guidance for parents about how to help their children, and *Bullying and Teasing: Helping Children Who Stutter*, which contains strategies for minimizing the likelihood that children who stutter will experience bullying and inappropriate teasing.

- *Posters and other materials* can also be used by speech-language pathologists and teachers in classrooms and therapy settings to minimize the possibility that children who stutter will be singled out or bullied in school. Examples include the Friends' Kids poster, which features children who stutter sharing messages of hope and encouragement, as well as the NSA's *Stutter Buddies* poster, which depicts popular newsletter characters modeling different ways of coping successfully with stuttering. In addition, Friends, the NSA, and the SFA have created posters highlighting *Famous People Who Stutter*, to remind members that people who stutter have reached great heights in their lives, regardless of the fact that they stuttered.

- *Videotapes, CDs, and DVDs* highlight the stuttering experience from the perspective of individuals who stutter. For example, the SFA has produced several helpful videotapes, and more recently, DVDs, that provide information for people whose lives are affected by stuttering. Although the majority of these materials are geared toward professionals, a new DVD, *Stuttering: for Kids by Kids,* provides an entertaining and informative overview of stuttering for young children. Video offerings from self-help groups are more limited, although the *NSA* has recently produced *Transcending Stuttering: The Inside Story* (Schneider, 2004), which uniquely describes the types of positive changes that people who stutter may experience during their lives. Groups such as the NSA and Friends also sell materials produced by other organizations to make it easier for members to gain access to information about stuttering.

Other Services

Finally, self-help and similar organizations have other means of supporting the cause of people who stutter. Examples include:

- *Toll-free hotlines and email addresses* give people the opportunity to get information about stuttering. Hotlines can be used by people who stutter, families of children who stutter, teachers and speech-language pathologists, the media, and others who are interested in learning more about stuttering and stuttering self-help services. For Friends, the number is 866–866–8335; for the NSA, it is 800–937–8888 (800 We-Stutter); and for the SFA, the number is 800–992–9392.

♦ *Research facilitation* provides opportunities for members to interact with scientists who are investigating stuttering, as well as to read descriptions of research projects that members can join if they wish. For example, the NSA's Research Committee (NSARC) receives and reviews requests from investigators seeking to recruit participants for research studies. The committee facilitates interactions between scientists and members for approved projects through mailings and emails, announcements in NSA newsletters, and direct contact at group meetings. The NSARC also hosted a joint symposium for people who stutter, clinicians, and scientists that aimed to improve communication about stuttering (Yaruss & Reeves, 2002). The SFA is also active in supporting research on stuttering. It provides regular updates on stuttering research in its newsletters, as well as support for research and related activities. A summary of the SFA's research activities is available on the organization's Web site.

♦ *Miscellaneous services.* In addition to the specific tasks described above, self-help and related organizations also provide other services to their members on a daily basis by maintaining and facilitating contact among members, answering inquiries from the public and the media for stories and news items about stuttering, developing promotional and public service announcements that increase public awareness and understanding about stuttering, responding to inaccurate or misleading stories with up-to-date information about stuttering, and generally seeking to correct misconceptions about stuttering so that people who stutter can get the most out of their lives without encountering discrimination and misunderstanding.

Although many of the functions described in the preceding paragraphs are designed to help support group participants and to provide public advocacy about stuttering, stuttering self-help groups also spend considerable effort and energy supporting speech-language pathologists. This is because clinicians are among the primary sources of new members for self-help groups (Yaruss et al., 2002). Furthermore, if self-help groups wish to improve the treatment of people who stutter, they must work directly with the clinicians who provide that treatment. Therefore, self-help organizations have increasingly sought to partner with speech-language pathologists and to enhance interactions between self-help and speech therapy. That interaction is the focus of the next section of this chapter.

♦ Interactions between Self-Help and Speech Therapy

Although stuttering self-help and mutual aid groups have been formally available for nearly 30 years, the community of speech-language pathologists has only recently begun to explore, in earnest, the many ways that self-help groups and professionals can partner with one another to improve treatment for individuals who stutter. It is safe to say that the relationship between consumer and professional groups was less cordial during the early years of the stuttering self-help movement. Gregory (1997) expressed the distrust that at least some speech-language pathologists apparently felt toward self-help groups, citing the belief that people participating in such groups were not taking "constructive action" (p. 405) to help themselves overcome stuttering. Of course, at least some members of stuttering self-help groups have also expressed their concerns about the speech-language pathology profession in various forums.

In recent years, however, there have been notable improvements in the relationship between self-help group participants and speech-language pathologists (e.g., Manning, 2001; Reeves, in press), and this trend is consistent with that described for other disorders (Adamsen & Rasmussen, 2001). Support for this statement is reflected in the many ways that speech-language pathologists and people who stutter now come together to collaborate on solutions to shared concerns. For example, speech-language pathologists have played an increasingly active role in the stuttering community, by serving on the boards of directors of prominent self-help groups, by partnering in the development of support and educational materials, and by attending and participating in workshops and conferences hosted by self-help groups. Indeed, at a recent national stuttering conference hosted by a support group, speech-language pathologists made up more than 20% of the participants. Conversely, a growing number of self-help group members have played active and vital roles in professional activities, by serving on committees of the American Speech-Language-Hearing Association (ASHA), by participating in the profession's recognition of clinicians who are specialists in stuttering, and by presenting invited workshops and seminars at ASHA conventions. Self-help organizations have worked directly to foster and develop this relationship by preparing materials designed to meet the specific needs of speech-language pathologists, by hosting continuing education workshops, and by facilitating research efforts. The efforts of one self-help group to enhance the work of speech-language pathologists were recognized in 2002 when ASHA presented the NSA with its prestigious Distinguished Service Award. The SFA has also been the recipient of this award, recognizing the excellent support that this organization has provided to speech-language pathologists over many years.

Further evidence for the growing collaboration and alignment between professionals and members of the self-help community can be seen in the fact that this chapter on stuttering self-help groups appears in a text on the treatment of stuttering. Although self-help has been mentioned in several earlier texts (e.g., Manning, 2001), this may be the first time that an entire chapter in an academic text has been devoted to self-help groups for persons who stutter. Even the authorship of this chapter, which includes a speech-language pathologist who is not a person who stutters (Yaruss), a speech-language pathologist who stutters and who is also active in the self-help community (Quesal), and a prominent member of the stuttering self-help community who is not a speech-language pathologist (Reeves), reflects the growing bond between the self-help and professional communities.

Thus, despite an admittedly rocky start, the relationship between the professional and consumer communities now appears to be significantly improved, moving toward a stronger partnership between two groups that share common interests and goals. Clinicians can, therefore, begin to consider whether and how they should participate in this partnership. When one begins to explore options for developing such partnerships, however, some questions may arise. For example, when considering how people who are receiving stuttering therapy might learn about stuttering self-help groups, it is reasonable to ask whether it is appropriate for clinicians to refer their clients to self-help groups directly, as part of the educational counseling that is provided in therapy. If the clinician is going to make a direct referral, another question might relate to *which* clients should be referred to self-help groups and in what capacity (e.g., receiving newsletters only, attending local chapter meetings, or going to annual conferences). Other questions relate to the specific topics that should be addressed in therapy vs. self-help and that should be addressed through self-help, whether and how families should be involved in self-help, and how treatment and self-help participation should be scheduled (e.g., should clients complete therapy before joining a self-help group or should they participate in both opportunities simultaneously).

Unfortunately, relatively little empirical evidence can be found in the stuttering literature to provide answers to these questions. It is clear that some people who stutter do participate in self-help groups while they are still in therapy (Yaruss et al., 2002), and some clinicians inform their clients about self-help as a matter of standard practice (e.g., Reardon & Reeves, 2002; Reardon-Reeves & Yaruss, 2004). Still, questions about whether self-help and treatment should be pursued simultaneously and whether some people are more likely to benefit from self-help than others remain largely unanswered. In an attempt to provide some guidance to clinicians trying to determine how they should partner with self-help groups, the next section proposes several service-and-support delivery models that highlight possible interactions between self-help and therapy for people who stutter.

◆ Service-and-Support Delivery Models Incorporating Self-Help and Speech Therapy

When considering ways to integrate self-help with treatment for people who stutter, numerous possibilities come to mind. Although it is not known for certain, it is our experience and opinion that most people who stutter receive only treatment (i.e., they do not participate in self-help at all).

A much smaller number of people may participate only in self-help groups without receiving treatment. Others may participate in self-help groups only after they have completed treatment (whether successfully or unsuccessfully), and still others might participate in a self-help group while they are receiving treatment and continue with the self-help group after treatment has ended. The latter situation may reflect the experience of most current self-help members, based on survey results mentioned above (e.g., Yaruss et al., 2002) as well as a recent census of NSA members (McClure & Yaruss, 2003). Nevertheless, many respondents in the Yaruss et al. (2002) survey reported that their interest in receiving treatment actually increased as a result of their participation in self-help. This suggests that some people might return to treatment after spending some time in self-help, though others may participate in treatment and self-help in a recursive or iterative fashion, given the finding that most respondents in the Yaruss et al. (2002) survey had received treatment several times throughout their lives. A summary of these and other possible service-and-support delivery models is shown in **Table 14–2**.

The possible interactions between self-help and treatment become even more complex, in light of the fact that there are different forms of treatment (e.g., "traditional" face-to-face treatment sessions, medication, electronic fluency devices, etc.), different therapy settings (e.g., school or clinic, private practice, hospital), different therapy schedules (i.e., intensive, extended) and formats (e.g., individual or group), and different types of self-help groups (e.g., those managed by professionals, those that incorporate practice of specific techniques by support groups [as defined by Borkman, 1999], and mutual aid groups). There are also many ways that people can be involved in self-help groups, ranging from simply reading a brochure to regularly receiving newsletters to participating in online discussion groups to attending local chapter meetings (whether occasionally or frequently) to attending annual conferences. Thus, there is no single way in which people who stutter participate in both treatment and self-help.

Because of the wide variety of possible interactions between self-help and treatment, and because every person who stutters is unique, in terms of his or her experiences and goals for treatment (e.g., Travis, 1927; Van Riper, 1973), it seems appropriate for clinicians to determine whether or not to recommend self-help for their clients who stutter on an *individual* basis. Some clients may benefit from self-help group participation, regardless of whether they are in treatment, whereas others may not. And, of course, self-help groups are not for everyone. Just as people find benefits from different types of treatment, and just as some people prefer not to participate in treatment at all, there are many people who, for whatever reason, do not wish to participate in a self-help group. It is worth noting that none of those surveyed in the studies of stuttering self-help groups that were reviewed earlier reported negative consequences as a result of their group participation. It is likely that this is simply due to the nature of the surveys that were administered, though a similar lack of negative findings has been found in other surveys of self-help participants (e.g., Kyrouz & Humphries, 2002).

Table 14–2   Service-and-Support Delivery Options Involving Self-Help and Treatment*

Model	Service-and-Support Options
Solo	Treatment only Self-help only
Sequential	Treatment followed by self-help Self-help followed by treatment
Simultaneous	Treatment and self-help beginning and ending at the same time
Sequential/simultaneous	Treatment followed by both treatment and self-help Self-help followed by both self-help and treatment
Simultaneous/sequential	Treatment and self-help together followed by treatment only Treatment and self-help together followed by self-help only
Iterative or recursive	Treatment and self-help interacting over time

*Note that the intensity and nature of the treatment can vary, as can the degree of self-help group participation.

Still, clinicians should be flexible in considering whether and when to refer clients to self-help groups, and they should be sure to consider each client's goals in combining treatment and self-help. For example, some people who stutter may seek out self-help for the camaraderie they experience in being with other people who stutter, whereas others may be interested primarily in providing support to other people who stutter. Some clients may be looking for a place to practice speech techniques, and others may be hoping to find a place where they do not have to use their techniques at all. Still others may be in the stage of treatment where they are still learning about stuttering, or they may be experiencing difficulty adjusting to the fact that they stutter. If they are relatively new to the process of adjusting to stuttering, they may benefit from meeting and interacting with people who exhibit a range of different speech characteristics and attitudes about stuttering. As indicated by the findings of the surveys discussed earlier, people participate in self-help groups for all of these reasons and more. As a result, there are a variety of reasons that clinicians might, or might not, wish to recommend self-help groups for individual clients who stutter. The next section examines some of these reasons in more detail, taking into account the nature of stuttering and the ways that self-help groups can serve as an adjunct to various approaches to stuttering therapy.

◆ Self-Help as an Adjunct to Stuttering Therapy

As many authors have acknowledged, stuttering can be described as a broad-based, multidimensional disorder that can affect many aspects of a person's life (see reviews in Yaruss, 1998; Yaruss & Quesal, 2004). Although preschool-age children may not experience negative consequences associated with their stuttering, many school-age children, adolescents, and adults do experience negative communication attitudes, as well as difficulty achieving their goals in life, because of their stuttering. The varied experiences that people who stutter has contributed to the numerous disagreements among experts regarding the nature and treatment of the disorder (see, e.g., Bloodstein, 1993, 1995). Elsewhere, the present authors have attempted to formalize the description of speakers' varied experience of the stuttering disorder based on the World Health Organization's *International Classification of Functioning, Disability, and Health* (ICF; WHO, 2001). Specifically, it can be said that school-age children, adolescents, and adults experience, to varying degrees: (1) an impairment in body function that affects their ability to produce fluent speech; (2) negative affective, behavioral, and cognitive (self)-reactions to their stuttering; (3) negative reactions by people in their environments (including factors such as discrimination for adults who stutter, or bullying and teasing for young children who stutter); and (4) limitations in their ability to perform daily activities or restrictions in their opportunity to participate fully in their lives (Yaruss, 1998, 2001; Yaruss & Quesal, 2004).

The ICF model can be used not only to describe the nature of stuttering, but also to describe the goals of various treatment approaches (Yaruss, 2001). For example, some treatment programs appear to focus primarily on modifying speech behaviors (*impairment*), whether through fluency-shaping techniques such as prolonged speech or through manipulation of the length and complexity of utterances (J.C. Ingham, 1999; R.J. Ingham, 1984; O'Brian, Onslow, Cream, & Packman, 2003; Ryan, 1974). Other treatments are more focused on the speaker's *reactions* to stuttering or on the *limitations* the speaker experiences in daily interactions (e.g., Cooper, 1997; Starkweather & Givens-Ackerman, 1997). Of course, many treatment programs draw from several different techniques to help people who stutter achieve gains in several domains (see discussions in Guitar, 2005; Manning, 2001; Shapiro, 1999), and it can be seen that these treatments address multiple components of the ICF model.

Just as the ICF can be used to help describe different approaches to treatment, it can also be useful in describing the potential role of self-help groups for individuals who stutter. It can also help to identify which aspects of the disorder might be more easily addressed through self-help groups and which might be better addressed through treatment. In the following sections, potential benefits of self-help group participation are considered individually for the four components of the ICF model.

Impairment

The impairment of stuttering relates to the difficulties speakers experience in producing speech smoothly and fluently. One way that self-help groups can help people address their fluency concerns is to provide them with a forum for practicing speech techniques, particularly along a hierarchy from easier to harder situations, to achieve generalization of treatment effects. Of course, many individuals receiving therapy aimed at improving fluency engage in such practice within their treatment sessions, and this is not a primary focus of self-help groups. Still, it can be useful for people receiving speech therapy to have ready access to a group of individuals who can help them as they extend their practice beyond the therapy setting. Self-help groups can provide such camaraderie. At the same time, research has shown that people seek self-help groups not just to practice their speech techniques, but also to have a place where they can communicate freely, without worrying about whether or not they stutter. Thus, it seems that the primary benefits of stuttering self-help may be realized in domains other than the stuttering impairment.

Affective, Behavioral, and Cognitive Self-Reactions

The negative reactions that people may experience as part of the stuttering disorder can include: (1) *affective* reactions, such as feelings of embarrassment, anxiety, shame, and guilt about stuttering; (2) *behavioral* reactions, such as tension or struggle during stuttering, avoidance, or circumlocution; and (3) *cognitive* reactions, such as negative thoughts, low self-esteem, and reduced self-confidence (e.g., Cooper, 1987; Murphy, 1999; Murphy, Yaruss, & Quesal, in press-a). These are the areas in which self-help groups are most widely recognized to provide benefits, not only for people who stutter but for people experiencing a wide variety of health and other concerns (Kyrouz & Humphries, 2002). Findings from the surveys referenced throughout this chapter confirm that many people who stutter do indeed experience gains in these areas through their participation in self-help. Sheehan (1970), for example, wrote that people who stutter "can do things for each other in groups that no individual therapist can accomplish...The discovery that you are not alone, that your experiences are shared and sharable with others like you, can be in itself enormously therapeutic" (p. 297). As will be discussed in more detail in the next section, such benefits are seen not only by adults who stutter, but also by teenagers and school-age children. Even parents of children who stutter can come to the realization that they are not alone in facing stuttering, and this can help them make the same therapeutic gains that their children experience. By meeting with others who have had similar experiences, and by finding out that they are not the only ones struggling with stuttering, individuals who stutter and their families can begin to come to terms with the disorder and feel less anxious or concerned about their own (or their child's) speaking difficulties. (In fact, one of the primary slogans of the NSA is, "If you stutter, you're not alone.")

Of course, such benefits can be gained from treatment programs that incorporate group interactions (Conture & Melnick, 1999; Kelly & Conture, 1991). Still, given widely reported findings that many speech-language pathologists are not comfortable treating individuals who stutter (e.g., Cooper & Cooper, 1985, 1996; St. Louis & Durrenberger, 1993), combined with the many challenges associated with caseload management and service delivery that clinicians face when working in school settings (see review in Yaruss, 2002), it is clear that such supportive treatment groups are not available to many people currently enrolled in therapy for stuttering, particularly in school settings. Thus, the need to share common experiences becomes particularly important for people who do not have access to supportive group interactions within their formal treatment setting. It seems appropriate, then, for clinicians to refer their clients who stutter to self-help groups to facilitate changes related to speakers' negative reactions to stuttering, particularly if they do not provide such group interaction through treatment. This is true even if changes in affective, behavioral, and cognitive reactions to stuttering are targeted in therapy, for again, group interaction, such as that provided through self-help, can assist with generalization of therapy gains into real-world settings. This includes gains related to the speaker's negative reactions to stuttering.

Environmental Reactions and Influences

The reactions of people in the speaker's environment can have a significant impact on the experience of people who stutter. This is true not only for children and adults who stutter, but also for their families. For children, in particular, considerable attention has been paid to the role that parents can play in treatment, and several approaches to treatment for young children directly involve parents (e.g., Conture & Melnick, 1999; Gottwald & Starkweather, 1995; Harris, Onslow, Packman, Harrison, & Menzies, 2002; Hill, 2003; Lincoln & Onslow, 1997; Onslow, Andrews, & Lincoln, 1994; Onslow, Costa, & Rue, 1990; Rustin, Botterill, & Kelman, 1996; Starkweather, Gottwald, & Halfond, 1990; Chapter 5, this volume). In fact, because the majority of treatment programs for young children who stutter are actually administered by parents in the child's real-world environment, it is particularly important for parents to address their own affective, behavioral, and cognitive reactions to their child's stuttering (see Logan & Yaruss, 1999; Yaruss & Reardon-Reeves, 2006). The effect of the environment on school-age children has also been well-documented, particularly in relation to the likelihood of bullying by classmates and the difficulties the child may experience in academic settings (Blood & Blood, 2004; Davis, Howell, & Cook, 2002, Langevin, Bortnick, Hammer, & Wiebe, 1998; Langevin, Kully, & Ross-Harold, this volume; Murphy & Quesal, 2002; Murphy, Yaruss, & Quesal, in press-b; Yaruss, Murphy, Quesal, & Reardon, 2004). Although some treatment approaches definitely do address these concerns, not all children (or their families) receive comprehensive therapy that meets these important needs.

Self-help groups can also play a major role in helping to reduce negative reactions of those in a speaker's environment, in part by providing information about the disorder through their advocacy efforts, and in part by helping others understand what it is like to be a person who stutters. Self-help groups such as the NSA and Friends, as well as the SFA, are particularly focused on helping parents of children who stutter learn to minimize their own fears and anxieties. This, in turn, can help children who stutter to feel less concerned about their speaking difficulties (e.g., Logan & Yaruss, 1999; Murphy et al., in press-a; Yaruss & Reardon-Reeves, 2006). Such groups have also focused on the school-age child's experience of stuttering, with booklets, posters, and other resources aimed at "normalizing" (Murphy, 1999) the child's experience of stuttering. Again, some therapy approaches address these types of goals, though must do not. Participation in a self-help group can be seen as a direct way of supporting the client's attainment or maintenance of such treatment goals outside of the therapy setting. For those treatment approaches that do not specifically address these broader aspects of the speaker's experience of stuttering, it may be particularly useful for clinicians to refer their clients to self-help groups so they can receive benefits in these important domains.

Activity Limitation/Participation Restriction

Ultimately, the impact of the stuttering disorder on the lives of school-age children, adolescents, and adults who stutter involves more than just the speaking difficulties and the negative emotional or cognitive reactions. A key aspect of the speaker's experience of stuttering relates to the limitations in what speakers can do, or restrictions in their ability to participate fully in their daily lives (Yaruss & Quesal, 2004). Examples of the types of limitations reported by people who stutter include difficulties in holding conversations with other people, talking on the phone or giving presentations in work settings (for adults), and reading out loud or answering questions in class (for school-age children or adolescents). If speakers experiences challenges in these areas of their daily interaction, they may experience a broader reduction in their satisfaction with communication in general, and a reduced quality of life overall (Yaruss & Quesal, 2006). Here, again, results of surveys indicate that self-help groups can be helpful in minimizing these negative consequences of the stuttering disorder. Specifically, survey respondents have indicated that participating in self-help groups helps them feel an increased sense of confidence and well-being, regardless of whether or not they were participating in treatment at the time or whether these broader aspects of the disorder were specifically targeted in the therapy they had received. Thus, if clinicians wish to help clients achieve a greater sense of self-confidence, well-being, and quality of life, it seems appropriate to refer school-age children, adolescents, and adults, as well as parents of preschool children, to self-help groups, both during and after therapy.

In sum, self-help groups can provide benefit for people who stutter within all of the domains defined by the WHO for describing disorders such as stuttering. In some cases, clients may receive these benefits as part of a comprehensive approach to therapy. In situations where it is not possible to provide broad-based treatment (or in situations where clinicians are unable to provide treatment at all, e.g., due to a lack of third-party reimbursement), then clinicians can expand the influence and benefits of their treatment by encouraging their clients to participate in self-help groups. This will allow clients to experience gains in aspects of the disorder that, for whatever reason, are not directly addressed in the clinical setting. Furthermore, even if treatment does address broader aspects of the disorder, clinicians may still find that their clients benefit from self-help group participation as a way of enhancing generalization and supporting clients' long-term maintenance of improvements.

◆ Specific Recommendations for Integrating Stuttering Treatment and Self-Help

The previous sections of this chapter have discussed the rationale and general benefits that stuttering self-help groups can provide when used as an adjunct to stuttering treatment. This final section provides specific recommendations for clinicians who are considering referring their clients to self-help groups. These are discussed by age group for all of the specific populations that speech-language pathologists treat (excluding preschool children, who are not generally in need of *self-help* groups for their stuttering, though they may benefit from treatment groups for stuttering, as noted above). The section begins with a review of self-help options for adults, then continues with a discussion of self-help for teenagers and school-age children, and ends with a review of self-help options for parents of school-age and preschool children. In addition, the benefits of self-help group participation for speech-language pathologists is presented. A summary of these key recommendations is presented in **Table 14–3**.

Adults Who Stutter

As discussed above, adults who stutter come to therapy with widely varying needs and goals. Clinicians can facilitate their clients' attainment of individual goals, both in and out of treatment, by giving them the opportunity to learn about all aspects of the stuttering disorder. The more knowledge a speaker has about stuttering, the more likely he or she will be to achieve mastery of treatment techniques and to maintain therapy gains over time. Therefore, it is recommended that adults who stutter become educated about all of their options for participating in self-help. They should be given information about the self-help and other groups that address the needs of adults who stutter (presently these include, Speak Easy International and the NSA, in addition to materials from the SFA that are relevant for adults who stutter), and they should be informed about the various services (e.g., booklets and books, videotapes, etc.) provided by these organizations. Most notable among these services are local support chapters (at the time of this writing, the NSA has more than 80 local chapters around the country for adults who stutter), newsletters, and annual conferences. Many individuals who stutter report that these resources can have life-changing effects (Ahlbach & Benson, 1994; Hood, 1998). Of course, not all clients will choose to take advantage of these opportunities. This is to be expected, for self-help is not for everybody, just as treatment is not for everybody. Some clients may prefer to attend treatment only, whereas others may opt for self-help instead of treatment after

Table 14–3   Key Goals and Recommendations for Self-Help Group Participation for Various Age Groups

Age Group/Population	Relevant Goals	Recommendations
Adults	Receive support from other adults Learn about stuttering (and treatment)	Local chapters Annual conferences and workshops Newsletters and online contacts
Teenagers	Receive support from other teenagers Enhance motivation and optimism	Local chapters Annual conferences and workshops Newsletters and online contacts
School-age children	Minimize isolation and reduce shame Enhance motivation and optimism Learn about stuttering (and treatment)	Youth and family workshops Local chapters Annual conferences and workshops Newsletters and online contacts
Parents of children who stutter	Reduce fear and anxiety Learn about stuttering and treatment Receive support from other parents	Materials (booklets, Web sites, newsletters) Youth and family workshops Local chapters and annual conferences
Speech-language pathologists	Expand understanding of stuttering Increase knowledge of treatment options Reduce anxiety about stuttering therapy	Continuing education workshops Annual conferences and workshops Materials (booklets, Web sites, newsletters)

learning of the benefits (and low cost) of self-help groups. It is the authors' belief that this is simply part of providing individualized treatment options (Yaruss, 2004), and clinicians are encouraged not to view self-help as being in competition with their treatment. At the same time, clinicians may find, as highlighted in the surveys summarized above, that many clients are actually *more* motivated and willing to work toward therapy goals after participating in a self-help group. As people learn more about their disorder, they often begin to minimize their adverse reactions, and they find that they can overcome the negative consequences of the disorder (as others in their self-help group may have done). This can, in turn, give them a sense of optimism and hope that they were previously lacking, and this can improve their motivation for therapy. Finally, it is worth noting that some adults who stutter may initially be reluctant to consider self-help, though as they progress in therapy, they may find that they are more open to acknowledging their stuttering and interacting with and learning from others who stutter. As a result, the timing of a clinician's recommendation that a client participate in self-help groups may need to be considered carefully.

Teenagers Who Stutter

Teenagers who stutter face several difficult challenges, not least of which is dealing with the fact that they are "different" from their friends in a very obvious and important way (i.e., in their ability to communicate freely and effortlessly). Many teens realize that they are nearing the age when they will be attending college or participating in job interviews, and this may dramatically increase their anxiety about stuttering. Furthermore, some teenagers are coming to terms with the fact that they have not yet "outgrown" the disorder, and their hopes for a rapid, spontaneous recovery have largely faded.

The threat of having to face new situations may instill a new sense of urgency or motivation in some clients, so the teenage years may present a unique opportunity for clinicians to work toward more advanced goals, both in and out of treatment. Self-help groups can help teens see the benefits of learning therapy techniques and overcoming their concerns about stuttering by introducing them to adults who stutter who have successfully achieved their goals in life. Teens can also minimize their sense of isolation by meeting others who have shared similar experiences. Therefore, even though many teens will find value in newsletters and online interactions, it is the face-to-face interactions that are particularly recommended with clients in this age range. Participation in local chapters, such as the NSA's growing Teens Who Stutter (TWST) groups, as well as attendance at annual conferences, such as those offered by Friends and the NSA, are strongly recommended. These events provide the best chance for teens who stutter to meet other teens and adults who stutter. Teens may receive additional benefits from hearing the message of motivational keynote speakers, such as those featured at conferences and workshops, for these speakers can help teens figure out for themselves what their goals will be, both in and out of therapy. This can help them take greater responsibility for their own success.

School-Age Children Who Stutter

The majority of research on self-help groups for stuttering has focused on the needs of adults who stutter, though children who stutter can benefit from participating in self-help groups as well. Many school-age children who stutter face significant challenges because their speaking difficulties set them apart from other children. This is an age when communication with one's peers becomes a particularly important part of daily interaction. Thus, children who stutter may be at increased risk for experiencing isolation from others. They may also experience a growing anxiety about facing difficult speaking situations. Unfortunately, however, many school-age children do not yet possess the motivation or drive that is necessary to achieve success in therapy. As a result, they may be unwilling or unable to put the necessary effort into their speech practice or homework, even though they fear their stuttering and feel certain that they would rather not stutter.

Participating in stuttering self-help can help school-age children on several levels. Many school-age children who stutter may never have met another person who stutters. Meeting other children through a support group can help children see that they "are not alone" in facing their speaking difficulties. Moreover, the support group environment gives children the opportunity to see that other people cope with stuttering in a variety of ways. Meeting other people who stutter can also help children realize that they are not as different from others as they may have believed themselves to be. This can help to further minimize the shame or isolation they feel (Murphy, 1999). Some children who stutter may wonder whether they will ever be able to achieve their goals in life, so they may be relieved to meet adults who stutter who are successfully working as firefighters, doctors, veterinarians, lawyers, engineers, college professors, etc. (Meeting successful people who stutter can also be very helpful for the parents, for they, too, may harbor concerns about whether their children will be able to achieve goals such as going to college or getting a job.) Again, some treatment programs may provide these types of interactions, though it is probably fair to say that the majority of children receiving treatment in a typical school setting do not have access to these important and potentially life-changing experiences.

At present, there are relatively few standing self-help groups for school-age children, though the NSA has recently introduced a new initiative, called NSA Kids, that dramatically expands a local chapter program specifically geared to this age group. In addition, both the NSA and Friends host "youth and family" workshops around the country, as well as their annual conferences. These events bring children who stutter, their families, and their speech-language pathologists together for an extended period of education, self-help, and support. Both NSA and Friends also offer moderated, protected chat rooms or listservs where school-age children can develop friendships with other children across the nation, as well as newsletters specifically for children who stutter (e.g., the NSA's *Stutter Buddies* newsletter and *Reaching Out,* published by Friends). These newsletters can serve as a useful therapy resource, as well, for they often contain ideas about how to help school-age children achieve their goals in therapy. It is the present authors' strongly held belief that the school-age years represent the most important time for children who stutter to be exposed to the self-help community, so clinicians are encouraged to give all of their school-age clients the opportunity to learn about and, if they choose, to participate in stuttering self-help groups.

Parents of Children Who Stutter

Helping parents come to terms with stuttering can be one of the most challenging aspects of a clinician's job. In many settings, it can be difficult for clinicians to even have the opportunity to meet with parents to discuss treatment options, let alone provide specific support for parents' concerns. In school settings, for example, clinicians cannot easily write treatment goals in their individualized education plans (IEPs) that address the needs of parents. Similar restrictions may exist in settings that depend on third-party reimbursement, such as hospitals or clinics. The lack of contact parents may have with clinicians, combined with a lack of understanding about the nature and treatment of the disorder, can compound parents' concerns about their children's well-being. This can lead to increased anxiety and fear about stuttering.

As noted above, the SFA has, for many years, published booklets and videotapes designed to minimize parents' concerns about stuttering by educating them about the problem, as well as by training speech-language pathologists who serve parents and their children. Two well-known examples include *If Your Child Stutters: A Guide for Parents* (Ainsworth & Fraser, 2005) and *Stuttering and Your Child: Questions and Answers* (Conture, 2005). The self-help groups have also sought to educate parents. For example, the NSA publishes a newsletter specifically written for parents of young children who stutter, as well as a 60-page booklet designed to help parents minimize their fears and concerns so they will be better able to participate in making appropriate treatment decisions for their children (Yaruss & Reardon-Reeves, 2006). In addition to providing education, self-help groups also provide personal support and interaction so parents can see that they are not alone in facing their child's stuttering. Thus, self-help groups involve parents in their family and youth programs, workshops, and annual conferences, as described above. Through the new NSA Kids program, the NSA has started to expand its local chapters for children and their families. Parents who choose to take advantage of these opportunities can find tremendous camaraderie and comfort through these events and resources, as they begin to meet other parents who understand their concerns.

It has been the present authors' experience that educated and accepting parents make better partners in the therapy process, regardless of the type of therapy that is being offered. This partnership ultimately translates to better outcomes for the child, both in and out of therapy. Self-help groups are one helpful way for parents to obtain this education, acceptance, and support. Self-help groups also provide parents with useful information about stuttering through their toll-free hotlines and Web sites. Having access to an informed and trusted source where parents can receive accurate and timely guidance and support can help them feel more empowered to deal with the wide variety of issues that face them. Because of the relatively limited contact that many clinicians may have with parents of children who stutter, it is recommended that clinicians provide information about stuttering self-help groups to *all* of the parents they work with. This way, parents can choose for themselves whether stuttering self-help will be meaningful for them. If they choose to participate, this serves not only to reduce their anxiety; it can also place them within a broader network of individuals who can answer their questions about stuttering and help them through the difficult task of dealing with their children's speaking difficulties.

Clinicians for Those Who Stutter

Although this chapter has focused primarily on the reasons that speech-language pathologists should refer their clients to self-help groups, it is also true that speech-language pathologists themselves can find benefits from participating in stuttering self-help groups. As noted above, self-help groups have made a concerted effort in recent years to reach out to clinicians and improve the relationship between the consumer and professional communities, through the creation of information materials that can be used in therapy and the presentation of CE workshops.

Another compelling reason for speech-language pathologists to participate in stuttering self-help groups is the increased knowledge about the disorder—and reduced discomfort with stuttering—that clinicians gain by interacting with people who stutter. The reluctance and reduced confidence that many speech-language pathologists feel about working with people who stutter has been well-documented (Brisk, Healey, & Hux, 1997; Cooper & Cooper, 1985, 1996; Kelly, et al, 1997; St. Louis & Durrenberger, 1993). At least some of this discomfort can be traced to the lack of training that many student clinicians receive regarding stuttering (Mallard, Gardner, & Downey, 1988; St. Louis & Lass, 1980). As training requirements in the area of fluency disorders diminish even further (Yaruss, 1999; Yaruss & Quesal, 2002), discomfort with stuttering is only likely to become more widespread.

Clinicians can help themselves become better equipped to help people who stutter by overcoming their own discomfort about the disorder. As demonstrated throughout this chapter, one very helpful way for people to come to terms with stuttering, whether they are living with it or treating it, is to interact with people who stutter. Therefore, the present authors suggest that speech-language pathologists who work with people who stutter consider participating in self-help groups to determine for themselves whether they find benefits. Aside from receiving training through CE workshops, clinicians can also learn about stuttering self-help by attending an annual conference or local chapter meetings, or by reading newsletters and participating in online discussion groups. All of these activities can help speech-language pathologists better understand the perspectives of people who stutter and, ultimately, provide better treatment for their clients who stutter.

◆ Conclusion

The purpose of this chapter has been to describe the role that self-help groups can play in the treatment of children and adults who stutter. To date, little formal research has been conducted, though anecdotal evidence and a few surveys suggest that people who stutter do receive benefits from their participation in self-help groups. In addition, research on self-help groups conducted in other disorder areas (e.g., Katz, 1993; Katz & Bender, 1976, 1987; Kyrouz & Humphries, 2002) has clearly demonstrated self-help groups can play an important role in helping people face a wide variety of challenges. The overall goal of the chapter has been to argue that, regardless of the specific therapy approach that is employed, there are compelling reasons for speech-language pathologists to consider referring their clients, young and old, to self-help groups for stuttering.

Given the wide range of services offered by today's support groups, it is clear that many people who stutter can benefit in some fashion from participating in self-help groups, whether it be through reading newsletters or participating in local chapter meetings or attending annual conferences and workshops. Thus, for the present authors, the question is not *whether* to offer individuals who stutter information about self-help groups, but *how* to offer such information so clients will have the opportunity to determine for themselves whether self-help group participation will be valuable for them. Clinicians are encouraged to explore the possibilities of combined service-and-support delivery models that may give children and adults who stutter and their families their best opportunity to achieve gains, both in and out of the therapy room. Experience to date suggests that clients will not be the only ones to benefit from the support they gain through self-help. Clinicians will also benefit from their partnership and collaboration with the broader community of people who are concerned about the well-being of people who stutter.

References

Adamsen, L., & Rasmussen, J. (2001). Sociological perspectives on self-help groups: Reflections on conceptualization and social processes. Journal of Advanced Nursing 35(6), 909–917.

Ahlbach, J., & Benson, V. (Eds.), (1994). To say what is ours. Anaheim Hills, CA: National Stuttering Project.

Ainsworth, S., & Fraser, J. (2005), If your child stutters: A guide for parents (6th ed.). Memphis, TN: Stuttering Foundation of America.

Andrews, G., Guitar, B., & Howie, P. (1980). Meta-analysis of stuttering treatment. Journal of Speech and Hearing Disorders 45, 287–307.

Banks, E. (2000, Summer). Self-help and the new health agenda. Self-help 2000. The Newsletter of the National Self-help Clearing House 1–2.

Blood, G. W. (1993). Treatment efficacy in adults who stutter: Review and recommendations. Journal of Fluency Disorders 18, 303–318.

Blood, G. W., & Blood, I. M. (2004). Bullying in adolescents who stutter: Communicative competence and self-esteem. Contemporary Issues in Communication Science and Disorders 31, 69–79.

Bloodstein, O. (1993). Stuttering: The search for a cause and a cure. Boston: Allyn & Bacon.

Bloodstein, O. (1995). A handbook on stuttering (5th ed.). San Diego, CA: Singular Publishing Group.

Boberg, E. (1981) Maintenance of fluency. New York: Elsevier.

Borkman, T. J. (1999). Understanding self-help/mutual aid: Experiential learning in the commons. New Brunswick, NJ: Rutgers University Press.

Bradberry, A. (1997). The role of support groups and stuttering therapy. Seminars in Speech and Language 18, 391–399.

Brisk, D. J., Healey, E. C., & Hux, K. A. (1997). Clinicians' training and confidence associated with treating school-age children who stutter: A national survey. Language, Speech, and Hearing Services in Schools 28, 164–176.

Conture, E. G. (1996). Treatment efficacy: Stuttering. Journal of Speech and Hearing Research 39, S18–S26.

Conture, E. G., (Ed.). (2005). Stuttering and your child: Questions and answers (3rd ed.). Memphis, TN: Stuttering Foundation of America.

Conture, E. G., & Melnick, K. (1999). Parent-child group approach to stuttering in preschool and school-age children. In M. Onslow & A. Packman (Eds.), Early stuttering: A handbook of intervention strategies (pp. 17–51). San Diego, CA: Singular Press.

Cooper, E. B. (1987). The chronic perseverative stuttering syndrome: Incurable stuttering. Journal of Fluency Disorders 12, 381–388.

Cooper, E. B. (1997). Fluency Disorders. In T. A. Crowe (Ed.), Applications of counseling in speech-language pathology and audiology. Baltimore: Williams & Wilkins.

Cooper, E. B., Cooper, C. S. (1985). Clinician attitudes towards stuttering: A decade of change (1973–1983). Journal of Fluency Disorders 10, 19–33.

Cooper, E. B., & Cooper, C. S. (1996). Clinician attitudes towards stuttering: Two decades of change. Journal of Fluency Disorders 21, 119–136.

Cordes, A. K. (1998). Current status of the stuttering treatment literature. In A. K. Cordes & R. J. Ingham (Eds.), Treatment efficacy for stuttering: A search for empirical bases (pp. 117–144). San Diego, CA: Singular Publishing Group.

Craig, A. (1998). Relapse following treatment for stuttering: A critical review and correlative data. Journal of Fluency Disorders 23, 1–30.

Davis, S., Howell, P., & Cook, F. (2002). Sociodynamic relationships between children who stutter and their non-stuttering classmates. Journal of Child Psychology and Psychiatry 43, 141–158.

Diggs, C. (1990). Self-help for communication disorders. ASHA 32(1), 32–34.

Gottwald, S. R., & Starkweather, C. W. (1995). Fluency intervention for preschoolers and their families in the public schools. Language, Speech, and Hearing Services in Schools 2, 117–126.

Gregory, H. H. (1997). The speech-language pathologist's role in stuttering self-help groups. Seminars in Speech and Language 18, 401–410.

Graham, C. G., & Conture, E. G. (2007). An indirect approach for early intervention for children who stutter. In: Conture, E. G. & Curlee, R. (Eds.). Stuttering and Related disorders of fluency. (pp. 77–99). New York: Thieme.

Guitar, B. (2005). Stuttering: An integrated approach to it's nature and treatment (3rd ed.). Baltimore: Williams & Wilkins.

Harris, V., Onslow, M., Packman, A., Harrison, E., & Menzies, R. (2002). An experimental investigation of the impact of the Lidcombe Program on early stuttering. Journal of Fluency Disorders 27, 203–214.

Hill, D. (2003). Differential treatment of stuttering in the early stages of development. In H. Gregory (Ed.), Stuttering therapy: Rationale and procedures (pp. 142–185). Boston: Allyn & Bacon.

Hillis, J. W., & McHugh, J. (1998). Theoretical and pragmatic considerations for extraclinical generalization. In A. K. Cordes & R. J. Ingham (Eds.), Treatment efficacy for stuttering: A search for empirical bases (pp. 243–292). San Diego, CA: Singular Publishing

Hood, S. B. (Ed.). (1998). Advice to those who stutter (2nd ed.). Memphis, TN: Stuttering Foundation of America.

Hunt, B. (1987). Self-help for stutterers—Experience in Britain. In L. Rustin, H. Purser, & D. Rowley (Eds.), Progress in the treatment of fluency disorders (pp. 198–214). London: Taylor & Francis.

Ingham, J. C. (1999). Behavioral treatment of young children who stutter: An extended length of utterance method. In R. F. Curlee (Ed.), Stuttering and related disorders of fluency (2nd ed.) (pp. 80–100). New York: Thieme.

Ingham, R. J. (1984). Stuttering and behavior therapy: Current status and experimental foundations. San Diego, CA: College Hill.

Ingham, R. J., & Onslow, M. (1987). Generalization and maintenance of treatment benefits for children who stutter. Seminars in Speech and Language 8, 303–326.

Jezer, M. (1997). Stuttering: A life bound up in words. New York: Basic Books.

Katz, A. H. (1993). Self-help in America: A social movement perspective. New York: Twayne.

Katz, A. H., & Bender, E. I. (1976). The strength in us: Self-help groups in the modern world. New York: New Viewpoints.

Katz, A. H., & Bender, E. I. (1987). Self-help groups in western society: History and prospects. Journal of Applied Behavioral Science 12, 265–282.

Kelly, E. M., & Conture, E. G. (1991). Intervention with school-age stutterers: A parent-child fluency group approach. Seminars in Speech and Language 12, 309–322.

Kelly, E. M., Martin, J. S., Baker, K. E., et al. (1997). Academic and clinical preparation and practices of school speech-language pathologists with people who stutter. Language, Speech, and Hearing Services in Schools 28, 195–212.

Krall, T. (2001). The International Stuttering Association—objectives, activities, outlook: Our dreams for self-help and therapy. In H-G. Bosshardt, J. S. Yaruss, & H. F. M. Peters (Eds.), Fluency disorders: Theory, research, treatment, and self-help. Proceedings of the 3rd World Congress on Fluency Disorders (pp. 30–40). Nijmegen, The Netherlands: Nijmegen University Press.

Krauss-Lehrman, T., & Reeves, L. (1989). Attitudes toward speech-language pathology and support groups: Results of a survey of members of the National Stuttering Project. Texas Journal of Audiology and Speech Pathology 15(1), 22–25.

Kyrouz, E., & Humphries, K. (2002). A review of research on the effectiveness of self-help mutual aid groups. In B. J. White & E. J. Madera (Eds.), American Self-Help Clearinghouse Self-Help Group Sourcebook (7th ed.). Cedar Knolls, NJ: American Self-Help Group Clearinghouse.

Langevin, M., Bortnick, K., Hammer, T., & Wiebe, E. (1998). Teasing/bullying experienced by children who stutter: Toward development of a questionnaire. Contemporary Issues in Communication Science and Disorders 25, 12–24.

Lincoln, M., & Onslow, M. (1997). Long-term outcome of early intervention for stuttering. American Journal of Speech-Language Pathology 6(1), 51–58.

Logan, K. J., & Yaruss, J. S. (1999). Helping parents address attitudinal and emotional factors with young children who stutter. Contemporary Issues in Communication Science and Disorders 26, 69–81.

Mallard, A. R., Gardner, L. S., & Downey, C. S. (1988). Clinical training in stuttering for school clinicians. Journal of Fluency Disorders 13, 253–259.

Manning, W. H. (2001). Clinical decision making in fluency disorders (2nd ed.). San Diego, CA: Singular Publishing.

McClure, J. A., & Yaruss, J. S. (2003). Stuttering survey suggests success of attitude-changing treatment. The ASHA Leader 8, 19.

Murphy, W. P. (1999). A preliminary look at shame, guilt, and stuttering. In N. Bernstein Ratner & E. C. Healy (Eds.), Stuttering research and practice: Bridging the gap (pp.131–143). Mahwah, NJ: Lawrence Erlbaum Associates.

Murphy, W. P., & Quesal, R. W. (2002). Strategies for addressing bullying with the school-age child who stutters. Seminars in Speech and Language 23, 205–211.

Murphy, W., Yaruss, J. S., & Quesal, R. W. (in press-a). Enhancing treatment for school-age children who stutter I: reducing negative reactions through desensitization and cognitive restructuring. Journal of Fluency Disorders.

Murphy, W., Yaruss, J. S., & Quesal, R. W. (in press-b). Enhancing treatment for school-age children who stutter II: Reducing bullying through role-playing and self-disclosure. Journal of Fluency Disorders.

O'Brian, S., Onslow, M., Cream, A., & Packman, A. (2003). The Camperdown Program: Outcomes of a new prolonged speech treatment model. Journal of Speech, Language, and Hearing Research 46, 933–946.

Onslow, M., Andrews, G., & Lincoln, M. (1994). A control/experimental trial of an operant treatment for early stuttering. Journal of Speech and Hearing Research 37, 1244–1259.

Onslow, M., Costa, L., & Rue, S. (1990). Direct early intervention with stuttering: Some preliminary data. Journal of Speech and Hearing Disorders 55, 405–416.

Ramig, P. (1993). The impact of self-help groups on persons who stutter: A call for research. Journal of Fluency Disorders 18, 351–361.

Reardon-Reeves, N. A., & Yaruss, J. S. (2004). The Source for Stuttering: Ages 7–18. East Moline, IL: Lingui Systems.

Reardon, N., & Reeves, L. (2002). Stuttering therapy in partnership with support groups: the best of both worlds. Seminars in Speech and Language, 23, 213–218.

Reeves, P. L. (2006). The role of self-help/mutual aid in addressing the needs of individuals who stutter. In N. Bernstein Ratner & J. Tetnowksi (Eds.). Current Issues I. Stuttering Research and Practice: Volume 2 (pp. 255–278). Mahwah, NJ: Lawrence Erlbaum.

Rustin, L., Botterill, W., & Kelman, E. (1996). Assessment and therapy for young disfluent children: Family interaction. San Diego, CA: Singular.

Ryan, B. P. (1974). Programmed stuttering therapy for children and adults. Springfield, IL: Thomas.

Schneider, P. (2004). Transcending stuttering: The inside story [DVD]. New York: National Stuttering Association.

Shapiro, D. (1999). Stuttering intervention: A collaborative journey to fluency freedom. Austin, TX: PRO-ED.

Sheehan, J. G. (1970). Stuttering: Research and therapy. New York: Harper and Row.

Starkweather, C. W. (1995). The electronic self-help group. In C. W. Starkweather & H. F. M. Peters (Eds.), Stuttering: Proceedings of the 1st World Congress on Fluency Disorders (pp. 499–503). Nijmegen, the Netherlands: Nijmegen University Press.

Starkweatherm C, W., & Givens-Ackerman, J. (1997). Stuttering. Austin, Tx: PRO-ED.

Starkweather, C. W., Gottwald, S. R., & Halfond, M. H. (1990). Stuttering prevention: A clinical method. Englewood Cliffs, NJ: Prentice-Hall.

St. Louis, K. (Ed.). (2001). Living with stuttering: Stories, basics, resources and hope. Morgantown, WV: Populore Publishing Company.

St. Louis, K. O., & Durrenberger, C. H. (1993). What communication disorders do experienced clinicians prefer to manage? ASHA 35, 23–31.

St. Louis, K. O., & Lass, N. J. (1980). A survey of university training in stuttering. Journal of the National Student Speech Language Hearing Association 10, 88–97.

Stuttering Foundation of America. (n.d.). Stuttering Foundation of America: A history. Memphis, TN: Stuttering Foundation of America.

Thomas, C., & Howell, P. (2001). Assessing efficacy of stuttering treatments. Journal of Fluency Disorders 26, 311–333.

Travis, L. E. (1927). Stuttering. Chicago: The Classroom Teacher, Inc.

Van Riper, C. (1973). The treatment of stuttering. Englewood Cliffs, NJ: Prentice-Hall.

World Health Organization. (2001). International classification of functioning, disability, and health. Geneva: World Health Organization.

Yaruss, J. S. (1998). Describing the consequences of disorders: Stuttering and the International Classification of Impairments, Disabilities, and Handicaps. Journal of Speech, Language, and Hearing Research 49, 249–257.

Yaruss, J S. (1999). Current status of academic and clinical education in fluency disorders at ASHA-accredited training programs. Journal of Fluency Disorders 24, 169–184.

Yaruss, J. S. (2001). Evaluating treatment outcomes for adults who stutter. Journal of Communication Disorders 34(1–2), 163–182.

Yaruss, J. S. (2002). Facing the challenge of treating stuttering in the schools. Seminars in Speech and Language 23, 153–159.

Yaruss, J. S. (2004). Documenting individual treatment outcomes in stuttering therapy. Contemporary Issues in Communication Science and Disorders 31, 49–57.

Yaruss, J. S., Murphy, W. P., Quesal, R. W., & Reardon, N. A. (2004). Bullying and teasing: Helping children who stutter. New York: National Stuttering Association.

Yaruss, J. S., & Quesal, R. W. (2002). Academic and clinical education in fluency disorders: An update. Journal of Fluency Disorders 27, 43–63.

Yaruss, J. S., & Quesal, R. W. (2004). Stuttering and the International Classification of Functioning, Disability, and Health (ICF): An update. Journal of Communication Disorders 37, 35–52.

Yaruss, J. S., & Quesal, R. W. (2006). Overall Assessment of the Speaker's Experience of Stuttering (OASES):Documenting multiple outcomes in stuttering treatment. Journal of Fluency Disorders, 31, 90–115.

Yaruss. J. S., Quesal, R. W., Reeves, L, et al. (2002). Speech treatment and support group experiences of people who participate in the National Stuttering Association. Journal of Fluency Disorders 27, 115–135.

Yaruss, J. S., & Reardon-Reeves, N. (2006). Young children who stutter: Information and support for parents (4th ed.). New York: National Stuttering Association.

Yaruss, J. S., & Reeves, L. (2002). Pioneering stuttering in the 21st century: The first joint symposium for scientists and consumers. (Summary Report and Proceedings). Anaheim, CA: National Stuttering Association.

Yaruss, J. S., & Soifer, A. (1998). Preliminary analysis of the outcomes of an adult stuttering treatment group. In E. C. Healey & H. F. M. Peters (Eds.), Proceedings of the 2nd World Congress on Fluency Disorders (pp. 257–261). Nijmegen, The Netherlands: University of Nijmegen Press.

15

A Critical Review of the Effect of Drugs on Stuttering

Keith G. Saxon and Christy L. Ludlow

The purpose of this chapter is to assist clinicians with making decisions regarding adding drugs to a therapeutic regimen for the treatment of stuttering. The chapter begins with a review of methods for rating the scientific evidence on treatments. Some of the pitfalls of research design and placebo conditions to consider when reviewing the scientific literature are discussed. A critical review of the currently available evidence on the effects of various medications on stuttering is provided. We hope that this chapter will assist readers with making informed decisions based on the scientific evidence available on whether a medication might be considered for a particular client. The bases for therapeutic decisions depend on the patient's difficulties at the time of treatment, which may change at different times in the life of the same individual.

When considering neuropharmacological agents for the treatment of stuttering, we need to understand the mechanism of a drug when administered either alone or as an adjunct to behavioral intervention. In many disorders, including stuttering, knowledge in several areas is necessary to make the optimal therapeutic choice. Our understanding of the mechanisms involved in stuttering come from brain imaging, genetics, behavioral, motoric, and speech-language studies as well as longitudinal studies of the development and recovery from stuttering, and responses to known treatments. Various treatment alternatives are available and one approach may not be equally effective for all persons who stutter. Further, persons who stutter may have additional difficulties for which a neuropharmacological intervention may or may not be appropriate; for example, in adults who also suffer from depression or children with attention deficit/hyperactivity disorder (ADHD). As with the treatment of all disorders, therapeutic decisions should attempt to provide the best fit for each individual patient.

◆ Evaluating Evidence from Clinical Studies or Trials

Rating the Strength of Evidence

The strength of the evidence provided by a clinical study or trial depends upon the quality of the research design. The reader should review the trial design before considering the evidence regarding a treatment. There are multiple classification systems for evidence-based reviews of the results of clinical trials. A recent review of such systems found 19 systems were adequate for assessing study quality (West, et al., 2002). In clinical research the gold standard is a random controlled trial (RCT), which has the following characteristics:

- Subjects are randomly assigned to different treatment groups so the investigator cannot unconsciously place those patients most likely to recover into the experimental treatment group.

- A control group (often a placebo) is available for comparison with the new treatment.

- The evaluation of the outcome of treatment is independent from the experimenters.

- The participants, evaluators, and experimenters are blinded to who is getting the placebo and who is getting the new experimental treatment.

Eight systems for evaluating the results of clinical trials were found by West et al. (2002) as acceptable for classifying treatment studies with reference to RCTs. For this review, we will use the framework employed by the American Academy of Neurology, Therapeutics and Technology Assessment Subcommittee, September 1999 (Goodin & Edlund, 1999). Each level of evidence (described below) will support judgments at different levels of certainty regarding the probable benefit of a new treatment for a disorder.

In this system, studies are given a class designation based on the quality of the research design (**Table 15–1**). For example, a Class I study is a large RCT with objective and blinded assessment of the outcome of a treatment. Class I studies provide a greater level of evidence than lower class studies (Level A being the most informative and Level U being the least). Several studies are needed to reach a level of evidence before a conclusion can be reached on whether a treatment is beneficial or not with a high level of certainty. For establishing that a particular treatment is beneficial, several Class I studies are needed (**Table 15–1**). On the other hand, Class III studies can only provide Level C evidence that can only reach a "possible benefit" as a level of certainty.

- Level A evidence can establish a treatment as *beneficial*.

- Level B evidence can determine that a treatment is *probably* beneficial.

- Level C evidence can only determine that a treatment might *possibly* be useful.

- Level U evidence can only indicate that the effects of a treatment are *unknown*.

Table 15–1   Classifications of Studies, Levels of Evidence Provided, and Certainty of Conclusions Reached

Class of Study	Control Groups	Outcome Measures	Design	Level of Evidence	Certainty of Conclusion
Class I	Random assignment to control group	Objective and blinded	Large prospective	Level A	Beneficial or not
Class II	Equivalent control group	Blinded	Small prospective	Level B	Probably beneficial or not
Class III	Control group	Independent assessment	Crossover designs	Level C	Possibly beneficial or not
Class IV	Uncontrolled	Patient reports	Case series	Level U	Unknown

Class I studies are well-designed RCTs involving many centers. Level A evidence requires several published Class I studies that are:

1. Prospective (the study was designed beforehand);

2. Have patients randomly assigned between control and experimental treatment groups;

3. Use masked (blinded) measures of effectiveness;

4. Assess outcomes reflecting a patient's ability to meet his or her needs for daily living with treatment (for children, being able to participate in classroom and play activities may be relevant);

5. Have adequate statistical power (an adequate sample size to test the hypothesis) and account for dropouts (Jones, Gebski, Onslow, & Packman, 2002);

6. Control sources of bias (on the part of the participants or the experimenters in favor of the new treatment); and

7. Use inclusion/exclusion criteria to define a large representative sample of the patient population.

Level A evidence requires that several RCTs are available in the literature on the treatment for a particular condition with at least one study being conducted across multiple centers. Several supportive Class I clinical trials are usually required before the Food and Drug Administration (FDA) will approve a new drug as a treatment for a disorder.

Level B evidence requires Class II prospective trials with similar control and experimental groups from a representative population with masked (blinded) outcome assessment where:

1. Primary outcomes are clearly defined;

2. Exclusion/inclusion criteria are clearly defined;

3. Adequate accounting for dropouts (subjects leaving the study before they have completed it) and adequate numbers of participants in treatment groups or conditions to have minimal potential for bias; and

4. Information on relevant baseline characteristics for the groups showing that they were substantially equivalent or that statistical adjustment for baseline differences has been adequate.

Level B evidence may also include RCTs in a representative population that lack one of *criteria* 1 through 4 (Class II trials).

Level C evidence includes all other controlled trials, Class III trials, in a representative population where the outcome assessment is independent of patient treatment. Class III trials can include well-defined natural history controls or patients serving as their own control in a crossover design where the same persons undergo two phases, a medication phase and a placebo phase. Patient bias is difficult to prevent in crossover designs because side effects are more evident during the active drug condition, leading the patients to expect more benefit in that condition.

Level U evidence includes all Class IV studies, including uncontrolled trials, case series, case reports, or expert opinions.

Different Classes of Research Provide Different Levels of Evidence

When developing and evaluating a new treatment, research studies usually follow a sequence from uncontrolled Class IV trials through Class III, II, and I, studies that address different questions. Initially, the aim is to determine whether or not a new drug is safe to give to patients in an uncontrolled Class IV study. Class III studies are aimed to identifying which dosage does not have too many side effects and yet provides some benefit. Only Class II and I trials, mentioned above, will determine if a new treatment is beneficial in a significant proportion of persons with the disorder. As research on a new drug progresses from Class IV through to Class I, the strength of the evidence increases regarding whether or not it is beneficial for a particular disorder from Level U (unknown) to Levels C, B, and finally A.

Class IV trials are usually small and uncontrolled, and they may involve the first use in humans or in persons with a particular disorder. If the drug or device already has been found effective for a particular disorder, that is, it has been approved and labeled by the FDA for that disorder or indication, then a Class IV study might be conducted to determine whether it is safe to use in a different patient disorder. For example, if the drug was already shown to be beneficial for persons with depression, then a Class IV study may examine whether it is safe to use in persons who stutter who are not depressed, which would be a new "off-label" indication. Off-label studies often require FDA approval or a waiver for the use of the medication for the treatment of a different disorder. Class IV studies usually only have 10 to 20 participants, are not blinded, and therefore are inherently biased (e.g., both the participants and the experimenter knows who does and does not receive the drug under study). Sources of bias include both the patients and the investigators, who usually are both eager to have the new treatment be beneficial. Further, the measures may not be made independent from the investigators, and there may be no control condition or group. Such studies do not provide evidence regarding treatment benefit and contribute only to Level U evidence. However, they are able to report on side effects and any adverse effects of the treatment in that disorder, a necessary first step.

Class III trials are usually prospective (that is, designed in advance) and aimed at determining an effective dose for using the new treatment with persons having a particular disorder. Groups may be compared at different drug dosages, with a baseline and/or placebo condition. These are referred to as crossover designs when the same individuals are compared at different drug dosages, or in a placebo and drug phase, often with a random ordering of the two phases between patients. As mentioned above, crossover designs are often biased because participants will experience side effects during the drug or at higher dosages and expect a greater benefit in that phase. This potential for bias can only be reduced when different groups of individuals receive different drug dosages, a "between subjects" design, which requires larger numbers of participants. For safety reasons, the participants, but not the investigators, may be blinded, so that if the high-dose condition/group has significant side effects (adverse events), that high-dose condition/group (arm) of the study can be stopped. Class III trials usually contribute only to Level C evidence because they are not well controlled. Some Class III trials may include a nontreated comparison group/condition and blinded measurement. When the investigators are blinded, an independent Data Safety Monitoring Committee (DSMC) is needed for monitoring the study. The DSMC reviews the unblinded data to assure that patients are not being harmed or that the study is stopped if one treatment arm shows a clear benefit over the other. Often Class III studies have a sample size of between 20 and 40 participants.

Class II studies are prospective trials aimed at comparing a new treatment with the established treatment for a disorder. Class I trials involve multiple centers to allow for an adequate representative sample size of between 100 and 500 patients. Because both the patients and the investigators are blinded, an independent DSMC is essential to review the un-blinded data on a regular basis to assure that patients are not being harmed or if one treatment arm should be stopped. The goal is to measure the new treatment's effectiveness relative to the best treatment currently available, which in stuttering would be behaviorally oriented speech therapy. Only one small Class II study has compared the effects of neuropharmacological treatments with the gold standard, speech therapy (P.G. Wells & Malcolm, 1971). Most medication studies in stuttering are either small Class II trials with various levels of control or Class III crossover studies reporting on a small number of persons' responses to a medication in comparison with their response to a placebo.

Evidence from Treatment Combinations May Be More Relevant to Clinical Practice

Other fields have confronted the issue of combining behavioral and neuropharmacological interventions. One disorder, ADHD, may serve as an example. The National Institute of Mental Health

Collaborative Multi-site Multimodal Treatment Study of Children with ADHD randomly assigned more than 500 children to one of four treatment groups: (1) medication management; (2) intensive behavioral management; (3) a combination of the first two treatments; and (4) a control consisting of the current standard of care, medications (The MTA Cooperative Group, 1999; Hinshaw, et al., 2000; Taylor, 1999; Wells, et al., 2000). This multicenter Class I trial provided Level A evidence for clinical decisions in managing ADHD.

The evaluation of the potential benefit of combined treatments is particularly relevant to the design of future medication trials in stuttering. Most medication treatment trials have been conducted in adults who stutter and have evaluated the effects of medications alone, although their clinical use is more likely to be as an adjunct to speech therapy. For example, a medication may allow those persons with other disorders besides stuttering to achieve a greater benefit from speech therapy when the two therapies are combined—a situation more relevant to real-life intervention decisions. On the other hand, maximizing a given treatment prior to adding another can be preferred; that is, first studying the effects of a medication in subjects who have already achieved maximum benefit from speech therapy allows clearer assessment of a medication's therapeutic effects. In either case, an initial approach might be to evaluate the use of medications as an adjunct to speech therapy in adults prior to using similar designs in children.

Study Design Factors Can Strengthen or Weaken Evidence

Participant characteristics Many factors influence the relative strength of the evidence provided by an empirical study. The more alike the subjects are in their characteristics, such as sex, age, severity of disease, and presence or absence of other disease entities, the more predictable the results will be for others with similar characteristics. In medication trials, the drug effects are altered by pharmacokinetics, that is, how the drug is metabolized by different individuals. This may be influenced by certain characteristics such as genetic phenotype, sex, time of testing relative to menses, liver function, renal function, percent body fat, hydration, and even sleep (Gallin, 2002).

Carryover effects Carryover effects refers to when a subject moves from one treatment to another, that is, elements of the initial treatment linger and combine, in uncontrolled ways, with the elements of the subsequent treatment. Carryover effects may, therefore, interfere with the main effects of the medication in crossover designs. Residual pharmacological or psychological effects from the first medication may alter the effects of the second, producing a difference in the effects of a medication between groups assigned to two different treatment orders. Randomly assigning patients to two groups, one receiving drug A before B and the other B before A is one approach to balancing two different drug orders. Carryover effects of one drug to another can also be dealt with by determining how a drug is metabolized, its excretion time, and half-life, when timing the crossover washout time period between two drugs (i.e., the time the effects of Drug X takes to dissipate in a person's system before one can begin to independently assess the influence of Drug Y). On the other hand, crossover designs reduce some of the between-patient variability when the same subjects are in both treatment groups. Parallel group designs, where subjects are placed in one treatment arm and compared with other subjects in a different treatment arm, often require larger numbers of research participants to measure a treatment difference because of between-subject variance.

Outcome measures Similarly, treatment outcome measures also can play a role in the ability to measure a treatment difference. The more reliably the behavioral outcome can be measured with a minimum amount of variance from experimenter to experimenter (inter-rater reliability) or from time to time (intra-rater reliability), the better the estimate of the treatment effect (effect size).

Statistical power Statistical power depends on the intra- and inter-subject variability, the effect size of the benefit from a medication, and the number of subjects studied. Low power increases the chance of missing a significant treatment effect. By controlling other factors that can contribute to stuttering besides the medication effects, such as holidays, stress, or changes in lifestyle, it is more likely that the medication effect will not be masked by other factors.

Experimenter/participant bias An important concern is to reduce experimenter and participant bias. Double-blinding (masking) the experiment where neither the subject nor the experimenter knows who is receiving the experimental medication, a placebo, or a control substance, while not always possible, is considered a stronger design. Participants and experimenters are naturally biased to want a new treatment to be beneficial and may have previously held beliefs against older treatments. Besides blinding both the experimenters and the participants, a placebo treatment control group is often important to determine the degree to which a benefit is influenced by expectation.

The Placebo Effect in Clinical Trials

Benson, among many others, has studied and defined the placebo effect and discussed three elements: (1) the client's beliefs; (2) the clinician's beliefs; and (3) the client-clinician relationship (Benson, 1997). The bane of every investigator and the friend of every clinician, placebo effects must be assessed and managed in every clinical drug trial where Level A evidence is sought. Placebo, Latin for "I shall please," is ubiquitous in research, and has been demonstrated to affect not only subjective rating of symptoms and function, but also physiological measures including blood pressure, airway resistance, and gastrointestinal function (Gay, Rendell, & Spiro, 1994). Placebo effects can be found even in neurodegenerative diseases such as Parkinson's disease where patients have significant motor control disorders (Shetty, Friedman, Kieburtz, Marshall, & Oakes, 1999) It stands to reason, therefore, if placebo frequently effects the above conditions and disorders, it is powerful in stuttering research.

A specific treatment effect is defined as the difference between the treatment improvement and that created by placebo. The larger the placebo effect, the less difference can be discerned between the placebo and the treatment, possibly leading to "ceiling effects," leaving no room for further improvement in symptoms beyond the placebo benefit.

Placebo responses also often vary considerably among participants, as some persons are more suggestible than others. In addition, the placebo and the treatment response may interact: As some persons receive some relief from a treatment they become more suggestible to placebo benefits. This response may vary greatly as the patient group is large and more heterogeneous. For example, participants may vary in other disorders that might be amenable to medication effects (Fries, et al., 2006) in addition to differences in background, education, social-economic status, cognitive style, etc. The greater the individual variation, the less the statistical power (Liu, Zhao, Shaffer, Icitovic & Chase, 2005).

Several strategies have been tried to limit placebo effect. One is to identify and exclude "placebo responders." "Run-in" is one technique: a short period before the actual trial takes place, high placebo responders are identified and removed from the trial, and those participants with lesser placebo responsiveness are stratified to statistically correlate their results. That is, equal proportions of persons with low placebo responsiveness would be assigned to each group, those receiving the experimental treatment and those receiving the placebo. At least in the psychiatric literature, run-in has been criticized as a time-waster, deceptive, and unhelpful. (Montgomery, 1999; Schweizer & Rickels, 1997; Trivedi & Rush, 1994) Lengthened trials may work to increase the treatment versus placebo response differences because placebo responses tend to relapse over time. Studies have shown that subjects report improvements when they perceive side effects. With regard to drug treatment, control of appearance, taste, and side effects is useful in successfully blinding the subject and investigator. The strategy of using an active placebo to deliver side effects has several drawbacks. The active placebo could potentially exacerbate the underlying symptom making the treatment drug look better than it should, a false-positive (that is, indicating improvement from the treatment drug when none really occurred). On the other hand, when an the active placebo is effective in relieving a symptom, it may make it difficult to quantify changes resulting from the treatment drug.

The effectiveness of double-blinding designs in eliminating bias and placebo effects may be checked by giving questionnaires to the participants and the study staff and asking when they thought the placebo and drug were given. An effective double-blinding would theoretically have the participants getting the correct answer 50% of the time. Even in a perfectly blinded study, if the therapeutic agent is clearly effective, correct responses may be skewed in the direction of the therapeutic agent.

Gordon et al. (1995) used positive controls with a placebo and therapeutic agent in a crossover design—a design where the participant receives active medications in both phases—to provide information about the efficacy of one class of drugs for stuttering in contrast with another class. In a positive control study, a drug of a different class, not expected to have the same therapeutic effect as the test drug, is used. This design can help determine whether the response to the test medication is specific to stuttering and not because the side effects are alerting subjects that they are taking an active drug.

♦ The Effects of Drugs on Stuttering

Neurotransmission in the Central Nervous System

Although perhaps obvious, it is important to keep in mind that drugs generally function by altering the communication, or "neurotransmission," between neurons at synaptic junctions in the central nervous system. Thus, a basic understanding of neurotransmission is required to interpret the actions of various pharmacological agents or drugs. Vast amounts of literature cover the large scope and depth of knowledge in neuropharmacology, the study of the effects of drugs on neuronal function. Knowledge in this field moves rapidly as new discoveries occur almost daily. The present introduction to the pharmacological treatment of stuttering covers only the general principles and may be outdated as new knowledge develops. The following overview is drawn heavily from two sources: Chapter 8 in *Fundamental Neuroscience* (Deutch & Roth, 1999) and *Goodman's* & *Gilman's The Pharmacological Basis of Therapeutics* (Hardman & Limbird, 2001).

As mentioned above, neurotransmission occurs via synaptic junctions between neurons. In the simplest situation, involving two neurons, for one neuron, the presynaptic neuron, to produce a response in another neuron, the postsynaptic neuron, the following events must occur. First, a particular neurotransmitter substance is synthesized in the *presynaptic neuron* and then moved into vesicles within the presynaptic neuron. The vesicle must bind itself to the presynaptic membrane and in the event of an action potential (an electrochemical event) in the presynaptic neuron, the vesicle will open to allow the transmitter to be released into the synaptic junction (or "gap") between the two neurons. Once the neurotransmitter is released into the synaptic junction, it must be recognized by specific proteins in the membrane of the *postsynaptic neuron,* referred to as receptors. Once the neurotransmitter is taken up (i.e., "uptake") by the postsynaptic receptor, ion flux will occur across postsynaptic membrane producing an action potential. After being released into a synaptic junction by the presynaptic neuron, the neurotransmitter is broken down by enzymes, and the by-products are taken back up into the presynaptic neuron or by adjacent glia (white matter supporting cells), referred to as reuptake, and are reprocessed back into neurotransmitter to be clustered into vesicles in the presynaptic neuron for the entire neurotransmission process to re-occur.

Abnormalities at the synapse may lead to a variety of neurological disorders. Several mechanisms are involved in regulating the level of neurotransmitter released or present in the synaptic junction. If certain enzymes are not present either in the synaptic junction or in the glia, then neurotransmitters may not be broken down and can accumulate in the synaptic junction. Similarly, if postsynaptic receptors do not take up or bind the neurotransmitter, then the neurotransmitter may accumulate in the synaptic junction. Further, if transport molecules required for neurotransmitter reuptake into the presynaptic neuron are absent or not functioning, then neurotransmitter can accumulate in the synaptic junction and increase the excitability of the postsynaptic neuron. Alternatively, if a postsynaptic receptor is inactivated, then the postsynaptic neuron is less likely to fire, resulting in reduced neurotransmission.

Interference with neurotransmission may yield both immediate and long-term changes and can alter neurotransmission in different ways. Because of the complexity of synaptic neurotransmission, neuropharmacological agents may influence neurotransmission at one or more of the steps in the process. Drugs can work to influence several postsynaptic receptor sites, which are either excitatory or inhibitory in nature. Drugs can also work to influence the channels through which ions pass, facilitating or blocking ion flow as well as changing synthesis or reuptake of a neurotransmitter. As is described below there are different classes of neurotransmitters in the central nervous system, and different classes of drugs alter the function of some of these neurotransmitters. Most drugs that are commercially available have multiple actions, however, altering more than one neurotransmitter in the brain. **Table 15–2** provides a listing of many of the medications discussed below, the neurotransmitter systems they affect, their drug class, and their synaptic action.

Evidence on the Use of Drugs for the Treatment of Stuttering

In the following review using MEDLINE searches and previous reviews (Brady, 1991; Ludlow & Braun, 1993; Maguire, Yu, Franklin, & Riley, 2004), the present authors identified 75 reports of effects of neuropharmacological agents in adults who stutter. The large majority were Class IV uncontrolled studies and case reports. None were Class I studies, 4 were Class II, and 11 were Class III. In reviewing the evidence available for a drug class, only studies contributing to the highest level of evidence on the use of a drug for the treatment of stuttering were included in the evidence table **(Table 15–3)** and used to assign a level of evidence (A, B, C, or U). For example, if Class II studies were available on a particular drug, Class IV studies regarding that drug usually were not included.

Drugs that Affect the Catecholamine Neurotransmission System

The catecholamine system includes norepinepherine, epinephrine, and dopamine. These neurotransmitters are excitatory in effect. Drugs have been developed to both augment and block these

Table 15–2 Neurotransmitter Systems, Drug Classes, and Examples of Drugs and Their Actions

Neurotransmitter	Drug Class	Examples Generic (Brand name)	Actions
Dopamine	Dopamine enhancers	Levodopa (L-Dopa®)	Biosynthesis of dopamine
Dopamine	Antipsychotic	Haloperidol (Haldol®)	D2 receptor blocker
Dopamine	Antipsychotic	Olanzapine (Zyprexa®)	D1-D4 receptor blocker and serotonin 2 blocker
Dopamine	Antipsychotic	Clozapine (Clozaril®)	D1-D5 receptor blocker, adrenergic, cholingeric, histaminergic and serotonin antagonist
Norepinephrine	Antidepressants	Desipramine (Norpramin®)	Norepinephrine reuptake blocker
Serotonin	Antidepressants	Clomipramine (Anafranil®)	Serotonin selective reuptake blocker
	Antidepressants	Paroxetine (Paxil®)	Serotonin selective reuptake blocker
	Antidepressants	Fluoxetine (Anafranil®)	Serotonin selective reuptake blocker
γ-aminobutyric acid (GABA)	Antianxiety	Diazepam (Valium®)	Receptor agonist
	Antianxiety	Alprazolam (Xanax®)	Receptor agonist
	Antispasmodic	Baclofen (Lioresal®)	Increased inhibition of motor neurons
Channel blockers	Antiarrhythmatic®	Verapamil (Verelan®)	Calcium channel blockers

Table 15–3 Evidence Table of Studies of Different Neuropharmacological Agents in Stuttering

Author, Year	Drug/Class	Blind	Control	Placebo Effects	Cohort Size	Dropout Rate %	Follow-up & Rx	Duration	Fluency change	Rate	Class
Haloperidol											
Wells & Malcolm, 1971	Haloperidol	Double	Random assignment to placebo and combined therapy groups	40% inc. in symptoms	36	33	10/36	4 and 8 weeks	p = .01	83%	II
Swift, Swift & Arellano 1975	Haloperidol	Double	Random assigment	0.1% 4.6% worse in reading	19	10.5	90 days 3/4	3 weeks	85%	p<.05	II
T. J. Murray, Kelly, Campbell, & Stefanik, 1977	Haloperidol	Double	Crossover	16%	26	31	27.7 1/26	3 months	61%	Inc.	III
Rantala & PetriLarmi, 1976	Haloperidol	Double	Crossover	20%	66	12	–		NS	Inc.	III
Rosenberger, Wheelden, & Kalotkin, 1976	Haloperidol	Double	Crossover	27%	8	0	–	6 or 12 weeks	NS	Inc.	III
Burns, Brady, & Kuruvilla, 1978	Haloperidol	Double	Acute crossover; apomorphine placebo and haloperidol	0%	12	0	NA	Acute only	p = .05	80%	III
Prins, Mandelkorn, & Cerf, 1980	Haloperidol	Double	Crossover	In some subjects	14	29	–	2 months	p = .04	p = .009	III
Other **Dopamine Antagonists**											
Maguire, Riley, Franklin, & Gottschalk, 2000	Dopamine antagonist risperidone	Double	Placebo control	14.5%	16	0	––	6 weeks	p = .01 p = .001	Not measured	II

(Continued)

Table 15–3 Evidence Table of Studies of Different Neuropharmacological Agents in Stuttering (*Continued*)

Author, Year	Drug/Class	Blind	Control	Placebo Effects	Cohort Size	Dropout Rate %	Follow-up & Rx	Duration	Fluency change	Rate	Class
Maguire, Riley, et al., 2004	Olanzapine	Double	Placebo control	14.0% SSI 1% SSS	24	4%	23/24	12 weeks	33%SSI $p = 0.04$ 22% SSS	Not measured	II
Maguire et al., 1999	Dopamine antagonist risperidone	No	Placebo control	0%	21	0	—	6 weeks	$p < .05$ severity NS % duration	Not measured	III
Rothenberger, Johannsen, Schulze, Amorosa, & Rommel, 1994	Dopamine antagonist tiapride	No	Crossover 2 dose levels	NA	10	29%	—	20 weeks	$p = .014$	Inc.	IV
Norepineprine Reuptake Inhibitor											
Stager, Ludlow, Gordon, Cotelingham, & Rapoport, 1995b	Tricyclics chlomipramine & desipramine	Double	Crossover	No comparison	16	11	2/16 DMI desipramine	12 weeks	DMI vs placebo	NS NS	III
Serotonin Selective Reuptake Inhibitors											
Gordon, et al., 1995 (same study as Stager 1995b)	Tricyclics chlomipramine & desipramine	Double	Crossover	Not reported	17	2	CMI 50% at 12 months	10 weeks	CMI superior to DMI; $p < .05$; patient ratings	NS	III
Stager, Ludlow, Gordon, Cotelingham, & Rapoport, 1995a	Longterm	Double	Crossover; chlomipramine vs placebo	No comparison	5	0	NA	8 months	NS	NS	III
Schreiber & Pick, 1997	SSRI paroxitene	No	No	No	3	0	—	NA	100%	NA	IV

(Continued)

Table 15–3 Evidence Table of Studies of Different Neuropharmacological Agents in Stuttering (*Continued*)

Study	Agent										
Boldini, Rossi, & Placidi, 2003	SSRI paroxitene	No	No	No	1	0	—	NA	Improved	Inc.	IV
Calcium Channel Blockers											
Brady, Price, McAllister, & Dietrich, 1989	Verapamil	Double	Crossover	NS	10	0	9/10	3 weeks	.007	0.002	III
Brumfitt & Peake, 1988	Verapamil	Double	Crossover	NS	16	12.5%	—	6 weeks	NS	NS	III
Zachariah 1980	Verapamil	Single	Placebo control	15%	70	0%	50	6 days	84% subjective improvement.	Not measured	IV

DMI, desipramine; *inc.*, increase; *%SSI*, stuttering severity instrument; *%SSS*, self-assessment of stuttering severity.

typically excitatory effects through a variety of mechanisms. Most of the neuropharmacological research on stuttering has focused on dopaminergic neurotransmission, likely because of early case reports; some persons were placed on dopaminergic blockers for other disorders, such as schizophrenia or Tourette's syndrome, with a concomitant change noted in their stuttering. Others have observed increases in stuttering following the administration of L-dopa, a synthetic form of dopamine. Anderson, Hughes, Rothi, Crucian, and Heilman (1999) reported increased stuttering during periods following levodopa therapy in a man with Parkinson's disease. Likewise, Louis, Winfield, Fahn, and Ford (2001) reported on two patients with Parkinson's disease whose stuttering increased with levodopa therapy.

Dopaminergic Agents   Dopamine (dihydroxyphenylethylamine) is present in a variety of neurons in the central nervous system. There are at least five different dopamine receptor types. Pharmacologial agents have been developed to block the D1 and D2 receptors, which are closely associated with psychotic illnesses including schizophrenia. Haloperidol (Haldol®) is a D2 receptor blocker known to reduce neurotramission in dopaminergic neurons in the striatum, frontal cortex, medulla, and midbrain, and it was initially developed as an antipsychotic agent but has found a variety of applications over time. Side effects induced with chronic use of haloperidol include involuntary movements (dyskinesia), fatigue, dry mouth, blurring vision, drowsiness, anxiety, depression, and facial tics. Because of the nontrivial side effects, haloperidol and other D2 receptor antagonists are in limited use today.

Seven studies, most crossover designs (**Table 15–1**), compared the use of haloperidol versus an inactive placebo to reduce stuttering (Burns, Brady, & Kuruvilla, 1978; T. J. Murray, Kelly, Campbell, & Stefanik, 1977; Prins, Mandelkorn, & Cerf, 1980; Rantala & Petri-Larmi, 1976; Rosenberger, Wheelden, & Kalotkin, 1976; Swift, Swift, & Arellano, 1975; Wells, 1974; Wells & Malcolm, 1971). As mentioned, all but two of these seven studies were crossover designs; only two involved random assignment to different groups. Six reported on their placebo effects, which ranged from a 40% increase in stuttering symptoms to a 27% decrease in stuttering symptoms, that is, findings demonstrated the high variability in stuttering behavior under placebo (**Table 15–1**).

The Wells study (Wells & Malcolm, 1971) is most notable in that it included six groups controlling for three experimental factors: haloperidol (the experimental drug), orphenadrine co-administered to reduce the side effects of haloperidol, and speech therapy used both in combination and alone. The six groups were as follows:

Group 1. Haloperidol and orphenadrine and speech therapy

Group 2. A placebo for haloperidol and orphenadrine and speech therapy

Group 3. A placebo for haloperidol, a placebo for orphenadrine, and speech therapy

Group 4. Haloperidol and orphenadrine without speech therapy

Group 5. A placebo for haloperidol and orphenadrine and speech therapy

Group 6. A placebo for both medications without speech therapy

Unfortunately only six subjects were included in each of the six groups. Only group 1 with all three factors (i.e., the two drugs and speech therapy) and group 4 with both medications and no speech therapy showed improvement. This Class II study and the Swift study (Swift et al., 1975) (see **Table 15–3**) indicate that haloperidol *is probably effective* in the treatment of stuttering. The authors strongly suggest that Class II studies are needed to examine the interaction *between* medication and speech therapy. However, given the severity of the side effects of haloperidol, some of which can be long lasting (e.g., tardive dyskinesia, a disorder much more disabling than stuttering), it is not recommended for use in the management of stuttering. That is, haloperidol's numerous negative side effects nullify its positive main effect.

Other drugs with dopamine antagonist effects include: tiapride (Rothenberger, Johannsen, Schulze, Amorosa, & Rommel, 1994), risperidone (Risperdal®), and clozapine (Clozaril®). Maguire and colleagues conducted one unblinded Class III (Maguire et al., 1999) and one blinded Class II (Maguire, Riley, Franklin, & Gottschalk, 2000) randomized double-blind placebo-controlled trial of risperidone. More recently, olanzapine (Zyprexa®), which is a receptor blocker for serotonin2, another neurotransmitter system, as well as being a dopamine D1–D4 receptor blocker, was found beneficial on three speech measures in a placebo-controlled double-blind Class II trial involving random assignment of 24 adults between treatment and placebo groups (Maguire, Riley et al., 2004). Because two of these are Class II trials with random assignment to treatment and placebo groups, the evidence demonstrates that these newer dopamine antagonists *are probably effective* in the treatment of stuttering. No significant side effects were reported, indicating that further research would be warranted, particularly in combination with speech therapy and using Class II randomized group comparisons.

On the other hand some case reports show serious transient side effects with the use of other serotonin and dopamine receptor blockers. Pimozide (Orap®) induced significant depression and other side effects in a double-blind crossover study (Bloch, et al., 1997); four of seven participants developed depression (four major, one minor depression); one developed akathesia (inability to sit still); and three developed mild parkinsonism. In addition, clozapine (Clozaril®), which interferes with D_1-D_5 receptors and is also an adrenergic, cholinergic, histaminergic, and serotinergic antagonist, induced stuttering in four different case reports (Duggal, Jagadheesan, & Nizamie, 2002; Ebeling, Compton, & Albright, 1997; Supprian, Retz, & Deckert, 1999; Thomas, Lalaux, Vaiva, & Goudemand, 1994).

Given that two Class II trials show some stuttering benefit with dopamine receptor blockade, the evidence suggests that these agents *probably benefit* stuttering. Although statistical significance has been reached on measures of stuttering severity with these pharmaceutical agents, the clinical significance of these speech changes to participants' lives and communication abilities is still unclear. However, it would seem that the degree of clinical benefit relative to the side effects usually prohibits persons from continuing on these medications long term, making them a less viable treatment option. Short-term use in conjunction with speech therapy would seem like a more viable option to explore, beginning with small Class III trials. Studies examining outcomes, both in comparison with speech therapy or in combination with speech therapy, are needed to determine whether dopamine receptor blockade might be beneficial for treatment of stuttering.

Norepinephrine Reuptake Inhibitors   Norepinephrine is another catecholamine neurotransmitter contained in specific neurons in the central nervous system as well as in postganglionic sympathetic neurons in the peripheral nervous system. Reuptake inhibitors for norepinephrine were developed as antidepressants, they and have been used in a few studies in adults who stutter. Imipramine and desipramine are two examples of this drug class. Desipramine (Norpramin®) was used in a double blinded crossover Class III study comparing it with clomipramine (see below) and was not beneficial on measures of stuttering severity (Stager, Ludlow, Gordon, Cotelingham, & Rapoport, 1995b). Only 6 of 16 participants reported that they were improved from baseline, but few experienced side effects. Although only one Class III study is available for this class of medications, it is *possible* that this class of medications may *not* be beneficial in the treatment of stuttering.

Serotonin Selective Reuptake Inhibitors (SSRI)

These medications interfere with the action of plasma membrane transporter molecules, which are needed for the reuptake of serotonin from the synaptic junction. Because reuptake is blocked, serotonin increases in the synaptic junction leading to increased postsynaptic neuronal excitation. Examples of this drug class include clomipramine (Anafranil®), paroxotine (Paxil®), and fluoxetine

(Prozac®). A double-blinded, crossover controlled Class III study compared clomipramine (Anafranil®) and desipramine with placebo (Gordon et al., 1995). Seventeen participants underwent a baseline and placebo phase before being randomly assigned to one of two medication orders, 5 weeks of one medication, 2 weeks of placebo washout, and 5 weeks of the other medication. One report found decreases in stuttering frequency and severity (Stager et al., 1995b). In another report, clomipramine had a significant improvement over desipramine on subjects' visual analogue scales, indicating a decrease in their perceived stuttering severity, thoughts about stuttering, resistance to stuttering, judgment of others' reactions to their stuttering, and expectancy of stuttering (Gordon et al., 1995). Fifty percent of the subjects (8/16) chose to continue on clomipramine after the study. In a separate report, five were followed up for 8 months with a modest benefit on stuttering that was less than the initial 6-week benefit (Stager, Ludlow, Gordon, Cotelingham, & Rapoport, 1995a).

Paroxetine (Paxil®) is an SSRI that produced such significant adverse effects in adults who stuttered that an investigational study of the medication had to be stopped for safety reasons (Bloch, Stager, Braun, & Rubinow, 1995). During withdrawal from paroxetine, two men who had previously had brief episodes of minor depression had significant mood changes. In one, hypomania, hyperactivity, aggression, optimism, and talkativeness occurred between 2 days and 1 week after withdrawal. The other developed suicidal impulses, became irritable, dizzy, short-tempered, and homicidal 2 weeks after withdrawal. These symptoms abated after 2 and one-half weeks. The authors interpreted them as reactions to depletion of central serotonin after reuptake was no longer blocked.

On the other hand, paroxetine benefited acquired stuttering (see Chapter 17 in this volume for a detailed discussion/description of acquired stuttering) and depression in a few case reports (Schreiber & Pick, 1997), and other case studies have also found that paroxetine benefited patients with both obsessive-compulsive disorders and stuttering (Boldrini, Rossi, & Placidi, 2003; M. G. Murray & Newman, 1997). Some SSRIs, however, have been reported to have induced stuttering. Both Sertraline (Zoloft®) and fluoxetine (Prozac®) have induced stuttering in individual cases (Christensen, Byerly, & McElroy, 1996; Guthrie & Grunhaus, 1990).

Given that only one Class III study (Gordon et al., 1995) showed benefit with disappointing results in the long term (Stager et al., 1995a), it is *unknown* whether or not this (SSRI) class of medications could be helpful in stuttering. The significant side effects with some of these agents (Bloch et al., 1995) suggest that caution must be used in administering these medications to persons who stutter.

GABA Agonists

γ-Aminobutyric acid (GABA), an amino acid, is the major inhibitory neurotransmitter in the brain. There are at least two different types of GABA receptors, $GABA_A$ and $GABA_B$. The $GABA_A$ receptor contains the chloride ion channel, resulting in the influx of this negatively charged ion following neurotransmission. Benzodiazepines modulate $GABA_A$; some examples are diazepam (Valium®) and alprazolam (Xanax®), both well-known medications used for anxiety disorders. Baclofen (Lioresal®), a $GABA_B$ receptor agonist affecting G proteins, is known to increase inhibition of motor neurons and has been used to treat spasticity. To date, there are no controlled studies of the use of GABA receptor agonists in stuttering, and it is unknown whether these would benefit persons who stutter.

Channel Blockers

Following an uncontrolled report of benefit of verapamil (Verelan®) in stuttering (Zachariah, 1980), calcium channel blockers were examined in the 1980s in stuttering. One Class III double-blinded placebo controlled crossover study reported more modest improvement with only two participants continuing on the medication over 30 months (Brady, Price, McAllister, & Dietrich, 1989). Another Class III trial, however, found no significant benefit (Brumfitt & Peake, 1988). Overall, the few well-controlled trials of calcium channel blockers indicate that calcium channel blockers *possibly may not benefit* stuttering.

Summary

This evidence-based review of neuropharmacological treatment of stuttering has shown that:

1. *Haloperidol* is probably beneficial in the treatment of stuttering (but side effects are prohibitive to its use for treatment).

2. Other *dopamine receptor blockers*, have fewer side effects than haloperidol and are probably beneficial in the treatment of stuttering, and they need to be evaluated in comparison with speech therapy and in combination with speech therapy. Because fewer significant side effects were reported, this class of drugs would appear to be a fertile area for exploration.

3. *Neuroepinephrine reuptake inhibitors* are possibly not beneficial in stuttering.

4. It is presently unknown whether *SSRIs* alter stuttering (although side effects may be prohibitive).

5. *Calcium channel blockers* are possibly not beneficial in the treatment of stuttering.

These conclusions take into account the outcomes reported and the level of certainty of the evidence after controlling for bias and placebo effects. However, this analysis only considers short-term side effects in that sufficient numbers of participants were willing to continue taking the medications for the trials to be completed and provide useful results. Very limited long-term data are available, and only one study examined the potential for combining medications with speech therapy.

In conclusion, no Class I clinical trials are currently available to demonstrate that neuropharmacological agents are beneficial in persons who stutter. However, it must be recognized that if this classification method were applied to all treatment for stuttering in adults (i.e., behavioral as well as pharmaceutical), no Class I multiple-center random controlled clinical trials are available that demonstrate that other treatments are beneficial for stuttering in chronically affected adults. We recommend that placebo controlled, randomized clinical trials be conducted examining whether speech therapy alone or in combination with neuropharmacological agents are beneficial for chronic adult stuttering. Only Class I and Class II studies provide adequate controls for placebo effects and should be considered the preferred designs for therapeutic trials in stuttering.

References

Anderson, J. M., Hughes, J. D., Rothi, L. J., Crucian, G. P., & Heilman, K. M. (1999). Developmental stuttering and Parkinson's disease: the effects of levodopa treatment. Journal of Neurology, Neurosurgery, and Psychiatry 66(6), 776–778.

Benson, H. (1997). The nocebo effect: History and physiology. Prev Med 26(5 Pt 1), 612–615.

Bloch, M., Stager, S., Braun, A., Calis, K. A., Turcasso, N. M., Grothe, D. R., et al. (1997). Pimozide-induced depression in men who stutter. Journal of Clinical Psychiatry 58(10), 433–436.

Bloch, M., Stager, S. V., Braun, A. R., & Rubinow, D. R.(1995). Severe psychiatric symptoms associated with paroxetine withdrawal [letter]. Lancet 346, 57.

Boldrini, M., Rossi, M., & Placidi, G. F. (2003). Paroxetine efficacy in stuttering treatment. International Journal of Neuropsychopharmacology 6(3), 311–312.

Brady, J. P. (1991). The pharmacology of stuttering: A critical review. American Journal of Psychiatry 148, 1309–1316.

Brady, J. P., Price, T. R., McAllister, T. W., & Dietrich, K. (1989). A trial of verapamil in the treatment of stuttering in adults. Biological Psychiatry 25, 626–630.

Brumfitt, S. M., & Peake, M. D. (1988). A double-blind study of verapamil in the treatment of stuttering. British Journal of Disorders of Communication 23, 35–40.

Burns, D., Brady, J. P., & Kuruvilla, K. (1978). The acute effect of haloperidol and apomorphine on the severity of stuttering. Biological Psychiatry 13, 255–264.

Christensen, R. C., Byerly, M. J., & McElroy, R. A. (1996). A case of sertraline-induced stuttering. Journal of Clinical Psychopharmacology 16(1), 92–93.

Deutch, A. Y., & Roth, R. H. (1999). Neurotransmitters. In M. J. Zigmond, F. E. Bloom, S. C. Landis, J. L. Roberts, & L. R. Squire (Eds.), Fundamental neuroscience (pp. 193–234). New York: Academic Press.

Duggal, H. S., Jagadheesan, K., & Nizamie, S. H. (2002). Clozapine-induced stuttering and seizures. American Journal of Psychiatry 159(2), 315.

Ebeling, T.A., Compton, A.D., & Albright, D. W. (1997). Clozapine-induced stuttering. American Journal of Psychiatry 154(10), 1473.

Fries, S., Grosser, T., Price, T. S., Lawson, J. A., Kapoor, S., DeMarco, S., et al. (2006). Marked interindividual variability in the respone to selective inhibitors of cyclooxygenase-2. Gastroenterology 130(1), 55–64.

Gallin, J. (2002). Principles and practice of clinical research. San Diego, CA: Academic Press.

Gay, T., Rendell, J. K., & Spiro, J. (1994). Oral and laryngeal muscle coordination during swallowing. Laryngoscope 104, 341–349.

Goodin, D., & Edlund, W. (1999). Process for developing technology assessment. St. Paul., MN: American Academy of Neurology.

Gordon, C. T., Cotelingam, G. M., Stager, S., Ludlow, C. L., Hamburger, S. D., & Rapoport, J. L. (1995). A double-blind comparison of clomipramine and desipramine in the treatment of developmental stuttering. Journal of Clinical Psychiatry 56, 238–242.

Guthrie, S., & Grunhaus, L. (1990). Fluoxetine-induced stuttering [letter] [see comments]. Journal of Clinical Psychiatry 51, 85.

Hardman, J., & Limbird, L (Eds.). (2001). Goodman & Gilman's the pharmacological basis of therapeutics. New York: McGraw Hill.

Hinshaw, S. P., Owens, E. B., Wells, K. C., Kraemer, H. C., Abikoff, H. B., Connors, C. K., et al. (2000). Family processes and treatment outcome in the MTA: negative/ineffective parenting practices in relation to multimodal treatment. Journal of Abnormal Child Psychology 28(6), 555–568.

Jones, M., Gebski, V., Onslow, M., & Packman, A. (2002). Statistical power in stuttering research: A tutorial. Journal of Speech, Languge, and Hearing Research; 45(2), 243–255.

Louis, E. D., Winfield, L., Fahn, S., & Ford, B. (2001). Speech dysfluency exacerbated by levodopa in Parkinson's disease. Movement Disorders 16(3), 562–565.

Liu, W., Zhao, W., Shaffer, M. L., Icitovic, N., & Chase, G. A. (2005). Modelling clinical trials in herterogenous samples. Statistics in Medicine 24(18), 2765–2775.

Ludlow, C. L., & Braun, A. R. (1993). Research evaluating the use of neuropharmacological agents for treating stuttering: Possibilities and problems. Journal of Fluency Disorders 18, 169–182.

Maguire, G. A., Gottschalk, L. A., Riley, G. D., Franklin, D. L., Bechtel, R. J., & Ashurst, J. (1999). Stuttering: neuropsychiatric features measured by content analysis of speech and the effect of risperidone on stuttering severity. Comprehensive Psychiatry 40(4), 308–314.

Maguire, G. A., Riley, G. D., Franklin, D. L., & Gottschalk, L. A. (2000). Risperidone for the treatment of stuttering. Journal of Clinical Psychopharmacology 20(4), 479–482.

Maguire, G. A., Riley, G. D., Franklin, D. L., Maguire, M. E., Nguyen, C. T., & Brojeni, P. H. (2004). Olanzapine in the treatment of developmental stuttering: a double-blind, placebo-controlled trial. Annals of Clinical Psychiatry 16(2), 63–67.

Maguire, G. A., Yu, B. P., Franklin, D. L., & Riley, G. D. (2004). Alleviating stuttering with pharmacological interventions. Expert Opinion on Pharmacotherapy 5(7), 1565–1571.

Montgomery, S. A. (1999). The failure of placebo-controlled studies. ECNP Consensus Meeting, September 13, 1997, Vienna. European College of Neuropsychopharmacology. European Neuropsychopharmacology 9(3), 271–276.

MTA Cooperative Group. A 14-month randomized clinical trial of treatment strategies for attention-deficit/ hyperactivity disorder. (1999) Multimodal Treatment Study of Children with ADHD. Arch Gen Psychiatry 56(12), 1073–1086.

Murray, M. G., & Newman, R. M. (1997). Paroxetine for treatment of obsessive-compulsive disorder and comorbid stuttering. American Journal of Psychiatry 154(7), 1037.

Murray, T. J., Kelly, P., Campbell, L., & Stefanik, K. (1977). Haloperidol in the treatment of stuttering. British Journal of Psychiatry 130, 370–373.

Prins, D., Mandelkorn, T., & Cerf, F. A. (1980). Principal and differential effects of haloperidol and placebo treatments upon speech disfluencies in stutterers. Journal of Speech and Hearing Research 23, 614–629.

Rantala, S. L., & Petri-Larmi, M. (1976). Haloperidol (Serenase) in the treatment of stuttering. Folia Phoniatrica et Logopedica (Basel) 28, 354–361.

Rosenberger, P. B., Wheelden, J. A., & Kalotkin, M. (1976). The effect of haloperidol on stuttering. American Journal of Psychiatry 133, 331–334.

Rothenberger, A., Johannsen, H. S., Schulze, H., Amorosa, H., & Rommel, D. (1994). Use of tiapride on stuttering in children and adolescents. Perceptual and Motor Skills 79(3 Pt 1), 1163–1170.

Schreiber, S., & Pick, C. G. (1997). Paroxetine for secondary stuttering: Further interaction of serotonin and dopamine. Journal of Nervous and Mental Disease 185(7), 465–467.

Schweizer, E., & Rickels, K. (1997). Placebo response in generalized anxiety: Its effect on the outcome of clinical trials. Journal of Clinical Psychiatry 58(Suppl 11), 30–38.

Shetty, N., Friedman, J. H., Kieburtz, K., Marshall, F. J., & Oakes, D. The placebo response in Parkinson's disease. Parkinson Study Group. Clinical Neuropharmacology 22(4), 207–212.

Stager, S. V., Ludlow, C. L., Gordon, C. T., Cotelingham, M., & Rapoport, J. (1995a). Maintenance of fluency following long term clomipramine treatment. Proc 1st World Congr on Fluency Dis.

Stager, S. V., Ludlow, C. L., Gordon, C. T., Cotelingham, M., & Rapoport, J. L. (1995b). Stuttering speakers' fluency changes following a double-blind trial of clomipramine and desipramine. Journal of Speech and Hearing Research 38, 516–525.

Supprian, T., Retz, W., & Deckert, J. (1999). Clozapine-induced stuttering: Epileptic brain activity? American Journal of Psychiatry 156(10), 1663–1664.

Swift, W. J., Swift, E. W., & Arellano, M. (1975). Haloperidol as a treatment for adult stuttering. Comprehensive Psychiatry 16, 61–67.

Taylor, E. (1999). Development of clinical services for attention-deficit/hyperactivity disorder. Archives of General Psychiatry 56(12), 1097–1099.

Thomas, P., Lalaux, N., Vaiva, G., & Goudemand, M. (1994). Dose-dependent stuttering and dystonia in a patient taking clozapine. American Journal of Psychiatry 151(7), 1096.

Trivedi, M. H., & Rush, H. (1994). Does a placebo run-in or a placebo treatment cell affect the efficacy of antidepressant medications? Neuropsychopharmacology 11(1), 33–43.

Wells, K. C., Epstein, J. N., Hinshaw, S. P., Conners, C. K., Klaric, J., Abikoff, H. B., et al. (2000). Parenting and family stress treatment outcomes in attention deficit hyperactivity disorder (ADHD): An empirical analysis in the MTA study. Journal of Abnormal Child Psychology 28(6), 543–553.

Wells, P. G. (1974). Haloperidol in the treatment of stutter. Medical Journal of Australia 2(16), 491.

Wells, P. G., & Malcolm, M. T. (1971). Controlled trial of the treatment of 36 stutterers. British Journal of Psychiatry 119, 603–604.

West, S., King, V., Carey, T. S., Lohr, K. N., McKoy, N., Sutton, S. F., et al. (2002). Systems to rate the strength of scientific evidence. Evidence Report/Technology Assessment (Summary) 47, 1–11.

Zachariah, G. (1980). Verapamil in the management of stuttering. Antiseptic: Journal of Medicine and Surgery 77, 87–88.

Section V

Intervention: Related, Less Common Fluency Problems

16

Understanding and Treating Cluttering

Kenneth O. St. Louis, Florence L. Myers, Klaas Bakker, and Lawrence J. Raphael

The purpose of this chapter is to provide readers with a brief but comprehensive summary of cluttering, placing assertions and principles within the context of current status of research evidence. After reviewing the history of cluttering and providing a working definition of cluttering, the chapter covers epidemiology, co-existing disorders, etiology, diagnosis, and therapy. The reader should gain a better understanding of this little-known fluency disorder and how to manage cluttering individuals clinically.

◆ Current View of Cluttering

Cluttering has been variously described as the "orphan" of speech-language pathology (Daly, 1986; Weiss, 1964), but we believe it is time to retire that image. It suggests that the field of speech-language has disavowed involvement in the assessment and treatment of cluttering, but the following developments indicate an emerging change.

Approximately a decade ago, the *Journal of Fluency Disorders* published a special edition on cluttering. Likewise, a brochure on cluttering is widely circulated to consumers by the Stuttering Foundation of America (SFA) (St. Louis, 1998). Furthermore, individuals who clutter[1] have recently found their voice as well through a listserv on the Internet. Thus, cluttering now appears "on the map" of fluency disorders, a goal of the present authors and several other collaborators (Myers, St. Louis, Bakker, et al., 2002a, 2002b). Recent textbooks on stuttering have included substantial discussions of cluttering (e.g., Conture, 2001; Manning, 2001; Shapiro, 1999; Silverman, 2004) and—like the current book—entire chapters are now devoted entirely or substantially to cluttering (e.g., Bennett, 2006;

---

[1]In this chapter, we use the terms "person/individual/client who clutters" as well as the direct label of "clutterer" interchangeably. We fully recognize that many prefer person-first language only, but refer to research that clearly shows that "clutterer" or "stutterer" are viewed no more negatively than "person who clutters/stutters (Dietrich, Jensen, & Williams, 2001; St. Louis, 1999).

Curlee, 1999; Curlee & Siegel, 1997; Daly, 1996; Georgieva, 2004; Guitar, 2006; Ramig & Dodge, 2005). Nevertheless, although cluttering has achieved recognition as a disorder of some importance, its status as a clinical entity is questioned by some writers (e.g., Ryan 2001).

This new-found—or more precisely as we shall explain later—"rediscovered" respectability of cluttering in the field of fluency disorders invites a different metaphor. Accordingly we propose that cluttering be compared with a partly completed jigsaw puzzle (a metaphor also suggested by Daly, 1986). To assemble a complete and cohesive picture of cluttering, there is general agreement among those who have treated or studied cluttering about numerous pieces that fit together as part of the puzzle. By contrast, there are doubts about where other pieces may fit or if they even belong in the puzzle. Some of the pieces are literally missing. Important goals of future empirical research are to resolve doubts about if and where the questionable pieces fit and the identity of the missing pieces.

Perhaps the greatest challenge in assembling a cluttering puzzle has been the ongoing effort to discover which pieces are needed for the creation of a logical and empirically based definition of the disorder. The progress made thus far has focused research by clinicians and scientists on what they interpret as an identifiable fluency disorder and to develop a small but valid and reliable knowledge base. What sets this more recent knowledge apart from the sizable proportion of previous literature is that we can be reasonably confident that it describes one disorder rather than a large number of loosely related—or possibly unrelated—disorders.

◆ Historical Background

Table 16–1 presents a retrospective list of the names of contributors to the literature of cluttering. It is not meant to be exhaustive but, rather, to provide an historical perspective of this intriguing but less than well understood disorder.

What is immediately clear in **Table 16–1** is that the term "cluttering" is not new. In the medical specialty of phoniatrics in Europe in the first half of the 20th century, numerous physicians described fluency disorders that were suggestive of cluttering and stuttering. Unfortunately the terms they used were often interchangeable. For example, George Lewis (1907), one of several now-infamous "stammering school" specialists in the United States in the early 20th century, wrote that:

> . . . stuttering is engendered by nervous weakness and a poor physical condition generally, and manifests itself in lack of breath control and syllabication. The words and phrases are reiterated in nervous jerks. Stammering on the other hand, is caused by disturbance in the brain centers or by a peculiar sensitiveness which manifest itself in excessive efforts to speak (p. 25).

The first use of the term cluttering, in 1877 has been attributed to Adolph Kussmaul, a German lexicographer (Weiss, 1964).

Throughout the past 50 years, practitioners of phoniatrics and logopedics in Europe focused more strongly on the nature and clinical treatment of cluttering than did North American clinical speech-language pathologists or speech and hearing scientists (e.g., Luchsinger & Arnold, 1965), although there were exceptions (e.g., Van Riper, 1971; Weiss, 1964). During this period in the United States and Canada, the tenets of behavioral psychology and empiricism had profound effects on the practice of speech-language pathology, one of which was the exclusion of disorders for which reliable identification criteria had not been established. Cluttering was thus largely ignored, both in the laboratory and the clinic, and became relatively unfamiliar to scientists and clinicians during the middle and latter half of the 20th century. During this period, few references to cluttering were included in the North American literature, and most of these mentioned the work of European contributors (Hahn, 1943, 1956). Some popular texts (mainly concerned with stuttering) did not mention cluttering at all (Ingham, 1984; Sheehan, 1970; Wingate, 1976). By contrast, Van Riper (1971, 1982) reviewed some of the existing literature and postulated his now well-known Track II, a subgroup of stutterers that likely have co-existing cluttering.

Table 16–1 Selected Contributions to Cluttering from the Literature

Name	Selected Contributions to Cluttering
Kussmaul (1877)	First popularized the word "cluttering" in Germany
Freund (1952); Weiss (1967)	Similar positions, hereditary, and other connections between cluttering and stuttering; cluttering is the basic disorder and stuttering emerges from it in some cases
Luchsinger & Landolt (1955)	Reported likelihood of electroencephalogaphy (EEG) abnormalities in clutterers
Seeman & Novak (1963)	Hypothesized basal ganglia etiology and generalized motor deficit in cluttering
Langova & Moravek (1964)	Research to document organic nature of cluttering through investigations of clutterers and stutterers with EEG, delayed auditory feedback (DAF), and either stimulants or antianxiety drugs
Luchsinger & Arnold (1965)	Hypothesized hereditary influences and organic influences on cluttering
Arnold (1970)	Hypothesized that when language endowment and lateralized language are low (as in cluttering), musical ability is high and mathematical ability is low
de Hirsch (1970)	Hypothesized lack of maturation of the nervous system as an etiological factor in cluttering
Van Riper (1971)	Described Track II stutterers with a cluttering component
Becker & Grundmann (1971); Becker, Slassova, Asantiani, Beljakowa, & Hey (1977)	Hypothesized that a brain-injured subgroup of stutterers also manifested symptoms of cluttering, dysarthria, and tachylalia; found prevalence of cluttering to be ~1.5% in elementary schoolchildren
Dalton & Hardcastle (1977)	Considered speech of clutterers to be "over-coarticulated"
Daly (1986)	Neuropsychological tests indicate that an organic subgroup of stutterers are likely to manifest cluttering
Preus (1981)	Studied 100 adolescent stutterers and corroborated Van Riper's notion of a Track II stutterer
St. Louis (1992)	Advanced a working definition of cluttering as a fluency disorder that is not stuttering but also a rate disorder
Myers (1992)	Hypothesized that clutterers exceed their own individual capacities for rate; therefore, speech rate, language, and articulation do not function in synergy in cluttering and are exacerbated by a defective self-monitoring and self-regulatory system
Bakker (1996)	Inability to agree on a definition and to measure cluttering objectively and quantitatively are hindrances to further scientific advances

♦ Working Definition of Cluttering

Following is the most recently revised version of our working definition of cluttering. (See St. Louis, 1992, and St. Louis, Raphael, Myers, & Bakker, 2003, for earlier versions.) This definition reflects our best collective judgment of what cluttering is but will be further modified when and if data indicate a need to do so. *Cluttering is a fluency disorder characterized by a rate that is perceived to be abnormally rapid, irregular, or both for the speaker (although measured syllable rates may not exceed normal limits). These rate abnormalities further are manifest[2] in one or more of the following*

---

[2]The phrase "are manifest in" implies that the rate problems observed in cluttering cause the other symptoms. If we had indicated "are associated with," the reader could assume that there is simply a correlational connection between rate and disfluency, rate and excessive coarticulation, and so on. Recognizing that we may not be entirely correct, we believe it is important to advance a definition that clearly advances the centrality of rate problems in cluttering.

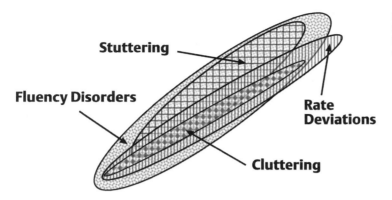

Figure 16–1 Hypothesized relationship between cluttering, stuttering, fluency disorders, and rate deviations.

symptoms: (a) an excessive number of disfluencies, the majority of which are not typical of people who stutter; (b) the frequent placement of pauses and use of prosodic patterns that do not conform to syntactic and semantic constraints; and (c) inappropriate (usually excessive) degrees of coarticulation among sounds, especially in multisyllabic words.

The definition indicates that cluttering is a *fluency disorder* even though it refers to a central problem of *rate* that underlies abnormalities in the integrity of articulatory coordination or that is associated with excessive normal disfluencies. This working definition also suggests a broader interpretation of *fluency disorder* than the one advanced in 1992 by the first author, a fluency disorder that is not stuttering (i.e., the excessive disfluencies) with a rapid and/or irregular speaking rate (St. Louis, 1992). These relationships are displayed in **Fig. 16–1** and are further clarified in a subsequent section. In the current and previous versions, we believe that cluttering, like stuttering, should still be considered to be—at least for the sake of clinical expediency—primarily a *fluency disorder*, partly for the reason that caseloads are often categorized by this generic term (see below). Nevertheless, we added the possibility of deviations in pauses, prosody, and coarticulation, all of which can affect the perception of rate and fluency. These deviations were added to our working definition of cluttering (St. Louis, 1992) because we have sometimes observed clutterers without excessive disfluencies, but with irregular pauses or deletions of weak syllables as the only—or primary—rate-related symptoms.

We believe that a good definition must function like an effective fisherman's net. It must catch the desired fish but fail to catch any fish or other items that are not desired. The message from this seemingly simple analogy turns out not to be simple at all. It requires the identification of those critical features of the condition or those symptoms without which a person would not be regarded as a clutterer. Moreover, it must also *not* include symptoms that may—but do not necessarily—accompany the essential symptoms. For instance, there is the question of whether or not the definition of cluttering should include a language component or an awareness component because problems in these areas are common in cluttering. As likely as they are to occur in clinical cases, we must ask, "Could a person who clutters manifest the other essential symptoms and not have any measurable or perceptible language or awareness difficulties?" If so, then these symptoms would not be necessary to the definition, even though they may occur in a large majority of cases. In essence, then, the critical features must be derived logically as much as empirically.

This will explain differences between our working definition and other definitions contained in the literature, most of which were derived from clinical treatment experience.[3] For example, a Task

---

[3]The authors of this chapter are not in complete agreement on this issue. The second author prefers to view cluttering as a spectrum disorder with resultant "subgroups," depending on where "derailment" occurs along the communication chain as a function of attempting to speak faster than the speaker is capable. One subgroup may have excessive disfluencies, another may produce excessive disfluencies with articulatory anomalies, and another may manifest noncohesive linguistic output. This clinically oriented perspective, derived from symptoms and self-appraisals of a majority of cluttering clients—though not every single one—illustrates the difficulty of generating a definition consisting only of essential features.

Force of the Special Interest Division of the American Speech-Language-Hearing Association on Fluency and Fluency Disorders offered the following definition: "Cluttering is a fluency disorder characterized by a rapid and/or irregular speech rate, excessive disfluencies, and often other symptoms such as language or phonological errors and attention deficits" (American Speech-Language-Hearing Association, 1999, p. 35). Weiss (1964; 1967) defined cluttering as one of several manifestations of an underlying condition he called "central language imbalance."

◆ Epidemiology

Prevalence and Incidence

Very limited data—and no recent studies—exist regarding the prevalence of cluttering. Becker and Grundmann (1971) reported that 1.5% of 7- and 8-year-olds in a German school manifested cluttering. Among groups of stutterers, the reported percentages of those who also cluttered have varied. Freund (1952) reported that in 121 cases of stuttering he had seen in his private practice, 22% also cluttered. This was equal to the percentage of co-existent cluttering and stuttering in 392 school-children he had also treated. Of Freund's 121 private clients, 51% of the pure stutterers had relatives with fluency disorders compared with 93% of the stutterers who also cluttered. As noted, Preus (1981) reported 32% of 100 adolescent stutterers also manifested some cluttering symptoms. Pure clutterers appear to be rare (Dalton & Hardcastle, 1977, 1989; St. Louis & Myers, 1997). Daly (1996) speculates that ~5% of all fluency disorders are pure clutterers. Filatova (2002) tested 55 fluency-disordered children between the ages of 7 and 16 and found that 7% were pure clutterers. We raise the possibility that all types of cluttering may be underdiagnosed because: (1) relatively few clinicians are as knowledgeable about cluttering as they are about stuttering; (2) few clutterers self-refer for services; and (3) some clutterers do not believe they have a speech disorder, and hence they do not seem to have a concern.

At present we do not have accurate estimates of the lifetime incidence of cluttering. Without: (1) a specific, commonly accepted, and empirically supported definition; and (2) either a major longitudinal research study of cluttering or replicated probability samples from the population, it is impossible to obtain such estimates.

Onset and Course

There is little information about the onset of cluttering, although several authors suggest it is later than for stuttering, often after the age of 7 (e.g., Diedrich, 1984). Our experience generally supports this supposition, even though we have evaluated a few preschool children who clearly cluttered. Among several explanations, it is possible that cluttering may manifest itself when language and thought become relatively more sophisticated with age. Accordingly, we suggest that cluttering is unlikely to be observed in toddlers using one- and two-word utterances compared with the early elementary-school-age child who has much to say and uses lengthier and more complex utterances. Obviously, empirical research regarding the onset of cluttering is much needed at this point.

Recovery with and without Therapy

Do clutterers recover spontaneously or as a consequence of therapy? To answer this question we must await new information that may enable us to fit together more pieces of the cluttering puzzle. Historical reports (e.g., Weiss, 1964) suggest that the prognosis for cluttering is not generally regarded to be as good as it is for stuttering. Case studies presented in a special edition of the *Journal of Fluency Disorders* suggest that prognoses ranged from quite poor (Thacker & Austen, 1996) to intermediate (e.g., St. Louis, Myers, Cassidy, et al., 1996) to good (e.g., Craig, 1996; Daly & Burnett,

1996; Langevin & Boberg, 1996). Our clinical experience leads us to hypothesize that the likelihood of improvement is related to clutterers' degree of self-awareness.

◆ The Nature of Cluttering

Cluttering Usually Co-exists with Other Disorders

A review of the literature yields dozens of symptoms that characterize cluttering or that differentiate it from stuttering and other conditions. In an extensive review of co-existing communication disorders, St. Louis, Ruscello, and Lundeen (1992) described cluttering as a condition that nearly always co-exists (or co-occurs) with symptoms of other disorders. For example, St. Louis and Hinzman (1986) identified 65 different symptoms for cluttering identified in six well-known references on the disorder. Given this state of affairs, it is not surprising that people who clutter manifest such a wide range of symptoms, some of which suggest different disorders. Two questions arise: "Which disorders are most likely associated with cluttering and which ones are not?" and "Are the relationships between the various symptoms causally or noncausally related to cluttering?" We can answer the first question in terms of general or agreement or disagreement in the literature, but a great deal of further research will be necessary to answer the second question. The following sections describe co-existing symptoms for which there is: (1) general agreement of common co-existence; and (2) a reasonable theoretical rationale to assume that co-existence might explain more about the nature of cluttering. We further submit that the first group of disorders characterized by consensus agreement should be considered in the typical clinical management of cluttering individuals.

Co-existing Disorders: General Agreement

The right side of **Fig. 16–2** (identical to **Fig. 16–1**) illustrates the hypothesized relationships, explained below, between fluency disorders, rate deviations, stuttering, and cluttering and reflects our working definition of cluttering. The left side of **Fig. 16–2** shows those disorders coexisting with cluttering that

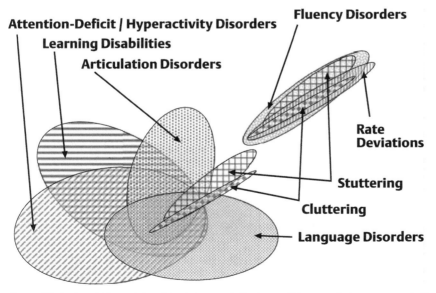

Figure 16–2 Co-existing relationships between cluttering and five speech, language, and other disorders.

are generally agreed by clinicians. The ensuring text summarizes important assumptions and dimensions of these relationships.

Fluency Disorder   In our view, cluttering—like stuttering—should continue to be categorized as a fluency disorder (e.g., St. Louis & Myers, 1997), even though an excess of perceived disfluencies may not be salient symptoms in the speech of those who clutter. The overlapping relationship among fluency disorders, stuttering, and cluttering, recognizes the possibility that there may be other fluency disorders beyond cluttering and stuttering, for example, neurogenic stuttering, psychogenic stuttering, and others, yet to be defined.

Rate Deviations   We hypothesize that speaking rate is usually—but not in every case—a component of speech fluency, which explains the small part of the ovals in **Figs. 16–1** and **16–2** representing rate deviations that is not included within the category of fluency disorders. The nonoverlapping rate deviations[4] would include, for example, individuals who simply speak much faster or slower than normal.

Our definition states that clutterers always manifest a deviation of rate as well as a fluency disorder, that is, the cluttering oval falls entirely within the ovals for rate deviations and fluency disorders. In addition, as we have defined them, clutterers can manifest one or two rate deviations (not shown in **Figs. 16–1** and **16–2**). The first is speaking at a rate that is judged by the listener to be too rapid; the second is speaking at a rate that is judged to be too irregular.

Our own preliminary research, described later, suggests that although clutterers may (or may not) be able to produce syllables as rapidly as normal controls (Raphael, Bakker, Myers, St. Louis, & MacRoy, 2004; Raphael et al., 2005), clinicians, researchers, and listeners often perceive their speech as "too fast" (e.g., St. Louis, 1996; St. Louis & Hinzman, 1986; St. Louis, Myers, Faragasso, Townsend, & Gallaher, 2004). Later, we will suggest that clutterers may manifest a rate that is *relatively* too fast for their own speech production capabilities.

It is quite common to observe otherwise normally speaking individuals who talk faster than nearly everyone else (e.g., St. Louis & Myers, 1997). Such individuals are often difficult to understand for the sole reason that listeners have difficulty comprehending speech at the speed at which it is produced. When a rapid speaking rate occurs in isolation, we agree with Weiss (1964) that it is not a typical speech disorder. The traditional term for excessively rapid rate is tachylalia, but the term denotes and connotes a *disorder*. For such individuals—whom we would *not* regard as clutterers—we prefer the more neutral term, excessively rapid speech (ERS). (We hasten to add that although they may not have a disorder per se, individuals with ERS could potentially benefit from speech therapy to reduce their rate to a level that others can more easily understand.)

A caveat is in order here. Apparently due to the fact that ERS should not be uniformly regarded as abnormal, Weiss (1964), Daly and Burnett (1999), and others have taken the position that excessive speaking rate should not be regarded as an obligatory symptom of cluttering. While agreeing with the logic of their position, we nonetheless believe that rate problems are central to cluttering.

The second way in which rate may appear deviant is in terms of its variability or as an excessively irregular or jerky rate. This is a perceptual judgment for which little objective data currently exist. However, clutterers tell us that they often stop talking "in midstream" while trying to collect their thoughts. Irregularity of rate may be associated with pauses that do not coincide with thought or linguistic junctures. Our own preliminary research, described below, suggests that clutterers are more variable in diadochokinetic (DDK) tasks than controls (Bakker, Raphael, Myers, St. Louis, & MacRoy, 2004).

Stuttering   Cluttering can and often does co-exist substantially with stuttering. (These two disorders are shown in the same proportional relationships in both **Figs. 16–1** and **16–2**.) As noted, in

---

[4]We use the term "rate deviations" rather than "rate disorders" because, as will be clarified later, excessively rapid speakers (ERS) are often not considered to have speech disorders, per se.

his description of stuttering "tracks," Van Riper (1971, pp. 108–111) identified individuals who manifested both stuttering and cluttering as Track II stutterers. His data gleaned from case files suggested that ~14% of stuttering clients could be classified as Track II. In Van Riper's discussion, he entertained the idea that they were clutterers, but based on such late-developing symptoms as avoidance and run-away repetitions in some cases, he considered them to be a subgroup of stutterers. Preus (1981) carefully studied 100 adolescent stutterers and reported that 32% of them also had "cluttering symptoms" (i.e., rapid speech, omission of sounds and syllables due to excessive coarticulation, and jumbled or insufficiently pre-programmed syntax), and 8% could be accurately classified as Track II stutterers, according to his more strict criteria.

A relatively large proportion of the cluttering literature has been—and continues to be—devoted to differentiating cluttering and stuttering (e.g., Filatova, 2002; Froeschels, 1955; Georgieva & Miliev, 1996). Unfortunately, this literature suffers from the lack of a universally agreed on and empirically supported definition of cluttering. The available literature as a whole suggests that the essential difference between these clinical populations centers on the speaker's level of preparedness for saying intended utterances. Stutterers know what they want to say but are interfered in their attempt to produce various words, whereas clutterers do not necessarily know all of what they want to say—or how—but say it anyway.

Part-word repetitions, prolongations, and blocks are typically produced by stutterers, whereas excessive but *normal* disfluencies often characterize the speech of clutterers. These include interjections, revisions, word repetitions, phrase repetitions, and unfinished words. It should be noted that word repetitions, especially one-syllable words, can also be symptoms of stuttering, especially as initial symptoms among young children who stutter.

Equally important, cluttering does not appear to engender nearly the degree of concern about saying particular sounds or words as stuttering does; the clutterer may even be quite unaware of many of the disfluencies or rate symptoms acutely noticed by others. A recent listserv for adults who clutter, although very likely not a representative sample, reveals that individuals who regard themselves as clutterers do experience concern and anxiety about speaking that appears to be more situational than word-specific. It is often reported that clutterers do not acquire and manifest the kinds of accessory behaviors such as eye blinks that often accompany stuttering.

Articulation Disorders   Our working definition suggests that inconsistent misarticulations, especially deletion of sounds in multisyllabic words, may be a consequence of persons who clutter attempting to speak faster than they are able. Virtually all speakers neutralize or change various phonemes, especially in fast speech and notably when they occur in unstressed syllables, for example, "D'ya wanna go?" for "Do you want to go?" Clutterers, however, exceed the normal qualitative and quantitative limits of these changes; they tend to delete or neutralize syllables that standard speakers do not neutralize (e.g., "explation" for "explanation" or "inbi-ity" for "inability"). As noted, these articulatory symptoms may occur in segments of speech that are devoid of perceived disfluencies. For example, Martin, Kroll, O'Keefe, and Painter (1983) reported a spectrographic study of one adolescent clutterer whose speech was often produced without distinct vowel formants, release bursts for stops, or aperiodic energy for fricatives.

In addition, conventional articulation disorders, such as consistent substitutions or distortions of various phonemes such as /s/, /r/, or /l/, are reported to be quite common among clutterers (e.g., Daly & Burnett, 1999; Froeschels, 1955). It is interesting that from a rare sample of six *nonstuttering* first through sixth graders, carefully selected from a large database (Hull, Mielke, Willeford, & Timmons, 1976) for verified rapid or irregular speaking rates and for excessively disfluent speech, four, or two-thirds, of them also manifested articulation disorders[5] (St. Louis et al., 1992).

---

[5]It should be noted that articulation disorders are also quite common in stuttering (e.g., Blood, Ridenour, Qualls, & Hammer, 2003; St. Louis, Murray, & Ashworth, 1991). About 40% of stutterers manifest articulation disorders, and that percentage can be higher if young elementary-age stutterers are considered (St. Louis, 1991).

Language Disorders   It is clear that there is considerable overlap between articulation and language disorders (St. Louis et al., 1992). As discussed earlier, one of the most debated issues in cluttering is the extent to which language disorders should—or should not—be considered part of its definition (e.g., Daly, 1992–93; Daly & Burnett, 1999; Myers, 1996; Weiss, 1964). To date we have seen a few cluttering children with no obvious language problems, so, for that reason, we consider language disorders to be common co-existing problems rather than obligatory symptoms. Nevertheless, language disorders are common in cluttering (Myers, 1996). For example, Pitluk (1982) found near significant differences between four 9- to 12-year-old clutterers and four normal speaking controls on an expressive language test for aphasia. The small group of cluttering individuals produced less concise and more redundant descriptions as well as fewer self-corrections than the normal speakers. Using the same large database mentioned above (Hull, et al., 1976), a group of 24 first through sixth graders (controlled for sex, grade, and location) with "possible cluttering" (i.e., abnormal "fluency" ratings, deviant "articulation" ratings, but not "stuttering" classifications) was found to manifest important differences in language compared with 24 normal speakers (St. Louis, Hinzman, & Hull, 1985). Although the mean length of utterances were virtually identical, the "possible cluttering" group had less complete (i.e., a lower percentage of utterances with both a noun phrase and verb phrase) and less complex (i.e., number of verbs per utterance) than the normal control group. Mazes (Loban, 1976), or verbiage consisting of false starts, disfluent speech, and words irrelevant to the message being conveyed are common in cluttered speech as well (e.g., St. Louis & Myers, 1997). When mazes are prevalent, our clinical experience suggests that they are frequently linguistically and/or cognitively motivated.

Clutterers often manifest pragmatic and narrative problems (Myers, 1996). Based on the authors' experience, they frequently have difficulty maintaining cohesive and coherent conversations. Teigland (1996) reported that three young clutterers were more likely than control subjects to manifest pragmatic language problems on a task involving taking the listener's perspective into account.

Attention Deficit/Hyperactivity Disorders   With increasing recent awareness and diagnoses of attention deficit/hyperactivity disorders (ADHD) (Volkmar, 2003), this condition is frequently reported to co-exist with cluttering. The diagnostic criteria for ADHD (American Psychiatric Association, 1994) include symptoms of: (1) inattention (e.g., "fails to pay attention to details or makes careless mistakes," "does not follow through on instructions or fails to finish school work," or "is easily distracted by external stimuli"); or (2) hyperactivity/impulsivity (e.g., "fidgets with hands or feet/squirms in seat," "talks excessively," or "interrupts or intrudes"). Among other criteria, these symptoms must be present before the age of 7 years, be manifest in at least two settings, and show clear evidence of "clinically significant impairment in social, academic, or occupational functioning." Numerous ADHD symptoms (American Psychiatric Association, 1994) have been reported to be characteristic of many clutterers by various authors (e.g., Daly, 1992–93; St. Louis, 1996; St. Louis & Hinzman, 1986). By contrast, even though controlled data are lacking, we suspect that most individuals diagnosed with ADHD do not clutter.

Specific Learning Disabilities   Guidelines for the diagnosis of learning disabilities (LD) from the 1997 Individual with Disabilities Education Act include failure to achieve commensurate with age and ability and a severe discrepancy between achievement and intellectual ability in such areas as oral expression, listening comprehension, or mathematics calculation. Importantly, these discrepancies cannot result primarily from: (1) a visual, hearing, or motor impairment; (2) mental retardation; (3) emotional disturbance; or (4) environmental, cultural, or economic disadvantage (Council for Exceptional Children, 2002).

Like ADHD, specific LD have been reported to co-exist with cluttering (e.g., Daly, 1986; Tiger, Irvine, & Reis, 1980), especially difficulties in expression, reading, and writing. In addition, although corroborating data are anecdotal, lower than average skills in such areas as handwriting (e.g., Roman, 1963; Weiss, 1964) and music (e.g., Langova & Moravek, 1970; Luchsinger & Arnold, 1965) have also been reported as co-existing with cluttering symptoms.

The co-existence of LD with ADHD (**Fig. 16–1**) is supported by questionnaire data, In a telephone survey of nearly 80,000 US households, 3.3% of 6- to 11-year-old children were diagnosed with ADHD (or ADD), 4.2% with LD, and 3.5% with both ADHD and LD (Centers for Disease Control, 2002).

Co-existing Disorders: Possible Theoretical Relevance

Central Auditory Processing Disorders   Preus (1992, 1996) suggested a possible link between cluttering and central auditory processing disorders (CAPD). In a recent symposium on cluttering that, among other purposes, explored potential links of cluttering to other disorders (Myers et al., 2002a, 2002b), Katz, who is well known for his pioneering work in CAPD, speculated that cluttering may be associated with central auditory processing. Molt (1996) reported that three children who cluttered, compared with controls, evidenced abnormalities on both a central auditory test battery and on scalp-recorded auditory event-related potentials. Wolk (1986) summarized the case study of a young adult who cluttered who had normal auditory discrimination but manifested difficulties in identifying dichotically presented syllables, compared with data from previous studies of normal speakers.

The theoretical relevance of CAPD to cluttering is that the speech of individuals with CAPD includes many of the same symptoms as cluttered speech. In the symposium mentioned above, Katz asserted that symptoms common to CAPD and cluttering, such as rapid speech, omission of weak syllables, excessive disfluencies, and excessive verbal revisions, suggest that common brain functions may be involved. Clearly, this possibility is strongly deserving of controlled, empirical clinical studies.

Basal Ganglia Syndrome   In the same symposium (Myers, et al., 2002a, 2002b), Wiig speculated about the overlap of symptoms between several so-called basal ganglia syndromes wherein a person's brain "executive function" (Royall, Lauterbach, Cummings, Reeve, Rummans et al., 2002) does not function normally. Behavioral dimensions of this executive function include the skills of behavioral regulation, initiation of action, planning and organization, monitoring, responding to feedback and shifting, and working memory. *Wiig* identified several disorders that may share common deficits, such as Tourette's syndrome, autism, pervasive developmental delay, Asperger's syndrome, obsessive compulsive disorder, LD, ADHD, mood disorders, and other anxiety disorders. Individuals who clutter seem to manifest several difficulties in executive function, which may explain why so many of these disorders co-exist with cluttering (e.g., Thacker & Austen, 1996).

Apraxia of Speech   Another disorder that is sometimes mentioned by clinicians as possibly co-existing with cluttering is apraxia of speech, or more accurately, developmental apraxia of speech (DAS). DAS is a disorder with putative neurological and genetic etiology characterized especially by inconsistent misarticulations that are not related to normal phonological development. DAS affects longer and more complex words more than shorter, simple words, and the speaker often appears to be groping for the right articulation, frequently attempting a difficult word several times (National Institute on Deafness and Other Communication Disorders, 2006). Diedrich (1984) presented a differential diagnostic table showing that DAS shared 9 of 12 symptoms with cluttering. Given difficulties in defining and diagnosing both disorders, we are uncertain about the possible nature of a link or overlap between DAS and cluttering.

Subgroups of Cluttering   At this time, we are reasonably comfortable differentiating pure cluttering from cluttering co-existing with stuttering (Daly & Burnett, 1999; St. Louis & Myers, 1997). Pending a great deal of careful epidemiological research on cluttering, it would be premature to speculate about specific subgroups of clutterers. Nevertheless, we agree with Dalton and Hardcastle (1977) that anecdotal and historical reports (e.g., Luchsinger & Arnold, 1965) suggest yet-to-be-identified subgroups. The reports of co-existing—and overlapping—conditions especially would suggest the need for research for further refining the diagnostic classification of cluttering.

◆ Possible Models of Cluttering Etiology

Current models attempting to explain etiology belong to at least one of four categories: (1) theories that refer to CNS integrity; (2) theories that involve cognitive processing capabilities; (3) genetic models; and (4) models that are common to both stuttering and cluttering.

Central Nervous System Function Models

The integrity of the central nervous system (CNS) has been the focus of a wide range of explanations for cluttering. The earliest explanations targeted integrity of the CNS in its entirety (e.g., Cabanas, 1954; de Hirsch, 1961). Early clinical investigations, for example, reported that subclinical electroencephalogram (EEG) abnormalities were most frequently observed among persons who clutter, and to a lesser degree among persons who both clutter and stutter, but the likelihood of these same observations among pure stutterers was indistinguishable from that of normals (e.g., Landolt & Luchsinger, 1954; Luchsinger & Landolt, 1951, 1955; Moravek & Langova, 1962). Importantly, these abnormalities did not result in localization-specific conclusions. Nevertheless, one location has been specifically suggested based on the early EEG research; Seeman (1970) predicted the presence of microscopic lesions in the striatal cortex, which is the general location of the basal ganglia.

Unfortunately the above-cited researchers predated development of localization specific and temporally sensitive brain-imaging technologies, and so they were forced to use crude and early forms of clinical EEG instead. Such would have been possible with current evoked response potential strategies, which are time-linked with specific linguistic or other stimuli. Moreover, such research would shed light on the temporal aspects of how specific cognitive responses unfold in response to stimulus conditions. Despite these promising potentials, these methodologies appear to have not been used with persons who clutter.

More recent research (Dalton & Hardcastle, 1989; Darley, Aronson, & Brown, 1975) implicated the basal ganglia in cluttering on the basis of similarities between some (but certainly not all) of the characteristics of the speech of clutterers and those who suffer from hypokinetic dysarthria (Lebrun, 1996). More recently, Wiig (in Myers et al., 2002a, 2002b) suggested a link between cluttering and certain forms of learning disability and attention-related disturbances based on studies employing new brain imaging technologies.

Cognitive Processing Capabilities Models

A different venue of etiological explanations involves integrity of cognitive processing. Specific cognitive processes implicated in cluttering so far are: (1) linguistic processing (e.g., Daly & Burnett, 1999; Weiss, 1964); (2) attention (St. Louis & Myers, 1997); (3) central auditory processing (Molt, 1996; Myers, et al., 2002a, 2002b); (4) motor-speech related functions (Dalton & Hardcastle, 1989; de Hirsch, 1961); and (5) multiple cognitive systems-related explanations (e. g., Daly & Burnett, 1999; Myers, 1992). Clearly, linguistic processing notions have received the most attention in cognitive processing-related cluttering explanations. However, no studies have yet supported the notion that presumed linguistic processing differences among persons who clutter are associated with actual brain differences. Again, evoked response methodologies have not to date been used to study cognitive or linguistic process differences of those who clutter. Rather, linguistic processing differences were interpreted as a congenital characteristic of the language system of persons who clutter (Weiss, 1964).

Proponents of the linguistic processing viewpoint have suggested that cluttering is a linguistic syndrome (e.g., Daly, 1992–93; Daly & Burnett, 1999). However, if cluttering were associated with deviant linguistic processing, one might assume that there should be parallels with clinical facts known about aphasia such as, for example, symptoms associated with Broca's or Wernicke's aphasia, even though disruptions could conceivably be "subclinical" and serve mainly to exacerbate or cause a variety of cluttering symptoms. In the absence of such parallels, the linguistic interpretation of cluttering needs to identify aberrant linguistic behaviors unlike those that are typical of aphasia but perhaps more like those that characterize developmental child language disorders or relative inefficiencies compared with the performance levels of normal speakers.

A synergistic framework proposed by Myers (1992) provides a parallel model to that of Daly and Burnett (1999). This model describes how the problems of persons who clutter originate from a tendency to produce speech at a rate too fast for the individual to handle. When this happens, the timing of various communication events (e.g., encoding of thought units into language or linguistic units into articulatory gestures) are neither well-synchronized nor integrated. By-products of this dissynergy include disfluencies, poor speech intelligibility, and compromises in narrative and discourse skills.[6]

Genetic Models

There appears to be widespread consensus (e.g., Daly & Burnett, 1999; St. Louis & Myers, 1995, 1997; Weiss, 1964) that cluttering reflects a possible genetic predisposition for disfluent speech. There is evidence that cluttering runs in families, and possibly even in the same families where there are disproportionately many persons who stutter (Luchsinger & Arnold, 1965; Weiss, 1964). Moreover, the literature suggests that cluttering is four times more likely among males than females (Arnold, 1960), which is suggestive for a genetic explanation as well. Yet, based on preliminary research, we are currently uncertain that the 4:1 ratio will be confirmed by future research (e.g., Raphael et al., 2005; St. Louis & McCaffrey, 2005).

Cluttering-Stuttering Models

We noted earlier that cluttering and stuttering often co-exists in the same individual. Several authors have suggested possible links between cluttering and stuttering (e. g., Freund, 1952; Weiss, 1964). Moreover, as noted above, Van Riper (1971, 1982) recognized a developmental Track II in stuttering that contains convincing similarities to the developmental course of cluttering. Although not a specific indication of a possible etiology of cluttering, the apparent association between the disorders suggests a potential relatedness of their respective etiologies. This is not to say, however, that cluttering and stuttering are the same disorders. Our research, described below, suggests that cluttering and stuttering disfluencies are probably not the same, although preliminary data (Myers, St. Louis, Lwowski et al., 2004) suggest that clutterers may not manifest more disfluencies than normal speakers.

♦ Recent Studies of Cluttering

Speech Production of Clutterers

Rate

An acoustic study of syllable rate of the severely cluttered, conversational utterances of an adolescent clutterer (Bakker, Raphael, Myers, & St. Louis, 2000) highlighted several procedural issues that create challenges to the objective study of cluttering. Among them was the fact that if the count of

---

[6]There are parallels between Myers synergism model for cluttering and the model of Zackheim and Conture (2003)who suggested, relative to stuttering, that the "match" between the dynamically, rapidly changing linguistic components of an utterance (e.g., length and complexity) and the relatively static, slowly changing linguistic maturity (i.e., MLU) of a speaker appears to influence the fluency of the utterance. There are also parallels to linguistic "dissociations" observed in stuttering (Anderson, Pellowski, & Conture, 2005).

syllables actually produced, determined from spectrograms, was used as the basis for calculations, then the clutterer's rate fell within the normal range of syllables per second even though the individual's speaking rate was perceived as very fast. It was clear that the speaker was omitting entire syllables or sounds.[7] In many cases the omitted syllables could be reasonably inferred from the morphological or syntactic context and from the acoustic information that was present in the speech signal. When the omitted syllables were included in the total count of "intended" syllables, the syllable rate was much higher and exceeded normal limits.

Needless to say, however reasonable the interpolations of omitted material might have been, they constituted the sort of "mind-reading" that seemingly compromises the collection of objective, replicable data. Accordingly, the authors constructed a protocol intended to elicit utterances of predetermined content. These utterances included DDK syllable trains (e.g., /p^t^k^/), multisyllabic words modeled on the DDKs (e.g., "pattycake,"), and other reading and conversational tasks.

To date, the authors have been recruiting clutterers and matching each of them to an ERS (a nonclutterer who speaks excessively rapidly), and to a normal-speaking control. Initial data analyses so far have been primarily focused on the DDKs and analogous real words spoken by clutterers and their sex- and age-matched normal controls. Relative to speaking rate, one of the most interesting findings has been that at their self-selected, "comfortable" speaking rates, a majority of clutterers produced somewhat fewer syllables per second than their matched controls. (Raphael et al., 2004, 2005). Participants also were asked to produce the DDK and analogous words at their maximum rate—and then "even faster." Some clutterers produced more syllables per second in the faster of these two maximum rates than their matched controls in these conditions, but most did not.

These findings seem at first to be counterintuitive. On the other hand, the findings may not be surprising if we posit that clutterers speak at a rate faster than they can handle. The DDK task eliminates many factors that potentially tax their ability to articulate speech. For example, DDKs do not make the same demands of speakers to map cognitive on to formulative processes that are typically the case during conversational speech. That is, DDK productions do not require the speaker to quickly and spontaneously convert preverbal thought/intention into an integrated code or plan used to orally express the speaker's intention. Rather, with DDK, the speaker engages in something more akin to parroting rather than formulating speech or language, with the focus of effort during DDK production on articulation, not on conveying a message. Thus, given that clutterers may not be skilled at producing speech rapidly, when they have the opportunity to select a comfortable—for them—articulatory rate, it may well be that they select one that they can handle.

Regarding accuracy of rate imitation, preliminary analysis (Raphael et al., 2004, 2005) of the slow, modeled rate for matched pairs of participants reveals that the clutterers are not as accurate as the controls in matching the experimenter's rate. On average, the clutterers exceeded the modeled rate of the experimenter to a much greater extent than the controls.

Disfluency

Preliminary studies by the authors indicate that clutterers exhibit predominantly typical or "normal" disfluencies. Using the *Systematic Disfluency Analysis* (Campbell & Hill, 1994), Myers, St. Louis, Raphael, Bakker, and Lwowski (2003) studied the disfluencies of 10 clutterers during conversational speech. More than 90% of the disfluencies were "more typical" disfluencies (interjections, revisions, hesitations, word repetitions, phrase repetitions, and unfinished words), and two-thirds

---

[7]More precisely, in addition to omission of syllables we have observed "elision" of sounds. Eliding sounds refers to the type of omission one hears in contractions but that may result in the same number of syllables as an unelided form. For example, "How are you doing?" has the same number of syllables as "How're you doing," because the syllabic /r/ takes the place of the full word "are." Synonyms of elision might be "contraction" or "compression."

were interjections, revisions, and hesitations. Importantly, wide variability in overall frequency of disfluency per participant was observed across clutterers. Not surprisingly, typical rather than atypical disfluencies occurred also in the speech of age- and sex-matched controls (Myers, St. Louis, Bakker, Lwowski, & Raphael, 2004) as well as ERS speakers (Myers, St. Louis, Lwowski et al., 2004). Based on emerging data, when comparing clutterers to typical speakers, there appear to be similarities in kind or types of disfluencies.[8]

The common occurrence of interjections and revisions may have implications for the nature of fluency breakdowns in cluttering. According to Starkweather (1987), interjections reflect a "more mature form of normal disfluency" compared with word or phrase repetitions. Logan and LaSalle (1999) postulated that revision behaviors may reflect "conceptual" or "formulative" breakdowns in language encoding.

Myers, Stueber, & St. Louis (1997) reported on the prevalence of contiguous disfluencies (or clusters) exhibited by two clutterers studied earlier (Myers & St. Louis, 1996). Analysis of speech samples showed that the more severe clutterer exhibited a greater number of clusters as well as longer cluster sequences, compared with the less severe clutterer. However, both subjects shared similar types of disfluencies in the clusters; specifically, interjections, unfinished words, and revisions composed the three most commonly occurring disfluencies.[9]

Differences in frequency of disfluencies between clutterers and stutterers have not been extensively studied. Rieber, Smith, and Harris (1976) reported that adult clutterers produced nearly 40% more disfluencies (both those typically referred to as "normal disfluencies" and as "stutterings" or "dysfluencies" [American Speech-Language-Hearing Association, 1999]) in the first trial of an oral reading task than stutterers did. Furthermore, on repeated trials, cluttering and stuttering groups manifested the adaptation effect for the combined disfluency categories. Both groups also produced many more disfluencies in longer than shorter words and at the beginning of words as compared with the ends of words. Unlike previous research with stuttering (e.g., Conway & Quarrington, 1963), neither clutterers nor stutterers manifested the most disfluencies in the initial words of the sentences.

Listener Perception of Cluttered Speech

St. Louis, Myers, and Faragasso et al. (2004) asked listeners to rate short speech samples from two young clutterers reported earlier (Myers & St. Louis, 1996) who had been investigated in a single-subject study of treatment using delayed auditory feedback (DAF) (St. Louis et al, 1996). In the 2004 study, listeners were asked to listen to and judge perceptual dimensions of "naturalness" (derived from Martin, Haroldson, & Triden, 1984), "disfluency," "rate," "articulation," and "language," all on 9-point scales. Samples from these two boys were different but averaged ~3.5 to 5 scale values out of a possible 9, where 1 stood for "excellent" or "highly natural" and 9 stood for "very poor" or "highly unnatural." For both clutterers, rate and naturalness received the least favorable ratings. This was followed by articulation, which was somewhat more favorably rated, and finally by disfluency and language, which were most favorably rated. The above-described study (St. Louis, Myers, Faragasso et al. 2004) also investigated the interactions among cluttering severity, the speech task (e.g., oral reading vs monologue vs conversation), the perceptual task of listeners, and even geographic differences among groups of judges, indicating multifaceted, interactive influences on perceptual ratings. Data from the same investigation (Myers & St. Louis, in press) indicated that perceptual judgments of rate and disfluency were reasonably—but not highly—correlated with objective counts of syllables per minute and disfluencies per 100 syllables reported earlier (St. Louis et al., 1996). Accordingly, the perceptual judgments showed that one clutterer improved under DAF whereas the other did not.

---

[8]Interestingly, DeNil, Sasisekaran, Van Lieshout, and Sandor (2005) reported that individuals with Tourette's syndrome manifest different disfluencies from stuttering that are—perhaps not coincidentally—similar to cluttering.

[9]The nature of these clusters was quite different than those reported by LaSalle and Conture (1995) for children who stutter.

Self-Awareness of Cluttering

The present authors have just begun to investigate clutterers' self-awareness of their own communication, using scaled ratings as well as interviews. Our preliminary findings indicate that there is great variability in degree of self-awareness in clutterers compared with typical speakers (Raphael, Myers & St. Louis, et al., 2003). Normal speakers appear to be more aware of their speech skills and the limitations thereof, whereas clutterers show more variability in self-awareness of speech rate and clarity, ranging from denial that there is a problem to acknowledging compromises in speech rate and clarity. It has been our clinical experience that some clutterers profess no ongoing awareness of their speech rate or irregularities (even after some success in therapy), whereas other clutterers are aware and self-modify when they sense that the speaking situation calls for clearer and slower speech (e.g., when their speech is recorded for later examination). It is our conjecture, however, that sustained monitoring and modulation of speech output requires concerted vigilance on the part of clutterers; these skills do not come "naturally" nor "automatically" to them, especially when speaking extemporaneously on topics of great excitement and complexity.

♦ Treatment of Cluttering

Evaluation

Special Considerations

The foregoing indicates that a wide range of disorders and problems may co-exist with cluttering. Accordingly, the clinical evaluation of cluttering should take account of most of the potential areas wherein weakness or problems have been consistently reported. These should include all symptoms of cluttering, whether essential or optional (e.g., Daly, 1986; Weiss, 1964).

We continue to promote a team approach to evaluation with suspected clients with cluttering (St. Louis & Myers, 1995, 1997). The speech-language pathologist should lead the team if there is good reason to suspect that cluttering will emerge as a primary diagnosis. Other members might involve the classroom teacher, the client's LD or ADHD specialist, an audiologist, and possibly a (pediatric) neurologist (if medication has or may be prescribed) or neuropsychologist (if significant brain dysfunction is suspected). Typically, the evaluation for cluttering will include most or all the components of a stuttering evaluation but may require considerable additional time to cover other areas of concern. We recommend setting aside at least 2 hours for interview and testing with each client, even if that means scheduling more than one evaluation appointment, for example, in a school setting. In the relatively unlikely event that a preschool child has suspected cluttering, the suggested evaluation and subsequent treatment suggestions will need to be modified.

Case History

The primary focus of the evaluation is to obtain information on the person's rate, fluency, articulation, language, and awareness. If possible, a case history questionnaire from any diagnostic textbook in speech-language pathology, with additional questions about stuttering (e.g., Bennett, 2006; Conture, 2001; Gregory, 2003; Guitar, 2006; Manning, 2001; Ramig & Dodge, 2005; Shapiro, 1999; Silverman, 2004) should be mailed out to the client or parent prior to the evaluation appointment. In this way, questions for an effective interview can be planned in advance. The case history should document: the onset; course; co-existing problems; past and current treatment or advice (including well-meant but ineffective assistance); pre-, peri-, and postnatal history; general, motor, and language developmental landmarks; family history of fluency and other disorders; relevant medical and pharmacological history; school history; social history; and other relevant areas. Standard practice indicates that the interview and subsequent testing should be audio- or videotape-recorded for later verification and analysis.

Performance on Speech and Language Tasks

As in stuttering evaluations, speech should be sampled generously in a wide range of tasks. We recommend rote tasks (e.g., counting, days of the week, memorized material); imitation (e.g., single-syllable words, multisyllabic words, sentences); oral reading (if the client can do so); monologue; and conversation (e.g., small talk and topics that evoke excitement or special interest for the client). Some clutterers normalize when placed before a microphone or camera (e.g., Daly & St. Louis, 1998). Therefore, ample speaking time or opportunities must be provided for the client to become sufficiently accustomed to the recording equipment to foster "letting down his guard" and manifesting cluttering. Given that clutterers often manifest articulation and language difficulties, we advocate administering an articulation test and age-appropriate, norm-referenced tests of language comprehension and production. In addition, it is important to obtain a spontaneous language/narrative sample, to obtain such measures as mean length of utterance (MLU), as standardized tests of speech-language do not always reflect spontaneous conversational usage of speech and language.

Computer-Based Cluttering Assessment Tool

Among the challenges of cluttering severity measurement are: (1) a lack of precise and behaviorally explicit definitions of cluttering; (2) the nature of cluttering itself (which varies in form, and from moment to moment); and (3) the multidimensional nature of symptoms thought to be part of a cluttering problem with the possibility that the combination of such dimensions may vary among clients. These challenges, which depend on observation of specific behaviors, suggest that the development of rigorous assessment protocols will be unlikely or impractical in the foreseeable future.

One possible solution may be to measure cluttering in a molar/perceptual, rather than a molecular/ behavioral way. This would imply gathering of perceptual information, rather than counting and/or timing of specific and operationally defined behavioral features. The experimental *Cluttering Assessment Program* (Bakker, 2005)[10] (**Fig. 16–3**) employs two possible tacks to cluttering severity measurement: (1) percentage talking time cluttered, as a molar/perceptual severity estimate; and (2) responses to a set of visual analog scales which in a previous investigation (St. Louis, Myers, Faragasso et al., 2004) were found to represent relevant features for the description of cluttering severity.

To determine the percentage of talking time that is cluttered, the clinician marks talking time (including both cluttered and noncluttered segments) with the left button of the computer mouse. The right mouse button is simultaneously pressed when speech is cluttered. When using a wireless mouse, this assessment can be conducted in real-time while ensuring that the clinician-client interaction is as natural as possible.[11] Percent talking time cluttered expresses the proportion of speech that is judged to be cluttered.

The second part of the *Cluttering Assessment Program* involves use of a set of computerized visual analog scales (**Fig. 16–4**) for perceptually rating the performance of the client. To mark one's responses, the cursor is moved to the desired location on the scoring bar and the mouse button is pressed to leave a mark. This is instantly interpreted by the computer as a percentage score (on the visual analog scale) as well as on a 1 through 9 scale such as often is used in perceptual measures of fluency disorders as in the case of "speech naturalness" (Martin, et al., 1984).

---

[10]The *Cluttering Assessment Program* is available as freeware at http://www.stutteringhomepage.com.

[11]A Macintosh-compatible version of the program does not exist at this time, and its development is limited by the fact that Macintosh computers utilize only one mouse button.

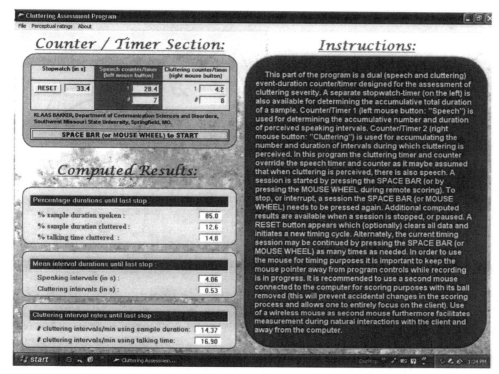

Figure 16–3 Scoring tool for percentage talking time cluttered and other related quantified measures in the *Cluttering Assessment Program*.

Self-Awareness Measures

As noted above, clutterers are often reported to be less aware of their speech difficulties than individuals who stutter (e.g., Daly & Burnett, 1999; St. Louis & Myers, 1997). At least, it seems that they are aware of different aspects of speech and language than stuttering clients. Finally, little is known about specific areas of concern for those who clutter. Accordingly, if the clients are old enough, we suggest that they be asked to fill out the following self-appraisal questionnaires: the *Self-Awareness of Speech Index* (*SASI*) (St. Louis & Atkins, 2005) (revised from the *Speech Awareness Questionnaire* [Atkins & St. Louis, 1988]); the *Perceptions of Speech Communication* (*PSC*) (Daly & Burnett, 1999) (adapted by Daly [1978] from Woolf's [1967] *Perceptions of Stuttering Inventory* wherein "stuttering" is replaced by "speech" or "speech difficulty"); and the *St. Louis Inventory of Life Perspectives and Speech/Language Difficulty* (*SL♦ ILP-SL*) (St. Louis, 2005) (adapted similarly from the *St. Louis Inventory of Life Perspectives and Stuttering* [St. Louis, 2001]). Copies of the SASI and SL♦ILP-SL are provided in **Appendixes 16–1** and **16–2**. To date, none of these instruments is standardized, but each can be used as a criterion-referenced tool. Low scores on the SASI would suggest that clutterers' degree of awareness of their own speech is compromised and might suggest that awareness should be targeted in therapy. Low scores on the PSC would likely confirm that clutterers do not experience significant difficulties with respect to avoidance, struggle, and expectancy often observed in stuttering. Moderate to high scores on the PSC might indicate significant concern about the cluttering. High scores on many items in the SL♦ ILP-SL would indicate that clients experience significant suffering, disability, and handicap as a result of their cluttering. Other items provide the clinician important information about how much clients may wish to be treated, to interact with other clutterers, or to rate their own health status.

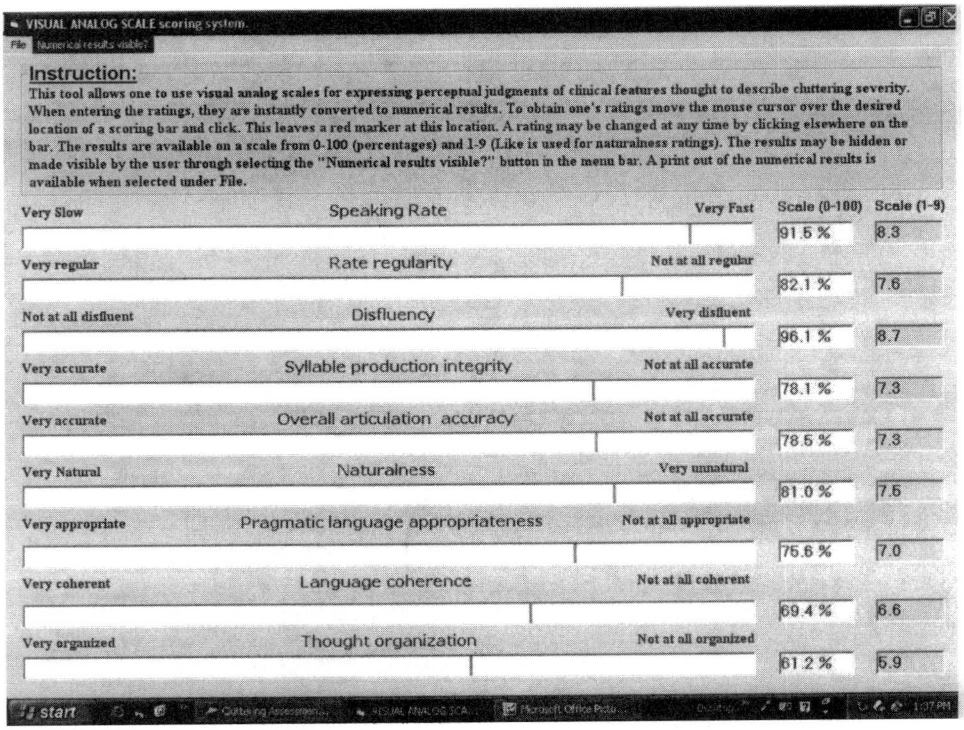

Figure 16–4 Scoring tool with perceptually based visual analog scales, each expressing a clinical aspect of cluttering severity in the *Cluttering Assessment Program*.

Other Potential Tasks and Measures

Because clutterers are frequently reported to have oral motor difficulties (e.g., Daly & St. Louis, 1998; Raphael et al., 2005), central auditory difficulties (Molt, 1996; Preus, 1996), LD (Tiger et al., 1980; Daly, 1986); St. Louis & Myers, 1997), ADHD (St. Louis & Myers, 1997), and difficulties such as handwriting (Daly & Burnett, 1999), we recommend a battery of tests covering areas besides speech and language. This battery should include: an oral examination, an audiological evaluation including pure tones and tympanometry (including central auditory tests, if possible), and samples of motor skill. Motor tasks should allow evaluation of general coordination, level of activity (e.g., fidgeting), handwriting, and DDK tasks (e.g., DDK sequences in the *Oral Speech Mechanism Screening Examination-3* [St. Louis & Ruscello, 2000]). If LD is suspected, psychoeducational testing of such areas as reading comprehension, spelling, writing, mathematical skills, and other academic areas may be useful. Similarly, psychological assessments of attention and distractibility are also warranted. If diagnoses of LD and/or ADHD have already been made, it is likely that reports from previous evaluation reports from school or other psychometrists can be requested. Finally, referrals to—or reports from—neurologists or neuropsychologists are important if neurological damage is suspected or if pharmacological treatment is a possibility. To date, there is no clear evidence that cluttering should be treated with drugs, but it is worth noting that one recent case study was reported indicating that cluttering was reduced in a 52-year-old woman by bethanachol, a cholinergic agent (Brady, 1993).

Table 16–2   Overview of a Range of Clinical Signs, Ranging from Diagnostic Significance to Occasional Presence, Associated with Cluttering and a Selection of Related Disorders (not intended for differential diagnosis)

Key

FD—Fluency Disorder
RD—Rate Deviation
Cl—Cluttering
St—Stuttering
ArtD—Articulation Disorder
LangD—Language Disorder
ADHD—Attention Deficit/Hyperactivity Disorder
LD—Learning Disability

X—Important sign that is important for inclusion in the category (sometimes in combination with other Xs)

x—Sign frequently present but is not necessary for inclusion in the category

?—Sign that may or may not be present and is not necessary for inclusion in the category

Sign	FD	RD	St	Cl	ArtD	LangD	ADHD	LD
Excessive typical disfluencies	X		?	X		x		x
Excessive atypical disfluencies	X		X	?				
Excessively rapid rate	X	X		X				
Excessively slow rate		X	x					
Excessively irregular rate	X	X	x	X		?	?	?
Atypical pauses	X	x	x	X		x	?	?
Pragmatic errors			?	x		X	x	x
Semantic errors						X		x
Syntactic/morphological errors			?	x	x	X		x
Lexical (word finding) errors	x			x		X		x
Mazes	?	x	?	x		x	?	?
Phonological errors				?	X	x		
Consistent developmental misarticulations			x	x	X	x		
Excessive neutralization of vowels		x		X	?			
Excessive "over-coarticulated" (collapsed) syllables		x		X	?			
Atypical coarticulation patterns	X	x		X	?			
Distractible				x			X	x
Hyperactive				x			X	x
Reading difficulties				x		x	x	X
Writing difficulties				x		x	x	X
Mathematical difficulties						x	?	X

Summary

Cluttering may be present in pure form or it may exist with other disorders or problems. In the latter case, we recommend including any co-existing diagnoses in any written clinical summaries that are prepared. **Table 16–2** summarizes obligatory and optional diagnostic signs for various conditions often observed in clutterers. (Readers should note that this table is not a comprehensive diagnostic tool and is not intended to be used for the purposes of differential diagnosis.)

Therapy

On the assumption that clutterers speak at a rate faster than they can easily, fluently, and accurately manage, we propose a synergistic model (Myers, 1992) for treatment as various parts of the communication system can be affected by an excessive rate. When inappropriately rushing both the planning and production of their speech-language, people who clutter may not be allowing themselves enough time to encode or convert their thoughts into cohesive plans to permit accurate, fluent speech or language production. In many instances, the excessive rate affects the speaker's articulation so that speech intelligibility suffers. In still other instances, the speech of clutterers contains interjections, incomplete phrases, and revision behaviors, reflecting discoordination (or dyssynergy) between the language and speech processes.[12]

Given the centrality of rate, we advocate a *systems approach* to the clinical management of cluttering based on our belief that a system that is well-timed allows for synergy among the component parts. Analogous to a speeding train, when the speech and language system is ill-timed by going too fast, or in a jerky or disorganized manner, "derailment" occurs.[13] Derailment can be manifested at the articulatory or linguistic level. Derailment can also occur at the higher or more "central" level of thought organization. The adage that "haste makes waste" often applies to cluttering. Clinical management of cluttering, therefore, aims to increase the coordination (synergy) and timing (synchrony) of the communication system to reduce the "waste" or "mistakes" due to an overly charged system. Modulating the tempo of output should be a primary goal. As many clutterers experience difficulties in sensing this modulation, we propose that an equally if not more important goal of therapy is to heighten the clutterer's awareness of his or her haste and the behavioral ramifications (communication derailments) thereof. After all, one needs to sense what one is doing before one can channel one's energy to self-correct. The following therapy strategies represent a compendium of clinical strategies considered by the authors (Myers & Bradley, 1992, St. Louis & Myers, 1995, 1997; St. Louis, Myers, Bakker, & Raphael, 2004, 2005) as well as by others (e.g., Daly, 1996). We recommend that clinicians use their knowledge of individual clients to select and use those techniques for which there is good reason to assume will be helpful and effective. This is not a list that should be applied to all clients, but elements selected according to the individual needs of each client.

To Increase Awareness and Self-Monitoring Skills

◆ Use audio and videotaped speech to monitor and self-correct.

◆ Tape-record client's speech on a digital tape recorder and play it back: (1) at a fast speed to show how cluttering sounds; and (2) at a slow speed to show how it might be improved (reorder wherein these functions preserve the vocal frequency).

◆ Heighten client's sensory awareness of movements first during nonspeech motor acts such as rate of moving arms or hands or when walking, then during speech motor acts.

◆ Use various types of computer-generated visual feedback of speech rate (e.g., comparing client's tracing with clinician's model on a Visi-Pitch screen [Kay Electronics, Pine Brook, NJ]).

◆ Give "speeding tickets" (for children) following episodes of rapid speech.

◆ Use feedback from listener (e.g., facial expressions, verbal indications of communication breakdown due to clutterer's poor speech, and linguistic coherence).

◆ Provide opportunities to monitor and provide feedback to other clutterers in group sessions.

To Improve Rate (as well as Articulation and Speech Intelligibility)

◆ Slow overall rate using DAF.

◆ Use syllable-timed speech (e.g., metronome) as an intermediary technique (this approach alone would not facilitate natural sounding speech).

---

[12]The dyssynergy model is similar to the dissociation idea more recently discussed by Anderson, Pellowski, and Conture (2005) for stutterers, that there can be dissociation between thought and formulation, dissociation among elements of formulation, dissociation between formulation and production, and dissociation among elements of production.

[13]See Conture (2001, p. 41) for a pictorial metaphor of timing problems for stuttering.

- Prolong vowels because they are easy focal points to prolong, thereby reducing rate.

- Attend to word endings and unstressed vowels and syllables.

- Use more distinct and more deliberate articulatory gestures (e.g., wider excursion of articulators).

- Impose pauses for breath groups.

- Mark reading passages with "stop signs" wherever there are periods and commas.

- Use analogy of speedometer to regulate rate.

- Use self-imposed phrasing to help with organization of speech and language or thought.

- Aim for greater prosodic variations (assuming that greater prosodic variations will slow the rate and produce more natural-sounding speech).

- Give added stress to accented syllables.

- Read and/or recite poetry with "interpretation" to increase prosodic variations and pauses and to increase overall effectiveness of speech delivery.

- Use skits and plays to: (1) increase awareness of partner's turn in conversation; and (2) highlight pauses imposed by lines from different speakers to automatically stop clutterer from perseverating and festinating (i.e., going faster and faster).

- Use music to impose slower and/or more varied prosody (e.g., smooth, easy, and slow lullabies vs fast staccato beat of a march).

- If group therapy, have clients take turns "conducting" speech and/or singing depending on their "composition" (legato, allegro, pianissimo); have children sing or recite a lullaby for softer, gentler, slower speech or a march for more rhythmic and deliberate cadence.

- Shadow the speech of slow and effective speakers.

To Improve Linguistic and Narrative Skills

- Teach clients elements of story grammar (i.e., episodes, problem resolution).

- Help clients to sequence thoughts if they report several thoughts coming at once.

- Increase turn-taking skills to reduce tendency to interrupt and improve skills for appropriate adjacency and contingency.

- Increase semantic classification and categorization skills for word-finding difficulties.

- Increase speed and accuracy of word retrieval (e.g., naming drills).

- Formulate ideas using appropriate syntactic structures.

- Increase cohesion of extended talk (e.g., through appropriate use of relational terms such as "although" and "however").

To Improve Fluency Skills

- Review audio- and videotapes for use of fillers, revisions, incomplete phrases, and other disfluencies.

- Have client transcribe his or her own maze behaviors (e.g., use the systematic disfluency analysis (SDA) [Campbell & Hill,1994] system and point out inefficiencies in client's information output due to excessive maze behaviors).

- Use aforementioned strategies for rate and language to decrease disfluencies as well.

To Improve Meta-Cluttering Skills

♦ Point out specific attributes of client's cluttering behaviors (e.g., difficult to understand, dropping of sounds and syllables).

♦ Differentiate reactions of self and others to the client's cluttering.

♦ Compare the nature of thought and language organization after moments of clarity with moments of incoherence.

♦ Compare sensory feedback associated with fast rate, irregular rate, and slower rate.

♦ Discuss with client the relative effectiveness of different therapy approaches.

♦ For clutterers who also stutter, talk about behaviors associated with one's moments of cluttering compared with stuttering.

♦ Identify effects of speaking rapidly and propulsively on general body state (e.g., "Do you feel more tense when you talk fast?").

♦ Compare effects on clutterer when others speak rapidly versus more slowly.

♦ Explore jointly client's reactions when speaking to someone who is difficult to follow because of poor speech intelligibility or poor narrative and pragmatic skills.

♦ Use analogies from animal kingdom (e.g., stride of a racehorse vs hippopotamus or penguin) or engines (e.g., car skidding on ice, derailment of speeding train, or the synergism of a Porsche engine).

To Improve Phonatory and Respiratory Behaviors

♦ Mark passages with pauses for breath intake.

♦ Heighten client's awareness when exceeding optimum number of words per breath group.

To Improve Family, Friend, and Employer Support

♦ Obtain feedback, during moments of clear speech and poor communication, from family and friends.

♦ Recommend participation in group speaking activities (e.g., oral presentations at school, Toastmasters ([www.toastmasters.org], or other monitored activities at home or school).

To Improve Collaboration with Other Team Members

♦ Consult with—or refer to—ADHD or LD specialist if school-age clutterers have significant attention, activity, distractibility, or academic problems; coordinate therapy plans around ADHD and/or LD goals if relevant.

♦ Consult with—or refer to—psychologist if adult clutterers have significant ADHD-related problems.

♦ Consult with—or refer to—mental health specialist if clutterers manifest problems in social adjustment.

♦ Consult with—or refer to—pediatric or general neurologist if clutterers have pharmacological issues.

To Foster Transfer and Maintenance   It is one matter to help the clutterer become a slower, more fluent, and more intelligible speaker while speaking in an ideal situation such as with the clinician. It is quite another for the person to make those changes permanent in all communicative situations.

To foster transfer and/or maintenance, the clinician should program specific activities and assignments designed specifically for each client's needs. Following are a few suggestions that may assist in this process.

Daly (1992) outlined a procedure for preparing "anchor" tapes or CDs for cluttering clients wherein very short samples of the person's seriously cluttered speech, slightly cluttered speech, and noncluttered speech are recorded. The client is asked to listen to the tape every day, and even several times a day, to: (1) help maintain awareness of what goes wrong in cluttering; (2) serve to "recalibrate" the targets of good speech; and (3) provide consistent reminders to practice. Whether or not "anchor" tapes are used, activities to promote daily speaking practice in a new and controlled way is extremely useful. Some clutterers have found that self-help groups for stuttering, such as National Stuttering Association chapters, are a good place for them to practice and feel the support of others. It is likely that clutterers who might benefit from attending a stuttering support group will need to educate the stutterers about cluttering and how its treatment and maintenance challenges may be different from those faced by the stutterers. This can be accomplished by the clutterer, perhaps in conjunction with a visit by his or her clinician. Another source of support that has recently emerged is an online support group for cluttering individuals that can be accessed at cluttering@yahoogroups.com.

◆ Conclusion

A fitting metaphor for cluttering is that of an unfinished jigsaw puzzle, both in terms of the pieces that have been fitted and the actual pieces that are yet to be fitted or even included in the overall puzzle. Cluttering is considered to be a fluency disorder with a central problem of rate, possibly with the speaker attempting to speak faster than he or she is able. The cause of cluttering is not known but it is likely that neurological, linguistic, cognitive, and genetic factors play a role. Numerous other disorders typically—though not always—co-exist with cluttering, and these disorders should be carefully considered in evaluation and treatment.

References

American Psychiatric Association. (1994). Diagnostic and statistical manual of mental disorders (4th ed.). Washington, DC: Author.

American Speech-Language-Hearing Association, Special Interest Division 4; Fluency and Fluency Disorders. (1999 March). Terminology pertaining to fluency and fluency disorders: Guidelines. ASHA 41(Suppl. 19), 29–36.

Anderson, J. D., Pellowski, M. W., & Conture, E. G. (2005). Childhood stuttering and dissociations across linguistic domains. Journal of Fluency Disorders 30, 219–253.

Arnold, G. E. (1960). Studies in tachyphemia: I. Present concepts of etiologic factors. Logos 3, 25–45.

Arnold, G. E. (1970). An attempt to explain the causes of cluttering with LLMM theory. Folia Phoniatrica 22, 247–260.

Atkins, C. P., & St. Louis. K. O. (1988). Speech awareness questionnaire (SAQ). Communiqué (Journal of the West Virginal Speech-Language-Hearing Association), 8–11.

Bakker, K. (1996). Cluttering: Current scientific status and emerging research and clinical needs. Journal of Fluency Disorders 21, 359–365.

Bakker, K. (2005). Cluttering Assessment Program. Software. Author. Available at http://www.stutteringhomepage.com.

Becker, K. P., & Grundmann, K. (1971). Investigation on incidence and symptomatology of cluttering. Folia Phoniatr (Basel) 22, 261–271.

Becker, K. P., Slassova, N. A., Asatiani, N. M., Beljakowa, L. J., & Hey, W. (1977). Stottern. Berlin: VEB Verlag Volk und Gesundheit.

Bakker, K., Raphael, L. J., Myers, F. L., & St. Louis, K. O. (2000). Acoustic and perceptual-phonetic analyses of cluttered and noncluttered speech. Paper presented at the Annual Convention of the American Speech-Language-Hearing Association, Washington, D.C.

Bakker, K., Raphael, L. J., Myers, F. L., St. Louis, K. O., & MacRoy, M. (2004). DDK production variability in cluttered speech. Poster presented at the Annual Convention of the American Speech-Language-Hearing Association. Philadelphia, PA.

Bennett, E. M. (2006). Working with people who stutter: A lifespan approach. Upper Saddle River, NJ: Pearson Merrill Prentice-Hall.

Blood, G. W., Ridenour, V. J., Qualls, C. D., & Hammer, C. S. (2003). Co-occurring disorders in children who stutter. Journal of Communication Disorders 36, 427–448.

Brady, J. P. (1993). Treatment of cluttering. New England Journal of Medicine 329, 813–814.

Cabanas, R. (1954). Some findings in speech and voice therapy among mentally deficient children. Folia Phoniatrica 4, 34–37.

Campbell, J. G., & Hill, D. G. (1994). Systematic disfluency analysis. Evanston, IL: Northwestern University.

Centers for Disease Control. (2002). Attention deficit disorder and learning disability: United States, 1997–1998. Vital and health Statistics, Series 10, Volume 206. Available at http://www.ldonline.org/ld_indepth/add_adhd/add_ld_1997_1998.html. Accessed January 23, 2006.

Council for Exceptional Children. (2002). Public policy & legislative information: IDEA '97 regulations. Retrieved January 23, 2006, from http://www.cec.sped.org/idea/idea2.html.

Conture, E. G. (2001). Stuttering: Its nature, diagnosis, and treatment. Needham Heights, MA: Allyn & Bacon.

Conway, J., & Quarrington, B. (1963). Positional effects in stuttering of contextually organized verbal material. Journal of Abnormal and Social Psychology 67, 299–303.

Craig, A. (1996). Long-term effects of intensive treatment for a client with both a cluttering and stuttering disorder. Journal of Fluency Disorders 21, 329–335.

Curlee, R. F. (Ed.). (1999). Stuttering and related disorders of fluency (2nd ed.). New York: Thieme.

Curlee, R. F., & Siegel, G. M. (Eds.). (1997). Nature and treatment of stuttering: New directions (2nd ed.). New York: Allyn & Bacon.

Dalton P, & Hardcastle W. (1977). Disorders of fluency and their effects on communication. New York: Elsevier-North Holland.

Dalton P, & Hardcastle W. (1989). Disorders of fluency and their effects on communication (2nd ed.). London: Elsevier-North Holland.

Daly, D. A. (1978). Perceptions of Speech Communication. Author Ann Arbor, MI.

Daly, D. A. (1986). The clutterer. In K. O. St. Louis (Ed.), The atypical stutterer (pp. 155–192). New York: Academic Press.

Daly, D. A. (1992). Helping the cluttering: Therapy considerations. In F. L. Myers & K. O. St. Louis (Eds.), Cluttering: A clinical perspective (pp. 107–124). Kibworth, Great Britain: Far Communications. (Reissued in 1996 by *Singular*, San Diego, CA.)

Daly, D. A. (1992-93). Cluttering: A language-based syndrome. Clinical Connection 6, 4–7.

Daly, D. A. (1996). The Source for stuttering and cluttering. East Moline, IL: LinguiSystems.

Daly, D. A., & Burnett, M. L. (1996). Cluttering: Assessment, treatment planning, and case study illustration. Journal of Fluency Disorders 21, 239–248.

Daly, D. A., & Burnett, M. (1999). Cluttering: Traditional views and new perspectives. In R. F. Curlee (Ed.), Stuttering and related disorders of fluency (2nd ed.) (pp. 222–254). New York: Thieme.

Daly, D. A., & St. Louis, K. O. (1998). Videotaping clutterers: How to do it and what to look for. In E. C. Healey & H. F. M. Peters (Eds.), 2nd World Congress on Fluency Disorders Proceedings (pp. 233–235). International Fluency Association.

Darley, F. L., Aronson, A. E., & Brown, J. R. (1975). Motor speech disorders. Philadelphia: Saunders.

de Hirsch, K. (1961). Studies in tachyphemia. Diagnosis of developmental language disorders. Logos 4, 3–9.

de Hirsch, K. (1970). Stuttering and cluttering. Developmental aspects of dysrhythmic speech. Folia Phoniatrica 22, 311–324.

Diedrich, W. M. (1984). Cluttering: Its diagnosis. In H. Winitz (Ed.), Treating articulation disorders: For clinicians by clinicians (pp. 307–323). Baltimore: University Park Press.

Dietrich, S., Jensen, K. H., & Williams, D. E. (2001). Effects of the label "stuttering" on student perceptions. Journal of Fluency Disorders 26, 55–66.

DeNil, L. F., Sasisekaran, J., Van Lieshout, P. H. H. M, & Sandor, P. (2005). Speech disfluencies in individuals with Tourette Syndrome. Journal of Psychosomatic Research 58:97–102.

Filatova, J. (2002). [Psycho-pedogogic criteria in identifying cluttering in school-age children.] Unpublished doctoral dissertation, Moscow Pedagogical State University, Moscow.

Freund, H. (1952). Studies in the interrelationship between stuttering and cluttering. Folia Phoniatrica 4, 146–168.

Froeschels, E. (1955). Contribution to the relationship between stuttering and cluttering. Logopaedie en Phonatrie 4, 1–6.

Georgieva, D., (Ed.). (2004). Fluency Disorders: New Research Perspectives. Sofia, Bulgaria: Grafis. (In Bulgarian)

Georgieva, D., & Miliev, D. (1996). Differential diagnosis of cluttering and stuttering in Bulgaria. Journal of Fluency Disorders 21, 249–260.

Gregory, H. H. (2003). Stuttering therapy. Boston: Allyn & Bacon.

Guitar, B. (2006). Stuttering: An integrated approach to its nature and treatment (3rd ed.). Philadelphia: Lippincott Williams & Wilkins.

Hahn, E. F. (1943). Stuttering: Significant theories and therapies. Stanford, CA: Stanford University Press.

Hahn, E. F. (1956). Stuttering: Significant theories and therapies (2nd ed.). Stanford, CA: Stanford University Press.

Hull, F. M., Mielke, P. W., Willeford, J. A., & Timmons, R. J. (1976) National Speech and Hearing Survey. Final Report for Grant OE-32–15–0050–5010 (607). No 50978, Office of Education, Washington, D.C.

Ingham, R. J. (1984). Stuttering and behavior therapy: Current status and experimental foundations. San Diego, CA: College-Hill Press.

Kussmaul, A. (1877). Speech disorders. In Cyclopedia of the practice of medicine. New York: William Wood & Co.

Landolt, H., & Luchsinger, R. (1954). (Paraphasia praecox, stuttering and chronic orgains psychosyndromes: Results of EEG and logopathological studies). Dtsch Med Wochenschr 79, 1012–1015.

Langevin, M., & Boberg, E. (1996). Results of intensive stuttering theapy with adults who clutter and stutter. Journal of Fluency Disorders 21, 315–327.

Langova, J., & Moravek, M. (1964). Some results of experimental examinations among stutterers and clutterers. Folia Phoniatrica 16, 290–296.

Langova, J., & Moravek, M. (1970). Some problems of cluttering. Folia Phoniatrica 22, 325–336.

LaSalle, L. R., & Conture, E. G. (1995). Disfluency clusters of children who stutter: Relation of stutterings to self-repairs. Journal of Speech and Hearing Research 38, 965–977.

Lebrun, Y. (1996). Cluttering after brain damage. Journal of Fluency Disorders 21, 289–296.

Lewis, G. A. (1907). Home cure for stammerers. Detroit: Winn & Hammond.

Loban, W. (1976). The language of elementary school children. Champaign, IL: National Council of Teachers of English.

Logan, K. J., & LaSalle, L. R. (1999). Grammatical characteristics of children's conversational utterances that contain disfluency clusters. Journal of Speech, Language, and Hearing Research 42, 80–91.

Luchsinger, R., & Arnold, G. E. (1965). Voice-speech-language: Clinical communicology: Its physiology and pathology. Belmont, CA: Wadsworth.

Luchsinger, R., & Landolt, H. (1951). (EEG examination in stuttering with and without cluttering). Folia Phoniatrica 3, 135–150.

Luchsinger, R., & Landolt, H. (1955). Cluttering, the so-called stuttering with cluttering, and their relation to aphsia; electroencephalographic findings and study of speech pathology. Folia Phoniatrica 7, 12–43.

Manning, W. H. (2001). Clinical decision making in fluency disorders (2nd ed.). Vancouver: Singular.

Martin, R. R., Haroldson, S. K., & Triden, K. A. (1984). Stuttering and speech naturalness. Journal of Speech and Hearing Disorders 49, 53–58.

Martin, R. E., Kroll, R. M., O'Keefe, B. M., & Painter, C. (1983). Cluttered speech: Spectrographic analysis. Paper presented at the Annual Convention of the American Speech-Language-Hearing Association, Cincinnati, OH.

Molt, L. F. (1996). An examination of various aspects of auditory processing in clutterers. Journal of Fluency Disorders 21, 215–225.

Moravak, M., & Langova, J. (1962). Some electrophysiological findings among stutterers and clutterers. Folia Phoniatrica 14, 305–316.

Myers, F. L. (1992). Cluttering: A synergistic framework. In F. L. Myers & K. O. St Louis (Eds.), Cluttering: A clinical perspective (pp. 71–84). Kibworth, Great Britain: Far Communications. (Reissued in 1996 by Singular, San Diego, CA.)

Myers, F. L. (1996). Cluttering: A matter of perspective. Journal of Fluency Disorders 21, 175–186.

Myers, F. L., & Bradley, C. L. (1992). Clinical management of cluttering from a synergistic framework. In F. L. Myers & K. O. St. Louis (Eds.), Cluttering: A clinical perspective (pp. 85–105). Kibworth, Great Britain: Far Communications. (Reissued in 1996 by Singular, San Diego, CA.)

Myers, F. L., & St. Louis, K. O. (1996). Two youths who clutter, but is that the only similarity? Journal of Fluency Disorders 21, 297–304.

Myers, F. L., & St. Louis, K.O. (in press) Disfluency and speaking rate in cluttering: Perceptual judgments versus counts. Bulgarian Journal of Communication Disorders.

Myers, F. L., St. Louis, K. O., Bakker, K., Raphael, L. J., Wiig, E. et al. (2002a). Putting cluttering on the map: Looking ahead. Seminar presented at the Annual Convention of the American Speech-Language-Hearing Association, Atlanta, GA.

Myers, F. L., St. Louis, K. O., Bakker, K., Raphael, L. J., Wiig, E. et al. (2002b). Putting cluttering on the map: Looking back.

Seminar presented at the Annual Convention of the American Speech-Language-Hearing Association, Atlanta, GA.

Myers, F. L., St. Louis, K. O., Bakker, K., Lwowski, A., & Raphael, L. J. (2004). Disfluencies of cluttered and noncluttered speech. Poster presented at the Annual Convention of the New York State Speech-Language-Hearing Association, Albany, NY.

Myers, F. L., St. Louis, K. O., Lwowski, A., Bakker, K., Raphael, L. J., & Frangis, G. (2004). Disfluencies of cluttered and excessively rapid speech. Poster presented the Annual Convention of the American Speech-Language-Hearing Association. Philadelphia, PA.

Myers, F. L., St. Louis, K. O., Raphael, L. J., Bakker, K., & Lwowski, A. (2003). Patterns of disfluencies in cluttered speech. Poster presented at the Annual Convention of the American Speech-Language-Hearing Association, Chicago, IL.

Myers, F. L., Stueber, K. A., & St. Louis, K. O. (1997). Clustering of disfluencies in cluttering. Poster presented at the Annual Convention of the American Speech-Language-Hearing Association, Boston, MA.

National Institute on Deafness and Other Communication Disorders (NIDCD). (2006). Apraxia of speech. Retrieved January 23, 2006 from http://www.nidcd.nih.gov/health/voice/apraxia.asp.

Pitluk, N. (1982). Aspects of the expressive language of cluttering and stuttering schoolchildren. South African Journal of Communication Disorders 29, 77–84.

Preus, A. (1981). Identifying subgroups of stutterers. Oslo: Universitetsforlaget.

Preus, A. (1992). Cluttering upgraded. In F. L. Myers & K. O. St. Louis (Eds.), Cluttering: A clinical perspective (pp. 349–357). Kibworth, Great Britain: Far Communications. (Reissued in 1996 by Singular, San Diego, CA.)

Preus, A. (1996). Cluttering upgraded. Journal of Fluency Disorders 21, 349–357.

Ramig, P. R., & Dodge, D. M. (2005). The child and adolescent stuttering treatment and activity resource guide. Clifton Park, NY: Thompson Delmar Learning.

Raphael, L. J., Bakker, K., Myers, F. L., St. Louis, K. O., Fichtner, V., & Kostel, M. (2005). An update on diadochokinetic rates of cluttered and normal speech. Poster presented at the Annual Convention of the American Speech-Language-Hearing Association. San Diego, CA.

Raphael, L. J., Bakker, K., Myers, F. L., St. Louis, K. O., & MacRoy, M. (2004). Diadochokinetic rates of cluttered and normal speech. Paper presented at the Annual Convention of the American Speech-Language-Hearing Association. Philadelphia, PA.

Raphael, L. J., Myers, F. L., St. Louis, K. O., Bakker, K., Lwowski, A., Bileychvck, C., et al. (2003). Contrasting cluttered and normal speech: Acoustic and metacommunication analyses. Poster presented at the annual convention of the New York State Speech-Language-Hearing Association, Rye Brook, NY.

Rieber, R. W., Smith, N., & Harris, B. (1976). Neuropsychological aspects of stuttering and cluttering. In R.W. Rieber (Ed.), The Neuropsychology of language: Essays in honor of Eric Lenneberg. (pp. 45–66). New York: Plenum Press.

Roman, K. G. (1963). Studies in tachyphemia IV: The interrelationship of graphologic and oral aspects of language behavior. Logos 6, 41–58.

Royall, D. R., Lauterbach, E. C., Cummings, J. L., Reeve, A., Rummans, T. A., Kaufer, D. I., et al. (2002). Executive control function: A review of its promise and challenges for clinical research. Journal of Neuropsychiatry and Clinical Neuroscience 14, 377–405.

Ryan, B. P. (2001). Programmed therapy for stuttering in children and adults (2nd ed.) Springfield, IL: Charles C. Thomas.

Seeman, M., & Novak, A. (1963). Ueber die Motorik bei Polterern. Folia Phoniatr 15, 170–176.

Seeman, M. (1970). Relations between motorics of speech and general motor ability in clutterers. Folia Phoniatrica 22, 376–378.

Shapiro, D. A. (1999). Stuttering Intervention: A collaborative journey to fluency freedom. Austin, TX: PRO-ED.

Sheehan, J. G., (Ed.). (1970). Stuttering: Research and therapy. NY: Harper & Row.

Silverman, F. H. (2004). Stuttering and other fluency disorders (3rd ed.). Long Grove, IL: Waveland Press, Inc.

Starkweather, C. W. (1987). Fluency and stuttering. Englewood Cliffs, NJ: Prentice-Hall.

St. Louis, K. O. (1991). The stuttering/articulation disorders connection. In H. F. M. Peters, W. Hulstijn, & C. W. Starkweather (Eds.), Speech motor control and stuttering (pp. 393–399). Amsterdam: Elsevier.

St. Louis, K. O. (1992). On defining cluttering. In F. L. Myers & K. O. St. Louis (Eds.), Cluttering: A clinical perspective (pp. 37–53). Kibworth, Great Britain: Far Communications. (Reissued in 1996 by Singular, San Diego, CA.)

St. Louis, K. O. (1996) A tabular summary of cluttering subjects in the special edition. Journal of Fluency Disorders 21, 337–343.

St. Louis, K. O. (1998). Cluttering: Some guidelines. Memphis, TN: Stuttering Foundation of America.

St. Louis, K. O. (1999). Person-first labeling and stuttering. Journal of Fluency Disorders 24, 1–24.

St. Louis, K. O. (2001). Living with stuttering: Stories, basics, resources, and hope. Morgantown, WV: Populore.

St. Louis, K. O. (2005). St. Louis Inventory of Life Perspectives and Speech/Language Difficulty (SL♦ILP-S/L). Morgantown, WV: Populore.

St. Louis, K. O., & Atkins, CP. (2006). Self-Awareness of Speech Index (SASI). Morgantown, WV: Authors.

St. Louis, K. O., & Hinzman, A. R. (1986). Studies of cluttering: Perceptions of speech-language pathologists and educators of cluttering. Journal of Fluency Disorders 11, 131–149.

St. Louis, K. O., Hinzman, A. R., & Hull, F. M. (1985). Studies of cluttering: Disfluency and language measures in young possible clutterers and stutterers. Journal of Fluency Disorders 10, 151–172.

St. Louis, K. O., & McCaffrey, E. (2005). Public awareness of cluttering and stuttering: Preliminary results. Poster presented at the Annual Convention of the American Speech-Language-Hearing Association. San Diego, CA.

St. Louis, K. O., Murray, C. D., & Ashworth, M. S. (1991). Co-existing communication disorders in a random sample of school-aged stutterers. Journal of Fluency Disorders 16, 13–23.

St. Louis, K. O., & Myers, F. L. (1995). Clinical management of cluttering. Language, Speech, and Hearing Services in Schools 26, 187–195.

St. Louis, K. O., & Myers, F. L. (1997). Management of cluttering and related fluency disorders. In R. F. Curlee & G. M. Siegel (Eds.), Nature and treatment of stuttering: New directions (2nd ed.) (pp. 313–332). New York: Allyn & Bacon.

St. Louis, K. O., Myers, F. L., Bakker, K., & Raphael, L. J. (2004). Clinical and research perspectives on cluttering. In D. Georgieva (Ed.), Fluency Disorders: New Research Perspectives (pp. 246–288). Sofia, Bulgaria: Grafis. (In Bulgarian)

St. Louis, K. O., Myers, F. L., Bakker, K., & Raphael, L. J. (2005). Clinical management of cluttering. Neurologopedia 1, 47–59. (In Polish)

St. Louis, K. O., Myers, F. L., Cassidy, L. J., Michael, A. J., Penrod S. M., Litton, B. A. et al. (1996). Efficacy of delayed auditory feedback for treating cluttering: Two case studies. Journal of Fluency Disorders 21, 305–314.

St. Louis, K. O., Myers, F. L., Faragasso, K., Townsend, P. S., & Gallaher, A. J. (2004). Perceptual aspects of cluttered speech. Journal of Fluency Disorders 29, 213–235.

St. Louis, K. O., Raphael, L. J., Myers, F. L., & Bakker, K. (2003, November). Cluttering updated. The ASHA Leader 8–21, 4–5, 20–23.

St. Louis, K. O., & Ruscello, D. M. (2000). Oral Speech Mechanism Screening Examination (3rd ed.). Austin, TX: PRO-ED.

St. Louis, K. O., Ruscello, D. M., & Lundeen, C. (1992). Coexistence of communication disorders in schoolchildren. ASHA Monographs, No. 27.

Teigland, A. (1996). A study of pragmatic skills of clutterers and normal speakers. Journal of Fluency Disorders 21, 201–214.

Tiger, R., Irvine, T., & Reis, R. (1980). Cluttering as a complex of learning disabilities. Language, Speech, and Hearing Services in Schools 11, 3–14.

Thacker, A. J., & Austen, S. (1996). Cluttered communication in a deafened adult with autistic features. Journal of Fluency Disorders 21, 271–279.

Van Riper C. (1971). The nature of stuttering. Englewood Cliffs, NJ: Prentice-Hall.

Van Riper ,C. (1982). The nature of stuttering (2nd ed.). Englewood Cliffs, NJ: Prentice-Hall.

Volkmar FR. (2003). Changing perspectives on ADHD. American Journal of Psychiatry 160, 1025–1027.

Weiss, D. A. (1964) Cluttering. Englewood Cliffs, NJ: Prentice-Hall.

Weiss, D. A. (1967). Cluttering. Folia Phoniatrica 19, 233–263.

Wingate ME. (1976). Stuttering: Theory and treatment. NY: Irvington.

Wolk L. (1986). Cluttering: a diagnostic case report. British Journal of Disorders of Communication 21, 199–207.

Woolf, G. (1967). The assessment of stuttering as struggle, avoidance and expectancy. British Journal of Disorders of Communication2, 158–177

Zackheim, C. T., & Conture, E. G. (2003). Childhood stuttering and speech disfluencies in relation to children's mean length of utterance: A preliminary study. Journal of Fluency Disorders 28, 115–142.

Appendix 16.1   Self-Awareness of Speech Index (SASI)

Name   **Date**
Instructions: Please check (√) the appropriate box for each question. Work rapidly and do not look back or change your answers.

		Never	Rarely	Usually	Always
1	I notice differences in the way I say words as compared with the way other people say words.	❑	❑	❑	❑
2	I notice when other people use fillers when they talk, such as "uh," "ya know," and "um."	❑	❑	❑	❑
3	I try to copy the way other people say certain words.	❑	❑	❑	❑
4	I listen to whether someone else's voice is high-pitched or low-pitched.	❑	❑	❑	❑
5	I am aware of other people's accents as they talk.	❑	❑	❑	❑
6	I know when I repeat a sound, word, or phrase.	❑	❑	❑	❑
7	I notice pitch changes in my own voice.	❑	❑	❑	❑
8	I pay attention to how fast other people talk.	❑	❑	❑	❑
9	I notice repetitions of sounds, words, or phrases when other people talk.	❑	❑	❑	❑
10	I am aware of how other people say words.	❑	❑	❑	❑
11	I pay attention to how fast I talk.	❑	❑	❑	❑
12	I notice when I stumble over words.	❑	❑	❑	❑
13	I notice my own accent.	❑	❑	❑	❑
14	I am aware when I use fillers when I talk, such as "uh," "ya know," and "um."	❑	❑	❑	❑

Summary Form

Instructions: Count the number of checks in each of the 4 columns of the completed *SASI* form. Write the totals in the boxes in the 1st row. Multiply these numbers by the weights provided in the 2nd row and write Weighted Totals in the boxes in the 3rd row. Write the sum of these four numbers in the Grand Total box in the 4th row. On the line below, divide the Grand Total by 14 to determine the Average *SASI* Score. Round the Average *SASI* Score to the nearest tenth, e.g., 2.4.

	Never	Rarely	Usually	Always
Total Checks in Each Category	❑	❑	❑	❑
Weights (Multipliers)	×1	×2	×3	×4
Weighted Totals	❑	❑	❑	❑
Grand Total			❑	

Average *SASI* Score: _____ / 14 = _____
                              Grand Total

Additional copies of this form are available from Populore, PO Box 4382 Morgantown, WV 26504 USA. 866-667-8679.

Average *SASI* Scores can range from 1.0 (completely unaware of speech in oneself and others) to 4.0 (extremely aware of speech in oneself and others).

The Average *SASI* Score for 171 unselected college students (34% males and 66% females, with a mean age of 21 years [range = 18 − 44 years]) was 2.7, with individual *SASI* items ranging from 1.7 to 3.4 (Atkins & St. Louis, 1988).

Appenix 16.2   St. Louis Inventory of Life Perspectives and Speech/Language Difficulty (SL♦ILP-SL): A Taking Stock Self-Study Exercise

Name: **Age:**   **Date:**
Instructions: After each of the following questions, please *circle the number* **that best represents your opinion. Be as honest as you can. There are no right or wrong answers.**

1. Overall, how much DIFFICULTY, HANDICAP, OR SUFFERING do you experience from your speech or language difficulty *at this time?*

1	2	3	4	5	6	7	8	9	?
None				Moderate				Very Much	I Don't Know

2. Overall, how much does your speech or language difficulty NEGATIVELY AFFECT YOUR ABILITY TO INTERACT WITH OTHER PEOPLE *at this time?*

1	2	3	4	5	6	7	8	9	?
No Negative Effect				Moderate Negative Effect				Extreme Negative Effect	I Don't Know

3. Overall, how much do you FEEL ABLE OR UNABLE TO CONTROL YOUR SPEECH OR LANGUAGE DIFFICULTY *at this time?*

1	2	3	4	5	6	7	8	9	?
Completely Able to Control				Equally Able or Unable to Control				Completely Unable to Control	I Don't Know

4. Overall, how SEVERE is your speech or language difficulty *at this time?*

1	2	3	4	5	6	7	8	9	?
No Difficulty	Very Mild			Moderate				Very Severe	I Don't Know

5. Overall, how much do you FEEL A NEED OR DESIRE TO GET HELP for your speech or language difficulty *at this time?*

1	2	3	4	5	6	7	8	9	?
None				Moderate				Very Much	I Don't Know

6. HOW IMPORTANT A PROBLEM IS YOUR SPEECH OR LANGUAGE DIFFICULTY IN YOUR LIFE *at this time?*

1	2	3	4	5	6	7	8	9	?
Not Important At All				Moderate				Very Important	I Don't Know

7. HOW IMPORTANT A PROBLEM IS YOUR SPEECH OR LANGUAGE DIFFICULTY IN THE LIVES OF THE PEOPLE YOU LIVE WITH *at this time?*

1	2	3	4	5	6	7	8	9	?
Not Important At All				Moderate				Very Important	NA (e.g., I live alone) or I Don't Know

(Continued)

8. Overall, how much do you FEEL INCLINED TO ASSOCIATE WITH OTHER PEOPLE WITH SPEECH OR LANGUAGE DIFFICULTIES *at this time?*

1	2	3	4	5	6	7	8	9	?
Not At All				*Moderate*				*Very Much*	*I Don't Know*

9. Overall, how much do you FEEL INCLINED TO HELP OTHER PEOPLE WITH SPEECH OR LANGUAGE DIFFICULTIES *at this time?*

1	2	3	4	5	6	7	8	9	?
Not At All				*Moderate*				*Very Much*	*I Don't Know*

10. Overall, how is your PHYSICAL HEALTH *at this time?*

1	2	3	4	5	6	7	8	9	?
Very Poor				*Not Poor but Not Good*				*Excellent*	*I Don't Know*

11. Overall, how is your MENTAL HEALTH *at this time?*

1	2	3	4	5	6	7	8	9	?
Very Poor				*Not Poor but Not Good*				*Excellent*	*I Don't Know*

12. Overall, how SATISFIED WITH YOUR LIFE are you *at this time?*

1	2	3	4	5	6	7	8	9	?

13. How much did your *speech or* LANGUAGE DIFFICULTY AFFECT YOUR ANSWER ON THE PREVIOUS QUESTION, No. 12. above?

1	2	3	4	5	6	7	8	9	?
No Effect on #12				Moderate Effect on #12				Completely Determined #12	I Don't Know

Additional copies of this form are available from Populore, PO Box 4382, Morgantown, WV 26504 USA, 866-667-8679.

17

Etiology, Symptomatology, and Treatment of Neurogenic Stuttering

Luc F. De Nil, Regina Jokel, and Elizabeth Rochon

The sudden or gradual development of stuttering or stutter-like speech disfluencies in adults has been documented extensively in the clinical literature. Not only does the clinical management of this disorder pose specific challenges, it also provides an intriguing window into the neurological processes underlying speech fluency, speech production, and language formulation. The purpose of this chapter is to review and interpret the scientific and clinical literature on neurogenic stuttering and to formulate some clinically useful guidelines for assessment and treatment. After a brief discussion of terminology, we review available data on incidence and prevalence of neurogenic stuttering. This is followed by a more detailed discussion of the speech fluency characteristics in this population, including secondary behaviors and the presence or absence of emotional reactions and negative speech attitudes. Next, we will review assessment strategies, including a description of an assessment battery that we have found useful in our clinical work. Finally, we provide an overview of treatment strategies described in the literature and conclude with some final remarks on the importance, both theoretical and clinical, of larger-scale experimental investigations with this disorder population.

Although neurogenic stuttering is most typically described as occurring primarily in adults, and as such differentiated from developmental stuttering, there have been several reports suggesting that the onset of neurogenic fluency disorders may also be observed during childhood (Kuhar, 1986; Nass, Schreter & Heier, 1994). Two types of acquired stuttering are typically recognized: *neurogenic* and *psychogenic* (although psychogenic stuttering will not be reviewed in any detail as part of this chapter, we will include references to this literature when appropriate.) Neurogenic stuttering is generally diagnosed when the onset of stutter-like disfluencies occurs following a neurological event, such as head trauma or disease, which disrupts normal brain function. In the absence of any apparent disruption to neurological function, adult-onset stuttering is often considered to be of psychogenic origin. However, the differentiation between neurogenic and psychogenic stuttering is complicated and not always straightforward to make, as we will discuss later.

Developing a thorough understanding of acquired stuttering is important for several reasons. First, although the prevalence of acquired stuttering is generally considered to be low, it is not uncommon for clinicians, particularly those who work in medical settings, to come across such patients (Market, Montague, Buffalo, & Drummond, 1990; Stewart & Rowley, 1996). Second, acquired stuttering, similar to developmental stuttering, often poses a serious communication problem that affects a person's ability to interact with his or her environment. Therefore, patients with acquired stuttering—just as those with developmental stuttering—deserve to receive the best evidence-based fluency intervention. Third, although it is debatable whether acquired and developmental stuttering are similar or different speech fluency disorders (Canter, 1971; Helm-Estabrooks, 1993; Lebrun, Bijleveld, & Rousseau, 1990; Ringo & Dietrich, 1995; Rosenbek, Messert, Collins, & Wertz, 1978), a greater understanding of the relationship between neurological and/or psychological conditions and the onset of stutter-like disfluencies in adulthood holds promise for providing more insight into developmental stuttering. This latter point seems especially relevant for neurogenic stuttering given the recent advances in understanding the neural bases of developmental stuttering (De Nil, 2004).

The recognition that stuttering can have its onset in adulthood is not new. As early as the 19th century, clinical reports were published describing patients with stutter-like symptoms. For instance, Kussmaul (1877) provided a brief description of a young man who experienced what he called "Aphatisches Stottern" following a mild stroke. Pick (1899) also described a 63-year-old man with a stroke-induced acquired stutter. Despite these early reports, relatively few publications appeared until the early 1970s and most consisted of isolated clinical case studies. In 1971, Canter published an influential paper, to be discussed in more detail below, in which he presented diagnostic criteria for neurogenic stuttering and differentiated between three different types of acquired stuttering. Following this publication, acquired stuttering gained greater recognition among clinicians and researchers, leading to a significant increase in the number of published reports, again, however, consisting mostly of clinical case studies.

◆ Terminology

Even a cursory review of the literature in this area suggests that there is no shortage of terms used to refer to neurogenic stuttering. Authors have variously referred to neurogenic stuttering as: *late onset stuttering/stammering, acquired stuttering, adult-onset stuttering, neurological stuttering, cortical stuttering, sudden onset of stuttering, neurogenic stuttering, organic stuttering, stuttering associated with acquired neurological disorders (SAAND), and dysphatic stuttering*, among others. Although these various terms may be historically based or reflect personal author preferences, it cannot be excluded that they indicate the potential presence of subgroups within the larger population. Indeed, several authors have argued for the recognition of several subgroups within the larger category of neurogenic stuttering. For instance, Canter (1971), differentiated between dysarthric, apraxic, and dysnomic stuttering. More recently, Van Borsel (1997) argued for the following different types of late-onset stuttering: pharmacogenic, psychogenic, malingered, and neurogenic. Moreover, within the broader category of neurogenic stuttering, Van Borsel suggested that thalamic stuttering may constitute one of several different subtypes (Van Borsel, Van Der Made, & Santens, 2003). Helm-Estabrooks, Yeo, Geschwind, and Freedman (1986) described stuttering associated with distinct medical entities, such as stroke, head trauma, extrapyramidal disease, tumor, dementia, drug usage, and other causes. They also differentiated between transient and persistent neurogenic stuttering, which was believed to be associated with either multifocal unilateral (transient) or bilateral (persistent) lesions (Helm, Butler, & Canter, 1980). In this chapter, we will primarily use the term "neurogenic stuttering." Although it is clear that there are significant inter-individual differences among patients, we do not believe that the data as of yet are sufficiently extensive and robust to identify reliably distinct subgroups of people with acquired stuttering.

◆ Prevalence and Incidence of Neurogenic Stuttering

Other than general observations that neurogenic stuttering is a rare or uncommon disorder (Ringo & Dietrich, 1995), very little direct or reliable information is available regarding its prevalence or incidence. Market, Montague, Buffalo, and Drummond (1990) contacted ~150 clinicians in the United States, of which 100 responded that they had treated at least one patient with neurogenic stuttering during the last few years. Although the findings of Market et al. seem to indicate that neurogenic stuttering is not that rare, no information was provided about how the clinicians who were initially contacted for the survey were selected, nor was any information provided as to the average caseload of the clinicians who responded positively. Stewart and Rowley, (1996) reported results of a survey similar to the one used by Market et al. to study neurogenic stuttering in Great Britain. Of the 100 clinicians initially contacted, 36 completed surveys on patients with neurogenic stuttering. However, again it is unclear how the initially contacted clinicians were selected. One of the factors that complicates obtaining data on incidence and prevalence is the fact that neurogenic stuttering does not always persist but may be transient in nature (Helm-Estabrooks, 1993). This may decrease the likelihood that its presence is detected in the clinical environment, resulting in an underestimation of its occurrence when using survey tools. Some more direct evidence is available in a study by Ghika-Schmid, van Melle, Guex, and Bogousslavsky (1999). As part of a study of emotions in stroke patients, they followed unselected acute patients from the first 4 days to 3 months poststroke. Of the 53 patients followed during the study, one patient was reported to exhibit stuttering (no information was provided whether stuttering may have existed premorbidly in this patient). Although this would suggest an incidence rate of ~2% among stroke patients, it is unclear from the study how stuttering was defined or identified.

As pointed out earlier, the onset of neurogenic stuttering theoretically can occur at any age, but it is most typically identified when stuttering occurs first post-puberty. Surveying 81 patients with neurogenic stuttering, Market et al. (1990) reported a mean age of onset of 43.7 years. Similarly, in their survey of 36 patients, Stewart and Rowley (1996) observed a mean age of onset of 48.2 years. This corresponds closely with the mean age of 48.5 years reported by Mazzucchi, Moretti, Carpeggiani, Parma, and Paini (1981) in their study of 16 patients. In our own study of 12 patients with neurogenic stuttering, the mean age of onset was 49.42 years (Jokel & De Nil, 2003). However, it is not unusual to see acquired stuttering occur at a younger age. Callis-Landrum, DiDanato, Rosenfield, and Viswanath (1990) reported on 5 patients with a mean age of 30 years. Ludlow, Rosenberg, Salazar, Grafman, and Smutok (1987) reported on 10 subjects with chronic acquired stuttering following penetrating missile brain injuries. Although the mean age of this group at the time of the study was 34.9 years, all subjects were recruited for the study 15 years post-injury, dating the onset of acquired stuttering back to their late teens or early twenties. One of the patients we investigated developed acquired stuttering at the age of 17 years following a stroke. Moreover, a few authors have reported on potential neurogenic stuttering in children. Aram, Meyers, and Ekelman (1990) reported a higher frequency of stuttering disfluencies among children with unilateral brain lesions. Using a 3% cutoff for minimum frequency of stuttering disfluencies (Conture, 2001), 5 of the 33 young participants in the Aram et al. study (mean age at testing: 9.84 years for children with left-lateralized lesions and 7.00 years for those with right lateralized lesions) would be classified as stuttering. This would correspond to a 15% prevalence rate among children with unilateral brain lesions, compared with the 1% typically reported for developmental stuttering in the general population. Probably the youngest person reported to date as experiencing neurogenic stuttering was a 2-year-old girl who experienced an intense transient stuttering episode following a second stroke (Nass et al., 1994).

The prevalence of neurogenic stuttering tends to be biased toward male speakers. In the two survey studies mentioned before, Stewart and Rowley (1996) found 62% of the patients with acquired stuttering to be male. Market et al. (1990) reported that in their surveyed group 79% of the affected individuals were male. Among the five younger children with symptoms of neurogenic stuttering reported by Aram et al. (1990), none were girls although girls made up 36% of the total group of children with brain lesions.

Of particular interest is the timing of stuttering onset relative to the onset of the neurological disorder or lesion. Similar to developmental stuttering, which typically (but not always) is characterized by a gradual development, the precise onset of neurogenic stuttering in many patients is not easily determined. In some patients, the onset of neurogenic stuttering has been reported as occurring immediately or very shortly (within a few weeks) after the onset of the medical problem (Balasubramanian, Max, Van Borsel, Rayca, & Richardson, 2003; Rentschler, Driver, & Callaway, 1984; Stewart & Grantham, 1993; Van Borsel, Van Lierde, Cauwenberge, Guldermont, & Van Orshoven, 2001). Often this appears to be the case with neurogenic stuttering associated with cerebral vascular accidents. In others, the onset of stuttering occurred some time, often months, after the initial medical problem was first diagnosed (Mowrer & Younts, 2001; Van Borsel et al., 2003). In several of these patients, stuttering appeared following a second incidence or an aggravation of the medical condition (Chung, Im, Lee, & Lee, 2004; Helm-Estabrooks, 1993; Nass et al., 1994). In still other patients, stuttering was observed prior to the diagnosis, but obviously not the presence, of a neurological condition (Lebrun, Retif, & Kaiser, 1983). In many published case studies, however, the time of onset cannot be determined reliably because stuttering either developed gradually, and the moment of onset cannot be precisely determined, or was not reliably documented in the available medical history report. As such, we do not feel confident at the present time to draw any general and valid conclusions regarding a relationship between onset timing and etiological or speech fluency characteristics. It seems clear, however, that the longer the time interval is between the onset or diagnosis of the neurological condition and the reported onset of stuttering, the more problematic it will be to make a causal link between the two conditions, to the exclusion of possible other contributing factors, including psychological reactive behaviors. Clearly, this is an area that requires longitudinal studies based on direct observations of persons who develop neurogenic speech fluency problems.

◆ Characteristics of Neurogenic Stuttering

Etiology and Neuroanatomical Correlates

Neurogenic stuttering has been reported following various lesions or degenerative disease conditions and as such does not appear to be associated exclusively with a particular neurological disorder or disruption in any particular brain area. In a survey study of 100 cases of patients with neurogenic stuttering, Market et al. (1990) reported that 38.3% started to stutter following head trauma and 37% following ischemic accidents, for a total of 75.3% of all patients analyzed in their study. The remainder of their participants acquired stuttering following a variety of disease and trauma conditions, including neurodegenerative diseases (1.2%). Stewart and Rowley (1996) reported that 69.2% of the subjects in their sample (~25 patients) had a "neurogenic" origin, which presumably combined stroke, trauma, and neurodegenerative diseases. No further differentiation was made within this group.

Penetrating head lesions often result in more localized trauma and therefore potentially may yield more specific information on the role of certain cortical or subcortical brain areas in acquired stuttering. In one of the most extensive studies in this population, Ludlow et al. (1987) compared head injury patients with and without neurogenic stuttering. Brain areas more affected in patients with neurogenic stuttering included white matter tracts (internal and external capsule, low frontal white matter tracts), as well as subcortical nuclei (caudate and lentiform nuclei). The occurrence of stuttering was not related to lateralization or the size of the lesion.

In the case of neurogenic stuttering following stroke, several brain sites have been implicated, including subcortical regions such as thalamus and brain stem (Abe, Yokoyama, & Yorifuji, 1993; Van Borsel & Taillieu, 2000), basal ganglia (Nass et al., 1994), and cerebellum (Van Borsel & Taillieu, 2000), as well as cortical regions including temporal and parietal lobe (Ardila & Lopez, 1986; Bijleveld,

Lebrun, & Dongen, 1994; Helm-Estabrooks et al., 1986), supplementary motor area (Van Borsel, et al., 1998), and frontal cortex (Van Borsel & Taillieu, 2000). Similar to findings by Ludlow et al. (1987) in trauma patients, neurogenic stuttering following stroke can occur with either unilateral (left or right) or bilateral lesions.

Various neurodegenerative conditions, each affecting different areas of the brain, have been reported to be associated with neurogenic stuttering. They include Parkinson's disease (PD) (Hertrich, Ackermann, Ziegler, Kaschel, 1993; Leder, 1996; Louis, Winfield, Fahn, & Ford, 2001), which affects the basal ganglia and substantia nigra in the brain stem, and multiple sclerosis (Mowrer & Younts, 2001), which is characterized by myelin loss in various areas of the brain.

In addition to these disorders, one can find idiosyncratic case studies in which the onset of acquired stuttering is thought to be related to a neural disorder even though there is no demonstrable brain etiology. Such conditions include headache (Perino, Famularo & Tarroni, 2000), chronic pain (Andy & Bhatnagar, 1992), anorexia (Byrne, Byrne & Zibin, 1993), and myelography (Pimental & Gorelick, 1985). Whether or not these case reports truly represent neurogenic stuttering, or should rather be classified as possibly psychogenic in nature, remains an open question.

Overall, it seems that neurogenic stuttering can be associated with lesions or disease conditions in a wide variety of brain regions, and the conclusion by Alm (2004) that the "basal ganglia circuits through the putamen may play an important role in many cases of neurologic stuttering" (p. 335) certainly would seem to need further corroboration. The various brain structures in which lesions have been noted to be associated with the onset of neurogenic stuttering seem to suggest that the neurological origin needs to be sought in a disruption of neural circuitry rather than a lesion in one specific brain region. Such involvement of widespread brain areas in neurogenic stuttering may not necessarily come as a surprise given that speech production and language processes themselves are controlled by a widely distributed network of neural functions (Demonet, Thierry, & Cardebat, 2005). In this respect, the recent functional imaging research in developmental stuttering may provide some critical insights. During the past decade, several studies using positron emission tomography, functional magnetic resonance imaging, and magnetoencephalography have started to reveal the intricate network of unilateral and bilateral brain regions that differentiate between stuttering and nonstuttering individuals (for reviews, see Brown, Ingham, Ingham, Laird, & Fox, 2005; De Nil, 2004; Ingham, et al., 2004), including overactivations in primary and premotor cortex, anterior cingulate cortex, cerebellum, and deactivations in auditory cortex. Although some investigations have revealed atypical right hemisphere activation in adults with developmental stuttering, many studies have reported a general overactivation of regions in both the left and right hemisphere (De Nil, 2004). In addition, several recent studies have shown that developmental stuttering is characterized not only by functional but also by structural differences, especially in the frontolateral and auditory cortex (Foundas, Bollich, Corey, Hurley, & Heilman, 2001; Foundas et al., 2003; Sommer, Koch, Paulus, Weiller, & Buchel, 2002). At present, no similar functional or structural studies have been reported with persons with neurogenic stuttering, but this obviously is an area in need of investigation and may provide some powerful data relevant to our understanding of both developmental and neurogenic stuttering.

Speech Characteristics

As mentioned before, arguably one of the most influential articles on neurogenic stuttering has been published by Canter (1971). In this article, entitled "Observations on neurogenic stuttering: A contribution to differential diagnosis," the author distinguished between three subgroups of neurogenic stuttering: (1) *dysarthric* stuttering in which speech fluency breakdown is a result of "faulty motor execution," primarily in patients with PD and cerebellar lesions; (2) *apraxic* stuttering, seen in patients with verbal apraxia of speech who have lost the ability to translate phonemes into motor speech patterns; and (3) *dysnomic* stuttering, where stuttering is associated with word retrieval problems. Canter suggested that each of these subgroups of neurogenic stuttering could be characterized according to distinct features of speech disfluencies. Dysarthric stuttering may be more likely characterized by tense articulatory blocks, whereas apraxic stuttering may consist primarily of "probing repetitions" of a sound as well as silent speech blocks. Patients with dysnomic stuttering, in turn, may experience predominantly word or phrase repetitions, in addition to pauses, articulatory gropings, and interjections. Canter also suggested the following criteria as useful in the differential diagnosis of acquired stuttering: (1) repetitions and prolongations on final consonants; (2) moments of stuttering occurring primarily on /r/, /l/, and /h/; (3) disfluencies not systematically related to grammatical function (e.g., content vs function words); (4) disfluencies possibly inversely related to the level of propositionality, with choral speech and repetitions resulting in more disfluencies compared with self-formulated speech; (5) absence of an adaptation effect (i.e., no decrease in disfluency with repeated readings); (6)absence of marked anxiety about the disfluencies, although annoyance is possible; and (7) no secondary behaviors (e.g., avoidance or escape behaviors).

Subsequent reviews and case studies have shown that Canter's behavioral criteria may not be as clear-cut and generalizable as originally suggested. Indeed, Van Borsel (1997) concluded that "clinical symptomatology does not enable one to safely distinguish neurogenic stuttering from developmental stuttering." (p. 21). Nevertheless, Canter's criteria have been very influential and have proven to be useful in the identification and assessment of at least several patients with neurogenic stuttering. For instance, as recently as 1993, Helm-Estabrooks (1993, p. 260) listed the following six characteristics of neurogenic stuttering as helpful for differential diagnosis of psychogenic or developmental forms of the disorder: (1) disfluencies occur on grammatical (or function) words nearly as frequently as on substantive (or content) words; (2) the speaker may be annoyed but does not appear anxious; (3) repetitions, prolongations, and blocks do not occur only on initial syllables of words and utterances; (4) secondary symptoms such as facial grimacing, eye blinking, or fist clenching are not associated with moments of disfluency; (5) there is no adaptation effect; and (6) stuttering occurs relatively consistently across various types of speech tasks. It is clear that these criteria are essentially similar to the ones suggested by Canter more than 20 years earlier. Indeed, the first five characteristics are almost identical to ones identified by Canter, whereas the sixth criterion points to a lack of task-specific or situational variability.

Types of Speech Disfluency

Although, in our opinion, evidence to clearly delineate subgroups of neurogenic stuttering is still insufficient, a review of the literature reveals that the type and characteristics of speech disfluencies may be influenced by the underlying etiology. Stroke patients seem to be more likely to experience repetitions that involve short segments, such as sounds or syllables, as well as longer words and phrases. Analyzing the speech of a group of seven stroke patients, Rosenbek et al. (1978) reported that the majority of disfluencies (72%) consisted of sound, syllable, and single-syllable word repetitions, whereas on average only 14% of the disfluencies consisted of prolongations and no speech blocks were observed. Van Borsel et al. (2003) also reported on a patient who experienced a thalamic stroke and whose disfluencies consisted primarily of word and part-word repetitions as well as interjections.

Although repetitions also appear to be a predominant feature in patients with head injury, the nature of their repetitions appear to be different from those observed in stroke patients. Ludlow et al. (1987) described the speech in their patients as "shot from a gun, with intermittent and unpredictable bursts of rapid and unintelligible speech, uncontrolled repetitions or prolongations, and long silences without struggle" (p. 62), which raises the possibility that their speech may be characterized by some clutter-like symptoms. Similar observations were reported by Marshall and Neuburger (1987).

In some patients, the occurrence of repetitions appears to be task-specific, which seems to counter the observation by Helm-Estabrooks that disfluencies are relatively consistent across speech tasks (see above). For instance, Abe and colleagues (1993) described a male patient who suffered a bilateral medial thalamic and brain stem infarct and showed syllable repetitions but only during spontaneous speech and not during word repetition or reading. In contrast, analyzing the speech of patients with traumatic head injury, Jokel, De Nil, and Sharpe (in press) found that the proportional frequency of their disfluencies stayed constant regardless of the complexity of the reading material (words, sentences, paragraphs), although during spontaneous speech the frequency of stuttering disfluencies tended to be higher in monologue than in conversation. Jokel et al. also found that the frequency of stuttering disfluencies in stroke-induced neurogenic stuttering decreased as the reading material became more complex. This observation may suggest that with increasing complexity, disfluencies resulting from language deficiencies became more prominent compared with the core stuttering disfluencies. Thus, it would seem important to consider carefully the nature of the language and reading material when comparing data across studies and across speakers, at least in the case of stroke-induced stuttering. Observations such as these suggest that etiology may influence the nature of speech disfluencies and that a more detailed and careful analysis of the frequency and type of these disfluencies ultimately may have differential diagnostic value for various subgroups of neurogenic stuttering.

In contrast to stroke patients, disfluencies in patients with PD seem to consist more frequently of attempts to produce rapid movements, articulatory freezing, frequent prolongations, or silent blocks. These characteristics were described by Canter (1971) as part of dysarthric stuttering. As such, the disfluencies in this population may be reflective of their underlying motor deficits. Louis et al. (2001) described the speech of two patients with PD, one of whom displayed frequent pausing and occasional blocking, whereas the other patient displayed primarily "pressured speech" and freezing, as well as sound repetitions. In contrast, Leder (1996) observed a 29-year-old patient with PD whose stuttering was characterized by blocks and multiple repetitions, often involving 20 or more repeated units. Although such extremely long repetitions could be considered similar to palilalia (Christman, Boutsen, & Buckingham, 2004), Van Borsel (1997) has argued that such an interpretation is not correct because he considers stuttering repetitions in patients with PD as being very distinct from those seen in palilalia, which is characterized more by repetitions that primarily affect speech fragments longer than those typically seen in stuttering.

Localization of Speech Disfluencies within the Word/Sentence

The large majority of disfluencies in stroke-induced stuttering can be observed in word and syllable initial positions. For instance, repetitions in the patient reported by Abe et al. (1993) were restricted to initial syllables in words. Similarly, stuttering was restricted to initial parts or sounds of a word in a woman who experienced a right hemisphere stroke (Fleet & Heilman, 1985). Rosenbek et al. (1978) analyzed the speech of seven patients and observed disfluencies primarily in initial word positions, with only the most severe patients showing "some instances of medial position repetitions" (p. 87). In our own study of six stroke patients performing a reading and spontaneous speech task, 93 to 95% of their disfluencies occurred in word initial position (Jokel & De Nil, 2003; Jokel et al., in press). Nevertheless, at least some patients do show a higher than expected frequency on medial and final segments, as suggested by Canter (1971) and Helm-Estabrooks (1993). Mowrer and Younts (2001) reported on a 36-year-old patient with multiple sclerosis who showed excessive part- and whole-word repetitions that occurred primarily in initial, but also, albeit to a lesser extent, in medial and final positions. Interestingly, Hertrich et al. (1993) suggested that the nature of disfluencies may differ depending on the localization in the word or sentence. They presented a patient with PD who demonstrated disfluencies on initial as well as final words in phrases, but initial disfluencies tended to involve consonant-vowel segments, whereas final disfluencies were more likely to involve longer syllable-level segments. Although medial and final disfluencies can be observed in persons with neurogenic stuttering, it is important to keep in mind that such disfluencies are not completely absent in those with developmental stuttering (Camarata, 1988; Lebrun & Van Borsel, 1990; McAllister & Kingston, 2005)

Adaptation

One of the characteristics often associated with neurogenic stuttering is the presumed absence of a reading adaptation effect. This effect, often seen in persons with developmental stuttering, results in a pronounced reduction in the overall frequency of disfluency following repeated reading of a text (see Bloodstein, 1995, for review of theory and empirical data pertaining to adaptation). Both Canter (1971) and Helm-Estabrooks (1993) listed the lack of adaptation as one of the distinguishing characteristics of neurogenic stuttering. Because many published studies do not comment on reading adaptation, or do not adequately describe how it was assessed, it is hard to obtain reliable data on the percentage of patients who do or do not show the effect. It is clear, however, that adaptation may be more common than previously thought. In our own observations (Jokel & De Nil, 2003; Jokel et al., in press), four of six patients with stroke-induced stuttering were able to complete three successive readings of the Rainbow Passage. Of these four, three showed a reduction of more than 30% in the frequency of stuttering disfluencies over three consecutive readings. On the other hand, only two of five patients with head injury showed a similar disfluency reduction. Similar reports in the literature that adaptation may occur in neurogenic stuttering, whereas at the same time not all individuals with developmental stuttering show reading adaptation, question the usefulness of this criterion as a differential diagnostic tool for neurogenic stuttering. It is possible, nevertheless, that the presence or absence of adaptation may differentiate between different neurological disorders (Helm-Estabrooks, 1993; Hertrich, et al., 1993; McClean & McLean, 1985).

Secondary Behaviors

Developmental stuttering, especially in older children and adults, is characterized not only by speech disfluencies but often also by a complex set of secondary behaviors. Such concomitant behaviors may be learned or may reflect cognitive or other processes (Conture & Kelly, 1991). These behaviors can be such a prominent element of the person's stuttering profile that some therapeutic approaches have focused, sometimes exclusively, on their elimination as a way of minimizing the external manifestation of stuttering. In contrast, it has been suggested that the absence of secondary behaviors in people with neurogenic stuttering is one of the criteria that can be used for differential diagnostic purposes (Canter, 1971; Helm-Estabrooks, 1993). Not unexpectedly, the literature on this issue is inconsistent in its support. Ringo and Dietrich (1995) found that 37 of 53 case studies (70%) published prior to 1993 reported the absence of secondary behaviors. No information was available for another 26 cases. If one were to make the assumption that the reason for not including secondary behaviors in the description of these 26 case studies was that such behaviors were not prevalent in these patients, this would indicate that up to 80% of the patients with neurogenic stuttering included in this review did not show any evidence of secondary behaviors. Such a finding would provide strong support for the differential diagnostic value of this criterion. However, caution is in order as a review of both older and more recent literature reveals that although some clinical case studies are very detailed and comprehensive, many others are rather sketchy in their description of behavioral characteristics. Furthermore, even for those case reports that do comment on the presence or absence of secondary behaviors, it is not always clear how such behaviors were defined, or whether the presence or absence of secondary behaviors was ascertained following casual observation or after more careful examination over longer periods of time and in a variety of speech contexts. Nevertheless, the fact remains that for many carefully reported clinical case studies, investigators have commented on the lack of secondary behaviors in people with neurogenic stuttering (Dworkin, Culatta, Abkarian, & Meleca, 2002; Lebrun & Leleux, 1985; Leder, 1996; McClean & McLean, 1985; Mowrer & Younts, 2001). In our own analysis of the stuttering characteristics of six patients with traumatic brain injury, three showed secondary behaviors, whereas the other three did not. Secondary behaviors observed in these patients consisted of more frequent than usual eye blinking, facial grimacing, head bending, foot tapping, and limb or head movements associated with stuttered moments but incongruent with the linguistic or communicative context. This observation of secondary behaviors in about half of the patients is consistent with the conclusion reached by Rosenbek et al. (1978) who reported accessory features, such as eye blinking and facial grimacing in three of seven patients. Interestingly, the most severe patients in their group were the ones who demonstrated the presence of secondary behaviors. Such a link with severity was not apparent in our own patients. The presence or absence of secondary behaviors needs to be interpreted in light of the onset of stuttering relative to the onset of the neurological lesion/disease (see above), and the timing of the speech assessment relative to the onset of stuttering. In some adults who develop neurogenic stuttering the time between onset of stuttering and the fluency assessment on which the published report is based may not have been sufficiently long for learned secondary behaviors to develop fully in the patient.

Attitudes and Emotions

Clinicians working with children or adults with developmental stuttering know that psychological reactions to speaking often are a significant component of the profile presented by their clients. These reactions may reflect innate (trait), as well as situational (state) or acquired personality characteristics. Given their importance in determining how the person interacts with his or her environment, and the outcome of treatment, these psychological reactions often are a major focus of intervention (Guitar, 1998). This has been confirmed by research showing that children and adults with developmental stuttering often show significantly more negative speech attitudes and other emotional reactions toward their ability to communicate (De Nil & Brutten, 1990; Vanryckeghem, Hylebos, Brutten, & Peleman, 2001), as well as potential differences in terms of temperament (Anderson, Pellowski, Conture, & Kelly, 2003; Lewis & Golberg, 1997). In contrast, very little systematic research has been conducted regarding psychological reactions in people with neurogenic stuttering. Based on clinical observation, Canter (1971) and Helm-Estabrooks (1993) proposed that adults with neurogenic stuttering may be annoyed but seldom develop marked anxiety toward their speech disfluencies.

However, as was the case with secondary behaviors, it is not always clear how psychological states or traits such as "anxiety," or "annoyance" were defined or assessed in the various clinical case reports. A review of the literature seems to confirm that most authors either do not report on emotional reactions or comment on their absence. The latter is particularly true for persons who experience neurogenic stuttering following head injury. Generally, persons with head injury are reported to be aware of the disfluency but not anxious or overly concerned about it (Lebrun, et al., 1990; Lebrun & Leleux, 1985; McClean & McLean, 1985), not unlike what can be observed in young children close to the onset of developmental stuttering (Guitar, 1998). Grant, Biousse, Cook, and Newman (1999) reported on four patients with stroke-associated stuttering. For two of the patients, observations on their psychological reactions were specifically included. One person was reported to be unaware of his disfluencies, whereas the second one "did not specifically complain of stutter, although he noted difficulty speaking" (p. 626). Interestingly, these were also the two patients who did not have a history of stuttering in childhood.

To investigate the presence of speech-related attitudes and perceptions more systematically, we administered the S-24 (Andrews & Cutler, 1974), a speech attitude test commonly used in the assessment of developmental stuttering, to a group of 12 patients with neurogenic stuttering, six of whom had stroke-induced stuttering, whereas the other 6 were diagnosed with traumatic brain injury (Jokel et al., in press). The average S-24 score for the stroke patients was 18.3, which is nearly identical to the average score (19.2) reported by Andrews and Cutler for people with developmental stuttering and significantly higher than the average score (9.42) for nonstuttering individuals. The patients with traumatic brain injury obtained an average S-24 score of 16.8. This finding suggests that, although persons with neurogenic stuttering may not demonstrate or overtly exhibit high levels of anxiety in specific speech situations, they nevertheless may demonstrate the same negative self-reported perceptions as evidenced by those with developmental stuttering, especially in the case of chronic acquired stuttering. As a result, neurogenic stuttering may very well result in the same social and interpersonal negative self-perception consequences as developmental stuttering. A good example of the presence of emotional responses to neurogenic stuttering is a patient reported by Lebrun et al. (1983) who became more disfluent when tense or at meetings. Similarly, some of the patients that the first author has worked with showed clear social and professional withdrawal effects that were directly related to their speech disfluencies. Clearly, at least some persons with neurogenic stuttering experience communicative obstacles very similar to those commonly seen in developmental stuttering. This latter observation may be closely related to whether the neurological deficiency affects the person's cognitive and emotional integrity, and thus his or her expected reaction to potentially stressful situational or communicative experiences. It would be a mistake, therefore, to ignore the assessment and treatment of emotional reactions and/or self-perceptions for these clients.

Other Speech or Language Problems that Can Accompany Neurogenic Stutering

Although neurogenic stuttering may occur as the only speech disorder evidenced by the patient, often there will be concomitant speech or language problems. Mazzuchi et al. (1981) reviewed case histories of 16 adult persons with neurogenic stuttering. For five of the patients, the onset of neurogenic stuttering was preceded by traumatic head injury. Two of the five patients also experienced additional language problems, such as paraphasias, anomia, and transient expressive aphasia. One of these patients also showed memory deficits. The remaining 11 patients developed neurogenic stuttering following a transient ischemic attack or other cerebrovascular episode. Of these, eight showed either transient or more permanent aphasia symptoms, including anomia, paraphasias, and dysgraphia. Similarly, Helm-Estabrooks (1986) included aphasia and apraxia symptoms as possible concomitant behaviors of neurogenic stuttering resulting from either stroke or head trauma, although the observations reported by Mazzuchi et al. (1981) would suggest that they are more frequent than suggested by Helm-Estabrooks, at least in the case of stroke-induced stuttering. Of the 10 patients with acquired stuttering following a penetrating head injury reported by Ludlow et al. (1987), three were diagnosed with Broca's aphasia, which persisted 15 years post-injury, whereas another patient was observed to experience aphasia 2 months post-injury, but no longer at the time of follow-up testing. However, the persons with acquired stuttering differed significantly from the control groups (healthy subjects and/or patients with head injury but no stuttering) on the following measures: receptive syntax, sentence production, word fluency. Reviewing 60 individual published reports of patients with neurogenic stuttering, we found that 22 reports mentioned the presence of additional speech and/or language problems, including aphasia or aphasia-like symptoms (8), dysathria and/or apraxia (12), as well as some other atypical speech problems such as high pitched voice (1) and hypernasality (1). The remaining case studies either did not comment on concomitant speech or language problems (18) or reported the absence of such problems. In most cases, if additional speech or language problems were identified, they were related to the neurological lesion or disease. For instance, patients with cerebral vascular accidents tended to show additional signs of aphasia, whereas patients who developed neurogenic stuttering as a result of multiple sclerosis or Parkinson's disease tended to show more dysarthric characteristics.

♦ Assessment

As discussed above, neurogenic stuttering can manifest itself in many different ways depending on several factors, including the nature of the associated disorder, the underlying etiology, and the time since onset. Moreover, neurogenic stuttering often is not the only communication disorder the patient is experiencing. For instance, in addition to speech fluency problems, some patients may also exhibit aphasia or dysarthria. Other patients may exhibit other motor or cognitive problems or experience chronic pain that affects their performance. All of these conditions may influence the quantity and quality of the neurogenic stuttering and therefore should be part of an assessment and/or treatment planning. Consequently, the assessment of neurogenic stuttering needs to be a highly individualized process, with information gathered along several different dimensions and synthesized into a coherent clinical picture. Although it is impossible in this chapter to provide a detailed overview of the various speech, language, motor, cognitive, and other tests and procedures that can be used during this assessment, we will discuss some general strategies that we have found to be clinically viable.

Two basic diagnostic questions that a clinician needs to address during assessment are:

Is the stuttering developmental or acquired? In many cases, the differential diagnosis between developmental and neurogenic stuttering is relatively straightforward, especially if there is a clear neurological event preceding the onset of stuttering, a reasonable link between the event and the speech difficulties, and no evidence of premorbid stuttering. In some cases, however, the trauma of the disease condition may have triggered a re-occurrence or aggravation of a preexisting stuttering disorder (Grant et al., 1999; Helm-Estabrooks, et al., 1986; Marshall & Neuburger, 1987). This, of course, raises the question whether the condition can truly be called neurogenic stuttering, or should rather be classified as developmental stuttering or developmental stuttering with an acquired overlay. Although this may be a theoretically important question, given our current knowledge of neurogenic stuttering, the answer may not necessarily have a lot of clinical significance for treatment planning. Indeed, as we will discuss below, some of the most successful interventions for neurogenic stuttering are not all that different from the approaches typically used with developmental stuttering. One of the potentially differentiating features, as illustrated by the four cases described by Grant and colleagues (1999), may be the presence of speech-related emotions. As discussed before, of the four patients described in this article, only the two who had a history of stuttering prior to the stroke showed significant emotional reactions to their disfluencies.

Is the stuttering neurogenic or psychogenic? Mahr and Leith (1992) define the diagnostic criteria of psychogenic stuttering as follows: (1) a change in speech pattern suggesting stuttering; (2) a relationship to psychological factors as evidenced by an onset associated with emotional conflict and/or secondary gain; (3) the lack of evidence of an organic etiology; (4) a past history of mental health problems; (5) atypical disfluency features (stereotypical repetitions, no islands of fluency within conversational speech, and no secondary behaviors); (6) a perception of "la belle indifférence" in which the patient shows a lack of emotional responses to the disfluencies; and (7) interpersonal interactions of a somewhat unusual or bizarre quality (see also Van Borsel & Taillieu, 2000).

Given the limited experience with psychogenic stuttering, the criteria outlined by Mahr and Leith are useful guidelines for differentially diagnosing psychogenic from neurogenic stuttering. Our main caution is with the criterion regarding organic etiology. Although the absence of a clearly defined neurological event preceding the onset of stuttering is often regarded as an indication of possible psychogenic stuttering, caution should be used when arriving at this conclusion. First, the absence of a neurological condition, at least at the time of onset of disfluencies, does not preclude that the stuttering may be a precursor to a gradually developing medical condition (Lebrun et al., 1983; Leder, 1996). Second, the neurological problem may be present but not necessarily visible during routine examinations.

Although the absence of an organic lesion or disease (assuming it is not a yet undetected brain condition) typically is a strong indicator for a psychogenic origin, the presence of a brain condition also does not necessarily exclude the diagnosis of psychogenic stuttering. Indeed, there is no reason to believe that people who experience a potentially devastating neurological disease, or have suffered brain trauma, may not also develop a psychological reaction that may manifest itself as psychogenic stuttering (Baumgartner & Duffy, 1997; Van Borsel, 1997). Indeed, one might conjecture that it would be abnormal *not* to react with some degree of psychosocial concern to neurological disease and/or trauma.

An Assessment Battery for Acquired Stuttering in Adults

To obtain a more detailed understanding of the speech fluency problems in a person with suspected neurogenic stuttering, we have developed a battery of tasks and tests that afford us a more complete picture of the fluency problems (see **Table 17–1**). Depending on the unique nature of each client, not all of these tests and tasks need or can be administered (for instance, a person with aphasia may need task modifications or may not be able to complete the reading tasks and questionnaires). Additional speech and language tasks or tests, not included in **Table 17–1**, may need to be administered depending on the nature of the presenting problem. Nevertheless, the information

Table 17–1   Assessment Battery for Acquired Stuttering in Adults (ABASA)

A. Case History
   a. Medical history, including neuroimaging data (structural and functional)
   b. Social and occupational history
   c. Personal/family speech and language history and current status
   d. Detailed history and current status of disfluencies (onset and development)
   e. Self-reported awareness of stuttering severity and secondary behaviors

B. Testing of General Functions
   a. Language (BDAE, BNT, PALPA, GORT, TROG, PPVT, PPTT)
   b. Speech: ABA, Motor speech examination
   c. Cognition: MMSE

C. Speech Fluency Assessment
   a. Reading: single words, short sentences, paragraph
   b. Spontaneous speech: monologue, conversation (minimum 200 syllables)
   c. More automatized speech (counting, days, months, singing)
   d. Fluency-enhancing techniques (slowed speech, delayed auditory feedback)
   e. Speech situation checklist
   f. Stuttering severity (SSI)

D. Self-Assessment of Attitudes (S-24, LCB)

BDAE, Boston Diagnostic Aphasia Examination (Goodglass, Kaplan, & Barresi, 2001); *BNT,* Boston Naming Test (Goodglass, et al., 2001); *GORT,* Gray Oral Reading Test (Wiederholt & Bryant, 1992); *LCB,* Locus of Control for Behavior (Craig, Franklin, & Andrews, 1984); *MMSE,* Mini-Mental State Examination (Folstein, Folstein, & McHugh, 1975); *PALPA,* Psycholinguistic Assessments of Language Processing in Aphasia (Kay, Lesser, & Coltheart, 1992); *PPTT,* Pyramids and Palm Trees Test (Howard & Patterson, 1992); *PPVT-III,* Peabody Picture Vocabulary Test (Dunn & Dunn, 1997); S-24 (Andrews & Cutler, 1974); *SSI,* Stuttering Severity Instrument (Riley, 1994); *TROG,* Test for Reception of Grammar (Bishop, 1989).

obtained as part of the clinical assessment as outlined in this table allows us to make better informed clinical decisions regarding the need of further intervention, and the nature of such intervention. As such it can be considered to be an important component of evidence-based practice. In the next section we describe elements that we believe are essential components of a fluency assessment of individuals known or suspected to exhibit neurogenic stuttering.

Detailed Case History

A detailed medical and developmental case history, as well as medical imaging information, if available, relevant to the disease or trauma condition of the patient, is an essential component of the assessment of neurogenic stuttering. Special attention should be given to the time since onset of the neurological problem, probing the possible presence of developmental stuttering as well as other speech and language problems, and associated coping behaviors, prior to the onset of the disease or brain trauma. Often, patients or their relatives may not recognize the premorbid presence of disfluencies such as stuttering, especially if the current neurogenic stuttering is rather severe. Several textbooks on developmental stuttering include detailed case history forms that may be useful in this respect (Conture, 2001; Guitar, 1998). In addition, disease-specific case information should be included as well.

Speech Fluency Analysis

Such analysis should include more than an overall subjective estimate of frequency and severity of speech disfluencies. It is necessary to differentiate between disfluencies that occur in normal speech and those associated with stuttering (Conture, 2001; Guitar, 1998; Yaruss, 1998) because an overall higher frequency of typical disfluencies in the presence of infrequent stuttering disfluencies may nevertheless give the impression of stuttering in these patients (De Nil, Sasisekaran, Van Leishout, & Sandor, 2005). Also, whereas the overall frequency of disfluencies may stay relatively constant in a patient, the proportion of stuttering to normal disfluencies may change significantly across speech tasks differing in complexity (Jokel & De Nil, 2003; Jokel et al., in press).

The frequency and type of disfluencies should be determined in a variety of reading and spontaneous speech conditions, including monologue and conversation. Speech material should include simple (e.g., single words) and more complex utterances (e.g., sentences and continuous text). Such material is readily available to clinicians or can be found in several widely available neurogenic language tests (e.g., Goodglass, Kaplan, & Barresi, 2001). If possible, depending on the language abilities of the patient, speech samples should be sufficiently long (at least 200 syllables) to provide a representative sample of current speech (dis)fluency and to provide an overall impression of the variability in stuttering across word and phrase loci and grammatical structures. Propositional speech (e.g., story telling or conversation) should be compared with more automatic speech (e.g., counting or naming the days of the week) because persons with neurogenic stuttering are much more likely than people with developmental stuttering to experience significant disfluencies in the latter speech tasks (Helm-Estabrooks, 1993; Helm-Estabrooks at al., 1986). For the same reason, the influence of fluency enhancing techniques on the frequency and severity of disfluencies should be evaluated. This may include delayed auditory feedback (DAF) or masking, choral speech, paced or rhythmic speech, and slow speech. Often, but not always, people with neurogenic stuttering will not significantly improve their speech fluency (indeed, some may even show increased disfluency), under these conditions.

◆ Assessment of Other Speech, Language, Cognitive, or Sensorimotor Abilities

If possible, we would use questionnaires to assess speech-related attitudes and perceptions, such as the S-24 (Andrews & Cutler, 1974) and the Locus of Control for Behavior (Craig, Franklin, & Andrews, 1984). In addition, we routinely administer the Mini-Mental State Examination (Folstein, Folstein, & McHugh 1975) as a screening tool for overall cognitive functioning. As we have discussed above, persons with neurogenic stuttering often show concomitant speech and/or language deficiencies. It also is important, therefore, to test for such other deficiencies that may affect or aggravate the presence of disfluencies, or may be mistaken for stuttering disfluencies. They include aphasia, word-finding problems, oral or verbal apraxia, acquired dyslexias, memory problems, and general sensorimotor problems. Which specific tests should be administered clearly will depend on the nature of the underlying neurological disorder, as well as the presenting symptoms.

◆ Treatment

Not all patients with neurogenic stuttering require treatment. For some, the stuttering disfluencies are of a transient nature and slowly improve over the course of a few weeks or months (Helm et al., 1980). For other patients, the disorder may be more persistent. Published reports of (un)successful treatment of neurogenic stuttering include a variety of intervention approaches, including the use of fluency therapy typically used with developmental stuttering, externally supported fluency using DAF or pacing, medication, and surgery, among others. At present, there does not seem to exist a preferred intervention approach that is consistently effective for all or even a subgroup of persons with neurogenic stuttering.

Behavioral Fluency Treatment

For many clinicians, the use of intervention techniques typically used for developmental stuttering often is the first approach. Meghji (1994) reported on the successful use of speech therapy techniques on a 27-year-old woman who experienced adult-onset stuttering following administration of an antidepressant drug. Although the nature of the speech techniques was not described, the patient was reported to speak slowly and fluently after 4 treatment sessions. Nowack and Stone (1987) reported on the use of fluency techniques with two patients, including nonrepetitive release of voiceless airflow aimed at producing fluent but slurred speech, and relaxation. Both patients were reported to show improved fluency. Because both also were undergoing adjustments to their anticonvulsant medication at the time of treatment, it is difficult to determine whether it was the behavioral or the pharmacological treatment, or both simultaneously, that resulted in increased speech fluency. Mowrer and Younts (2001) reported on the use of continuous phonation and vowel prolongation in a 36-year-old male patient with multiple sclerosis. Significant and lasting improvement in the frequency of repetitions was observed after only 2 sessions, at which time the focus of therapy shifted toward omissions, morphological errors, and prosody. Because of the fast positive effect of treatment on the repetitions, the authors questioned whether these may have had a compensatory role in the patient's speech, but they reported that they had ruled out a psychogenic origin of the person's speech disfluencies. Therapy in this patient was discontinued after 27 weekly sessions. Rubow, Rosenbek, and Schumacher (1986) described the use of stress management in a disfluent stroke patient, consisting of breathing exercises, progressive relaxation, and cognitive reframing. Speaking tasks were gradually increased in complexity. After 60 sessions of treatment, the patient showed decreased muscle activity in response to stress and improved fluency on single words and during conversation.

Delayed Auditory Feedback

Several published reports have documented the use of DAF in neurogenic stuttering. Marshall and Neuburger (1987) described treatment outcomes for three head-injured patients. Each patient underwent 1 hour of DAF treatment two or three times per week. All three subjects showed reduction in stuttering behaviors on the tasks used in treatment, but there was no generalization to new tasks, or to speaking situations outside the clinic. Upon discontinuation of DAF, one patient was able to maintain a high level of fluency but the other two returned to their pretreatment disfluency level within 6 months after termination of treatment. Downie, Low, and Lindsey (1981) used DAF in a patient with Parkinson's disease, who benefited from using the instrument for about a year. Adaptation to the delayed feedback gradually occurred and the beneficial effect was lost.

Drug Treatment

The use of therapeutic drugs for the treatment of neurogenic stuttering has also been reported. Perino, and colleagues (2000) described a patient with migraines whose physical symptoms and acquired stuttering were effectively and promptly eliminated following an injection of sumatriptan, a prescription pain relief drug. Because stuttering in this patient started rather suddenly 3 hours prior to the hospital visit and promptly disappeared following injection, a diagnosis of psychogenic stuttering would need to be considered. However, the authors felt that a psychogenic nature could be ruled out given the negative results from an in-depth psychological examination. Baratz and Mesulam (1981) reported the effectiveness of anticonvulsants in controlling stuttering in a patient who had developed seizures following a motor vehicle accident. The administration of paroxetine, a drug commonly used for anxiety disorders, to a patient with acquired stuttering following a stroke completely eliminated stuttering within 1 month of starting the treatment (Turgut, Utku, & Balci, 2002). Although not strictly drug related, Byrne et al. (1993) reported on an anorexic male patient who developed stuttering following a bout of severe weight loss. The stuttering slowly improved in the hospital as the patient gradually improved his diet and gained weight. They attributed the improvement in fluency to a reestablishment of a more normal body metabolism resulting in a recovery of brain tissue. Reports of the success (or lack thereof) of drug treatment for neurogenic stuttering should be compared with the effects of such treatment in persons with developmental stuttering and may help formulate specific hypotheses regarding the physiological mechanisms underlying their (lack of) ameliorating fluency effect.

Surgical Intervention

Andy and Bhatnagar (1992) described four patients with adult-onset stuttering, two of whom were treated for chronic pain and one for chronic headaches and seizures, using chronically implanted electrodes for stimulation of the left centromedian nucleus of the thalamus. Thalamic stimulation resulted in elimination of the stuttering in two patients and significant reduction of stuttering in the other two. Improvement in fluency was maintained at the time of follow-up (between 5 and 8 years postsurgery).

◆ Conclusion

Neurogenic stuttering, although relatively rare, is increasingly a well-recognized disorder in the clinical caseload of speech-language pathologists, especially those working in hospital or medical settings. Much of the information about neurogenic stuttering, however, is still based on case studies of single patients. The question, of course, is to what extent at least some of these reported patients are representative of the population at large, or are reported because they present with an atypical clinical picture. Nevertheless, the number of published case studies, as well as an increasing number of reports on larger groups of patients, and systematic reviews of the literature, have slowly allowed us to formulate a more comprehensive understanding of the disorder. What emerges is a fluency disorder with some common characteristics but in which inter-individual differences may well outweigh these commonalities. This may come as no surprise based on the literature review contained within this chapter. Indeed, the characteristics of neurogenic stuttering often seem to be determined to a greater or lesser extent by the characteristics of the underlying neurological disorder and associated communication, cognitive, motor, and other deficits. As a consequence, assessment as well as treatment of fluency disorders for these clients needs to be individually tailored and often consists of well-informed trial and error to find an assessment/intervention approach that works with a particular client. Fortunately, because of the number of clinical case studies and review articles available in the literature, clinicians may be able to find one or more case reports on clients similar to their own to help them in the clinical decision process.

Given the increased recognition of acquired stuttering, and especially neurogenic stuttering, as a distinct fluency disorder, one hopes that the coming years will see the initiation and publication of well-designed and prospective studies with larger sample size, as illustrated by Ludlow et al. (1987). Such studies are needed not only to provide better guidance to those working in the clinical field, but also to provide theoretical as well as informational insights for researchers investigating developmental stuttering and other communication disorders, especially from a neurological perspective.

Acknowledgments   The preparation of this article was supported in part by grants to the first author from the Natural Sciences and Engineering Research Council of Canada and the Canadian Institutes of Health. We would like to thank Drs. Edward Conture and Richard Curlee (the editors) for their helpful comments on an earlier version of the manuscript, and Sophie Lafaille for her assistance in the preparation of the many drafts of this manuscript.

References

Abe, K., Yokoyama, R., & Yorifuji, S. (1993). Repetitive speech disorder resulting from infarcts in the paramedian thalami and midbrain. Journal of Neurology, Neurosurgery and Psychiatry 56, 1024–1026.

Alm, P. A. (2004). Stuttering and the basal ganglia circuits: a critical review of possible relations. Journal of Communication Disorders 37, 325–369.

Anderson, J. D., Pellowski, M. W., Conture, E. G., & Kelly, E. M. (2003). Temperamental characteristics of young children who stutter. Journal of Speech, Language, and Hearing Research 46, 1221–1233.

Andrews, G., & Cutler, J. (1974). Stuttering therapy: The relation between changes in symptom level and attitudes. Journal of Speech and Hearing Disorders 39, 312–319.

Andy, O. J., & Bhatnagar, S. C. (1992). Stuttering acquired from subcortical pathologies and its alleviation from thalamic perturbation. Brain and Language 42, 385–401.

Aram, D. M., Meyers, S. C., & Ekelman, B. L. (1990). Fluency of conversational speech in children with unilateral brain lesions. Brain and Language 38, 105–121.

Ardila, A., & Lopez, M. V. (1986). Severe stuttering associated with right hemisphere lesion. Brain and Language 27, 239–246.

Balasubramanian, V., Max, L., Van Borsel, J., Rayca, K. O., & Richardson, D. (2003). Acquired stuttering following right frontal and bilateral pontine lesion: A case study. Brain and Cognition 53, 185–189.

Baratz, R., & Mesulam, M. M. (1981). Adult-onset stuttering treated with anticonvulsants. Archives of Neurology 38, 132.

Baumgartner, J. & Duffy, J. R., (1997). Psychogenic stuttering in adults with and without neurologic disease. Journal of Medical Speech-Language Pathology 5, 75–95.

Bijleveld, H., Lebrun, Y., & Dongen, H. V. (1994). A case of acquired stuttering. Folia Phoniatrica Logopedica 46, 250–253.

Bishop, D. V. M. (1989). Test for reception of grammar (2nd ed.). London: Harcourt.

Bloodstein, O. (1995). A handbook on stuttering (4 ed.). Chicago: National Easter Seal Society.

Brown, S., Ingham, R. J., Ingham, J. C., Laird, A. R., & Fox, P. T. (2005). Stuttered and fluent speech production: An ALE meta-analysis of functional neuroimaging studies. Human Brain Mapping 25, 105–117.

Byrne, A., Byrne, M., & Zibin, T. (1993). Transient neurogenic stuttering. International Journal of Eating Disorders 14, 511–514.

Callis-Landrum, L., DiDanato, R., Rosenfield, D. B., & Viswanath, N. S. (1990, November). Acquired versus developmental stuttering: differences in speech characteristics. Presented at the American Speech and Hearing Association Convention, Seattle, WA.

Camarata, S. M. (1989). Final consonant repetition: A linguistic perspective, Journal of Speech and Hearing Disorders 54, 159–162.

Canter, G. J. (1971). Observations on neurogenic stuttering: A contribution to differential diagnosis. British Journal of Disorders of Communication 6, 139–143.

Christman, S. S., Boutsen, F. R., & Buckingham, H. W. (2004). Perseveration and other repetitive verbal behaviors: Functional dissociations. Seminars in Speech and Language 25(4), 295–307.

Chung, S. J., Im, J. H., Lee, J. H., & Lee, M. C. (2004). Stuttering and gait disturbance after supplementary motor area seizure. Movement Disorders 19, 1106–1109.

Conture, E. G. (2001). Stuttering. It's nature, diagnosis and treatment. Needham Heights, MA: Allyn and Bacon.

Conture, E. G., & Kelly, E. M. (1991). Young stutterers' non-speech behaviors during stuttering. Journal of Speech and Hearing Research 34, 1041–1056.

Craig, A. R., Franklin, J., & Andrews, G. (1984). A scale to measure locus of control of behavior. British Journal of Medical Psychology 57, 173–180.

Demonet, J. F., Thierry, G., & Cardebat, D. (2005). Renewal of the neurophysiology of language: Functional neuroimaging. Physiological Reviews 85, 49–95.

De Nil, L. F. (2004). Recent developments in brain imaging research in stuttering. In B. Maassen, W. Hulstijn, R. Kent, H. F. M. Peters, & P. H. H. M. Van Lieshout (Eds.), Speech motor control in normal and disordered speech. Proceedings of the Fourth International Speech Motor Conference (pp. 150–155). Nijmegen: Uitgeverij Vantilt.

De Nil, L. F., & Brutten, G. J. (1990). Speech-associated attitudes: Stuttering, voice disordered, articulation disordered, and normal speaking children. Journal of Fluency Disorders 15, 127–134.

De Nil, L. F., Sasisekaran, J., Van Lieshout, P. H. H. M., & Sandor, P. (2005). Speech disfluencies in individuals with Tourette's syndrome. Journal of Psychosomatic Research 58, 97–102.

Downie, A. W., Low, J. M., & Lindsay, D. D. (1981). Speech disorder in parkinsonism - usefulness of delayed auditory feedback in selected cases. British Journal of Disorders of Communication 16(2), 135–139.

Dunn, L. M., & Dunn, L. M. (1997). Peabody picture vocabulary test. (3rd ed.). Circle Pines, MN: American Guidance Service.

Dworkin, J. P., Culatta R. A., Abkarian, G. G., & Meleca, R. J. (2002). Laryngeal anesthetization for the treatment of acquired disfluency: A case study. Journal of Fluency Disorders 27, 215–226.

Fleet, W. S., & Heilman, K. M. (1985). Acquired stuttering from a right hemisphere lesion in a right- hander. Neurology 35, 1343–1346.

Folstein, M. F., Folstein, S. E., & McHugh, P. R. (1975). Mini-Mental State: A practical method for grading the state of patients for the clinician. Journal of Psychiatric Research 12, 189–198.

Foundas, A. L., Bollich, A. M., Corey, D. M., Hurley, M., & Heilman, K. M. (2001). Anomalous anatomy of speech-language areas in adults with persistent developmental stuttering. Neurology 57, 207–215.

Foundas, A. L., Corey, D. M., Angeles, V., Bollich, A. M., Crabtree-Hartman, E., & Heilman, K. M. (2003). Atypical cerebral laterality in adults with persistent developmental stuttering. Neurology 61, 1378–1385.

Ghika-Schmid, F., van Melle, G., Guex, P., & Bogousslavsky, J. (1999). Subjective experience and behavior in acute stroke: The Lausanne Emotion in Acute Stroke Study. Neurology 52, 22–28.

Goodglass, H., Kaplan, E., & Barresi, B. (2001). Boston diagnostic Aphasia examination. Baltimore: Lippincott, Williams & Wilkins.

Grant, A. C., Biousse, V., Cook, A. A., & Newman, N. J. Stroke-associated stuttering. Archives of Neurology 56, 624–627.

Guitar, B. E. (1998). Stuttering. An integrated approach to its nature and treatment. Baltimore: Williams & Wilkins.

Helm, N. A., Butler, R. B., & Canter, G. J. (1980). Neurogenic acquired stuttering. Journal of Fluency Disorders 5, 269–279.

Helm-Estabrooks, N. (1986). Diagnosis and management of neurogenic stuttering in adults. In The atypical stutterer (pp. 193–217). San Diego, CA: Academic Press, Inc.

Helm-Estabrooks, N. (1993). Stuttering associated with acquired neurological disorders. In R. F. Curlee (Ed.), Stuttering and related disorders of fluency (pp. 205–218). New York: Thieme.

Helm-Estabrooks, N., Yeo, R., Geschwind, N., & Freedman, M.(1986). Stuttering: Disappearance and reappearance with acquired brain lesions. Neurology 36, 1109–1112.

Hertrich, I., Ackermann, H., Ziegler, W., & Kaschel, R. (1993). Speech iterations in Parkinsonism: A case study. Aphasiology 7, 395–406.

Howard, D. & Patterson, K. E. (1992). The pyramids and palms test. Bury St. Edwards, UK: Themes Valley Test Company.

Ingham, R. J., Fox, P. T., Ingham, J. C., Xiong, J., Zamarripa, F., Hardies, L., et al. (2004). Brain correlates of stuttering and syllable production: Gender comparison and replication. Journal of Speech, Language, and Hearing Research 47, 321–341.

Jokel, R., & De Nil, L. F. (2003). A comprehensive study of acquired stuttering in adults. In K. L. Baker & D. T. Rowley (Eds.), Proceedings of the Sixth Oxford Dysfluency Conference (pp. 59–64). Oxford, UK: Kevin Baker.

Jokel, R., De Nil, L. F., & Sharpe, A. K. (2006) A comparison of speech disfluencies in adults with acquired stuttering associated with stroke and traumatic brain injury. Journal of Medical Speech-Language Pathology (in press).

Kay, J., Lesser, R., & Coltheart, M. (1992). PALPA: Psycholinguistic assessments of language processing in aphasia. Hove, UK: Lawrence Erlbaum Associates Ltd.

Kuhar, M. J. (1986). Neuroanatomical substrates of anxiety: a brief survey. Trends in Neuroscience, 9, 311–313.

Kussmaul, A. (1877). Ueber das sogenannte aphatische stottern als symptom verschiedenortlich localisirter cerebraler herdaffectionen. Arch Psychiatr Nervenkr 32, 447–469.

Lebrun, Y., Bijleveld, H., & Rousseau, J. J. (1990). A case of persistent neurogenic stuttering following a missile wound. Journal of Fluency Disorders 15, 251–258.

Lebrun, Y., & Leleux, C. (1985) Acquired stuttering following right brain damage in dextrals. Journal of Fluency Disorders 10, 137–141.

Lebrun, Y., Retif, J., & Kaiser, G. (1983). Acquired stuttering as a forerunner of motor-neuron disease. Journal of Fluency Disorders 8, 161–167.

Lebrun, Y., & Van Borsel, J. (1990). Final sound repetitions. Journal of Fluency Disorders 15, 107–113.

Leder, S. B. (1996). Adult onset of stuttering as a presenting sign in a parkinsonian-like syndrome: A case report. Journal of Communication Disorders 29, 471–478.

Lewis, K. E., & Golberg, L. L. (1997). Measurements of temperament in the identification of children who stutter. European Journal of Disorders of Communication 32, 441–448.

Louis, E. D., Winfield, L., Fahn, S., & Ford, B. (2001). Speech dysfluency exacerbated by levodopa in Parkinson's disease. Movement Disorders 16, 562–565.

Ludlow, C. L., Rosenberg, J., Salazar, A., Grafman, J., & Smutok, M. (1987). Site of penetrating brain lesions causing chronic acquired stuttering. Annals of Neurology 22, 60–66.

Mahr, G., & Leith, W. (1992). Psychogenic stuttering of adult onset. Journal of Speech and Hearing Research 35, 283–286.

Market, K. E., Montague, J. C., Buffalo, M. D., & Drummond, S. S. (1990). Acquired stuttering: Descriptive data and treatment outcome. Journal of Fluency Disorders 15, 21–33.

Marshall, R. C., & Neuburger, S. I. (1987). Effects of delayed auditory feedback on acquired stuttering following head injury. Journal of Fluency Disorders 12, 355–365.

Mazzucchi, A., Moretti, G., Carpeggiani, P., Parma, M., & Paini, P. (1981). Clinical observations on acquired stuttering. British Journal of Disorders of Communication 16, 19–30.

McAllister, J., & Kingston, M. (2005). Final part-word repetitions in school-age children: Two case studies. Journal of Fluency Disorders 30(3), 255–267.

McClean, MD., & McLean, A. (1985). Case report of stuttering acquired in association with phenytoin use for post-head-injury seizures. Journal of Fluency Disorders 10, 241–255.

Meghji, C. (1994). Acquired stuttering. Journal of Family Practice 39, 325–326.

Mowrer, D. E., & Younts, J. (2001). Sudden onset of excessive repetitions in the speech of a patient with multiple sclerosis - A case report. Journal of Fluency Disorders 26, 269–309.

Nass, R., Schreter, B., & Heier, L. (1994). Acquired stuttering after a 2nd stroke in a 2-year-old. Devopmental Medicine and Child Neurology 36, 73–78.

Nowack, W. J., & Stone, R. E. (1987). Acquired stuttering and bilateral cerebral disease. Journal of Fluency Disorders 12, 141–146.

Perino, M., Famularo, G., & Tarroni, P. (2000). Acquired transient stuttering during a migraine attack. Headache 40, 170–172.

Pick, A. (1899). Ueber das sogenannte aphatische stottern als symptom verschiedenortlich localisirter cerebraler herdaffectionen. Arch Psychiatr Nervenkr 32, 447–469.

Pimental, P. A., & Gorelick, P. B. (1985). Aphasia, apraxia and neurogenic stuttering as complications of metrizamide myelography: Speech deficits following myelography. Acta Neurologica Scandinavica 72, 481–488.

Rentschler, G. J., Driver, L. E., & Callaway, E. A.(1984). The onset of stuttering following drug overdose. Journal of Fluency Disorders 9, 265–284.

Riley, G. D. (1994). Stuttering severity instrument for children and adults (3rd ed.). Austin, TX: PRO-ED.

Ringo, C., & Dietrich, S. (1995). Neurogenic stuttering: an analysis and critique. Journal of Medical Speech-Language Pathology 3, 111–122.

Rosenbek, J., Messert, B., Collins, M., & Wertz, R. T. (1978). Stuttering following brain damage. Brain and Language 6, 82–96.

Rubow, R. T., Rosenbek, J. C., & Schumacher, J. G. (1986). Stress management in the treatment of neurogenic stuttering. Biofeedback and Self-Regulation 11, 77–78.

Sommer, M., Koch, M. A., Paulus, W., Weiller, C., & Buchel, C. (2002). Disconnection of speech-relevant brain areas in persistent developmental stuttering. Lancet 360, 380–383.

Stewart, T., & Grantham, C. (1993). A case of acquired stammering: the pattern of recovery. European Journal of Disorders of Communication 28, 395–403.

Stewart, T., & Rowley, D. (1996). Acquired stammering in Great Britain. European Journal of Disorders of Communication 31, 1–9.

Turgut, N., Utku, U., & Balci, K. (2002). A case of acquired stuttering resulting from left parietal infarction. Acta Neurologica Scandinavica 105, 408–410.

Van Borsel, J. (1997). Neurogenic stuttering: A review. Journal of Clinical Speech and Language Studies 7, 17–33.

Van Borsel, J., & Taillieu, C. (2000). Neurogenic stuttering versus developmental stuttering: An observer's judgement study. Journal of Fluency Disorders 25, 242.

Van Borsel, J., Van Der Made, S., & Santens, P. (2003). Thalamic stuttering: A distinct clinical entity? Brain and Language 85, 185–189.

Van Borsel, J., Van Lierde, K., Cauwenberge, P., Guldermont, I., & Van Orshoven, M. (1998). Severe acquired stuttering following injury of the left supplementary motor region: A case report. Journal of Fluency Disorders 23, 49–58.

Vanryckeghem, M., Hylebos, C., Brutten, G. J., & Peleman, M. (2001). The relationship between communication attitude and emotion of children who stutter. Journal of Fluency Disorders 26, 1–15.

Wiederholt, J. L., & Bryant, B. (1992). Gray oral reading test. Austin, TX: PROED.

Yaruss, J. S. (1998). Describing the consequences of disorders: Stuttering and the International Classification of Impairments, Disabilities, and Handicaps. Journal of Speech, Language, and Hearing Research 41, 249–257.

18

Self-Control and the Treatment of Stuttering

Patrick Finn

The purpose of this chapter is to discuss the importance of self-regulation to the management of stuttering and provide an overview of strategies based on self-control or self-management procedures that are available for clinicians to employ in the behavioral management of stuttering. The chapter will begin with a discussion of why self-control should be of interest to clinicians, and why it is relevant as a clinical management approach. Basic concepts and definitions of terms in this area are presented. Subsequently, the remainder of this chapter will provide an overview of self-control techniques and conclude with descriptions of how these techniques might be incorporated into treatment. Upon completing this chapter readers will hopefully come to appreciate the value of self-control techniques in the treatment of stuttering, understand how these techniques can be implemented inside and outside the clinic, and learn how to evaluate the success of employing these techniques. A glossary of the terms related to self-control that will be used throughout this chapter is included in **Appendix 18–1.**

◆ Why is Self-Control of Interest to Clinicians Treating Stuttering?

As a concept, self-control or self-regulation broadly refers to any effort by individuals to modify their behavior, thoughts, or feelings to achieve a selected goal or standard (Voh & Baumeister, 2004). This concept is believed to have played a long-standing and essential role in the management of persistent stuttering. Prins (1997), who has probably been the most forceful proponent of this view, has argued that self-regulation undergirds the two best-known approaches to managing persistent stuttering. The stutter modification approach, for example, is based on the premise that clients must learn to self-regulate their reactions to stuttering such as minimizing or eliminating avoidance and struggle behavior (Van Riper, 1973), whereas the speech modification approach is based on the view that replacement of stuttered with stutter-free speech depends on how well clients can learn to self-manage their speech behavior (Goldiamond, 1968).

Self-control also appears as a relevant theme in accounts from individuals whose persistent stuttering has been successfully managed. For example, individuals who had undergone stuttering treatment commented that self-responsibility and self-management were among the factors they believed were important in making the transition from unsuccessful to successful management of their stuttering (Plexico, Manning, & DiLollo, 2005). Similar themes have also been reported by individuals who recovered from stuttering without the benefit of professional help (Finn, 1998). For example, Finn (2004) reported that people with stuttering that improved during their adolescent years or later believed that the reasons for their untreated recovery were based on self-managed changes in their speech behavior, as well as changes in their views about themselves and their stuttering. Futhermore, the validity of these individual accounts has been buttressed by a recent systematic review of stuttering treatment research that strongly suggested that self-management may be the most critical element in the design of treatment for adults who stutter (Bothe, Davidow, Bramlett & Ingham, 2006).

Self-control also appears to be a relevant variable in preventing relapse and promoting long-term behavior changes. For example, based on an examination of variables that contributed to relapse from stuttering treatment, Craig (1998) argued that self-control strategies are more likely to prevent relapse and lead to improved, long-term outcomes. Similarly, Kirschenbaum and Tomarken (1982), in their examination of treatment failures across a variety of behavior problems, concluded that self-monitoring and coping skills were essential to long-term success. Furthermore, Kirschenbaum (1987) reported that self-regulation also appears to be an important factor in accounting for long-term success among nonclinical endeavors, such as college-level athletics and other sports. In sum, self-regulation seems to be an essential component for meeting and maintaining highly desired goals, treatment or otherwise, across a wide spectrum of human behavior.

♦ Self-Control as a Clinical Management Technique for Stuttering

From a clinical perspective, self-control or self-management broadly refers to techniques that are applied to deliberately modify one's own behavior to achieve self-selected outcomes or specified treatment goals. One way to conceptualize self-control in a treatment context is to view it as a clinician-guided, self-management process, in which clinical-management and client-management can be viewed as opposite ends of a continuum rather than discrete procedures (Kazdin, 2001). The clinician initiates the treatment program, helps the client to establish new behaviors, trains the client to use self-management skills, provides feedback, and assists with problem solving. Successful self-management is achieved when clients are sufficiently independent that they require minimal, if any, clinician contact as their treated behavior change is incorporated into their everyday lives and maintained across time.

Self-management procedures are also generally consistent with an evidence-based framework, which can be broadly characterized as an empirically driven, measurement-based, client-sensitive approach for selecting and applying treatments (Sackett, Straus, Richardson, Rosenberg, & Haynes, 2001). Such a framework suggests that selected treatments should result in a clinically significant or easily recognizable treatment change that is meaningful and valued by clients and relevant others, such as parents, spouses, or employers (Finn, 2003). A meaningful change for people seeking professional help is the changing of behavior that prompted them to seek treatment in the first place (Baer, 1988). From the perspective of an evidence-based framework, this should mean it is necessary to measure the behavior that represents the client's complaint. Building on this premise, Ingham and Cordes (1997a) proposed a three-factor model of stuttering treatment outcome evaluation that is based on speech performance, speaking situations, and time, which incorporates clients' self-judged acceptability of treatment changes in combination with clinician-based measures. Thus, as couched within an evidence-based framework, self-measurement—and, consequently, a self-control perspective—serves as a basis for determining the clinical significance of treatment change from the client's view.

In view of the importance of self-regulation to the management of stuttering, the goal of this chapter is to provide an overview of strategies based on self-control or self-management procedures that are available for clinicians to employ in the behavioral management of persistent stuttering. To achieve this goal, the remainder of this chapter is divided into two major sections: (1) an overview of self-control techniques that have been employed during the behavioral management of stuttering; and (2) descriptions of how they might be incorporated into the establishment, transfer, and maintenance of treatment.

◆ Self-Control Techniques for Treatment of Stuttering

Various self-control techniques have been described in the behavior modification literature (e.g., Kazdin, 2001). The following section summarizes some of the major techniques that have been used in stuttering treatment and suggests others that may be worth considering as part of a clinical management strategy.

Self-Selected Treatment Goals

There are several reasons why self-selected treatment goals are considered an important beginning for behavior change. First, clients are more likely to be motivated to change and adhere to long-term treatment regimens when they believe they have selected goals of personal importance (Maes & Karoly, 2005). Second, a clinically meaningful outcome is more likely if a clinician directly addresses the problems that compose a client's primary complaint (Baer, 1988). Third, clinicians who work within an evidence-based approach are required to carefully consider their client's personal concerns when selecting the most appropriate, empirically supported treatment approach (Sackett et al., 2001).

Clients are likely to have a wide variety of reasons for seeking treatment for their stuttering, and the clinician's task is to help clients understand their motivation for change and to describe their treatment goals specifically enough so that these goals can be adequately operationalized for treatment purposes. Client-selected treatment goals, like any clinician-selected goal, must be specific, realistic, and clinically relevant if they are going to be reasonably obtainable. However, clients who stutter may not have an adequate understanding of the nature of their disorder and its variability that would be appropriate for achieving these kinds of goals. Moreover, clients are unlikely to have systematically observed their own stuttering; therefore, they may not have sufficient self-knowledge for developing goals that can be operationalized for treatment purposes.

Maintaining a structured diary is one approach that might help clients systematically observe their stuttering and its variability, and obtain information appropriate for developing self-selected treatment goals (Watson & Tharp, 2007). Structured diaries are written records of clients' daily observations of their thoughts, behaviors, and feelings related to stuttering. Clients are instructed to record and organize their observations in terms of their antecedents (A), behaviors (B), and consequences (C) (**Fig. 18–1**).

Antecedents	Behavior	Consequences
A	B	C
9:30 AM: Introduce self at work meeting, felt physical tightening in throat and chest	Blocked when trying to say my name	Embarrassed, felt red-faced, colleague briefly looked away
1:00 PM: Lunch with friend	Didn't stutter once!	Feeling good!
3:00 PM: Ordering coffee at deli	Stuttered several times	Too tired to care, clerk didn't seem to notice.

Figure 18–1 An example of entries in a structured diary in which client records antecedents (A), behavior (B), and consequences (C).

Antecedents refer to settings' events that cue or stimulate behavior and can include environmental situations, physical events, thoughts, or feelings. For example, for many people who stutter, antecedents that trigger stuttering often consist of situations perceived to have communicative pressure, such as speaking to authority figures or talking on the phone. The behaviors that are triggered by antecedents will usually consist of some physical or motoric event such as stuttered speech, but they could also consist of cognitive or affective events, such as negative communication attitudes or anxiety related to speaking. Consequences are what happen *after* these behaviors, which for clients who stutter are likely to include negative feelings or thoughts that occur as a result of stuttering, like embarrassment, or certain physical behaviors such as leaving the speaking situation, or it could also include listeners' negative reactions to stuttering, such as teasing.

Recorded observations in a structured diary, especially over several days to a week, can serve as a basis for clients in collaboration with their clinicians to determine if there are patterns in their stuttering or reactions to stuttering. Based on these systematic self-observations, clients are better able to collaborate with their clinician in developing specific treatment goals. These goals can then be operationalized and defined in terms that make it clear how to measure them. Thus, the structured diary helps to develop self-selected goals that, in turn, can be used to develop measurement procedures for monitoring clients' treatment progress and outcome.

Self-Measurement

Definition and Considerations

Self-measurement—also known as self-monitoring or self-observation—refers to when clients systematically observe and record aspects of their own behavior, usually in an ongoing fashion across time (Cone, 1999). Self-measurement is considered a direct measure of behavior that can be tailored to the goals and problems of individual clients that presents two important advantages over other clinic-related measures. First, the measure is likely a more accurate representation of the behavior of clinical interest, because it can be obtained when the behavior actually occurs. In contrast, other client-based sources of information, such as clinic interviews or self-report questionnaires, are indirect measures because they rely on clients' recollections of behavior that occurred at a different time and place than when the information is obtained and are often less practical to administer continuously throughout treatment (Korotitsch & Nelson-Gray, 1999). Such retrospective measures are likely to be less accurate because people's memories are often biased representations of real events (Gilovich, 1991). Thus, self-report measures are likely to be limited representations of what actually occurs in a client's everyday life, which can be problematic with a variable disorder like stuttering.

A second advantage of self-measurement is that it can be obtained in the situations where stuttering behavior takes place. This is important because the most salient aspects of this behavior for clients are much more likely to occur in speaking situations outside the clinic that clinicians cannot readily observe and in which clients cannot always obtain a permanent record (e.g., audio- or video recording).

The main purposes of self-measurement in a clinical context are to describe clients' behavior, to evaluate treatment progress and outcome, and to serve as a therapeutic intervention (Foster, Laverty-Finch, Gizzo, & Osantowski, 1999). It can be used to record speech-related behaviors, thoughts, or feelings and the circumstances surrounding that behavior in the client's environment at any time of day. The structured diary is one example mentioned earlier that could be used by the client to help him or her describe stuttering behavior in its everyday context. But, this particular approach is recommended only for helping clients develop self-selected target behaviors because it is not practical as an ongoing measurement procedure, and only the most dedicated clients are likely to employ it for any extended period of time. Therefore, several practical issues need to be considered when clinically using self-measurement procedures.

First, clients are more likely to utilize self-measurements if they do not feel overburdened with self-monitoring too many behaviors, situations, or time periods. Second, the self-measurement procedure should be appropriate for the client's skill level, relatively easy to use, and nonobtrusive. Third, clinicians should not assume that clients know how to observe and record their own behavior. Therefore, the training methods for self-measurement should include: (1) a clearly defined target behavior; (2) explicit self-measurement instructions; (3) checking clients' understanding of definitions and instructions; (4) modeling and practicing the self-measurement procedure; and (5) periodic checks by clinicians to insure the continued accuracy of clients' self-measurements across time (Foster et al., 1999; Ingham & Cordes, 1997a).

Examples of Self-Measurement

Self-judgment of stuttering is instructive as an example of a self-measurement procedure, because it illustrates many of the above-mentioned points. First, it is a metric of stuttering that can be obtained in everyday speaking situations that provides a basis for evaluating treatment progress (e.g., Ingham et al., 2001) and facilitates the generalization of treatment gains (Ingham, 1982). Second, it is practical and easy to observe especially if the intervals of self-observation are relatively short (e.g., 1- to 3-minute intervals), the number of monitored speaking situations are manageable (e.g., three different weekly speaking situations), and speech samples can be audio-recorded without being obtrusive (e.g., telephone conversations). Third, it should not be assumed that people who stutter are accurate judges of their own stuttering. Problems with accuracy are well-documented by the disagreements found between self-judgments and listener-judgments of stuttering (e.g., Ingham & Cordes, 1997b). These differences can probably be resolved in the clinic, when the clinician and client rate the same speech samples and compare their results as a basis for developing an agreed-on definition of stuttering. However, if the basis for disagreement is related to a client's experience of stuttering as a loss of control, resolving this issue may be more challenging, because loss of control is a private event that is inaccessible to the listener. Nonetheless, if treatment reduces or eliminates a client's self-judged experience of loss of control during stuttering, then speaker-listener disagreements in this case may be a minor clinical concern (Ingham & Cordes, 1997a).

Self-judgments of stuttering may also be adopted as a treatment procedure. La Croix (1973), for example, reported that when self-counts of stuttering while speaking were employed as clinical procedures with two school-age males who stuttered, the frequency of their stuttering was dramatically reduced in the clinic and was reported to be reduced beyond clinic, as well. These ameliorative effects may be related to the highlighting or punishing effect that clients may experience with increased self-knowledge or awareness of their moments of stuttering (Siegel, 1970). It should be noted, however, that the therapeutic effects of self-judgments of stuttering may be transient and unpredictable, especially under laboratory conditions (Goldiamond, 1968; Ingham, Adams, & Reynolds, 1978; James, 1981a). Although this may limit its usefulness as a treatment technique, its utility as a measurement procedure for helping clients self-evaluate treatment benefits is not affected.

Self-rating of stuttering severity is another practical, convenient, and clinically relevant measure for evaluating treatment progress and outcome. Severity is a multidimensional concept that incorporates judgments of stuttering frequency, the duration of stutters, and the effort or struggle behavior associated with stuttering. Clinically, severity is often labeled using *categorical* terms, such as mild, moderate, or severe, but these terms are limited in their ability to describe stuttering variability across speaking situations and time. Perceptual rating scales are a flexible and clinically practical alternative because they involve measuring *degrees* of severity. For example, O'Brian, Packman, Onslow, and O'Brian (2004) recently described a 9-point stuttering severity scale, in which 1 represented *no stuttering*, 2 represented *mild stuttering*, and 9 represented *extremely severe stuttering*, that clinicians can use reliably and that correlates strongly with measures of stuttering frequency. Clients are also able to use it reliably to self-rate the severity of their stuttering in everyday speaking situations and produce severity ratings that are within reasonable levels of agreement with listener-based judgments of the same samples (O'Brian, Packman, & Onslow, 2004). Furthermore, the clinical utility of this rating scale has been demonstrated in treatment studies that employed this measure for conducting clinician and client evaluations of treatment progress and outcome (Hewat, O'Brian, Onslow, & Packman, 2001; O'Brian, Onslow, Cream, & Packman, 2003).[1]

Self-measurement procedures have been used clinically to evaluate characteristics of speech behaviors other than stuttering that are relevant to treatment progress and outcome. Speech naturalness, one of the most thoroughly researched scales, refers to a qualitative characteristic that appears to be related to how much treated speech sounds effortless and free from artificiality or constraint (Schiavetti & Metz, 1997). The clinical relevance of this variable was identified when researchers found that many stuttering treatment approaches characterized as "successful" often resulted in speech that was perceived as different from normal (Runyan & Adams, 1978, 1979). Subsequent research revealed that listeners were able to reliably distinguish between treated, stutter-free speech and normally fluent speech based on speech naturalness (Ingham, Gow, & Costello, 1985), using a 9-point rating scale in which 1 represented *highly natural sounding* and 9 represented *highly unnatural sounding* (Martin, Haroldson, & Triden, 1984). The clinical utility of this 9-point rating scale was demonstrated when it was shown that listener feedback based on this scale could be used to help clients self-manage their stutter-free speech so that it sounded more natural (Ingham, Martin, Haroldson, Onslow, & Leney, 1985; Ingham, Sato, Finn, & Belknap, 2001). People who stutter have also been highly dependable in self-rating their own speech naturalness (Finn & Ingham, 1994; Ingham, Ingham, Onslow, & Finn, 1989), and as a result, this variable or its variants have been included as a self-measurement procedure in various treatment approaches to help ensure that clients' speech is both stutter-free and natural sounding (e.g., Craig et al., 1996; Ingham et al., 2001; O'Brian et al., 2003).

Self-measurement procedures for evaluating clients' thoughts or feelings related to stuttering are rare in stuttering treatment, which is surprising because self-measurement is often the only method for directly measuring such private events (Korotitsch & Nelson-Gray, 1999). The potential barrier is that these events can only be experienced by the stutterer, but cannot be directly verified for their accuracy by an independent judge, such as the clinician. Methods that indirectly support the integrity of such self-measurement procedures, however, are possible. The convergent validity of self-measures could be evaluated by correlating measures of private events with measures of objective speech events. For example, treated stutterers sometimes complain that they attend too much to how they speak, such as focusing on fluency skills, rather than focusing on what they want to say (Cream, Onslow, Packman, & Llewellyn, 2003). Finn and Ingham (1994) attempted to operationalize this complaint by asking stutterers to self-rate how natural they felt about the amount of attention they were paying to the way they were speaking on a 9-point scale, in which 1 represented *highly natural* and 9 represented *highly unnatural*. Using this self-rating scale, it was found that stutterers' levels of cognitive effort were correlated with systematic variations in their levels of controlled fluency. Moreover, they were relatively consistent and valid judges of their levels of speech monitoring. Similar self-measurement procedures might prove useful for investigating other private events related to stuttering, such as speaking anxiety and avoidance behavior. Researchers have yet to investigate the clinical utility of such measures; nonetheless, clinicians should be encouraged to explore them with clients and report, if they can, on their viability in the literature.

In summary, self-measurement can be viewed as a foundation for many self-control procedures because it plays several critical roles. First, it provides clients with a basis for understanding their stuttering and evaluating treatment progress. Second, it is a useful tool for clients and clinicians to share quantifiable information about the client's behavior (O'Brian, Packman, & Onslow, 2004). Finally, it serves as the basis for other self-control techniques, such as those that will be discussed next.

---

[1] Steps for training clients to self-rate stuttering severity are available at http://www3.fhs.usyd.edu.au/asrcwww/downloads/ Camperdown_Tmt_Manual.pdf.

Self-Evaluation and Self-Consequation

Self-evaluation refers to clients comparing their performance with a self-selected target behavior or specified treatment standard. This plays an important role when clients are learning to self-manage their own treatment. For example, clients can be prompted during treatment to evaluate their speech performance at set intervals in terms of whether or not it was stutter-free and within a specified range for sounding natural (e.g., Ingham et al., 2001). The self-evaluation of their performance compared with these standards can determine the next step in the treatment protocol, such as moving them from establishment to the transfer phase. It should be clear that clients need the specific information that self-measurement procedures provide to adequately compare their performance against target performance and that self-measurement serves as the basis for their self-evaluation. As mentioned earlier, this means that target behaviors need to be operationalized and well specified; otherwise, self-evaluation will be impractical, if not impossible. Thus, self-measurement is a means for obtaining information about one's performance, and self-evaluation is the process of assessing or appraising that performance. These complementary procedures also serve as the foundation for self-consequation, another clinically important self-control technique.

Self-consequation refers to when clients are trained to administer consequences to themselves contingent on their achieving a specified target behavior rather than receiving consequences from a clinician (Kazdin, 2001). The advantage of training clients to administer their own consequences is that they can become their own treatment agents, and thus, can administer contingencies for behavior change beyond the clinic in everyday situations. As mentioned above, self-measurement and self-evaluation are usually required, as well, because clients will need to measure and evaluate their own behavior to determine if they have met the specific criteria necessary for consequation. Self-reinforcement and self-punishment are the two main forms of self-consequation that have been employed in stuttering treatment.

Self-reinforcement refers to clients rewarding themselves for achieving specified target behaviors (Watson & Tharp, 2007). Two different procedures can compose self-reinforcement. The first is self-determined reinforcement, which refers to clients determining for themselves the criteria for and amount of reinforcement they will receive. For this procedure, clinicians will probably need to help clients understand how to develop reinforcers and to understand that to maximize the treatment benefits of reinforcers; they must be received only if the target behavior has been met. Clients can also be instructed on the development, use, and flexibility of symbolic reinforcers, such as a point system, that can be incorporated into token systems (see Watson & Tharp, 2007). Clinician-controlled token systems have been employed during stuttering treatment with promising findings (e.g., Ingham & Andrews, 1973), but no investigations of clients' self-administered token systems have yet been reported.

The second procedure is self-administered reinforcement, which refers to clients administering rewards to themselves (Kazdin, 2001). Like any reward system, it is important that self-reinforcers are powerful enough to increase the likelihood that the rewarded behavior will be performed again in the future. Another important requirement is that clients must be free to reward themselves at any time and must not, therefore, be constrained by clinicians' pressures (Kazdin, 2001). It is unlikely, however, that such a requirement can be realistically accomplished in a treatment context (Hayes et al., 1985). Thus, it may be more practical to think of self-reinforcement as a procedure whereby a client controls the rewards, but the clinician will occasionally monitor and evaluate the client's performance to ensure the client's accuracy in achieving target behaviors. An example of this procedure, using a performance contingent maintenance schedule (see Ingham, 1980), is described in the last section of this chapter.

Shames and Florance (1986) described a unique use of self-administered reinforcement that has been integrated into several recent treatment approaches (e.g., Blood, 1995; Hillis, 1993). As part of a fluency shaping skills approach, clients are trained to engage in a 4-step process. The first step trains clients to self-instruct or signal themselves to perform monitored speech using an established, stutter-free speech pattern. The next step requires clients to self-monitor their performance in terms of target behavior criteria (e.g., extended phonation). The third step, self-evaluation, requires clients to evaluate the accuracy of their performance. The final step, self-consequation, has clients reward themselves with *unmonitored* speech, which means they speak without paying attention to the way they are speaking. Shames and Florance (1986) claimed that unmonitored speech would function as a reinforcer because it was based on the Premack principle, which states that behaviors that clients are more likely to perform can be used to reinforce behaviors they are less likely to perform. Thus—a high probability behavior—in this case, unmonitored speech, was used to reinforce a low probability behavior—monitored speech.

Self-punishment refers to clients' self-administration of an aversive stimulus contingent on the occurrence of an undesired behavior to decrease the frequency of future occurrences of that behavior (Kazdin, 2001). Generally speaking, punishment has not proven to be successful as a behavior modification approach (Watson & Tharp, 2007), but it has been quite effective in the treatment of stuttering. This has especially been the case with self-administered or self-initiated time-out (SITO) from speaking, which requires clients to stop speaking for a brief period of time, usually 1 to 3 seconds, contingent immediately whenever they stutter. It should be noted before going further, however, that even though SITO technically functions as a punisher, many clients do not perceive time-out as an aversive stimulus and have reported a variety of self-perceptions about time-out including that it helped them to relax, gave them time to think, or was an alerting signal (Adams & Popelka, 1971; James & Ingham, 1974). SITO, as a treatment strategy, has been demonstrated to have several advantages that clinicians should carefully consider. First, it is just as effective as clinician-administered time-out in reducing the frequency of stuttering (James, 1983a; Martin & Haroldson, 1982). Second, its benefits are more likely to generalize to nontreatment conditions than those from clinician-administered time-out (Martin & Haroldson, 1982). Third, the stutter-free speech resulting from time-out is relatively natural sounding (Hewat, Onslow, Packman, & O'Brian, 2006; Onslow, Packman, Stocker, van Doorn, & Siegel, 1997). In addition, several treatment outcome studies using SITO have found that its clinical benefits have been maintained 6 months or more posttreatment (Hewat et al., 2001; Hewat et al., 2005; James, 1981b).

There are also some disadvantages to SITO that should be mentioned. First, speakers often fail to self-consequate every instance of stuttering that is perceived by listeners, even though reductions in stuttering still occur (James, 1983a). Second, clients who are not as responsive to time-out may need to augment SITO with additional fluency skills (Hewat et al., 2006; James, Ricciardelli, Rogers, & Hunter, 1989).

A 5-stage treatment protocol for training SITO that clinicians might consider was outlined by Hewat and colleagues (2001)[2] and includes the following steps: (1) determining a client's responsiveness to clinician-administered time-out; (2) instructing the client on how to SITO, by pausing briefly for ~1 second after a stutter without any cues from the clinician; (3) using SITO first within, then beyond, clinic speaking situations; (4) learning to self-evaluate stuttering severity, using the 9-point severity scale described earlier; and (5) using SITO in everyday speaking environments and bringing audio recordings back to the clinic for evaluation and consultation with the clinician. Recent Phase II clinical trials have suggested that this procedure results in relatively stutter-free speech that is natural sounding (Hewat et al., 2006).

In summary, self-consequation is a flexible self-control procedure that can be integrated into the management of stuttering. Its chief advantage is that clients become their own clinicians, which has positive implications for long-term maintenance that will be discussed in more detail in the next section.

◆ Incorporating Self-Control Techniques into Stuttering Treatment

As discussed earlier, one way to conceptualize self-control in a treatment context is to view it as a clinician-guided, self-management process, in which client-management and clinician-management lie along a treatment continuum. Viewing self-management along such a continuum, however, does

---

[2] James (1983b) also presents a 5-step protocol for training a set of self-management skills for employing time-out from speacking.

not mean that clinicians should wait to introduce self-management strategies until the end of the treatment process. As already suggested, elements of self-control can be introduced even before treatment begins, such as during assessment when clients self-select their treatment goals. The following section provides an overview of how clinicians might consider incorporating self-control techniques into the establishment, transfer, and maintenance phases of treatment.

Establishment

The goal of establishment is to train clients to produce new behaviors accurately within the clinic environment. For treatments based on behavior modification, this typically consists of replacing stuttered with stutter-free, natural-sounding speech.

There are various approaches for achieving the establishment of stutter-free speech using behavior modification techniques that differ in terms of the degree to which they incorporate aspects of self-control. Examples of some of these approaches are briefly overviewed below, with an emphasis on the degree to which elements of self-control are included.

Prolonged speech and its variants are the most widely investigated and empirically supported techniques for establishing stutter-free speech (Bothe et al, 2006; Cordes, 1998). As a technique, prolonged speech relies largely on extended phonation, especially on vowel sounds, that is produced continuously, for the most part, within and between words. Additional components often include gentle onset, light articulatory contacts, and diaphragmatic breathing.

The basic approach for establishing and modifying prolonged speech has been based on a programmed instructional approach. This means that the stutter-free speech pattern typically begins with highly exaggerated, very noticeable prolongation at very slow speaking rates that is gradually shaped in a stepwise fashion to less exaggerated, barely noticeable prolongation performed at normal speaking rates. This stepwise approach, based on achieving specified criteria for each step, can be controlled by using either: (1) delayed auditory feedback that begins with long delays (e.g., 250 milliseconds) and decreases in 50 millisecond steps to no delay (0 milliseconds), (Ryan, 2001) or (2) specified speaking rates that begin very slow (40 syllables per minute [SPM])and are increased, usually in 30 syllable steps, to faster rates within a normal speaking range (e.g., 190 ± 20 SPM). Clients are sometimes provided with audiotaped models of prolonged speech at various speaking rates to guide their learning of the required behaviors (Ingham, 1987). As with many such approaches, this approach relies heavily on clinician feedback to clients concerning the accuracy of their performance, even though clients are often instructed to self-evaluate their own performance in terms of how well they are performing the target behaviors that compose prolonged speech (Boberg & Kully, 1994).

This basic approach has been modified in recent years, and in some cases dramatically changed, so that more self-control procedures have been incorporated into the establishment phase of treatment. Perhaps the most important change, in light of the unnatural sounding speech quality that often characterizes recently learned prolonged speech (Schiavetti & Metz, 1997), is the introduction of speech naturalness ratings, which are usually based on the 9-point scale described earlier (where 1 represents highly natural sounding and 9 represents highly unnatural sounding). Similar to the programmed instructional approach described above, prolonged speech is shaped in a stepwise fashion, but the criterion for each step no longer increases speaking rate but promotes more natural sounding speech (Ingham, 1987). Thus, once the prolonged speech pattern has been successfully shaped at a speaking rate of 100 ± 20 SPM, as described above, the criteria for the remaining steps are changed to decreasing speech naturalness ratings (e.g., 7 → 5 → 3) to a range that normal, nonstuttering speakers typically receive (1–3). The clinician establishes the criterion level of speech naturalness for each step, rates the client's naturalness, and provides the client with feedback. However, clients are instructed to self-regulate their prolonged speech pattern by exaggerating or minimizing its features in any way they wish, provided they maintain stutter-free speech and their target level of naturalness. Thus, when speech naturalness ratings are used as criteria, clients are clearly afforded an opportunity to self-regulate elements of their stutter-free speech. Overall, this modification to the basic, prolonged speech approach has resulted in favorable long-term treatment outcomes (e.g., Onslow, Costa, Andrews, Harrison, & Packman, 1996).

The establishment of prolonged speech ultimately depends on the client's ability to modify underlying physiological processes related to such factors as extending phonation intervals (e.g., prolonged vowels), gentle voice onsets, reducing the rate of articulatory movements (e.g., slowed speech rate), and sometimes reducing muscle tension (e.g., light articulatory contacts). This has led to another modification in the establishment phase that promotes the use of self-management skills.

Clinicians obviously do not have access to the underlying physiological processes that their clients are learning how to control. Thus, they have to rely on what they see and hear their clients do to evaluate the accuracy of their performance and provide appropriate feedback. This can be a difficult clinical task, and researchers have found that even experienced clinicians are not always able to provide accurate and reliable feedback on clients' production of these target behaviors (Onslow & O'Brian, 1998). Advances in technology, however, have helped to circumvent these issues.

Digital technology, for example, has allowed well-known self-control procedures, such as biofeedback (Schwartz & Andrasik, 2003), to become an integral part of the establishment process, especially for training prolonged speech. Biofeedback refers to clients being provided with information about their ongoing physiological processes (Kazdin, 2001). This information is displayed in real time so that clients can monitor moment-to-moment changes in these processes. Clients are instructed to modify the behaviors associated with these processes, and recent treatment studies have indicated that biofeedback procedures can be used successfully to teach clients how to control their phonatory behavior so that their speech is stutter-free and natural sounding (Ingham et al., 2001).

One example of an emerging biofeedback approach that has been tested empirically involves Modifying Phonation Intervals (MPI) (Ingham, 1999; Ingham et al., 2001). Accelerometer technology is used to provide clients with information about their phonatory behavior that, in turn, they utilize for learning a prolonged-like speech pattern. The accelerometer, which is about the size of a dime and is embedded in a neckband, detects vocal fold vibrations from the surface of the neck. The on-off durations of these vibratory patterns, or phonation intervals, are displayed in real time on a computer monitor so that clients receive ongoing feedback about this behavior while they are speaking. Clients are instructed to decrease the frequency of their short phonation intervals (i.e., intervals in the range of 20–130 milliseconds, depending on the individual client) in any way they can, while at the same time, producing stutter-free and natural sounding speech. The frequency of short phonation intervals that a client should not exceed is determined and pre-set into the computer's program by the clinician. The result is that clients learn to self-regulate a speech pattern that is akin to prolonged speech, but does not depend on highly exaggerated prolongation, and is also more natural sounding from the beginning of the establishment phase.

Clients are trained to produce this speech pattern during the establishment phase in progressively more difficult 1-to 3-minute training periods of self-generated speech, beginning with oral reading, followed by monologue, then conversation, and completed by speaking on the phone in the clinic to the clinician. Importantly, clients manage this stepwise progression by self-evaluating their speech at the end of each 1-to 3-minute training period in terms of two clinician-specified criteria: (1) the presence or absence of any stuttering; and (2) how natural sounding their speech was. To insure the accuracy of clients' self-assessments, the clinician periodically evaluates the clients' speech on the basis of the same criteria. This is especially critical when clients believe they are ready to progress to the next level of difficulty. In sum, clients learn to regulate and evaluate their own speech behavior, with the assistance of biofeedback, practically from the beginning of the establishment phase, which will be an important foundation for learning to self-manage their behavior beyond the clinic.

It should also be mentioned that there are other commercially available, computer-based biofeedback-like programs for training prolonged speech, such as Dr. Fluency™ (STS, Speech Therapy Systems, Ltd.) and the CAFET™ (Computer Technology for the Treatment of Stuttering). These programs were developed to provide clients with feedback related to variables that programmers believed were important to prolonged speech, such as gentle onset and diaphragmatic breathing, as well as reduced speaking rate. Unfortunately, the functional value of these variables and the programs' feedback procedures has not yet been adequately demonstrated. Other biofeedback procedures, indirectly related to prolonged speech, have focused on reducing levels of muscle tension in the lips and jaw, and clinical trials with school-age stutterers have been encouraging (Craig et al., 1996).

Recent developments in nonprogrammed approaches to training prolonged speech have also changed the extent to which self-control procedures are incorporated into the establishment phase. The Camperdown Program, for example, trains clients to produce stutter-free speech by presenting a video model of prolonged speech produced at 70 SPM[3] (O'Brian et al., 2003). Clients are first trained to accurately reproduce this model, and when this is achieved, they are instructed to use whatever elements of this new speech pattern they find most useful for controlling their stuttering. Clients then practice the target behavior in monologues and group conversations that include clinician feedback as needed. As a result, clients have considerable self-control over how and when they produce their treated speech behavior. It is important to add that clients are trained to self-evaluate the severity of their stuttering at the beginning of the establishment phase, using the 9-point stuttering severity scale that was described earlier. Later, during their group conversation phase, clients are also trained to self-rate their speech naturalness, using the same 9-point naturalness scale that has been mentioned throughout this chapter. Clients' progress through their different treatment phases are based on the clinician's evaluations of their speech behavior meeting the following clinician-specified criteria: (a) 1 to 2 on the stuttering severity scale; and (b) 1 to 3 on the speech naturalness scale. Initial clinical trials of the Camperdown Program have demonstrated considerable promise (O'Brian et al., 2003), but these positive findings have been marred somewhat by clients' notably high dropout rates.

In summary, self-control procedures have become increasingly integrated into the establishment phase of behavioral modifications of stuttering. It is believed that developing these self-management skills early in the treatment process may provide clients with a sense of empowerment that will help set the stage for the next treatment phase known as transfer.

Transfer

The goal of transfer is to train clients to generalize their clinic-established behavior changes to representative everyday speaking situations. This means that clinicians have to assist clients in learning to produce stutter-free, natural-sounding speech in nonclinic training situations because changes that occurred under establishment conditions will not necessarily generalize beyond those conditions.

Various strategies have been recommended for transferring behavior change during stuttering treatment (e.g., Ingham & Onslow, 1987). This chapter focuses only on strategies that emphasize the use of self-control procedures primarily because research findings have indicated that the use of such procedures is likely to facilitate generalization of treatment gains beyond the clinic (e.g., Ingham, 1982; Martin & Haroldson, 1982).

Probably one of the better-known strategies for promoting generalization is sequential modification, in which clients are trained to master target behaviors in progressively more difficult speaking situations. This procedure has a long been used in both the field of psychology (Wolpe, 1990) as well as stuttering (Brutten & Shoemaker, 1967) as an effective means to assist with transfer of behavior change. This programmed instructional approach shares elements with the establishment procedures described earlier. However, the clients rather than their clinician select and rank order the beyond-clinic situations in terms of their difficulty, which become the targets of transfer activities. Clients are likely to find that a structured diary is helpful for doing this because it provides information about the everyday situations they typically encounter, determines their level of concern with these situations, and reveals how frequently they occur. Ideally, these situations should be audio-recorded so that samples of the clients' speech are available for client- and clinician-evaluation.

---

[3]An electronic version of the video exemplar for 70 SPM is available at http://www3.fhs.usyd.edu.au/asrcwww/downloads/index.htm.

Clients can be instructed to self-manage their progress by evaluating their performance across several recordings of a specific speaking situation (e.g., speaking with work colleagues) until they have determined that they have mastered their target behaviors during at least three consecutive attempts (see Ingham, 1999). The clinician can provide guidance and feedback as necessary and corroborate clients' evaluations of their performance before proceeding to the next level of difficulty.

Another strategy for facilitating generalization is to modify the antecedents or stimuli that trigger stuttering in clients' beyond clinic speaking situations. As discussed earlier, behaviors are performed in the context of antecedents or setting events that cue or stimulate those behaviors. Clinicians can often assist in modifying such antecedents beforehand by carefully arranging in-clinic speaking activities during the establishment phase. For example, when clients learn target behaviors in a stepwise fashion, ranging from in-clinic oral readings to speaking on the phone, this sort of in-clinic progression may alter old antecedents that cued stuttering so that they become cues for target behaviors. Thus, speaking to strangers on the phone in-clinic, could be selected as the first transfer task. In addition, it allows clinicians to provide more support and guidance for clients as they make the first steps into the transfer phase. Similar modifications in antecedent control can be started during the establishment phase with in-clinic speaking activities that include face-to-face conversations of clients with strangers.

Of course, the ultimate goal of transfer is to modify the antecedent cues for stuttering that occur in clients' everyday lives. The structured diary is one way that everyday antecedents might be identified. Once clients become aware of how antecedents may be contributing to their stuttering, they can learn how to structure or modify them to maximize the likelihood that their target behaviors will occur instead. Perhaps the most challenging antecedents will consist of negative self-instructions or beliefs that some clients focus on when they are about to speak in certain situations. For example, before making a phone call, a client might tell him- or herself, "Here I go again, I just know I'm going to stutter. Why bother, I might as well hang up now!" Clients can be instructed that these kinds of self-defeating thoughts are simply increasing their expectation to stutter. However, once they have learned how to replace stuttered with stutter-free speech, they now have an alternative behavior. Thus, self-instructions can be modified so that they are positive and constructive. So, rather than clients thinking, "I can't do this!" they can think instead, "I can do this" and remind themselves how (Watson & Tharp, 2007). Clients can also count how often they engage in positive self-instructions, instead of negative self-instructions and reward themselves for making these kinds of modifications in their negative "self-talk."

A final example of a transfer strategy is training clients to mediate generalization, which involves their learning to self-manage the use of their target behaviors in everyday situations. The self-evaluation skills that were described during the establishment phase are essential here because when clients practice their target behaviors in beyond clinic settings, they need to self-evaluate their performance afterwards. For example, a college student could plan to practice his or her stutter-free, natural-sounding speech when asking the instructor a question during office hours, then self-evaluate his or her performance using the self-measurement tools described earlier and reward himself or herself accordingly afterwards. Similar to this example, Ingham (1982) demonstrated experimentally that self-evaluation training, combined with self-consequation, led to reductions in stuttering as clients' training was systematically introduced across different beyond-clinic speaking situations.

Clients can also be trained to construct X-Y line graphs for recording and displaying their self-measurement data across time and different speaking situations (Watson & Tharp, 2007). Readily available software programs, such as Microsoft Excel™ (Redmond, Washington), can be used to easily create, store, and view these graphs by both client and clinician. Visual inspection of graphic display can provide clients with a useful method for self-evaluating their patterns of change or variability over time, and it can also serve as a strong motivator. Thus, clients learn to self-evaluate their performance not only within specific situations but also across time. As many clinicians can attest, graphic displays of behavior changes across time can be informative, rewarding, and motivating. This is an experience that clients can share in as well when they mediate generalization and that may prove helpful during maintenance, the final phase of treatment.

Maintenance

The goal of maintenance is to promote durable behavior change across time in everyday speaking situations. This can be viewed as the phase during which clinician-management of behavior changes makes the complete transition to clients' self-management.

Self-evaluation and self-consequation are probably the most important self-control procedures that clients need to continue to use over time to maintain their treatment gains. These procedures have been demonstrated as highly effective when they have been included in a performance-contingent maintenance schedule (PCMS). PCMS refers to a telescoping maintenance schedule that begins after clients successfully complete the transfer phase (Ingham, 1980, 1999). The idea that guides the PCMS is that if clients and clinician agree that client performance is being maintained, then the time intervals between clinic visits are gradually increased in a stepwise fashion. In between clinic visits, clients self-evaluate their speech in everyday speaking situations, and if they determine their performance is satisfactory, they reward themselves by decreasing the frequency of their self-evaluations. On the other hand, if they determine that their performance is unsatisfactory, they increase the frequency of self-evaluations. Clients return to the clinic at agreed-on intervals with sample recordings of their speech so that the clinician can check on their performance. If the clinician and client agree that performance is satisfactory, the time interval until the next clinic visit is doubled (e.g., from a 2-week to a 4-week interval). Of course, when clients determine that their performance is unsatisfactory on more than several occasions, they request a meeting sooner with the clinician, rather than later, to resolve the problem. The basic premise underlying this approach, which has been well-supported by research (Ingham, 1980, 1982), is that as clients are increasingly successful in self-managing their maintenance, the clinician's management becomes less and less necessary.

As with any behavior change, it is likely that some clients will experience lapses when it appears that their old problem behaviors are occasionally resurfacing. Therefore, providing clients with coping strategies for dealing with such lapses is another strategy for promoting maintenance, and self-evaluation will play an important role in the development and implementation of these coping strategies.

Research has suggested that these lapses are most likely to occur when clients are in high-risk situations that elicit negative feelings (Marlatt, 1982). Based on the relapses that have occurred during long-term follow-ups by treatment outcome studies, it appears that clients may be most vulnerable within the first 4 to 12 months posttreatment (e.g., Boberg & Kully, 1994). The high-risk, high-stress posttreatment situations that were reported as likely to trigger re-occurrences of stuttering have included speech at work, such as talking at a meeting, undergoing a job interview, and having conversations on the telephone (Craig & Hancock, 1995). Therefore, clients should be trained to identify situations that are high-risk situations for them as individuals and to plan for how they will cope with lapses when they occur (Marlatt, 1982). Research on self-regulatory failure has consistently shown that lapses are more likely to become *re*lapses when clients react negatively and stop self-monitoring their behavior (Baumeister, Heatherton, & Rice, 1994, Kirschenbaum & Tomarken, 1982). This suggests that the most important foundation for any coping strategy is for clients to reinstate or continue to engage in self-measurement or self-evaluation of their behavior (Watson & Tharp, 2007).

Self-measurement provides clients with the information needed to problem solve and how to prevent lapses from becoming a relapse. Problem-solving skills usually consist of three basic steps: (1) identifying the concrete details of the problem; (2) generating a list of solutions and selecting the most viable option; and (3) implementing and evaluating the success of that solution (Watson & Tharp, 2007). People who stutter report that the three most common coping strategies they use include re-implementing therapy skills, seeking social support from family friends or a self-help group, and returning to the clinician for additional help (Craig & Hancock, 1995). Coping skills as a maintenance strategy have not yet been adequately evaluated for their long-term effectiveness, but there is evidence that suggests that they may have potential (e.g., Blood, 1995; Craig & Andrews, 1985) and should be investigated further.

◆ Conclusion

In closing, clinicians should understand that people with persistent stuttering appear to be able to learn to successfully self-regulate their problem over time to the point where they no longer consider it a handicap (Plexico et al., 2005), indicate that they feel like normal speakers (Boberg & Kully, 1994; Ingham et al., 2001), and may even consider themselves recovered from stuttering (Anderson & Felsenfeld, 2003; Finn, Howard, & Kubala, 2005). Most of the time, they report that they do not think about their stuttering, and some may, for all practical purposes, be considered normally fluent speakers, both by themselves and others (Finn, 1997; Finn et al., 2005). For those who report, from time to time, that they may still experience an occasional tendency to stutter, some have become, in many respects, quintessential self-managers (Finn, 2004; Finn et al., 2005). They describe how they have learned to identify situations that are likely to trigger problems and how they have become sensitive to the thoughts or feelings that might prompt it. And most important, when they have found themselves in these circumstances, they feel confident that they will be able to implement strategies for constructively dealing with or repairing their stuttering so that it is no longer a significant issue in their lives.

References

Adams, M. R., & Popelka, G. (1971). The influence of "time-out" on stutterers and their dysfluency. Behavior Therapy 2, 334–339.

Anderson, T. K., & Felsenfeld, S. (2003). A thematic analysis of late recovery from stuttering. American Journal of Speech-Language Pathology 12, 243–253.

Baer, D. M. (1988). If you know why you're changing a behavior, you'll know when you've changed it enough. Behavioral Assessment 10, 219–223.

Baumeister, R. F., Heatherton, T. F., & Rice, D. M. (1994). Losing control: How and why people fail at self-regulation. San Diego, CA: Academic Press.

Blood, G. W. (1995). POWER: Relapse management with adolescents who stutter. Language, Speech, and Hearing Services in Schools 26, 169–179.

Boberg, E., & Kully, D. (1994). Long-term results of an intensive treatment program for adults and adolescents who stutter. Journal of Speech and Hearing Research 37, 1050–1059.

Bothe, A. K., Davidow, J. H., Bramlett, R. E. & Ingham, R. J. (2006). Stuttering treatment research 1970–2005: I systematic review incorporating trial quality assessment of behavioral, cognitive, and related approaches. American Journal of Speech-Language Pathology 15, 321–341.

Brutten, G., & Shoemaker, D. J. (1967). The modification of stuttering. Englewood Cliffs, NJ: Prentice-Hall.

Cone, J. D. (1999). Introduction to the special section on self-monitoring: A major assessment method in clinical psychology. Psychological Assessment 11, 411–414.

Cordes, A. K. (1998). Current status of the stuttering treatment literature. In A. K. Cordes & R. J. Ingham (Eds.), Treatment efficacy for stuttering: A search for empirical bases (pp. 117–144). San Diego, CA: Singular Publishing.

Craig, A. (1998). Relapse following treatment for stuttering: A critical review and correlative data. Journal of Fluency Disorders 23, 1–30.

Craig, A., & Andrews, G. (1985). The prediction and prevention of relapse in stuttering: The value of self-control techniques and locus of control measures. Behavior Modification 9, 427–442.

Craig, A., & Hancock, K. (1995). Self-reported factors related to relapse following treatment for stuttering. Australian Journal of Human Communication Disorders 23, 48–60.

Craig, A., Hancock, K., Chang, E., McCready, C., Shepley, A., McCaul, A., et al. A controlled clinical trial for stuttering in persons aged 9 to 14 years. Journal of Speech and Hearing Research 39, 808–826.

Cream, A., Onslow, M., Packman, A., & Llewellyn, G. (2003). Protection from harm: The experience of adults after therapy with prolonged-speech. International Journal of Language and Communication Disorders 38, 379–395.

Finn, P. (1977). Adults recovered from stuttering without formal treatment: Perceptual assessment of speech normalcy. Journal of Speech, Language, and Hearing Research 40, 821–831.

Finn, P. (1998). Recovery without treatment: A review of conceptual and methodological considerations across disciplines. In A. K. Cordes & R. J. Ingham (Eds.), Treatment efficacy for stuttering: A search for empirical bases (pp. 3–28). San Diego, CA: Singular Publishing.

Finn, P. (2003). Evidence-based treatment of stuttering: II. Clinical significance of behavioral stuttering treatments. Journal of Fluency Disorders 28, 209–218.

Finn, P. (2004). Self-change from stuttering during adolescence and adulthood. In A. K. Bothe (Ed.), Evidence-based treatment of stuttering: Empirical bases and applications (pp. 117–136). Mahwah, NJ: Lawrence Erlbaum Associates Inc.

Finn, P., Howard, R., & Kubala, R. (2005). Unassisted recovery from stuttering: Self-perceptions of current speech behavior, attitudes, and feelings. Journal of Fluency Disorders 30, 281–305.

Finn, P., & Ingham, R. J. (1994). Stutterers' self-ratings of how natural speech sounds and feels. Journal of Speech and Hearing Research 37, 326–340.

Foster, S. L., Laverty-Finch, C., Gizzo, D. P., & Osantowski, J. (1999). Practical issues in self-observation. Psychological Assessment 11, 426–438.

Gilovich, T. (1991). How we know what isn't so: The fallibility of human reason in everyday life. New York: The Free Press.

Goldiamond, I. (1968). Stuttering and fluency as manipulatable operant response classes. In H. N. Sloane & B. D. MacAulay (Eds.), Operant procedures in remedial speech and language training (pp. 348–407). Boston: Houghton Mifflin.

Hayes, S. C., Rosenfarb, I., Wulfert, E., Munt, E. D., Korn, Z., & Zettle, R. D. (1985). Self-reinforcement effects: An artifact of social standard setting? Journal of Applied Behavior Analysis 18, 201–214.

Hewat, S., O'Brian, S., Onslow, M., & Packman, A. (2001). Control of chronic stuttering with self-imposed time-out: Preliminary outcome data. Asia Pacific Journal of Speech, Language, and Hearing 6, 97–102.

Hewat, S., Onslow, M., Packman, A., & O'Brien, S. (2006). A Phase II clinical trial of self-imposed time-out treatment for stuttering in adults and adolescents. Disabil Rehab 28, 38–42.

Hillis, J. W. (1993). Ongoing assessment in the management of stuttering: A clinical perspective. American Journal of Speech-Lang Pathology 2, 24–37.

Ingham, R. J. (1980). Modification of maintenance and generalization during stuttering treatment. Journal of Speech and Hearing Research 23, 732–745.

Ingham, R. J. (1982). The effects of self-evaluation training on maintenance and generalization during stuttering treatment. Journal of Speech and Hearing Disorders 47, 271–280.

Ingham, R. J. (1987). Residential prolonged speech stuttering therapy manual. Santa Barbara: Department of Speech and Hearing Sciences, University of California, Santa Barbara.

Ingham, R. J. (1999). Performance-contingent management in adolescents and adults. In R.F. Curlee (Ed.), Stuttering and related disorders of fluency (2nd ed.) (pp. 200–221). New York: Thieme.

Ingham, R. J., Adams, S., & Reynolds, G. (1978). The effects on stuttering of self-recording the frequency of stuttering or the word 'the'. Journal of Speech and Hearing Research 21, 459–469.

Ingham, R. J., & Andrews, G. (1973). An analysis of a token economy in stuttering therapy. Journal of Applied Behavior Analysis 6, 219–229.

Ingham, R. J., & Cordes, A. K. (1997a). Self-measurement and evaluating treatment efficacy. In R. F. Curlee & G. M. Siegel (Eds.), Nature and treatment of stuttering: New directions (2nd ed.) (pp. 413–437). San Diego, CA: Singular.

Ingham, R. J., & Cordes, A. K. (1997b). Identifying the authoritative judgments of stuttering: Comparisons of self-judgments and observer judgments. Journal of Speech, Language, and Hearing Reserach 40, 581–594.

Ingham, R. J., Gow, M., & Costello, J. M. (1985). Stuttering and speech naturalness: Some additional data. Journal of Speech and Hearing Disorders 50, 217–219.

Ingham, R. J., Ingham, J. C., Onslow, M., & Finn, P. (1989). Stutterers' self-ratings of speech naturalness: Assessing effects and reliability. Journal of Speech and Hearing Research 32, 419–431.

Ingham, R. J., Kilgo, M., Ingham, J.C., Moglia, R. A., Belknap, H., & Sanchez, T. (2001). Evaluation of a stuttering treatment based on reduction of short phonation intervals. Journal of Speech, Language, and Hearing Research 44, 1229–1244.

Ingham, R. J., Martin, R. R., Haroldson, S. K., Onslow, M., & Leney, M. (1985). Modification of listener-judged naturalness in the speech of stutterers. Journal of Speech and Hearing Research 28, 495–504.

Ingham, R. J., & Onslow, M. (1987). Generalization and maintenance of treatment benefits for children who stutter. Seminars in Speech and Language 8, 303–326.

Ingham, R. J., Sato, W., Finn, P., & Belknap, H. (2001). The modification of speech naturalness during rhythmic stimulation treatment of stuttering. Journal of Speech, Language, and Hearing Research 44, 841–852.

James, J. E. (1981a). Self-monitoring of stuttering: Reactivity and accuracy. Behavior Research and Therapy 19, 291–296.

James, J. E. (1981b). Behavioral self-control of stuttering using time-out from speaking. Journal of Applied Behavior Analysis 14, 25–37.

James, J. E. (1983a). Parameters of the influence of self-initiated time-out from speaking on stuttering. Journal of Communication Disorders 16, 123–132.

James, J. E. (1983b). Fluency training for stutterers. In: J. Hariman (Ed.) The therapeutic efficacy of the major psychotherapeutic techniques (pp. 48–57). Springfield, IL: Charles C. Thomas.

James, J. E., & Ingham, R. J. (1974). The influence of stutterers' expectancies of improvement upon response to time-out. Journal of Speech and Hearing Research 17, 86–93.

James, J. E., Ricciardelli, L. A., Rogers, P., & Hunter, C. E. (1989). A preliminary analysis of the ameliorative effects of time-out from speaking on stuttering. Journal of Speech and Hearing Research 32, 604–610.

Kazdin, A. E. (2001). Behavior modification in applied settings (6th ed.). Belmont, CA: Wadsworth/Thomson Learning.

Kirschenbaum, D. S. (1987). Self-regulatory failure: A review with clinical implications. Clinical Psychology Review 7, 77–104.

Kirschenbaum, D. S., & Tomarken, A. J. (1982). On facing the generalization problem: The study of self-regulatory failure. In P. C. Kendall (Ed.), Advances in cognitive-behavioral research and therapy, Vol. 1 (pp. 119–200). New York: Academic Press.

Korotitsch, W. J., & Nelson-Gray, R. O. (1999). An overview of self-monitoring research in assessment and treatment. Psychological Assessment 11, 415–425.

La Croix, Z. E. (1973). Management of disfluent speech through self-recording procedures. Journal of Speech and Hearing Disorders 38, 272–274.

Maes, S., & Karoly, P. (2005). Self-regulation assessment and intervention in physical health and illness: A review. Applied Psychology: An International Review 54, 267–299.

Marlatt, G. A. (1982). Relapse prevention: A self-control program for the treatment of addictive behaviors. In R. B. Stuart (Ed.), Adherence, compliance, and generalization in behavioral medicine (pp. 329–378). New York: Brunner/Mazel.

Martin, R. R., & Haroldson, S. K. (1982). Contingent self-stimulation for stuttering. Journal of Speech and Hearing Disorders 47, 407–413.

Martin, R. R., Haroldson, S. K., & Triden, K. A. (1984). Stuttering and speech naturalness. Journal of Speech and Hearing Disorders 49, 53–58.

O'Brian, S., Onslow, M., Cream, A., & Packman, A. (2003). The Camperdown Program: Outcomes of a new prolonged-speech treatment model. Journal of Speech, Language, and Hearing Reserach 46, 933–946.

O'Brian, S., Packman, A., & Onslow, M. (2004). Self-rating of stuttering severity as a clinical tool. American Journal of Speech-Lang Pathology 13, 219–226.

O'Brian, S., Packman, A., Onslow, M., & O'Brian, N. (2004). Measurement of stuttering in adults: Comparison of stuttering-rate and severity-scaling methods. Journal of Speech, Language, and Hearing Research 47, 1081–1087.

Onslow, M., Costa, L., Andrews, C., Harrison, E., & Packman, A. (1996). Speech outcomes of a prolonged-speech treatment for stuttering. Journal of Speech and Hearing Research 39, 734–749.

Onslow, M., & O'Brian S. (1998). Reliability of clinicians' judgments about prolonged-speech targets. Journal of Speech, Language, and Hearing Research 41, 969–975.

Onslow, M., Packman, A., Stocker, S., van Doorn, J., Siegel, G. M. (1997). Control of children's stuttering with response-contingent time-out: Behavioral, perceptual, and acoustic data. Journal of Speech, Language, and Hearing Research 40, 121–133.

Plexico, L., Manning, W. H., & DiLollo, A. (2005). A phenomenological understanding of successful stuttering management. Journal of Fluency Disorders 30, 1–22.

Prins, D. (1997). Modifying stuttering–The stutterers' reactive behavior: Perspectives on past, present, and future. In R. F. Curlee & G. M. Siegel (Eds.), Nature and treatment of stuttering (2nd ed.) (pp. 335–354). Needham Heights, MA: Allyn & Bacon.

Runyan, C. M., & Adams, M. R. (1978). Perceptual study of the speech of 'successfully therapeutized' stutterers. Journal of Fluency Disorders 3, 25–39.

Runyan, C. M., & Adams, M. R. (1979). Unsophisticated judges' perceptual evaluations of the speech of 'successfully treated' stutterers. Journal of Fluency Disorders 4, 29–38.

Ryan, B. P. (2001). Programmed therapy for stuttering in children and adults (2nd ed.). Springfield, IL: Charles C. Thomas.

Sackett, D. L., Straus, S. E., Richardson, W. S., Rosenberg, W., & Haynes, R. B. (2001). Evidence-based medicine: How to practice and teach EBM. Edinburgh, UK: Churchill Livingstone.

Schiavetti, N., & Metz, D. (1997). Stuttering and the measurement of speech naturalness. R. F. Curlee & G. M. Siegel (Eds.), Nature and treatment of stuttering: New directions (2nd ed.) (pp. 398–412). Needham Heights, MA: Allyn & Bacon.

Schwartz, M. S., & Andrasik, F. (2003). Biofeedback: A practitioner's guide (3rd ed.). New York: Guilford Press.

Shames, G., & Florance, C. L. (1986). Stutter-free speech: A goal for therapy. In G. H. Shames & H. Rubin (Eds.), Stuttering: Then and now (pp. 447–468). Columbus, OH: Charles E. Merrill.

Siegel, G. M. (1970). Punishment, stuttering and disfluency. Journal of Speech and Hearing Research 13, 677–714.

Van Riper, C. (1973). The treatment of stuttering. Englewood Cliffs, NJ: Prentice-Hall.

Voh, K. D., & Baumeister, R. F. (2004). Understanding self-regulation. In K. D. Voh & R. F. Baumeister (Eds.), Handbook of self-regulation: Research, theory, and applications (pp. 1–12). New York: The Guildford Press.

Watson, D. L., & Tharp, R. G. (2007). Self-directed behavior: Self-modification for personal adjustment (9th ed.). Belmont, CA: Wadsworth/Thomson Learning.

Wolpe, J. (1990). The practice of behavior therapy. New York: Pergamon Press.

Appendix 18–1   Glossary of Self-Control Terms Used in This Chapter

Self-administered reinforcement   Client administers reward to oneself rather than being clinician-administered

Self-administered time-out   Client stops self from speaking for brief period contingent on a behavior, such as stuttering. Synonym, self-initiated time-out

Self-consequation   Administer consequences to oneself contingent on achieving target behavior rather than receiving clinician-administered consequences

Self-control   (1) As a concept, usually used as a synonym for self-regulation; (2) as a clinical term, refers more broadly to techniques employed by any individuals for modifying their own behavior to achieve specific treatment goals. Synonym, self-management, self-regulation

Self-determined reinforcement   Client determines for self the criteria for and amount of reinforcement received during treatment

Self-evaluation   Compare one's performance with self-selected target or clinician-specified treatment goal

Self-management   Typically, a synonym for self-control, though its use in the literature is usually more specific to clinical applications than the term "self-control." Synonyms: self-control, self-regulation

Self-measurement   Client systematically observes and records aspect of own behavior, usually across time. Synonyms: self-monitoring, self-observation, self-judgment, self-rating

Self-punishment   Administer a stimulus to oneself contingent on occurrence of undesired behavior to decrease its frequency of occurrence

Self-regulation   As a broad concept, refers to any individual's effort to modify own behavior, thoughts, or feelings to achieve selected goal or standard. Synonym: self-control

Self-reinforcement   Broadly refers to rewarding oneself for achieving specified target behaviors

Self-selected goals   Treatment goals of personal importance that are specific, realistic, and clinically relevant

Index

Note: Page numbers followed by *f* and *t* indicate figures and tables, respectively.